CONCEPTS OF FITNESS and WELLNESS

with Laboratories

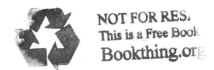

Charles B. Corbin

Arizona State University

Ruth Lindsey

Professor Emeritus
California State University-Long Beach

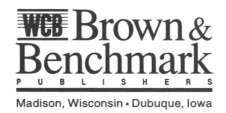

WCB Brown & Benchmark
PUBLISHERS

Madison, Wisconsin • Dubuque, Iowa

Book Team

Executive Editor *Ed Bartell*
Editor *Scott Spoolman*
Production Editor *Ann Fuerste*
Designer *Kristyn A. Kalnes*
Art Editor *Kathy Huinker-Timp*
Photo Editor *Robin Storm*
Permissions Coordinator *Karen L. Storlie*
Art Processor *Joyce E. Watters*
Visuals/Design Developmental Consultant *Marilyn A. Phelps*
Visuals/Design Freelance Specialist *Mary L. Christianson*
Publishing Services Specialist *Sherry Padden*
Marketing Manager *Pamela S. Cooper*
Advertising Manager *Jodi Rymer*

Brown & Benchmark

A Division of Wm. C. Brown Communications, Inc.

Executive Vice President/General Manager *Thomas E. Doran*
Vice President/Editor in Chief *Edgar J. Laube*
Vice President/Marketing and Sales Systems *Eric Ziegler*
Director of Production *Vickie Putman*
Director of Custom and Electronic Publishing *Chris Rogers*
National Sales Manager *Bob McLaughlin*

Wm. C. Brown Communications, Inc.

President and Chief Executive Officer *G. Franklin Lewis*
Senior Vice President, Operations *James H. Higby*
Corporate Senior Vice President and President of Manufacturing *Roger Meyer*
Corporate Senior Vice President and Chief Financial Officer *Robert Chesterman*

A Times Mirror Company

Library of Congress Catalog Card Number: 93-71948

ISBN 0-697-21611-X

Printed in the United States of America by Wm. C. Brown Communications, Inc., 2460 Kerper Boulevard, Dubuque, IA 52001

10 9 8 7 6 5 4 3 2

CONTENTS

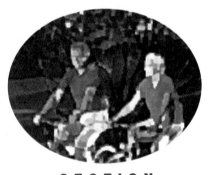
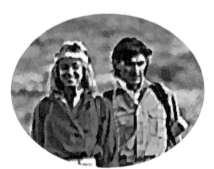
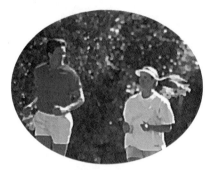
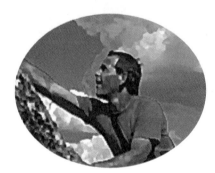

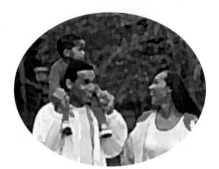

SECTION

V

Healthy Life-Styles 230

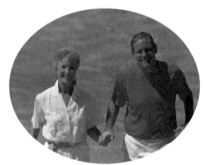

SECTION

VI

Wellness: Toward a Quality Life-Style 274

The Labs

Appendices

PREFACE

Over the last two decades, we have been committed to educational programs designed to encourage active, healthy living. We have found that an attractive, full-color presentation of materials in a format that is easy to understand goes a long way in promoting the desired end result. *Concepts of Fitness and Wellness* lives up to the high standards we have set.

This textbook is intended for an introductory college-level course dedicated to promoting healthy life-styles that result in optimal fitness and wellness. It grew out of another book, entitled *Concepts of Physical Fitness,* that focused on physical activity as a healthy life-style that contributes to physical fitness, health, and wellness. Over the years, however, it became increasingly clear that people who participated in regular physical activity also were interested in other behavioral changes that promote quality of life and feelings of well-being. *Concepts of Fitness and Wellness* is dedicated to providing information about a wide variety of healthy life-styles in addition to those covered in our fitness book. This NEW fitness and wellness book contains information about disease prevention (sexually transmitted diseases, cancer, and other important diseases related to life-style) as well as information concerning destructive behaviors such as use of tobacco and alcohol, and drug misuse and abuse. But more important, *Concepts of Fitness and Wellness* includes Concepts (chapters) on health promotion and the positive life-styles that can enhance quality of life. For example, a discussion of time management helps readers plan for recreation and leisure, as well as manage time, in order to have more opportunities to be with friends and loved ones. These supplement the more traditional wellness topics of physically active living, proper nutrition, and living a more relaxed life.

The NEW *Concepts of Fitness and Wellness* is for teachers and students who want more than a fitness book. The first section is an introduction to physical fitness and wellness, and sections II, III, and IV are devoted to physical fitness topics. The remaining two sections exemplify our commitment to the belief that wellness issues deserve much greater attention than they have received in other books of this type. Section V concerns life-style changes designed to enhance optimal health and wellness, and features Concepts on nutrition and stress management. A special Concept on consumer issues helps the reader use the best judgment when purchasing health products and services.

Section VI, *Wellness: Toward a Quality Life-style,* provides extensive information on the destructive habits of use and abuse of tobacco, alcohol, and other drugs. Disease and injury prevention are also discussed, with special emphasis on cancer and sexually transmitted diseases, including HIV/AIDS. Another Concept is dedicated to time management, to aid the reader in increasing positive living experiences such as meaningful recreation and quality time with friends and family. The final Concept is planning for life-style changes.

Among the important topics in the Concepts that precede those in the wellness sections are the health benefits of exercise, the amount of exercise necessary to develop optimal fitness, the facts about the FIT Formula, methods of self-evaluation, and exercises designed to build each fitness component. Other topics included in the fitness Concepts of the book are back care, body mechanics and posture, and stress management and relaxation. The steps in exercise program planning are outlined, and the reader is given information designed to aid in lifetime exercise adherence. Furthermore, exercise cautions discourage dangerous exercise that might result in injury or failure to adhere to a lifetime program.

Concepts of Fitness and Wellness contains the most up-to-date, scientific evidence available on topics of fitness and wellness. Because we are committed to scientific accuracy, a complete list of references is provided at the end of the book to document the points made in the text. We are also dedicated to making the book user-friendly. The book is organized in a unique way that has been shown to be very effective for learning. First, we use the term "Concept" rather than "Chapter" to indicate changes in topics. Webster defines concept as "an abstract idea generalized from particular instances."

The Concepts are presented in the following manner:

- Each Concept in the book begins with a conceptual statement, followed by an introductory paragraph.
- Health goals based on the Public Health Service's *Healthy People 2000* follow the introductory material.
- A glossary of terms is listed at the beginning of each Concept, then each term appears in boldface type when it occurs in the text for the first time. This gives the reader the opportunity to refer back to definitions if necessary.
- Factual information is presented in an outline format, followed by an explanation, discussion, and sample applications for the reader. Presenting information succinctly in this way allows for more information in less space and cuts through the verbiage often found in texts of this type.

- Suggested readings are listed at the end of each Concept to aid those who are interested in learning more.
- Laboratory experiences to accompany most of the Concepts appear at the end of the book. Labs and Concepts have been color coded with matching color tabs for easy identification.
- Also at the end of the book are appendices that contain supplemental exercise programs, charts of calories and nutrients in foods, and metric conversions of various rating charts.

Concepts of Fitness and Wellness is intended to help you make important decisions about a wide variety of fitness and wellness issues. We feel that the book will empower you to take responsibility for personal fitness and wellness by adopting and maintaining healthy life-styles. We hope that you will find the book interesting and useful, and that you will want to share its message with your family and friends.

A Note to Instructors

Concepts of Fitness and Wellness is an outgrowth of our earlier book, *Concepts of Physical Fitness*. This expanded book, with extensive NEW wellness information, contains many of the same features that has made the fitness book so successful over the past twenty-five years.

Using an outline format and presenting references at the end of the book (rather than at the end of each Concept) allows us to provide the most information in the least amount of space. This keeps the price down yet allows a full-color presentation that makes learning and reading more interesting.

Concepts of Fitness and Wellness is more than just a text; it is a full educational package. Many ancillary materials are available as part of the total educational package. The components of this package are:

- **Instructor's Manual (IM).** This revised manual includes: course objectives, suggestions for organization and scheduling lectures and labs, grading suggestions, lecture outlines (complete with visual aids), chapter objectives, key points, discussion questions, ideas for outside activities, audiovisual resources, sources of equipment, blackline masters for use in making overhead transparencies, and a test item file.
- **MicroTest III.** MicroTest III allows you to prepare custom exams using our prepared test bank along with your own test items. To improve the quality of our test items, we retained the services of a leading test expert, Dr. Weimo Zhu, to review and assist in writing the very best test items possible. MicroTest is available in IBM DOS, Windows, and MacIntosh versions.
- **Color Transparencies.** Two sets of transparencies are now available (on request). First, a NEW set of 50 color images is available. It includes a wide variety of transparencies including anatomical, physiological, fitness, and wellness images specifically for use with *Concepts of Fitness and Wellness*. A second set of 47 fitness and wellness transparencies supplements the NEW images.
- **Videos.** Videos continue to be available to instructors. The first tape focuses on physical fitness. It presents an overview of the administration of fitness tests found within the text, describes the concept approach, and features an aerobic dance routine. The second video focuses on wellness. It includes basic wellness definitions as well as a general wellness philosophy. Both tapes are perfect classroom tools for use in motivating students at an early stage in the course. They can be used in class prior to the presentation of those tests, or can serve as resource material for the instructor.
- **Computer Programs.** In addition to Testpak, several computer programs continue to be available in both IBM and MacIntosh formats. The computer assessment programs evaluate students in the areas of physical activity, target heart rate, heart disease risk, nutrition, and stress. Students enter information and receive instant feedback on their current status as well as ways to maintain or improve their levels of fitness.
- **Teacher's Resource Notebook (Binder).** A special notebook (binder) will be given free to each adopter of the text. This handy binder comes complete with tabbed dividers to contain such items as the Instructor's Manual, Transparencies, etc.

Acknowledgments

In the twenty-five years since the first edition of this book was published, many people have helped to make it successful. Many users have called or sent us suggestions that have been extremely helpful in improving subsequent editions. In addition, many people have reviewed manuscripts, served as consultants, or made suggestions for new labs or fact statements. The reviewers of this edition were: Ronnie Carda, Emporia State University; Bridgit A. Finley, Oklahoma City Community College; Carole J. Hanson, University of Northern Iowa; David Horton, Liberty University; John Merriman, Valdosta State College; Beverly F. Mitchell, Kennesaw State College; and Susan M. M. Todd, Vancouver Community College, Langara Campus. Other important individuals are listed in the Preface of the Instructor's Manual. Without their help, the book could not have been the success that it has proven to be over the years. We thank you all.

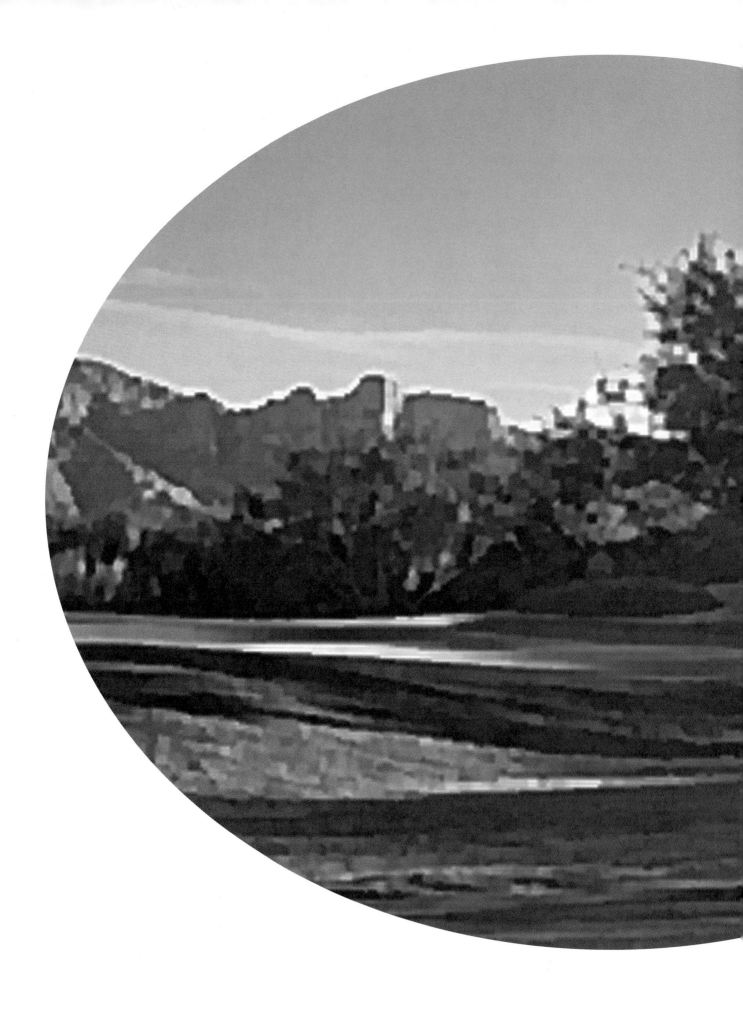

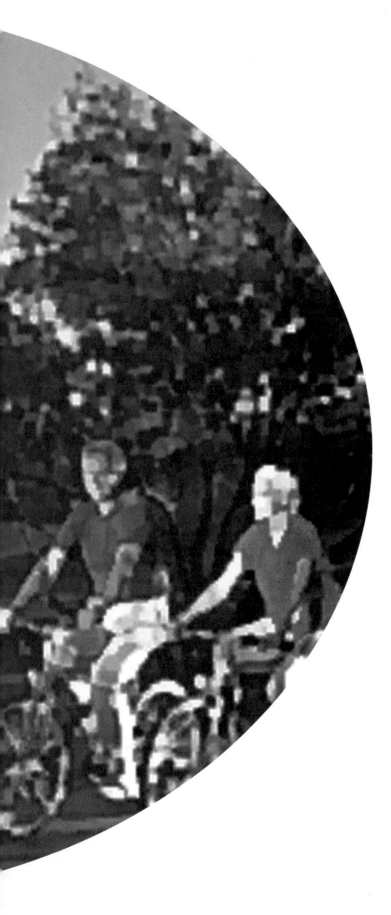

Introduction

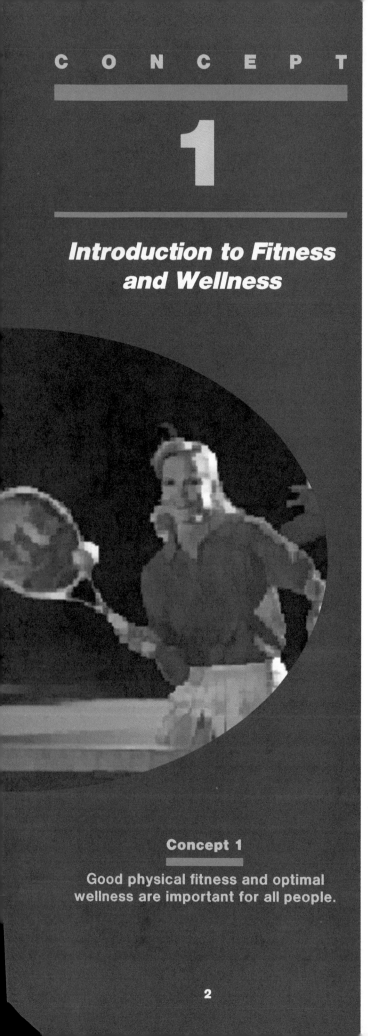

C O N C E P T

1

Introduction to Fitness and Wellness

Concept 1

Good physical fitness and optimal wellness are important for all people.

A Statement About National Health Goals

At the beginning of each concept in this book is a section entitled **Health Goals for the Year 2000.** Health goals that are relevant to that particular concept are presented. The health goals are abbreviated statements from the document *Healthy People 2000: National Health Promotion and Disease Prevention Objectives*. These goals, established by 22 expert groups representing more than 300 national organizations, are intended as realistic health goals to be achieved by the year 2000. The focus is on health as represented by a high quality of life and a sense of well-being. Although the goals are intended to improve the health of those in the United States, they seem important for all people in North America and in other cultures throughout the world. This book is written with achievement of these important health goals in mind.

Introduction

The human organism was designed to be active. Anthropologists indicate that the need to be active is associated with the "fight or flight" response. In search of food, primitive people sometimes had to fight with other predators or to flee for safety. In either case, the response was often vigorous activity. Even our more recent ancestors were required to do vigorous activity as a relatively major part of their normal daily routine. However, automation and technology have freed modern civilization from the exhausting physical labor required of earlier generations. The heavy physical work of the farmer and manual laborer is less and less likely to be a part of the normal daily routine of the average North American. Statistics indicate that in the past 100 years, the average workweek has been greatly reduced, thereby netting the average person many more hours of free time annually.

Even though physical exertion has become less necessary as a part of the normal work of many adults, the need for regular **exercise** has not decreased. If anything, it has increased.

Lack of regular physical activity results in poor **physical fitness.** Those who are not physically fit often suffer from **hypokinetic diseases** or conditions discussed later in this book.

In recent years many Americans have discovered that active living contributes significantly to good **health** and **wellness.** Regular physical activity is, however, only one of many different life-style patterns that can enhance health and quality of life. Recent scientific evidence suggests that a healthy life-style, more than any other single factor, is responsible for optimal wellness. The implication is that each of us can learn to alter our life-styles to foster lifetime fitness and wellness.

Health Goals for the Year 2000

▬ Increase the span of healthy life.
▬ Increase the physical activity levels of Americans.

Terms

Throughout the book, key terms are in bold type the first time they appear in the text. You may wish to check the definition of each term as you read.

Exercise
▬▬

Exercise, as used in this book, means human movement or physical activity. This term includes such formal activities as calisthenics; movements done in sports, dance, and games; as well as less formal activities, such as walking, jogging, and swimming. In this book, the terms *exercise, physical activity,* and *human movement* are used interchangeably and, in general, describe large muscle activities rather than highly specific, relatively nontaxing movements of small muscle groups.

Hypokinetic Diseases or Conditions
▬▬

Hypo means "under" or "too little," and *kinetic* means movement or activity. Thus, hypokinetic means "too little activity." A hypokinetic disease or condition is associated with lack of physical activity or too little regular exercise. Examples of such conditions include heart disease, low back pain, adult-onset diabetes, and obesity (see Concept 3).

Health
▬▬

Health is optimal well-being that contributes to quality of life. It is more than freedom from disease and illness, though freedom from disease is important to good health. Optimal health includes high-level mental, social, emotional, spiritual, and physical fitness within the limits of one's heredity and personal disabilities.

Illness
▬▬

Illness is the ill feeling and/or symptoms associated with a disease or circumstances that upset homeostasis.

Life-styles
▬▬

Life-styles are patterns of behavior or ways an individual typically lives.

Physical Fitness
▬▬

Physical fitness is the body's ability to function efficiently and effectively. It consists of health-related fitness and skill-related physical fitness, which have at least eleven different components, each of which contributes to total quality of life. Physical fitness is associated with a person's

ability to work effectively, to enjoy leisure time, to be healthy, to resist hypokinetic diseases, and to meet emergency situations. It is related to, but different from, psychological, sociological, emotional, and spiritual fitness, health, and wellness components. Although the development of physical fitness is the result of many things, optimal physical fitness is not possible without regular exercise.

Wellness
▬▬

Wellness is the integration of all parts of health and fitness (mental, social, emotional, spiritual, and physical) that expands one's potential to live and work effectively and to make a significant contribution to society. Wellness reflects how one feels (a sense of well-being) about life as well as one's ability to function effectively. Wellness, as opposed to illness (a negative), is sometimes described as the positive component of good health.

The Facts

Good health is of primary importance to most adults in our society.

When polled about important social values, 99 percent of American adults identified "being in good health" as one of their major concerns. The three concerns expressed most often were good health, good family life, and good self-image. The one percent who did not identify good health as an important concern had no opinion on any social issues. Among those polled, none felt that good health was unimportant.

Optimal health is more than freedom from disease.

During this century the life expectancy for the average person has increased by 60 percent. A child born in 1900 could expect to live only 47 years. A child born today can expect to live to the age of 73.7. Much of the increase in life span can be attributed to modern medical science. Many diseases that killed thousands in earlier times can now be easily treated. Pneumonia, which can be treated with antibiotics, is a good example.

As treatment for killer diseases became available, the emphasis shifted to disease prevention. Curing disease was still of concern, but the development of vaccines and other preventions for disease became central to the efforts of public health and medical experts. Many lives have been saved and much pain and suffering has been avoided as a result of the development of vaccines for diseases such as smallpox and polio.

As a result of the advances in **illness** treatment and prevention, an effort can now be made to focus on wellness. Wellness, or a sense of well-being, includes one's

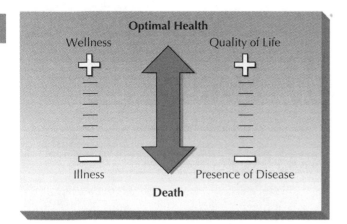

Figure 1.1

Wellness is an important part of optimal health.

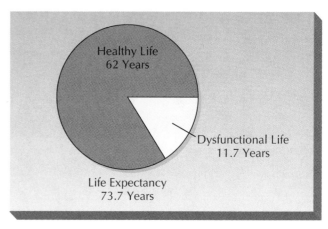

Figure 1.2

Years of healthy life as a proportion of life expectancy (U.S. population).

Source: *National Vital Statistics System and National Health Interview Survey.* Centers for Disease Central and Prevention, Atlanta, GA.

ability to live and work effectively and to make a significant contribution to society. It reflects how one feels about life as well as one's ability to function effectively. Wellness represents a quality of living component that is essential for optimal health.

As illustrated in figure 1.1, good health is partly associated with freedom from illness and disease. Disease treatment and prevention efforts are important to good health. However, as noted previously, a sense of well-being or wellness as reflected in quality living is critical to optimal health. Health promotion programs often go beyond disease treatment and prevention in that they contribute to optimal physical fitness and spiritual and emotional health, as well as other components that enhance the quality of life.

Increasing the span of healthy life is a principal health goal.

Consistent with the notion that optimal health includes a wellness dimension that is more than freedom from disease, the Public Health Service has adopted as its principal goal the increase in *healthy* span of life. It is true that the life expectancy is now 73.7 years, but the average person can expect to have only 62 years of *healthy* life (see fig. 1.2). The remaining 11.2 years are characterized as dysfunctional or lacking in the wellness component. Quality of life is diminished.

Lack of wellness is not, however, a problem exclusive to older people. Many young people fail to achieve wellness because of illness and/or less than quality living. Increasing the quality of life for people of all ages is as important as increasing the number of years lived. In addition to adding years to life, the goal is to add life to our years.

Life-style change, more than any other factor, is considered to be the best way of preventing illness and early death in our society.

When people in Western society die before the age of 65, it is considered to be early or premature death. The four major factors contributing to early death are noted in figure 1.3. Human biology, which includes hereditary predispositions to disease, accounts for only a small share of the causes of early death. Improvements in the environment and in the health-care system could substantially decrease early death, but by far the best way to decrease this problem is the promotion of healthy life-styles.

Healthy life-styles are critical to wellness.

Just as unhealthy life-styles are the principal causes of modern-day illnesses such as heart disease, cancer, and diabetes, healthy life-styles can result in an improved feeling of wellness that is critical to optimal health. In recognizing the importance of "years of healthy life," the Public Health Service also recognizes what it calls "measures of well-being." This "well-being" or wellness is associated with social, mental, spiritual, and physical functioning. Being physically active and eating well are two examples of healthy life-styles that can improve well-being and add years of quality living. Many of the healthy life-styles associated with good physical fitness and optimal wellness will be discussed in detail later in this book.

Regular physical activity is a healthy life-style that helps prevent hypokinetic diseases and conditions.

An increase in physical activity designed to improve physical fitness is a central goal in the plan designed to enhance the healthy life span of Americans by the year 2000.

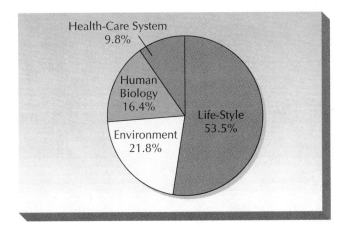

Figure 1.3

Percentage contribution of four sources to early death.

Source: K. E. Powell, K. G. Spain, G. M. Christianson, and M. P. Mollenkamp, "The Status of the 1990 Objectives for Physical Fitness and Exercise" in *Public Health Reports*, 19:101, 1989. U.S. Public Health Service.

Physical activity and physical fitness have been shown to reduce the risk of such hypokinetic illnesses as heart disease, hypertension, adult-onset diabetes, osteoporosis, obesity, mental health problems, some forms of cancer, and chronic musculoskeletal problems such as back pain. Exercise, fitness, and hypokinetic conditions will be discussed in detail in Concept 3.

Good physical fitness and regular physical activity are important to wellness.

Wellness is quality of life. Regular physical activity and good physical fitness have been shown to enhance quality of life in many ways. Physical fitness and exercise can help you look good, feel good, and enjoy life. Exercise helps keep body fat levels in normal ranges and is responsible for muscle development that can improve one's perception of self. Fitness and exercise have been associated with various mental and physical health benefits that help an in-dividual feel good and function effectively. Physical activity provides an enjoyable way to spend one's leisure time. Each of the wellness benefits of physical activity and physical fitness will be discussed in greater detail in the concepts that follow.

If optimal health is to be achieved, personal control of life-styles is necessary.

A recent poll indicates that 91 percent of adults would like to change their life-styles to make their lives more enjoyable and to change factors associated with wellness, such as reducing stress and tension. Unfortunately, many people feel that they do not have personal control over good health and wellness. For example, one survey suggests that most of the life-style changes deemed important by millions in our society ". . . will remain in the realm of fantasies, just beyond realization" (Harris & Associates 1987).

Experts have shown that people who feel that health is beyond personal control express such ideas as "Bad things (illness) can't happen to me and good things (wellness) are beyond my reach." Evidence is presented in this book to show that many of the most serious health problems in our society can happen to anyone, and that the risk of suffering from these problems can be greatly reduced by making life-style changes that are possible for all people. Adopting healthy life-styles not only helps in disease prevention but also can promote wellness, the quality of life component of optimal health.

Suggested Readings

Bruess, C., and G. Richardson. *Decisions for Health* 3d ed. Dubuque, IA: Wm. C. Brown Publishers, 1992.

McGinnis, J. M. "The Public Health Burden of a Sedentary Lifestyle." *Medicine and Science in Sports and Exercise* 24(1992)S196 (Supplement).

Public Health Service. *Healthy People 2000: National Health Promotion and Disease Prevention Objectives.* Washington, DC: U.S. Government Printing Office, 1991.

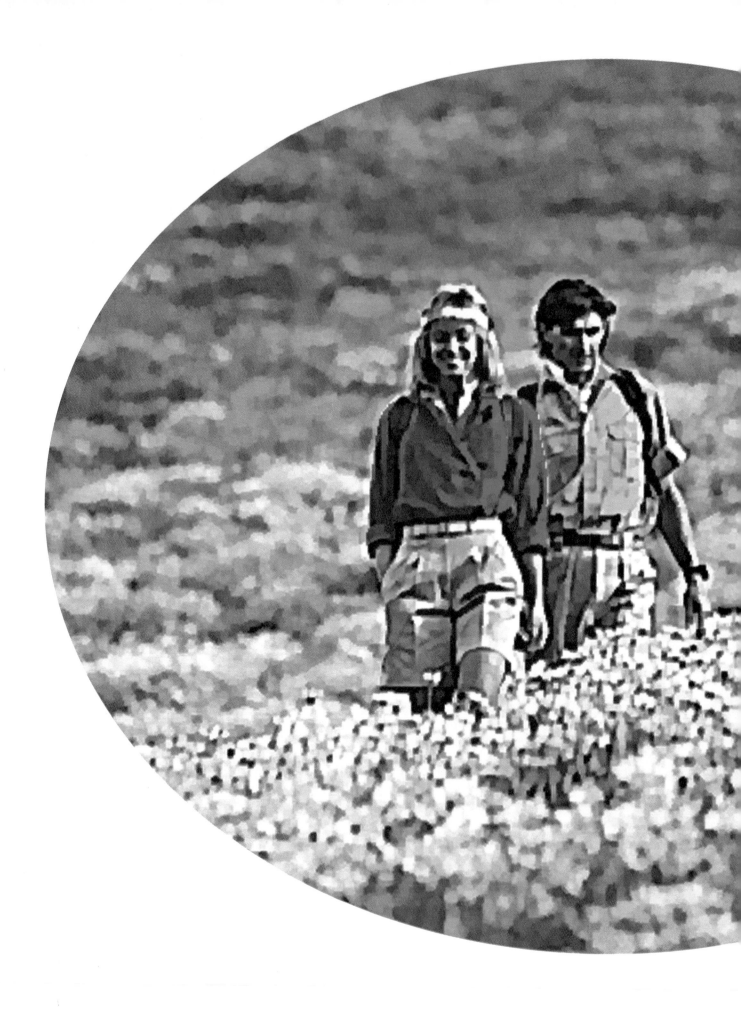

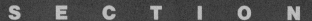

Foundations of Fitness and Exercise

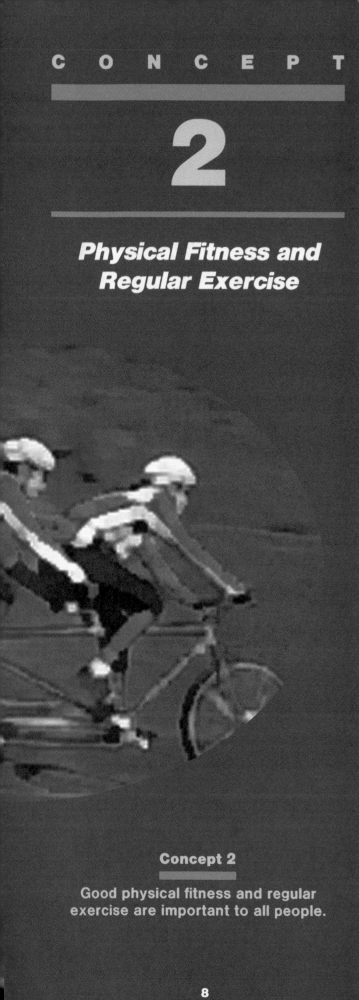

2

Physical Fitness and Regular Exercise

Concept 2

Good physical fitness and regular exercise are important to all people.

Introduction

Some people associate good **physical fitness** with being good at sports and games. It does take a certain degree of fitness to excel in these activities, but being able to perform specific skills may not be a good indicator of total physical fitness because some sports require only specific aspects of fitness.

Historically, physical fitness has often been misrepresented, at times identified exclusively with skill in sports, at other times identified too closely with only one of the many aspects of physical fitness. For example, in previous decades, fitness for men was often associated with muscle strength. This was evidenced by the popularity of programs such as Charles Atlas' Dynamic Tension Program advertised widely in magazines and comic books. In recent years, with the popularity of jogging and other forms of aerobic exercise, many people associated physical fitness almost exclusively with cardiovascular fitness. It is true that each of these is important, but it cannot be overemphasized that physical fitness is not a single entity but consists of a number of different characteristics, of which strength and cardiovascular fitness are only two. Each of the specific components of fitness is critical to developing optimal physical fitness and to achieving the benefits associated with being optimally fit.

Many factors contribute to good physical fitness, including heredity, maturation, environment, and life-styles such as nutrition. However, it is regular physical activity that is most important in physical fitness development. In fact, physical activity designed to promote physical fitness is the first and most prominent priority area listed among the health promotion goals in *Healthy People 2000*, a statement of goals for the nation for the year 2000.

Health Goals for the Year 2000

- Increase the proportion of people who do regular physical activity for cardiovascular fitness.
- Increase the proportion of people who do regular physical activity for strength, muscular endurance, and flexibility.
- Decrease the proportion of people who do no leisure-time physical activity.
- Reduce the prevalence of overfatness and increase physical activity among those who have excess body fatness.

Terms

Bone Integrity

Soundness of the bones associated with high density and absence of symptoms of deterioration.

Physical Fitness

Physical fitness is the entire human organism's ability to function efficiently and effectively. It is made up of at least eleven different components, each of which contributes to total quality of life. Physical fitness is associated with a person's ability to work effectively, to enjoy leisure time, to be healthy, to resist hypokinetic diseases, and to meet emergencies.

Health-Related Fitness Terms

Body Composition

The relative percentage of muscle, fat, bone, and other tissues of which the body is composed. A fit person has a relatively low, but not too low, percentage of body fat (body fatness).

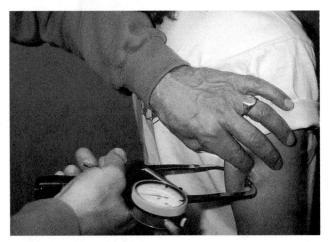

Body composition (fatness)

Cardiovascular Fitness

The ability of the heart, blood vessels, blood, and respiratory system to supply fuel, especially oxygen, to the muscles and the ability of the muscles to utilize fuel to allow sustained exercise. A fit person can persist in physical activity for relatively long periods without undue stress.

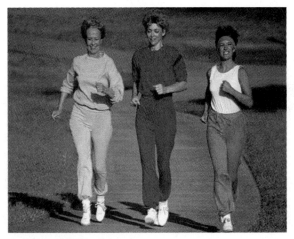

Cardiovascular fitness

Flexibility

The range of motion available in a joint. It is affected by muscle length, joint structure, and other factors. A fit person can move the body joints through a full range of motion in work and in play.

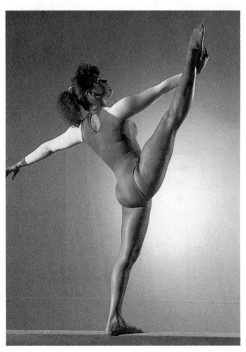

Flexibility

Muscular Endurance

The ability of the muscles to repeatedly exert themselves. A fit person can repeat movements for a long period without undue fatigue.

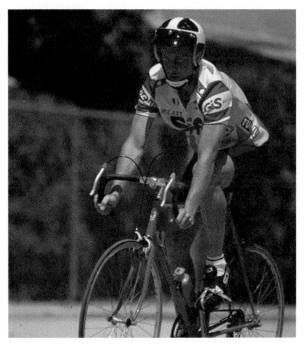

Muscular endurance

Strength

The ability to exert an external force or to lift a heavy weight. A fit person can do work or play that involves exerting force, such as lifting or controlling one's own body weight.

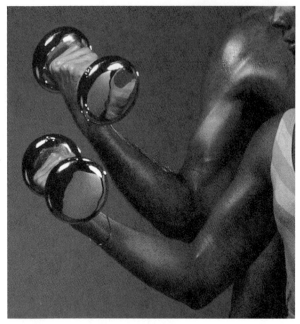

Strength

Skill-Related Fitness Terms

Agility

The ability to rapidly and accurately change the direction of the movement of the entire body in space. Skiing and wrestling are examples of activities that require exceptional agility.

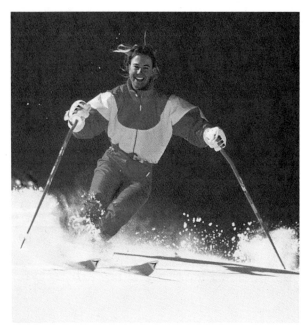

Agility

Balance

The maintenance of equilibrium while stationary or while moving. Water skiing, performing on the balance beam, or working as a riveter on a high-rise building are activities that require exceptional balance.

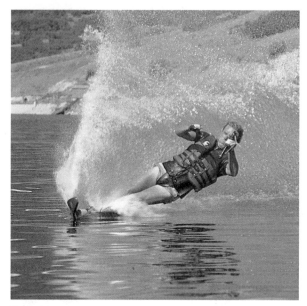

Balance

Coordination

The ability to use the senses with the body parts to perform motor tasks smoothly and accurately. Juggling, hitting a golf ball, batting a baseball, or kicking a ball are examples of activities requiring good coordination.

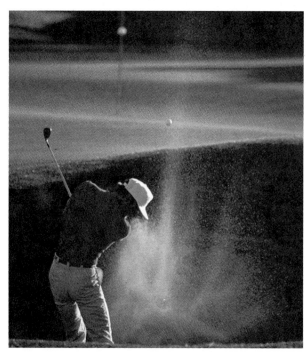

Coordination

Power

The ability to transfer energy into force at a fast rate. Throwing the discus and putting the shot are activities that require considerable power.

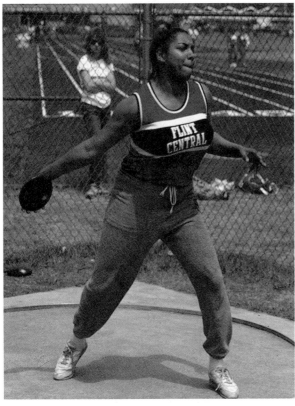

Power

Reaction Time

The time elapsed between stimulation and the beginning of reaction to that stimulation. Driving a racing car and starting a sprint race require good reaction time.

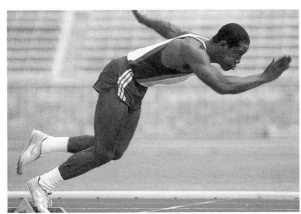

Reaction time

Speed

The ability to perform a movement in a short period of time. A runner on a track team or a wide receiver on a football team needs good foot and leg speed.

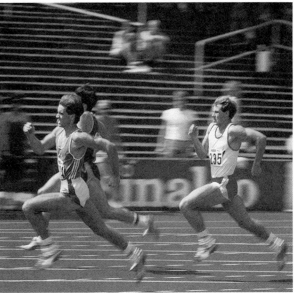

Speed

The Facts About Physical Fitness Components

Physical fitness consists of many components, each of which is specific in nature.

Physical fitness is a combination of several aspects rather than a single characteristic. A fit person possesses at least adequate levels of each of the health-related fitness components, and each of the skill-related fitness components. People who possess one aspect of physical fitness do not necessarily possess all of the other aspects.

Some relationship exists between different fitness characteristics, but each of the components of physical fitness is separate and different from the others. For example, people who possess exceptional strength do not necessarily have good cardiovascular fitness, and those who have good coordination do not necessarily possess good flexibility.

Body composition, cardiovascular fitness, flexibility, muscular endurance, and strength are the health-related components of physical fitness.

Because each fitness characteristic has a direct relationship to good health and lessens risk of hypokinetic disease, each is considered a part of health-related physical fitness.

Some experts consider **bone integrity** to be an additional part of health-related fitness.

Possessing a moderate amount of each component of health-related fitness is essential to disease prevention and health promotion. To some extent, having exceptionally high levels of health-related fitness is similar to having high level skill-related fitness. For example, moderate amounts of strength are necessary to prevent back and posture problems, whereas high levels of strength contribute most to improved performance in activities such as football and jobs involving heavy lifting.

Agility, balance, coordination, power, reaction time, and **speed** are often considered to be the main components of skill-related physical fitness.

Because each fitness characteristic is related to certain motor skills, such as those required in sports and in specific types of jobs, each is classified as a part of skill-related fitness. Skill-related fitness is sometimes called "sports fitness" or "motor fitness."

There is little doubt that there are other abilities that could be classified as skill-related fitness components. Also each part of skill-related fitness is multidimensional. For example, coordination could be hand-eye coordination such as batting a ball, foot-eye coordination such as kicking a ball, or any of many other possibilities. The six parts of skill-related fitness identified here are those that are commonly associated with successful sports and work performance. It should be noted that each could be measured in ways other than those presented in this book. Measurements are provided to help the reader understand the nature of total physical fitness and to help the reader make important decisions about lifetime physical activity.

Other Facts About Fitness and Exercise

Heredity influences physical fitness, total fitness, and optimal health.

There is good evidence that a person's potential to develop exceptionally high levels of physical fitness, especially skill-related physical fitness, is based on heredity. Just as physical fitness is influenced by heredity, so are other parts of total fitness and health. Predispositions to various diseases and health problems can be inherited.

Healthy life-styles are important to optimal health and quality of life.

Doing regular exercise is one of many healthy life-styles that contribute to optimal health and quality of life. Other life-style changes that can be made to help prevent disease and promote health are discussed in Concept 21. Unlike heredity, life-styles can be changed to improve fitness and health.

North Americans have become more active in recent years.

Adults in the United States have become more active in recent years. Since the Gallup Poll on exercise was begun in 1961, there has been a consistent increase in physical activity among adults. In 1961 only 24 percent of adults said they were active during their free time. Currently, more than half say they are active. Surveys in Canada show similar increases in adult physical activity. This indicates that the "fitness movement" is more than a fad. Regular exercise is becoming a part of the life-style of an increasing number of people.

Too many North Americans are not as active as they should be.

Though more adults are active than in the past, many who say they are active participate only occasionally. Research results indicate that most adults do not exercise enough to improve fitness and that many are totally inactive. Some current statistics, along with some goals for the year 2000, are presented in figure 2.1.

Some segments of the population are more fit and active than others.

In spite of the concerns of some about the fitness of our youth, children are the most active and fit segment of the population. Evidence indicates that teens are less active than children, and adults are less active than teens. Today, children have been shown to be as fit as children 30 years ago, with one exception: they are fatter than children of previous generations. There is concern that teens are less active than in past years. This fact is important because the teen years are a time when proper exercise and healthy life-styles can result in exceptional fitness gains.

Among the adult population, young middle-class males are most likely to be active. Women have become more active in recent years but are still less active than men. Older adults experience the same general benefits of regular physical activity that younger people do, but nearly twice as many are likely to be sedentary. People with disabilities and those with low incomes are also considerably less active than other adults.

Good physical fitness and regular exercise contribute to optimal health and wellness.

As noted in Concept 1, good fitness resulting from regular exercise reduces the risk of hypokinetic disease and contributes to wellness as evidenced by an improved quality of life. The health benefits of exercise and fitness will be outlined in greater detail in Concept 3.

Adults who do 30 minutes of exercise 5 days a week.

Currently = 22%

Goal = 30%

Adults who do cardiovascular fitness activity 3 days a week for at least 20 minutes a day.

Currently = 12%

Goal = 20%

People aged 6 and older who do regular strength, muscular endurance, and flexibility exercise.

Current = not known

Goal = 40%

People aged 6 and older who do no leisure-time physical activity.

Current = 24%

Goal = 15%

Figure 2.1

Physical activity and fitness goals for the year 2000.

Source: Data from the Public Health Service, *Healthy People 2000: National Health Promotion and Disease Prevention Objectives.* Washington, DC: U.S. Government Printing Office, 1991.

Industry has recognized the importance of exercise programs to employee fitness and productivity.

Realizing that many jobs are not as active as they were prior to automation, industry has taken steps to provide on-the-job exercise and fitness programs for their employees. More than one-half of all companies with 750 or more employees now have an exercise program. A national goal is to increase this number to 80 percent. Company officials endorse the fitness-in-industry movement because medical costs are skyrocketing, hypokinetic diseases such as back pain account for a billion-dollar annual loss in production, and absenteeism can be reduced considerably by offering employees an exercise and fitness program. Evidence indicates that such programs are cost-effective as well as popular among employees. One company official notes, "It's the best fringe benefit we've offered."

Many people are ignorant of the facts about exercise and physical fitness.

Unfortunately, many American adults hold misconceptions about health, fitness, and exercise. For example, more than 50 percent of inactive adults feel that such sports as baseball and bowling provide enough exercise to develop good health and physical fitness. Although the facts indicate otherwise, those who do not exercise regularly believe that they get all the exercise they need. Interestingly,

those who report that they participate in regular exercise are also the ones who are likely to feel that they do not get enough exercise for their own good.

The most popular forms of exercise among adults require very little skill or equipment and are easily accessible.

Surveys consistently show that walking, swimming, bicycling, aerobic dance, calisthenics, and jogging/running are among the most popular adult physical activities. All these can be done in or near the home for little or no cost. None requires a high degree of physical skill in order for a person to be successful or to enjoy the benefits associated with regular involvement. These activities are not often those that people value for their children, nor those in which they themselves were involved as children. And although football, baseball, basketball, gymnastics, and boxing are the activities adults most enjoy watching, they usually are not the ones in which they participate.

Regular exercise and good fitness can save money.

Studies show that sedentary living costs taxpayers huge amounts of money each year. It is projected that society could save $1,900 annually for each sedentary person who began regular exercise. The extra costs to taxpayers are the result of increased health insurance premiums, life insurance premiums, sick leave coverage, and disability insurance premiums.

Exercise can be important for many reasons, but it is not a cure-all, and if done improperly, it can be dangerous.

The many benefits of exercise are well documented in this book. However, certain types of exercise are contraindicated for certain people. Doing too much too soon can be dangerous for those who have not been involved in exercise on a regular basis. Those who exercise irregularly, such as the "weekend athlete" who exercises vigorously only on weekends or other special occasions, may be asking for trouble. There is some evidence that even avid exercisers can become overinvolved with their commitment to physical activity and develop an activity neurosis. This condition can develop if an individual becomes irrationally concerned about his or her need for involvement in exercise.

There is no single best form of exercise for all people.

Different people participate in different types of exercise for different reasons. This is as it should be. Each person has his or her own unique movement personality—no two people move in exactly the same way. Because movement personalities differ, there is a wide variety of leisure activities from which individuals can select. The choice of exercise and physical activities should be made only after carrying out the following steps:

- Assess your current health and physical fitness status to determine your individual needs.
- Examine your current interests. (Exercise should be enjoyable.)
- Acquire a knowledge and an understanding of the values of different activities.
- Determine which activities will best meet your needs and interests.
- Acquire skill and knowledge in the selected activities.

Exercise is for virtually everyone.

Exercise, whether it be sports or some other form of physical activity, should not be limited to those with good athletic ability. Regardless of age, sex, or athletic ability (if there is no serious medical limitation), there is some form of activity that everyone will find enjoyable and in which everyone can succeed.

Facts About Why People Do Not Exercise

The number one reason people give for not exercising is, "I don't have the time."

"I'm too busy!" This reason has been shown repeatedly to be the leading reason why people do not do regular exercise. Invariably, these people indicate that they know they should do more exercise and that they plan to in the future when "things are less hectic." For example, young people say that they will soon be established in a career and then they will have the time to exercise. Older people say that they wish they had taken the time to be active when they were younger.

Another major reason people do not exercise is, "It's too inconvenient."

Many who avoid exercise do so because it is inconvenient. They are exercise procrastinators. Specific reasons for procrastinating include: "It makes me sweaty"; "It messes up my hair"; and "I just can't find the energy." (It is interesting, though, that those who do exercise regularly report improvements in their appearance and a feeling of increased energy.)

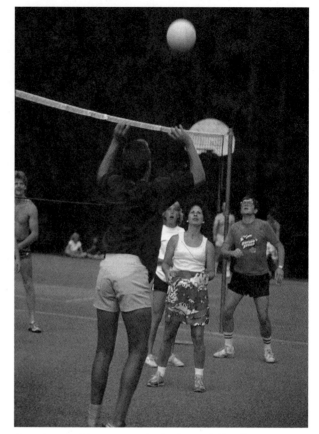

Exercise provides an opportunity for social involvement.

Large numbers of adults are not active because they "just don't enjoy exercise."

The reasons some people say they do not enjoy exercise include: "People might laugh at me"; "Sports make me nervous"; and "I am not good at physical activities." These people often lack confidence in their own abilities. In some cases, this is because of their past experiences in physical education or in athletics. With properly selected activities, even those who have never enjoyed exercise can get "hooked."

Poor health is a reason some people avoid exercise.

Some people avoid exercise because of health reasons. Though it is true that there are good medical reasons for not exercising, many people with such problems can benefit from exercise if it is properly designed for them.

Lack of facilities and bad weather are reasons some people do not exercise regularly.

Regular exercise is much more convenient if facilities are easy to reach and the weather is good. Still, recreational opportunities have increased considerably in recent years.

Furthermore, some of the most popular activities for building fitness require very little equipment, can be done in or near the home, and are inexpensive.

Some people do not perform regular exercise because they think they are too old.

As people grow older, many begin to feel that exercise is something they cannot do. For most people this is simply not true! Studies conducted over a period of years indicate that properly planned exercise for older adults is not only safe but also has many health benefits, including longer life, fewer illnesses, increased working capacity, and an improved sense of well-being.

Facts About Why People Do Exercise

The number one reason people exercise regularly is "for health and physical fitness."

Nearly all adults recognize the importance of exercise for good health and fitness. More than one national survey has shown that health and fitness is the single most important reason why people engage in regular exercise. Unfortunately, many adults say that a "doctor's order to exercise" would be the most likely reason to get them to begin a regular program. For some, however, waiting for a doctor's order may be too late.

Physical appearance is a common reason cited for doing regular exercise.

An important reason for exercising is to improve physical appearance. In our society, looking good is highly valued, thus physical attractiveness is another major reason why people participate in regular exercise. Of major importance to many adults is weight or fat control.

While the evidence suggests that exercise can be effective in helping you look your best, there is a danger of unrealistic expectations on the part of many people. Most would like to make a change in their appearance that is not likely to happen as a result of exercise alone.

Enjoyment is a major reason for exercising regularly.

A majority of adults say that enjoyment would be of paramount importance in deciding to exercise. This is not surprising, given statements from joggers that they began exercising for fitness but continue for such reasons as the "peak experience," the "runner's high," and "spinning free." In fact, movement can be an end in itself. Satisfaction can be derived from the mere involvement in the movement activity. The sense of fun, the feeling of well-being, and the general enjoyment associated with physical activity is well documented.

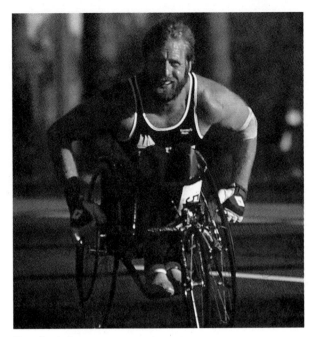
Exercise is for everyone.

Relaxation and release from tension are reasons given for doing regular exercise.

Relaxation and release from tension rank high as reasons why people do regular exercise. Exercise, such as walking, jogging, or cycling, is a way of getting some quiet time away from the stress of the job. For years, it has been recognized that exercise in the form of sports and games provides a catharsis, or outlet, for the frustrations of normal daily activities. Evidence indicates that regular exercise can help reduce depression and anxiety, both common symptoms in Western culture.

Physical activity can provide a way of meeting a challenge and developing a sense of personal accomplishment.

A sense of personal accomplishment associated with performing various physical activities is frequently a reason people exercise. In some cases, it is merely learning a new skill, such as racquetball or tennis; in other cases, it is running a mile or doing a certain number of sit-ups that provides this feeling of accomplishment. The challenge of doing something never done before is apparently a very powerful experience. Physical activities provide opportunities not readily available in other aspects of life.

An important reason many people exercise is the social experience of involvement.

Physical activity often provides the opportunity to be with other people. It is this social experience that many appreciate most about exercise. Frequent answers to the question, "Why do you exercise?" include: "It is a good way to spend time with other members of the family;" "It is a good way to spend time with close friends;" and "Being part of the team is a satisfying feeling." Physical activity settings can also provide an opportunity for making new friends.

The competitive experience is an important reason people participate in sports and physical activities.

"The thrill of victory" and "sports competition" are two reasons often given by people who participate in physical activities. For many, the competitive experiences can be very satisfying.

Suggested Readings

Bouchard, C., et al., eds. *Exercise, Fitness, and Health*. Champaign, IL: Human Kinetics Publishers, 1990.

Paffenbarger, R., et al. "Physical Activity and Physical Fitness as Determinants of Health and Longevity." In Bouchard, C., et al. *Exercise, Fitness, and Health*. Champaign, IL: Human Kinetics Publishers, 1990.

Physical Activity and Fitness Research Digest, published quarterly, contains articles of all kinds on exercise, sports, and fitness. Available from The President's Council on Physical Fitness and Sports.

Physician and Sportsmedicine, published monthly, contains articles of all kinds on exercise, sports, and fitness.

LAB RESOURCE MATERIALS

(For Use with Labs 2A and 2B, pages L-1–L-4)

Chart 2.1   The Physical Activity Questionnaire

The term "physical activity" in the following statements refers to all kinds of activities, including sports, formal exercises, and informal activities, such as jogging and cycling. Check your answers first, then read the directions for scoring at the end of the questionnaire.

	Strongly Agree	Agree	Undecided	Disagree	Strongly Disagree	Score
1. Doing regular physical activity can be as harmful to health as it is helpful.	☐	☐	☐	☐	☒	5
2. One of the main reasons I do regular physical activity is because it is fun.	☒	☐	☐	☐	☐	5
3. Participating in physical activities makes me tense and nervous.	☐	☐	☐	☐	☒	5
4. The challenge of physical training is one reason why I participate in physical activity.	☒	☐	☐	☐	☐	5
5. One of the things I like about physical activity is the participation with other people.	☒	☐	☐	☐	☐	5
6. Doing regular physical activity does little to make me more physically attractive.	☐	☐	☐	☐	☒	5
7. Competition is a good way to keep a game from being fun.	☐	☐	☐	☐	☒	5
8. I should exercise regularly for my own good health and physical fitness.	☒	☐	☐	☐	☐	5
9. Doing exercise and playing sports is boring.	☐	☐	☐	☐	☒	5
10. I enjoy taking part in physical activity because it helps me to relax and get away from the pressures of daily living.	☒	☐	☐	☐	☐	5
11. Most sports and physical activities are too difficult for me to enjoy.	☒	☐	☐	☐	☐	5
12. I do not enjoy physical activities that require the participation of other people.	☐	☐	☐	☐	☐	
13. Regular exercise helps me look my best.	☐	☐	☐	☐	☐	
14. Competing against others in physical activities makes them enjoyable.	☐	☐	☐	☐	☐	

Score the physical activity questionnaire as follows:

1. For items 1, 3, 6, 7, 9, 11, and 12, give one point for strongly agree, two for agree, three for undecided, four for disagree, and five for strongly disagree. Put the correct number in the blank to the right of the statements.

2. For items 2, 4, 5, 8, 10, 13, and 14, give five points for strongly agree, four for agree, three for undecided, two for disagree, and one for strongly disagree. Put the correct number in the blank to the right of the statements.

3. Determine each of the following seven scores by adding the numbers to the right of the items as indicated (two numbers for each score).

Health and fitness score   Item 1 _____ + Item 8 _____ = _____

Fun and enjoyment score   Item 2 _____ + Item 9 _____ = _____

Relaxation and tension release score   Item 3 _____ + Item 10 _____ = _____

Challenge and achievement score   Item 4 _____ + Item 11 _____ = _____

Social score   Item 5 _____ + Item 12 _____ = _____

Appearance score   Item 6 _____ + Item 13 _____ = _____

Competition score   Item 7 _____ + Item 14 _____ = _____

Total score _____

4. Determine your total score by adding each of the seven scores. Write your total score in the bottom blank.

5. Use chart 2.2 to determine your rating on each score.

Chart 2.2   Physical Activity Questionnaire *Rating Scale*

Classification	Each of Seven Scores	Total Score
Excellent	9–10	63–70
Good	7–8	50–62
Fair	6	42–49
Poor	4–5	30–41
Very poor	3 or less	29 or less

Chart 2.3   Physical Fitness Stunts

Prior to performing these stunts, a warm-up such as the one on pages 37 and 38 is recommended. The stunts are not meant to be good tests of fitness. Rather, they are used to help you better understand each component of fitness. Better tests are described later in the book. If you have a movement limitation that makes a stunt dangerous for you, do not perform it. Read about it or watch someone else do the stunt.

Item	Fitness Aspect	Pass	
1. *One-foot balance.* Stand on one foot; press up so that the weight is on the ball of the foot with the heel off the floor. Hold the hands and the other leg straight out in front for ten seconds.	Balance	Yes ☐	

Chart 2.3 *continued*

Item	Fitness Aspect	Pass	
2. *Standing long jump.* Stand with the toes behind a line; using no run or hop step, jump as far as possible. To pass, men must jump their height plus six inches. Women must jump their height only.	Power	Yes ☐	
3. *Paper ball pickup.* Place two wadded paper balls on the floor five feet away. Run, pick up the first ball, and return both feet behind the starting line. Repeat with the second ball. Finish in five seconds.	Agility	Yes ☐	5'
4. *Paper drop.* Have a partner hold a sheet of notebook paper so that the side edge is between your thumb and index finger about the width of your hand from the top of the page. When your partner drops the paper, catch it before it slips through the thumb and finger. Do not move your hand lower to catch the paper.	Reaction time	Yes ☐	
5. *Double heel click.* With the feet apart, jump up and tap the heels together twice before you hit the ground. You must land with your feet at least three inches apart.	Speed	Yes ☐	
6. *Paper ball bounce.* Wad up a sheet of notebook paper into a ball. Bounce the ball back and forth between the right and left hands. Keep the hands open and palms up. Bounce the ball three times with each hand (six times total), alternating hands for each bounce.	Coordination	Yes ☐	

Chart 2.3 *continued*

Item	Fitness Aspect	Pass
7. *Run in place*. Run in place for one and a half minutes (120 steps per minute). Rest for one minute and count the heart rate for thirty seconds. A heart rate of 60 or lower passes. A step is counted each time the right foot hits the floor. See page 59 for directions on counting pulse.	Cardiovascular fitness	Yes ☐
8. *Toe touch*. Sit on the floor with your feet against a wall. Keep the feet together and the knees straight. Bend forward at the hips. After 3 warm-up trials, reach forward and touch your closed fists to the wall. Bend forward *slowly;* do *not* bounce. Note: This is a test-stunt, not an exercise (see concept 18).	Flexibility	Yes ☐
9. *The pinch*. Have a partner pinch a fold of skin on the back of your upper arm halfway between the tip of the elbow and the tip of the shoulder. Use your textbook to measure the skinfold width. Men: No greater than the thickness of the textbook. Women: No greater than one and one-half the thickness of the textbook.	Body composition (body fatness)	Yes ☐
10. *Push-up*. Lie face down on the floor. Place the hands under the shoulders. Keeping the legs and body straight, press off the floor until the arms are fully extended. Women repeat once, men three times.	Strength	Yes ☐
11. *Side leg raise*. Lie on the floor on your side. Lift your leg up and to the side of the body until your feet are 24 to 36 inches apart. Keep the knee and pelvis facing forward. Do *not* rotate so that the knees face the ceiling. Perform 10 with each leg.	Muscular endurance and strength	Yes ☐

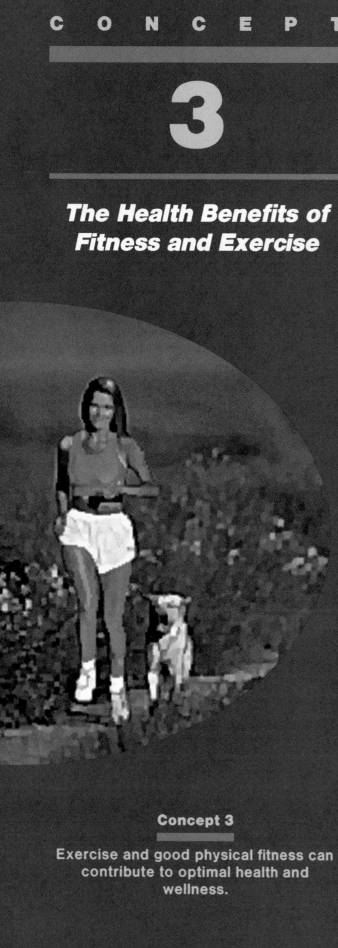

CONCEPT

3

The Health Benefits of Fitness and Exercise

Concept 3

Exercise and good physical fitness can contribute to optimal health and wellness.

Introduction

There are at least three major ways in which regular exercise and good physical fitness can contribute to optimal health and wellness (see figure 3.1) First, they can aid in **disease/illness prevention.** There is considerable evidence that the risk of hypokinetic diseases and conditions can be greatly reduced among those who do regular exercise and achieve good physical fitness.

Leading public health officials have suggested that "Physical activity is related to the health of all Americans. It has the ability to reduce directly the risk for several major **chronic diseases,** as well as to catalyze positive changes with respect to other risk factors for these diseases. . . . Physical activity may provide the shortcut we in public health have been seeking for the control of chronic diseases, much like immunization has facilitated progress against infectious diseases" (McGinnis 1992, p. S196).

Second, exercise and fitness can be a significant contributor to **disease/illness treatment.** Even with the best disease-prevention practices, some people will become ill. Regular exercise and good fitness has been shown to be effective in alleviating symptoms and rehabilitating after illness for such hypokinetic conditions as diabetes, heart attack, back pain and others.

Finally, exercise and fitness are methods of **health and wellness promotion.** They contribute to quality living associated with wellness, the positive component of good health. In the process they aid in meeting many of the nation's health goals for the year 2000.

Health Goals for the Year 2000

- Increase the span of healthy life.
- Reduce coronary heart disease deaths.
- Reduce cholesterol levels among adults.
- Reduce the incidence of overweight among adults.
- Reduce the proportion of adults with high blood pressure.
- Reduce stroke deaths.
- Reduce the incidence and deaths from diabetes.
- Reduce the incidence of chronic back conditions.
- Reverse the rise in cancer deaths.
- Reduce the prevalence of mental disorders.
- Reduce the adverse health effects of stress.
- Reduce the suicide rate.
- Reduce hip fractures among older people.
- Reduce hospitalization from asthma.

Terms

Acquired Aging

The acquisition of characteristics commonly associated with aging but that are, in fact, caused by immobility or sedentary living.

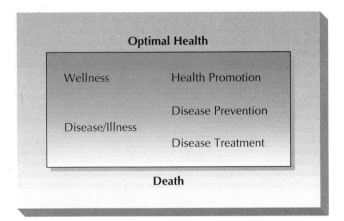

Figure 3.1
Contributors to optimal health and wellness.

Angina Pectoris

Chest or arm pain resulting from reduced oxygen supply to the heart muscle.

Arteriosclerosis

Hardening of the arteries due to conditions that cause the arterial walls to become thick, hard, and nonelastic.

Atherosclerosis

The deposition of materials along the arterial walls; a type of arteriosclerosis.

Chronic Disease

A disease or illness that is associated with life-style or environmental factors as opposed to infectious diseases (hypokinetic diseases are considered to be chronic diseases).

Collateral Circulation

Development of auxiliary blood vessels that may take over coronary blood circulation to the heart muscle in the event that one or more of the coronary arteries becomes obstructed or has diminished blood flow.

Congestive Heart Failure

The inability of the heart muscle to pump the blood at a life-sustaining rate.

Coronary Occlusion

The blocking of the coronary blood vessels.

Disease/Illness Prevention

Altering life-styles and environmental factors with the intent of preventing or reducing the risk of various illnesses and diseases.

Disease/Illness Treatment

Altering life-styles and use of medical procedures to aid in rehabilitation or reduction in symptoms or debilitation from a disease or illness.

Emotional Storm

A traumatic emotional experience that is likely to affect the human organism physiologically.

Fibrin

The substance that in combination with blood cells forms a blood clot.

Health and Wellness Promotion

Altering life-styles and environmental factors with the intent of improving quality of life.

High Density Lipoprotein (HDL)

A blood substance that picks up cholesterol and helps remove it from the body; often called "good cholesterol."

Hyperkinetic Condition

A disease/illness or health condition caused by or contributed to by too much exercise.

Hypertension

High blood pressure.

Lipids

All fats and fatty substances.

Lipoprotein

Fat-carrying protein in the blood.

Low Density Lipoprotein (LDL)

A core of cholesterol surrounded by protein; the core is often called "bad cholesterol."

Parasympathetic Nervous System

Branch of the autonomic nervous system that slows the heart rate.

Peripheral Vascular Disease

Lack of oxygen supply to the working muscles and tissues of the arms and legs resulting from decreased blood supply.

Stroke (Cerebrovascular Accident or CVA)

A condition in which the brain, or part of the brain, receives insufficient oxygen as a result of diminished blood supply; sometimes called apoplexy.

Sympathetic Nervous System

Branch of the autonomic nervous system that prepares the body for activity by speeding up the heart rate.

Time-Dependent Aging

The loss of function resulting from growing older.

Facts About Exercise, Fitness, and Disease Prevention/Treatment

Too many adults suffer from **hypokinetic diseases** (see definition on page 3).

In 1961, Kraus and Raab coined the term "hypokinetic disease." They pointed out that recent advances in medicine had been quite effective in eliminating infectious diseases but that degenerative diseases, characterized by sedentary or "take-it-easy" living, had increased in recent decades. In fact, heart disease is the leading cause of death in North America. High blood pressure, stroke, and coronary artery disease including heart attack afflict millions each year. The second leading medical complaint (headache is number one) is low back pain, and as many as one-half of all adults are considered to be obese. Studies now show that the symptoms of hypokinetic disease begin in youth. This suggests that the incidence of hypokinetic disease in our culture will not be reduced without considerable life-style change in people of all ages (see figure 3.2).

The link between regular physical activity and good health is now well documented.

People who exercise regularly can reduce their risk of death, regardless of the cause. Active people increase their life expectancy by two years compared to those who are inactive. One leading public health official indicates that increasing physical activity among the adult population would do wonders for the health of the nation because there are so many sedentary people who could benefit from active life-styles. "In fact, the national pattern of physical inactivity, in combination with the dietary patterns . . . ranks with tobacco use among the leading preventable contributors to death for Americans—well ahead of the contributions of infectious diseases" (McGinnis 1992, p. S197).

The Facts About Exercise and Cardiovascular Diseases

There are many types of cardiovascular diseases.

Hypertension (high blood pressure), **coronary occlusion** (heart attack), **atherosclerosis, arteriosclerosis, angina pectoris** (chest or arm pain), **stroke, peripheral vascular disease,** and **congestive heart failure** are among the more prevalent forms of heart disease. Evidence indicates that inactivity relates in some way to each of these types of disease.

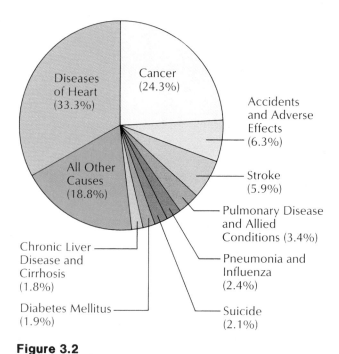

Figure 3.2

Major causes of death in the United States. The sum of data for the ten causes may not equal the total due to rounding.

Source: National Center for Health Statistics.

The various forms of cardiovascular disease are the leading killers in automated societies.

As noted in figure 3.2, cardiovascular diseases are the leading cause of death in the United States. Similar death rates are apparent in Canada, Great Britain, Australia, and other automated societies.

A wealth of statistical evidence indicates that active people are less likely to have coronary heart disease than sedentary people.

Much of the research relating inactivity to heart disease has come from occupational studies that show a high incidence of heart disease in people involved only in sedentary work. Even with the limitations inherent in these types of studies, the findings of more and more occupational studies present convincing evidence that the inactive individual has an increased risk of coronary heart disease.

Studies also indicate that people who are physically active in their leisure time have reduced risk of coronary heart disease if they expend a significant number of calories per week in strenuous sports and other activities. In fact, it was concluded that improving activity levels was among the best ways to reduce the risk of heart disease among adults.

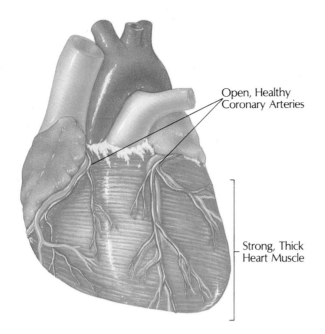

Figure 3.3

The fit heart muscle.

Recent evidence suggests that regular exercise can be a primary factor in reducing the risk of heart disease and early death from the heart disease.

The American Heart Association, after carefully examining the research literature said ". . . the body of research is now of sufficient strength to identify a sedentary lifestyle as a risk factor comparable to high blood pressure, high blood cholesterol, and cigarette smoke" (Cooper 1992). Also, one recent study of more than 15,000 college alumni shows that those who do regular exercise have lower death rates from heart disease than those who are inactive.

Recent decreases in the incidence of heart disease in the United States may be, in part, due to recent increases in activity levels of American adults.

Though heart disease is still present in epidemic proportions (one in three males will have a heart attack by age sixty), many experts feel that the increase in regular exercise by previously sedentary Americans is one reason for the modest decreases in heart disease in recent decades.

The Facts About Exercise and the Healthy Heart

There is evidence that regular exercise will increase the ability of the heart muscle to pump blood as well as oxygen.

A fit heart muscle can handle *extra* demands placed on it. Through regular exercise, the heart muscle gets stronger

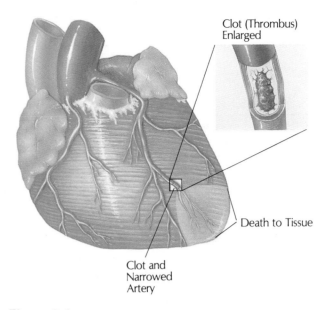

Figure 3.4

Heart attack.

and therefore pumps more blood with each beat, resulting in a slower heart rate and greater heart efficiency. Of importance is the fact that the heart is just like any other muscle—it must be exercised regularly if it is to stay fit. The fit heart has open, clear arteries free of atherosclerosis. (See figure 3.3.)

Contrary to popular belief, exercise does not cause "athlete's heart," nor does it injure the hearts of children.

The term *athlete's heart* is a misnomer. Though some investigators have found increases in heart size as a result of training, this is not the pathological increase in size associated with heart disease. There is no evidence that heavy exercise injures a normal heart.

Many parents suggest that strenuous exercise is harmful to their children. To be sure, overstrenuous activity for long periods may have deleterious effects, but regular activity has no harmful effect on children's hearts.

The Facts About Exercise and Heart Attack

Heart attack is the most prevalent and serious of all cardiovascular diseases.

A heart attack occurs when a coronary artery is blocked (see figure 3.4). A clot or thrombus is the most common cause. When a coronary occlusion or heart attack occurs, blood flow and oxygen to the heart muscle are cut off. If the coronary artery that is blocked supplies a major portion of the heart muscle, death will occur within minutes. Occlusions of lesser arteries may result in angina pectoris or a nonfatal heart attack.

Regular exercise reduces the risk of heart attack.

People who perform regular sports and physical activity have half the risk of a first heart attack compared to those who are sedentary.

There is evidence that regular exercise can improve coronary **collateral circulation** and thus reduce the chances of dying from a heart attack.

Within the heart, there are many tiny branches extending from the coronary arteries that supply blood to the heart muscle, as shown in figure 3.5. These interconnecting arteries can supply blood to any region of the heart as it is needed. If a person is relatively inactive, these interconnecting arteries are functionally closed. Though the evidence is not conclusive, the belief is that during regular exercise, these extra blood vessels are opened up to provide the heart muscle with the necessary blood and oxygen. For a person with atherosclerosis (research suggests most of us have some atherosclerosis beginning early in life) or a person who has suffered a heart attack, coronary collateral circulation may be very important. There is also evidence that the size of the coronary arteries increases as a result of exercise.

Improved coronary circulation may provide protection against a heart attack because a larger artery would require more atherosclerosis to occlude it. In addition, the development of collateral blood vessels supplying the heart may diminish the effects of a heart attack if one does occur. These "extra" (or collateral) blood vessels may take over the function of regular blood vessels during a heart attack.

The heart of the inactive person is less able to resist stress and is more susceptible to an **emotional storm** that may precipitate a heart attack.

The heart is rendered inefficient by one or more of the following circumstances: high heart rate, high blood pressure, and excessive stimulation. All of these conditions requires the heart to use more oxygen than is normally necessary and decrease its ability to adapt to stressful situations.

The "loafers heart" is one that beats rapidly because it is dominated by the **sympathetic nervous system,** which speeds up the heart rate. Thus, the heart continuously beats rapidly, even at rest, and never has a true rest period. Further, high blood pressure makes the heart work harder and contributes to its inefficiency.

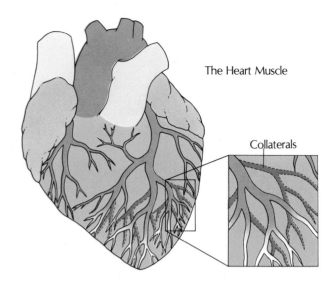

The Heart Muscle

Collaterals

Figure 3.5
Coronary collateral circulation.

Research indicates four things concerning exercise and the loafer's heart.

- Regular exercise leads to dominance of the **parasympathetic nervous system** rather than to sympathetic dominance; thus the heart rate is reduced and the heart works efficiently.
- Regular exercise helps the heart rate return to normal faster after emotional stress.
- Regular exercise strengthens the loafer's heart, making the heart better able to weather emotional storms.
- Regular exercise decreases sympathetic dominance and its associated hormonal effects on the heart, thus lessening the chances of altered heart contractibility and the likelihood of the circulatory problems that accompany this state.

Regular exercise is one effective means of rehabilitation for a person who has coronary heart disease or who has had a heart attack.

Not only does regular exercise seem to reduce the risk of developing coronary heart disease, but there is also evidence that those who already have the condition may reduce the symptoms of the disease through regular exercise. For those who have had heart attacks, regular and progressive exercise can be an effective prescription when carried out under the supervision of a physician. Remember, however, that exercise is not the treatment of preference for all heart attack victims. In some cases, it may be contraindicated.

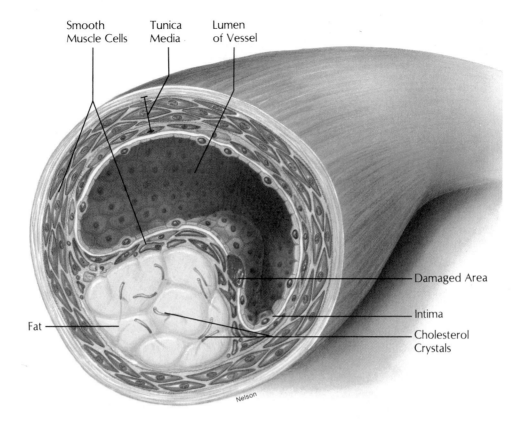

Smooth Muscle Cells · Tunica Media · Lumen of Vessel

Damaged Area

Intima

Cholesterol Crystals

Fat

Nelson

Figure 3.6

Atherosclerosis.

From Kent M. Van De Graaff and Stuart Ira Fox, *Concepts of Human Anatomy and Physiology*, 3d ed. Copyright © 1992 Wm. C. Brown Communications, Inc., Dubuque, Iowa. All Rights Reserved. Reprinted by permission.

The Facts About Exercise and Atherosclerosis

Atherosclerosis is implicated in many cardiovascular diseases.

Atherosclerosis is a condition that contributes to heart attack, stroke, hypertension, angina pectoris, and peripheral vascular diseases. Deposits on the walls of arteries restrict blood flow and oxygen supply to the tissues. Atherosclerosis of the coronary arteries, the vessels that supply the heart muscle with oxygen, is particularly harmful. If these arteries become narrowed, the blood supply to the heart muscle is diminished and angina pectoris may occur. Atherosclerosis increases the risk of heart attack because a clot is more likely to obstruct a narrowed artery than a healthy, open one.

Atherosclerosis, which begins early in life, is the result of a systematic build-up of deposits in an arterial wall.

Current theory suggests that atherosclerosis begins when damage occurs to the cells of the inner wall of the artery (intima). Substances associated with blood clotting are attracted to the damaged area. These substances seem to cause the migration of smooth muscle cells, commonly found only in the middle wall of the artery (media), to the intima. In the later stages, fats (including cholesterol) and other substances are thought to be deposited, forming plaques or protrusions (see figure 3.6) that diminish the internal diameter of the artery. Research indicates that the first signs of atherosclerosis begin in early childhood.

There is evidence that regular physical activity can help prevent atherosclerosis.

All of the ways in which regular exercise helps prevent atherosclerosis are not yet known. However, three of the most plausible theories are discussed below.

Lipid Deposit Theory

There are several kinds of fats in the bloodstream, including **lipoproteins,** phospholipids, triglycerides, and cholesterol. Whereas cholesterol is the most well-known fat, it is not the only culprit. Many blood fats are manufactured by the body itself, while others are ingested in high fat foods, particularly saturated fats (fats that are solid at room temperature). As noted earlier, blood **lipids** are thought to contribute to the development of athero-

Table 3.1
Cholesterol Goals (mg/100 ml)

	Total Cholesterol*	LDL-C	HDL-C	TC/HDL-C
Goal	180 or less	130 or less	55+	3.5 or less
Borderline	180–219	130–159	47–55	3.6–5.0
High risk	220+	160+	46 or less	5.0+

Source: Data from H. R. Superko, "The Role of Diet, Exercise, and Medication in Blood Lipid Management of Cardiac Patients" in *Physician and Sportsmedicine,* 16:67, 1988; and HDL data from B. Liebman, "Rating Your Risk" in *Nutrition Action,* 19:8, 1992.

Table 3.2
Blood Pressure Goals

	Blood Pressure Systolic	(mm/hg) Diastolic
Goal	120 or less	90 or less
Borderline	121–159	91–109
High risk	160+	110+

sclerotic deposits on the inner walls of the artery. One substance, called **low density lipoprotein (LDL)**, is considered to be a major culprit in the development of atherosclerosis. LDL is basically a core of cholesterol surrounded by protein and another substance that makes it water soluble. The theory is that regular exercise can reduce blood lipid levels, including LDL-C (the cholesterol core of LDL). People with high total cholesterol and LDL-C levels have been shown to have a higher than normal risk of heart disease (see table 3.1). New evidence indicates that a substance called apolipoprotein B (Apo B) combines with LDL to increase risk. A low Apo B level is desirable.

Protective Protein Theory

Whereas LDLs carry a core of cholesterol that is involved in the development of atherosclerosis, **high density lipoprotein (HDL)** picks up cholesterol (**HDL-C**) and carries it to the liver, where it is eliminated from the body. For this reason it is often called the "protective protein." High levels of HDL are considered to be desirable. When you have a blood test it is wise to determine the amount of HDL-C compared to the total amount of cholesterol (TC) in your blood. A low TC/HDL-C ratio is a good indicator of the protection you are receiving from HDL (see table 3.1). The theory is that people who do regular exercise have high HDL amounts, as evidenced by TC/HDL-C ratios, and therefore less heart disease. Just as Apo B together with LDL increases risk, another substance called apolipoprotein A-I (Apo A-I), attaches itself to HDL to help lower LDL levels. A high Apo A-I level is desirable.

Fibrin Deposit Theory

Fibrin is a sticky, threadlike substance in the blood that is important to the clotting process. The Fibrin Deposit Theory is that fibrin and other blood constituents involved in clotting may be involved in the development of atherosclerosis. Exercise has been shown to reduce fibrin levels in the blood. Although there is some evidence to support this theory, research results to date are not conclusive.

Exercise and Other Cardiovascular Diseases

Regular exercise and accompanying good physical fitness are associated with a reduced risk of high blood pressure.

Approximately 30 percent of adults have borderline or high-risk hypertension (see table 3.2). More men than women are likely to be hypertensive, as are more blacks than whites. Native Americans have a higher than normal incidence of hypertension, and the incidence for all groups increases as people grow older. A recent research summary indicates that the effects of physical activity on blood pressure are more dramatic than previously thought and are independent of age, body fatness, and other factors. Inactive, less fit individuals have a 30–50 percent greater chance of being hypertensive than active fit people. Regular exercise can also be one effective method of reducing blood pressure for those with hypertension. Goals for blood pressure are indicated in table 3.2.

Regular exercise can help reduce the risk of stroke.

Stroke is a major killer of adults. Those with high blood pressure and atherosclerosis are susceptible to stroke. Since regular exercise and good fitness are important to the prevention of both high blood pressure and atherosclerosis, exercise and fitness are considered helpful in the prevention of stroke.

Regular exercise is helpful in the prevention of peripheral vascular diseases.

There is evidence that people who exercise regularly have better blood flow to the working muscles and other tissues than inactive, unfit people. Since peripheral vascular disease is associated with poor circulation to the extremities, regular exercise can be considered one method of preventing this condition.

The Facts About Exercise, Health-Related, Fitness, and Other Hypokinetic Conditions

Active people who possess good muscle fitness are less likely to have back and other musculoskeletal problems than inactive unfit people.

Because few people die from it, back pain does not receive the attention given to such medical problems as heart disease and cancer. But back pain is considered to be the second leading medical complaint in the United States, second only to headaches. Only common colds and flu cause more days lost from work than this ailment. At some point in their lives, approximately 80 percent of all adults will experience back pain that limits their ability to function normally.

Many years ago, medical doctors began to associate back problems with the lack of physical fitness. It is now known that the great majority of back ailments are the result of poor muscle strength and endurance, and poor flexibility. Tests on patients with back problems show weakness and lack of flexibility in key muscle groups.

Though lack of fitness is probably the leading reason for back pain in Western society, there are many other factors that increase the risk of back ailments, including poor posture, improper lifting (see fig. 3.7) and work habits, heredity, and other disease states, such as scoliosis and arthritis. Some of these are discussed in greater detail in Concepts 16 and 17.

Obesity, as well as lesser degrees of fatness, is not a disease state in itself but is a hypokinetic condition associated with a multitude of far-reaching complications.

Obesity is associated with serious organic impairments, shortened life, psychological maladjustments, poor relationships with peers (especially among children), awkward physical movement, and lack of achievement in athletic activities. Obesity can be both a cause and an effect of physical unfitness. Those who are overfat have a higher risk of respiratory infections; are prone to developing high blood pressure, atherosclerosis, and disorders of the circulatory and respiratory systems; and have a greater than normal risk of some forms of cancer. The symptoms of adult-onset diabetes are associated with excessive fatness. (Fortunately, fat loss to normal levels is usually followed by remission of diabetic symptoms). Because exercise, together with sound nutritional management, is an effective means of lowering body fat, it can be helpful in reducing the risks of those conditions associated with fatness and obesity.

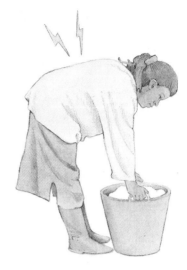

Figure 3.7

Back pain is a hypokinetic condition, but it may also be caused by incorrect lifting techniques.

Diabetes is often considered a hypokinetic condition because of the important role exercise plays in managing the disease.

By itself, exercise is not an effective treatment for Type I (insulin-dependent) diabetes. However, with proper medical supervision, exercise is encouraged for maintaining physical fitness for most diabetics. For those with Type II (noninsulin dependent, adult-onset) diabetes, regular exercise can help reduce body fatness and improve insulin sensitivity and glucose tolerance, all of which contribute to controlling the disease. Together with sound nutritional habits and proper medication, exercise can be useful in the management of diabetes.

Bone degeneration due to osteoporosis can be considered a hypokinetic condition.

Studies indicate that excessive bed rest can result in deterioration of the bones. When the long bones do not bear weight, they lose calcium and become porous and fragile. Even excessive sitting can result in bone deterioration, regardless of age. Bones are strengthened not only by bearing weight, but by the pull of active muscles. Regular exercise is as necessary for healthy bone development as it is for healthy muscle development. Osteoporosis commonly seen in older adults (especially in women) is caused by the decreased production of a specific hormone, and inadequate calcium intake, as well as by a lack of activity.

Common stress-related disorders can be considered hypokinetic conditions.

Some stress-related conditions prevalent in modern society are discussed in Concept 23; however, a few that are associated with inactive life-styles are noted here.

Insomnia is a condition that afflicts many people in our culture and one that is often stress-related. Results from a survey of American adults indicate that 52 percent feel regular exercise helps them to sleep better.

Depression is another stress-related condition experienced by many adults. Thirty-three percent of inactive adults report that they often feel depressed. For some, depression is a serious disorder that exercise alone will not cure; however, recent research does indicate that exercise, combined with other forms of therapy, can be effective in its treatment. For those with minor depression, exercise may also be helpful. One-third of very active people in one study felt that regular exercise helped them to better cope with life's pressures.

Even more common than depression and insomnia is the condition called *Type A behavior.* "Type A personalities" are stress-prone individuals with a greater than normal incidence of diseases. A Type A person is tense, overcompetitive, and worried about meeting time schedules. Regular exercise can be of special benefit to the Type A person, though noncompetitive exercise would probably be best.

In many cases, gastric ulcers may be a hypokinetic condition.

It has been theorized that gastric ulcers can be considered a hypokinetic condition because inactive individuals have a higher mortality rate from the condition than do active people. This conclusion must be considered tentative; however, the lower incidence of ulcers among active people, plus the fact that exercise can be effective in helping to manage stress and tension levels often associated with ulcer disease, suggest that regular exercise may be useful for some people in the prevention or management of gastric ulcer symptoms.

Some forms of cancer can now be considered as hypokinetic diseases.

The relationship between fitness, exercise, and cancer is not yet fully understood. However, preliminary evidence suggests that fit people who regularly exercise have increased protection against certain forms of cancer such as colon, reproductive system, and breast cancer. One possible reason for the reduced risk of colon/rectal cancer (the second most common cause of cancer deaths among males) is the reduced intestinal transit time among regular exercisers. Among women, nonathletes have been found to have a greater risk of breast cancer than athletes, though this finding needs further verification. For those who have cancer, there is evidence that exercise can help them lead more fulfilling and productive lives.

Hypokinetic diseases and conditions have many causes.

Regular exercise and good physical fitness are only two factors associated with the conditions described in this concept as hypokinetic diseases. Other healthy lifestyles cannot be overlooked in the prevention of these diseases.

Exercise, Physical Fitness, and Nonhypokinetic Diseases

Regular exercise can have positive effects on some nonhypokinetic conditions.

- Infections. Infectious diseases are not generally considered to be hypokinetic conditions. However, regular exercise that fosters physical fitness and good health may help you resist diseases resulting from lowered general resistance. On the other hand, when the body is fighting an infection, too much exercise can result in a lowered state of resistance.
- Arthritis. Many, if not most, arthritics are in a deconditioned state resulting from a lack of activity. The traditional advice that exercise is to be avoided by arthritics is now being modified in view of the findings that carefully prescribed exercise can improve general fitness and, in some cases, reduce the symptoms of the disease.
- Chronic Pain. There are many sources of pain that persist for long periods of time without relief; some are difficult to understand. Nevertheless, large numbers of adults are victims of chronic pain. Both aerobic exercise and resistance training are currently being prescribed as means of treating this problem.
- Premenstrual Syndrome (PMS). PMS, a mixture of physical and emotional symptoms that occur prior to menstruation, has many causes. However, current evidence suggests that changes in lifestyle, including involvement in regular exercise, may be effective in relieving PMS symptoms.

Exercise, Physical Fitness, and Aging

In many ways, **acquired aging** is similar to a hypokinetic condition.

Forced inactivity in young adults can cause losses in function (acquired aging) very much like those that are generally considered to occur with aging (**time-dependent aging**). Studies suggest that acquired aging is a product of a sedentary life-style. In Africa, Asia, and South America, where older adults (age sixty-five and older) maintain an active life-style, individuals do not acquire many of the characteristics commonly associated with aging in North America.

Regular exercise can significantly delay the aging process.

Regular physical activity in the elderly delays decline in physical abilities, improves quality of life, and enhances functional capacity. (Rousseau 1989, p. 116)

Adults are never "too old" to begin exercising.

Physical fitness for old age should begin in the early years in order to enjoy maximum benefits. If this does not occur for one reason or another, a person is never too old to begin exercising. Studies conducted over a period of years indicate that properly planned exercise for older people is not only safe, but also that older men and women are *not* significantly different from youth in their abilities to improve fitness through exercise. A review of recent research has concluded that:

> There is strong evidence that the decline in exercise capacity often observed in the elderly is neither inevitable nor, once it is developed, permanent. The activity levels of many older persons may decrease because of musculoskeletal difficulties or personal choice. These factors may exacerbate any decline in exercise capacity associated with normal aging (time-dependent). Unfortunately, this decline may endanger the older person's desire to maintain an independent life-style. The evidence of trainability of the cardiovascular system of the aging strongly suggests that exercise programs can contribute to the fulfillment of this desire. (Van Camp and Boyer 1989, p. 130)

Facts About Health and Wellness Promotion

Good health-related physical fitness and regular exercise are important to health promotion and feeling well.

Optimal health is more than freedom from disease. Regular exercise and good fitness help prevent illness and disease but also promote quality of life and feeling well. Good health-related fitness can help you feel good, look good, and enjoy life. Some of the health and wellness benefits of regular exercise are outlined in table 3.3 on page 30.

Good physical fitness can help an individual enjoy his or her leisure time.

A person who is not too fat, has no back problems, does not have to worry about high blood pressure, and has reasonable skills in lifetime sports is more likely to get involved and stay regularly involved in leisure time activities than one who does not have these characteristics. It is said that enjoying your leisure time may not add years to your life, but can add life to your years.

Good physical fitness can help an individual work effectively and efficiently.

A person who can resist fatigue, muscle soreness, back problems, and other symptoms associated with poor health-related fitness is capable of working productively and having energy left over at the end of the day. Surveys of employees who have the opportunity to improve fitness through involvement in employee fitness programs indicate that 75 percent have an improved sense of well-being. Employers indicate that absenteeism decreased by up to 50 percent among program participants. People with good skill-related fitness may be more effective and efficient in performing specific motor skills required for certain jobs.

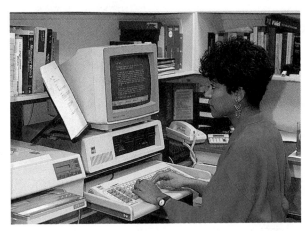

Fitness improves work efficiency.

Good physical fitness is essential to effective living.

Although the need for each component of physical fitness is specific to each individual, every person requires enough fitness to perform normal daily activities without undue fatigue. Whether it be walking, performing household chores, or merely feeling good and enjoying the simple things in life without pain or fear of injury, good fitness is important to all people.

Table 3.3

Health and Wellness Benefits of Regular Exercise

Major Benefit	Related Benefits	Major Benefit	Related Benefits
Improved cardiovascular fitness and health	• Stronger heart muscle • Lower heart rate • Possible reduction in blood pressure • Increased O_2 to brain • Reduced blood fat, including low density lipids (LDL) • Possible resistance to atherosclerosis • Increased work capacity • Possible improved peripheral circulation • Improved coronary circulation • Resistance to "emotional storm" • Reduced risk of heart attack • Reduced risk of stroke • Reduced risk of hypertension • Greater chance of surviving a heart attack • Increased protective high density lipids (HDL) • Increased oxygen carrying capacity of the blood	Reduction in mental tension	• Relief of depression • Improved sleep habits • Fewer stress symptoms • Ability to enjoy leisure • Possible work improvement
		Opportunity for social interactions	• Improved quality of life
		Resistance to fatigue	• Ability to enjoy leisure • Improved quality of life • Improved ability to meet some stressors
		Opportunity for successful experience	• Improved self-concept • Opportunity to recognize and accept personal limitations
		Improved sense of well-being	• Improved self-concept • Enjoy life—fun
		Improved appearance	• Better figure/physique • Better posture • Fat control
Greater lean body mass and less body fat	• Greater work efficiency • Less susceptibility to disease • Improved appearance • Less incidence of self-concept problems related to obesity	Reduced effect of acquired aging	• Improved ability to function in daily life • Better short-term memory • Fewer illnesses • Greater mobility • Greater independence • Greater ability to operate automobile
Improved strength and muscular endurance	• Greater work efficiency • Less chance of muscle injury • Reduced risk of low back problems • Improved performance in sports • Quicker recovery after hard work • Improved ability to meet emergencies	Improved flexibility	• Greater work efficiency • Less chance of muscle injury • Less chance of joint injury • Decreased chance of low back problems • Improved sports performance
		Other health benefits of exercise and physical activity	• Extended life • Decreased chance of adult-onset diabetes • Less chance of osteoporosis • Reduced risk of certain cancers

---

Good physical fitness may help you function safely and assist you in meeting unexpected emergencies.

Emergencies are never expected, but when they do arise, they often demand performance that requires good fitness. For example, flood victims may need to fill sandbags for hours without rest, and accident victims may be required to walk or run long distances for help. Also, good fitness is required for such simple tasks as safely changing a spare tire or loading a moving van without injury.

Table 3.4
Hypokinetic Disease Risk Factors

Factors That Cannot Be Altered

1. *Age*—As you grow older, your risk of contracting hypokinetic diseases increases. For example, the risk of heart disease is approximately three times as great after sixty than before. The risk of back pain and ulcer disease is considerably greater after forty.

2. *Heredity*—People who have a family history of hypokinetic disease are more likely to develop a hypokinetic condition. Heart disease, hypertension, ulcers, back problems, obesity, high blood lipid levels, and other problems have been shown to be more prevalent among those who have a family history of these conditions than among those with no family history. Black Americans are 45 percent more likely to have high blood pressure than whites; therefore, they suffer strokes at an earlier age with more severe consequences than whites.

3. *Sex*—Men have a higher incidence of many hypokinetic conditions than women. Although the number of women with heart disease is increasing, women still have only about half the incidence of the disease as men have; however, the incidence increases sharply in women after menopause.

Factors That Can Be Altered

4. *Body Fatness*—Having too much body fat is considered by many to be a hypokinetic condition because it may limit your ability to function efficiently and effectively. Even those who do not classify overfatness as a hypokinetic condition agree that it does increase the risk of other hypokinetic conditions. For example, loss of fat can result in relief from symptoms of adult-onset diabetes, can reduce problems associated with certain types of back pain, and can reduce the risks of surgery.

5. *Diet*—There is a clear association between hypokinetic disease and certain types of diets. The excessive intake of saturated fats, such as animal fats, is linked to atherosclerosis and other forms of heart disease. Excessive salt in the diet is associated with high blood pressure.

6. *Diseases*—People who have one hypokinetic disease are more likely to develop a second or even a third condition. For example, if you have diabetes, atherosclerosis, or high blood pressure, your risk of having a heart attack or stroke increases dramatically. People with poor posture have a high risk of experiencing back pain, and those with too much body fat have a greater than normal risk of diabetes. Although you may not be entirely able to alter the extent to which you develop certain diseases and conditions, reducing your risk and following your doctor's advice can improve your odds significantly.

7. *Regular Exercise*—As noted throughout this book, regular exercise can help reduce the risk of hypokinetic disease.

8. *Smoking*—Smokers have a much higher risk of developing and dying from heart disease than nonsmokers. The risk of heart attack is twice as great among young smokers as among young nonsmokers. (Most striking is the difference in risk between older women smokers and nonsmokers.) Smokers have five times the risk of heart attack as nonsmokers. Smoking is also associated with the increased risk of high blood pressure, cancer, and several other medical conditions. Apparently, the more you smoke, the greater the risk. To stop smoking even after many years can significantly reduce the hypokinetic disease risk.

9. *Stress*—There is evidence that people who are subject to excessive stress are predisposed to various hypokinetic diseases including heart disease and back pain. Statistics indicate that hypokinetic conditions are common among those in certain high-stress jobs and those having type A personality profiles.

Physical fitness is the basis for dynamic and creative activity.

Though the following quotation by former President John F. Kennedy is now more than thirty years old, it clearly points out the importance of physical fitness.

> The relationship between the soundness of the body and the activity of the mind is subtle and complex. Much is not yet understood, but we know what the Greeks knew: that intelligence and skill can only function at the peak of their capacity when the body is healthy and strong, and that hardy spirits and tough minds usually inhabit sound bodies. Physical fitness is the basis of all activities in our society; if our bodies grow soft and inactive, if we fail to encourage physical development and prowess, we will undermine our capacity for thought, for work, and for the use of those skills vital to an expanding and complex America.

The Facts About Risk Factors

There are many different positive life-styles that can reduce the risk of disease.

Many of the factors that contribute to optimal health and quality of life are also considered risk factors. Changing these risk factors can dramatically reduce the risk of hypokinetic diseases such as heart disease, obesity, back pain, and cancer, as well as other diseases such as infections and sexually transmitted diseases. Lack of exercise, poor nutrition, smoking, and inability to cope with stress are all risk factors associated with various diseases (see table 3.4).

Not all risk factors can be altered by life-style changes.

Some factors that can contribute to the increased risk of disease are not under your personal control. Three uncontrollable risk factors are: age, heredity, and sex. These factors that cannot be altered by life-style changes are presented in table 3.4.

> Altering risk factors can help reduce the risk of more than one adverse condition at the same time.

By altering the risk factors that are controllable, you can reduce the risk of several hypokinetic conditions. For example, controlling body fatness reduces the risk of diabetes, hypertension, and back problems. Altering your diet can reduce the chances of developing high levels of blood lipids, and thus reduce the risk of atherosclerosis.

> Risk reduction does not guarantee freedom from disease.

Reducing risk alters the probability of disease, but does not assure disease immunity.

> Certain heart disease risk factors are considered to be primary.

Some risk factors are more likely to contribute to heart disease than others. These are considered to be primary risk factors. Inactivity, high blood pressure (hypertension), particularly high systolic pressure, high blood fat levels (cholesterol and other fats), and smoking are considered to be primary risk factors. Others (noted in the questionnaire in Lab Resource Materials on page 33), such as age, exercise, and stress, are considered as secondary risk factors.

The Facts About Hyperkinetic Conditions

> Just as too little exercise can result in health problems, too much exercise can also contribute to illness and injury.

Hypokinetic means too little exercise. Conversely, hyperkinetic means too much exercise. Just as reasonable amounts of exercise can help reduce the risk of hypokinetic health problems, it has become apparent that excessive exercise can lead to hyperkinetic conditions that have negative effects on health and wellness. Several of the more common hyperkinetic conditions are described below.

Overuse Musculoskeletal Injuries

Evidence suggests that periodic rest is necessary to allow the body to recover from the stress of continuous and vigorous training. For example, runners who train seven days a week have more muscle and joint injuries than those who take at least one day a week off or reduce training levels several days a week. The most common overuse injuries are joint injuries to the foot, ankle, and knee; stress fractures in the lower extremities; and muscle/connective tissue injuries such as shin splints, strained hamstring muscles, and calf pain. These injuries are apparent among any type of exerciser who overdoes it. For example, dance aerobics instructors have been shown to be particularly likely to have overuse injuries. Tennis and baseball players often have similar problems, but their problems occur in different parts of the body (the arm and shoulder). The best way to prevent this type of hyperkinetic condition is periodic rest. Pain, the body's warning signal, is a good clue that the body needs rest.

Activity Neurosis

Activity neurosis is a compulsion to exercise. People with activity neurosis become irrationally concerned about their exercise regimen. They may exercise more than one time a day and rarely take a day off. The activity neurotic feels the need to exercise even when ill or injured. Musculoskeletal overuse injuries are especially common among activity neurotics. The excessive desire to exercise can also be the source of poor performance in other aspects of life, as well as a source of stress. Competitive athletes with this condition may have reduced performance, and among females, amenorrhea (no menstrual flow).

Anorexia Nervosa

Anorexia nervosa is an eating disorder associated with an obsessive desire to be lean. There is increasing evidence that many anorexics use compulsive exercise, as well as undereating, to keep body fat at low levels. For this reason anorexia nervosa can often be considered a hyperkinetic condition. This serious medical condition will be discussed in greater detail in Concept 13.

Body Neurosis

Body neurosis is an obsessive concern for having an attractive body. Among females, it is associated with an extreme desire to be lean. In some cases it can lead to anorexia. Among males, this condition is associated with an extreme desire to be muscular. Recent research indicates that increasing numbers of males are interested in leanness and a number of females are now compulsive about muscle mass gains. Those with body neurosis are often compulsive exercisers, though they are also more likely to be subject to nutritional quackery (use of quack dietary supplements) and in some cases resort to the use of anabolic steroids.

Suggested Readings

Blair, S. et al. "Bone Gain in Young Adult Women." *JAMA* 268(1992):2403.

Cooper, K. *Controlling Cholesterol.* New York: Bantam Books, 1988.

Corbin, C. B., and R. P. Pangrazi. "The Health Benefits of Exercise." *Research Digest for Physical Activity and Fitness* 1(1993):1.

International Society of Sport Psychology. "Physical Activity and Psychological Benefits: Position Statement." 20(1992):179.

Public Health Service. *Healthy People 2000: National Health Promotion and Disease Prevention Objectives.* Washington, DC: U.S. Government Printing Office, 1991.

LAB RESOURCE MATERIALS

(For use with Lab 3, page L-5)

Heart Disease Risk Factor Questionnaire

Circle the appropriate answer to each question.

	Risk Points				
	1	**2**	**3**	**4**	**Score**
Unalterable Factors					
1. How old are you?	30 or less	31–40	41–54	55+	_____
2. Do you have a history of heart disease in your family?	none	grandparent with heart disease	parent with heart disease	more than one with heart disease	_____
3. What is your sex?	female		male		_____
				Total Unalterable Risk Score	_____
Alterable Factors					
4. What is your percent of body fat?	F = 20%↓ M = 15%↓	25%↓ 20%↓	30%↓ 25%↓	35%↑ 30%↑	_____
5. Do you have a high-fat diet?	no	slightly high in fat	above normal in fat	eat a lot of meat and/or fried and fatty foods	_____
6. What is your blood pressure? (systolic, or upper, score)	120↓	121–140	141–160	160↑	_____
7. Do you have other diseases?	no	ulcer	diabetes	both	_____
8. Do you exercise regularly?	4–5 days a week	3 days a week	less than 3 days a week	no	_____
9. Do you smoke?	no	cigar or pipe only	less than ½ pack a day	more than ½ pack a day	_____
10. Are you under much stress?	less than normal	normal	slightly above normal	quite high	_____
				Total Alterable Risk Score	_____
				Grand Total Risk Score	_____

Chart 3.1 Heart Disease Risk *Rating Scale*			
Rating	**Unalterable Score**	**Alterable Score**	**Total Score**
Very high	9 or More	21 or More	31 or More
High	7–8	15–20	26–30
Average	5–6	11–14	16–25
Low	4 or Less	10 or Less	15 or Less

CONCEPT

4

Preparing for Exercise

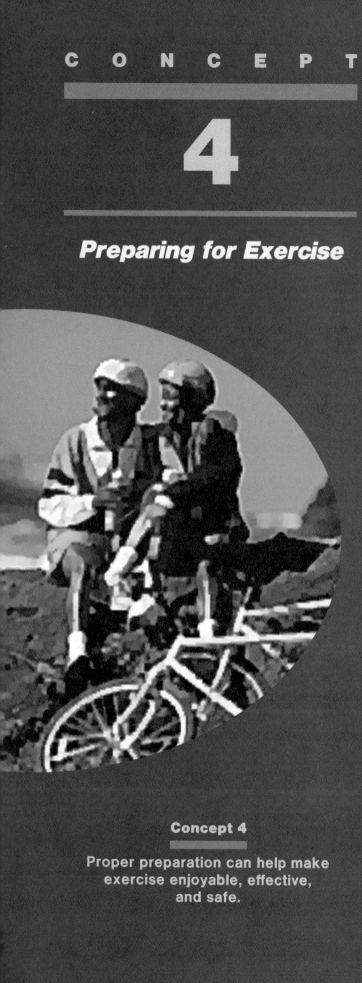

Concept 4

Proper preparation can help make exercise enjoyable, effective, and safe.

Introduction

More than at any other time in recent history, adults are engaging in some form of regular exercise during their free time. Unfortunately, all too often those who start an exercise program with good intentions drop out after a few days, weeks, or months. As noted in Concept 2, part of the problem is that people lack information concerning the correct way to exercise.

For those just beginning an exercise program, adequate preparation may be the key to persistence. It is hoped that a person armed with good information about preparing for exercise will become involved and stay involved with that exercise for a lifetime. To be effective, exercise must be something that is a part of a person's normal lifestyle. Some facts that will help you to prepare for exercise and make it part of your normal routine are presented in this concept.

Health Goals for the Year 2000

- Increase the proportion of people who do regular physical activity.
- Decrease the proportion of people who do no leisure-time physical activity.

Terms

Achilles Tendon

The long tendon that attaches the calf muscles to the heel bone on the back of the foot.

Cool-Down Exercise

Light to moderate tapering-off activity after vigorous exercise; often consisting of the same exercises used in the warm-up.

Dehydration

Excessive loss of water from the body, usually through perspiration, urination, or evaporation.

PAR-Q

This is an acronym for Physical Activity Readiness Questionnaire, designed to help you determine if you are medically suited to begin an exercise program.

Warm-Up Exercise

Light to moderate activity done prior to the workout. Its purpose is to reduce the risk of injury and soreness and possibly to improve performance in a physical activity.

Wind-Chill Factor

An index that uses air temperature and wind speed to determine the chilling influence of the environment on humans.

The Facts to Consider Before Beginning Exercise

Before beginning a regular exercise program, it is important to establish your medical readiness to participate.

There is no way to be absolutely sure that you are medically sound to begin an exercise program. Even a thorough exam by a physician cannot guarantee that a person does not have some limitations that may cause a problem during exercise. However, an exam is the surest way to make certain that you are ready to participate.

The American College of Sports Medicine, in its guidelines for evaluating health status for exercise participation, suggests that under certain circumstances people should have a preexercise exam, which includes an exercise test coupled with an EKG during exercise. Specifically, the college recommends a preexercise test for those forty-five years and over; for those thirty-five years and over who have a higher than normal risk of heart disease (see Lab 3 to check your risk); for those with symptoms of heart disease; and for those with known heart disease. Healthy people under forty-five need not have a preexercise exam but may wish to seek medical consultation when resuming exercise following injury or illness, when returning to an exercise program after an extended layoff, or when making significant modifications in exercise programs.

The British Columbia (Canada) Ministry of Health conducted extensive research to devise a procedure that would help people know when it was advisable to seek medical consultation prior to beginning or altering an exercise program. The goal was to prevent unnecessary medical examinations, while at the same time to give a reasonable assurance that regular exercise was appropriate for an individual. The research resulted in the development of the **PAR-Q** questionnaire. The **PAR-Q** consists of seven simple questions you can ask yourself to determine if medical consultation is necessary prior to exercise involvement. To help you decide whether to have a complete medical exam before you begin or modify your exercise program, or whether to adopt the American College of Sports Medicine guidelines, complete the PAR-Q provided in the Lab Resource Materials on page 42.

Young adults, such as college students, or older adults who plan to do intensive training (particularly for sports) may want to answer some additional questions concerning whether a medical exam is necessary before beginning (see chart 4.2).

It is important to dress properly for exercise.

The clothing you wear for exercise should be specifically for that exercise. It should be comfortable and not too tight or binding at the joints. Though appearance is important to everyone, comfort in exercise is more important than looks. Clothing should not restrict movement in any way. Preferably, the clothing that comes in direct contact with the body should be porous to allow for sweat evaporation. Some women, especially those who need extra support, should consider using an exercise bra, and men will need an athletic supporter. A warm-up suit over other exercise apparel is recommended because it can be removed during exercise if desired. Many exercise suits are nonporous so, by themselves, are not desirable for exercise.

Socks that fit properly should be worn during exercise. Tight-fitting socks can cause ingrown toenails, and loose-fitting socks can cause blisters. Sockless feet can result in blisters, abrasions, shoe odor, and excess wear on shoes.

Proper exercise footwear is important.

Most manufacturers now produce athletic shoes in six categories: running/jogging, walking, tennis, court, aerobic/fitness, and cross trainers. Many produce even more specialized shoes within each category. For example, many have separate court shoes for basketball and volleyball. For those who are highly dedicated to a specific activity, a specialized pair of shoes should be purchased. For those who do not specialize in one activity, the cross trainer is a good choice.

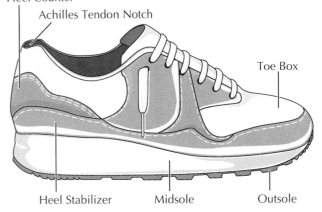

Proper exercise shoes are important.

The essential characteristics of all athletic shoes are listed below:

- Support. The heel counter and the heel stabilizer provide stability and control foot movement. The heel tab protects the **Achilles tendon** from trauma. A wide heel in running shoes provides stability and protects against ankle turns. For court games such as basketball, a high-top shoe is recommended for additional ankle support.
- Cushioning. It is generally agreed that good cushioning is important, especially in the heel and midsole. However, excessive cushioning is not recommended. Too much cushioning may increase

risk of injury by inhibiting the reflexes that help the body protect itself against the impact of the foot with the ground.

- Performance. A lightweight shoe requires less energy output over lengthy exercise periods. Good traction for a given sport is also important. For lengthy performances, a shoe that is at least partially made from a material that can breathe, such as nylon mesh, helps sweat evaporation and inhibits shoe weight gain.
- Fit. The toe box should be roomy enough so that you can wiggle your toes. Regardless of the type of shoe worn, exercise shoes should generally be one-half size larger than your regular shoes. If you wear two pairs of socks while exercising, you should wear two pairs when trying on the shoes. It is important to try on the shoes and move around in them before making a purchase. Make sure they feel good to you.

Probably the biggest mistake made in purchasing footwear is failure to replace shoes when they are worn out. The condition of the sole of the shoe is far less important than the breakdown of the heel (rundown to the inside or outside), or disproportionate wear that results in unusual movement patterns. It is better to replace shoes too soon than to risk injury from worn-out shoes.

Facts to Consider During Daily Exercise

There are three key components of the daily exercise program: the **warm-up exercise,** the workout, and the **cool-down exercise.**

The key component of a fitness program is the daily workout. Experts agree, however, that the workout should be preceded by a warm-up and followed by a cool-down.

The warm-up prior to exercise is recommended to prepare the muscles and heart for the workout.

There are two good reasons for warming up prior to exercise. The first is to prepare the heart muscle for exercise. The second is to stretch the skeletal muscles.

A warm-up designed to prepare the heart muscle for moderate to vigorous exercise should include approximately two minutes of walking, jogging, or mild exercise. Research shows that for some people, starting vigorous exercise abruptly is not wise. Apparently in some exercises, the increased blood flow to the heart and other muscles does not immediately increase when the exercise begins, at least not for all people. Adults who do this type of warm-up do not experience electrocardiogram abnormalities that are apparent in some people who do not warm up.

The skeletal muscle warm-up should include static stretching of the major muscle groups involved in the exercise that is to follow (see Concepts 8 and 9). It should be emphasized that even though warming up prior to an activity may help reduce the chance of muscle injury, it is not a substitute for a regular program of exercise designed to improve flexibility.

A warm-up that is suitable for walking, jogging, running, cycling, and even basketball is included here for your information and use. This warm-up can be used for other activities if stretching exercises for the major muscle groups involved in various activities are added. (Some good stretching exercises are described in Concept 9.) The cardiovascular warm-up is suitable for most activities, but other mild exercise (such as a slow, two-minute swim for swimmers or a slow, two-minute ride on a bicycle for cyclists) can be substituted.

Warm-up stretching can be done before or after the cardiovascular warm-up.

Some experts believe that the cardiovascular warm-up should precede the stretching warm-up because warm muscles are less apt to be injured by the stretch. Warm muscles also stretch farther. If you choose to stretch before the warm-up, make certain it is a gentle, static stretch. This is not the time for a flexibility workout. However, it is acceptable to begin your warm-up with stretching as long as static stretches are used.

There is a minimal and an optimal amount of exercise that should be included in a workout if improvements in health-related fitness are the goal.

Each component of health-related physical fitness has a "threshold of training" (minimal amount of exercise) necessary for improvement. Each component also has a "target zone"—that is, an optimal frequency, intensity, and time (duration) of exercise necessary to produce fitness gains. A properly prepared program includes exercise *above* the threshold level and *in* the target zone for *each part of health-related fitness.* The general concepts of threshold of training and exercise target zones are covered in greater depth in Concept 5. Specific threshold and target zone recommendations for each of the five components of health-related fitness are included in Concepts 6–13.

A cool-down after exercise is important.

Proper exercise planning is very important. One part of this planning is the organization of each exercise session. Each session should include a warm-up, a workout, and a cool-down. The warm-up has already been discussed. The workout, or actual exercise, is discussed in greater detail in later concepts. The cool-down is done immediately after the workout.

A Sample Warm-up and Cool-down for an Aerobic Workout

The exercises shown here can be used before an aerobic workout as a warm-up, or after workout as a cool-down. This sample program would be good before jogging, walking, or cycling. It includes slow cardiovascular exercise, as well as stretching for the lower and upper legs, the hip and back, and the trunk. If the activity you plan to do requires considerable use of different areas of the body, you should add stretching and circulatory exercises for those areas of the body (see Concept 9). Perform the exercises slowly. Do not bounce or jerk against the muscle. Hold each stretch for at least ten seconds. Perform each exercise at least once and up to three times. You may wish to have someone passively assist you in doing the exercise but, if so, you should read Concept 8 first.

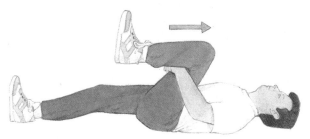

Figure 4.3

Leg hug (for the hip and back extensors).

Lie on your back. Bend one leg and grasp your thigh under the knee. Hug it to your chest. Keep the other leg straight and on the floor. Hold. Repeat with the opposite leg.

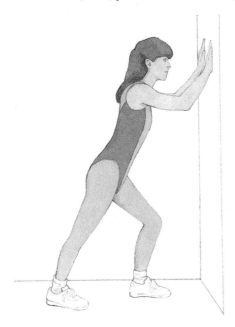

Figure 4.1

Calf stretcher for (1) gastrocnemius and (2) soleus.

Face a wall with your feet two or three feet away. Step forward on left foot to allow both hands to touch the wall. (1) Keep the heel of your right foot on the ground, toe turned in slightly, knee straight, and buttocks tucked in. Lean forward by bending your front knee and arms and allowing your head to move nearer the wall. Hold. (2) Bend right knee, keeping heel on floor. Hold. Repeat with the other leg.

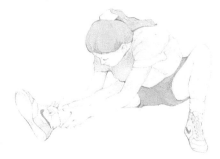

Figure 4.2

Back saver toe touch (for hamstrings).

Sit on the floor. Extend one leg and bend the other knee, placing the foot flat on the floor. Bend at the hip and reach forward with both hands. Grasp one foot, ankle, or calf, depending upon how far you can reach. Pull forward with your arms trying to touch your head to your knee. Keep your knee relatively straight. Hold. Repeat with the opposite leg.

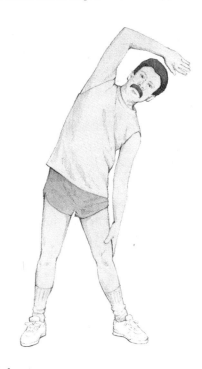

Figure 4.4

Side stretch.

With the feet apart approximately shoulder width, lean to one side. Reach down with the arm on that side and reach up over your head with the opposite arm. Let your body weight stretch the muscles as you lean downward. Do not twist or arch the back. Hold. Repeat to the other side.

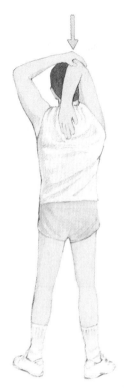

Figure 4.5

Zipper (for triceps and lower "pecs").

Lift right arm and reach behind head and down the spine (as if pulling up a zipper). With the left hand, push down on right elbow and hold. Reverse arm position and repeat.

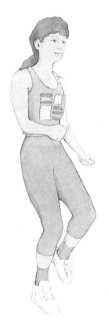

Figure 4.6

The cardiovascular warm-up.

Before you perform a vigorous workout, walk or jog slowly for two minutes. After exercise, do the same.

Like the warm-up, there are two principal components of a cool-down: static muscle stretching and an activity for the cardiovascular system. Although not all experts agree, some believe that static muscle stretching *after* the workout is more important than stretching before because it may help relieve spasms in fatigued muscles. Stretching done as part of the cool-down may be more effective for lengthening the muscles than stretching done at other times because the stretching is done when the muscle temperature is elevated and therefore is more likely to produce optimal flexibility improvements.

There is still some controversy about the best time to stretch and about the benefits of warming up and cooling down. However, given current evidence, both a warm-up and a cool-down seem wise.

A cardiovascular cool-down is also important. During exercise, the heart pumps a large amount of blood to the working muscles to supply the oxygen necessary to keep moving. The muscles squeeze the veins (see figure 4.7), which forces the blood back to the heart. Valves in the veins prevent the blood from flowing backward. As long as exercise continues, the blood is moved by the muscles back to the heart, where it is once again pumped to the body. If exercise is stopped abruptly, the blood is left in the area of the working muscles and has no way to get back to the heart. In the case of the runner, the blood pools in the legs. Because the heart has less blood to pump, blood pressure may drop. This can result in dizziness, and can even cause a person to pass out. The best way to prevent this problem is to taper off or slow down gradually after exercise. A cardiovascular cool-down should include approximately two minutes of walking, slow jogging, or any nonvigorous activity that uses the muscles involved in the workout.

The same program used for the warm-up may be used to cool down after exercise. For variety, you can choose some of the stretching exercises included in Concept 9.

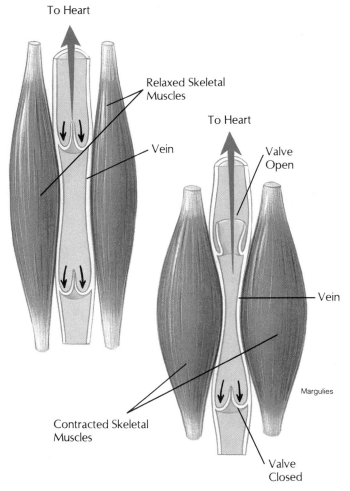

To Heart

Relaxed Skeletal Muscles

Vein

To Heart

Valve Open

Vein

Contracted Skeletal Muscles

Valve Closed

Margulies

Figure 4.7

The pumping action of the muscles.

From John W. Hole, Jr., *Human Anatomy and Physiology,* 6th ed. Copyright © 1993 Wm. C. Brown Communications, Inc., Dubuque, Iowa. All Rights Reserved. Reprinted by permission.

Facts About the Exercise Environment

Exercise in exceptionally hot or humid weather can be dangerous.

The normal human body temperature is 98.6 degrees. During vigorous exercise, or when the surrounding temperature is above this level, the body temperature begins to rise. If the body gets too hot, various heat problems can occur including heat cramps, heat exhaustion, and heat stroke (see table 4.1).

The body has its own methods of avoiding heat problems. The principal method of cooling is evaporation. During exercise, or even inactivity in hot weather, you perspire or sweat. Evaporation of the sweat results in cooling that helps keep the body temperature within normal limits. If the weather is both hot and humid, evaporation is a less effective means of cooling the body. Ex-

Table 4.1
Types of Heat-Related Problems

Problem	Symptoms	Severity
Heat cramps	Muscle cramps especially in muscles most used in exercise.	Least severe
Heat exhaustion	Muscle cramps, weakness, dizziness, headache, nausea, clammy skin, paleness.	Moderate severity
Heat stroke	Hot, flushed skin; dry skin (lack of sweating); dizziness; fast pulse; unconsciousness; high temperature.	Extremely severe

cessive sweating or lack of fluid replacement (drinking water) can result in **dehydration.** A person who is dehydrated stops sweating so evaporation can no longer be used to cool the body. The body diverts blood to the blood vessels in an attempt to cool the body by exchanging heat directly with the environment. This can result in the most dangerous type of heat problem—heat stroke.

When exercising in hot and humid environments, special precautions should be taken to prevent heat-related problems.

- Limit or avoid exercise in hot or humid environments. The apparent temperature is a combined value determined by both temperature and humidity. When the apparent temperature is below 90 degrees (32.2 degrees Celsius), exercise is safe for most people. Caution should be used when exercising at apparent temperatures ranging from 90 degrees to 100 degrees (37.7 degrees Celsius). Above 100 degrees apparent temperature is the danger zone, and exercise should be done with extreme care, limited, or canceled. (See table 4.2).
- Replace fluids regularly. Drink water at regular intervals *during* exercise. Drink water before and after exercise. For exercise lasting more than one or two hours, simple carbohydrate (glucose, fructose, or sucrose) in concentrations less than 5 percent are considered beneficial to performance and body cooling. Salt in drinks is generally considered unnecessary.
- Gradually expose yourself to exercise in hot and humid environments. The body gets better at handling heat and humidity with repeated exposure. Too much at once is especially dangerous.
- Dress properly for exercise in the heat and humidity. Wear white or light colors that reflect rather than absorb heat. Porous clothes allow the passage of

air to cool the body. Rubber, plastic, or other nonporous clothing is especially dangerous. A hat or porous cap can help when exercising in direct sunlight.
- Rest at regular intervals, preferably in the shade.
- Watch for signs of heat stress. If signs are present, stop immediately.

If overheating occurs, take immediate steps to cool the body.

- Get out of the heat—stop exercise.
- Remove excess clothing.
- Drink cool water.
- Immerse the body in cool water.
- If symptoms of heat stroke are present, seek immediate medical help.
- Statically stretch cramped muscles.

Exercise in exceptionally cold and windy weather can be dangerous.

Exercise in the cold is not considered to be as dangerous as exercise in the heat because you can always add clothing to keep warm. However, extreme cold can be dangerous to the exerciser because of a drop in body temperature or frostbite. A combination of wind and cold temperatures (**wind-chill factor**) poses the greatest danger.

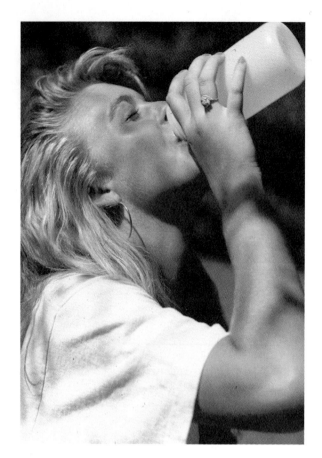

It is important to replace water during exercise.

Table 4.2

Exercise in the heat (apparent temperatures). (To read the table, find the air temperature on the bottom, then find the humidity on the left. Find the apparent temperature where the columns meet.)

Legend:
- □ = Safe Zone
- ▨ = Caution Zone
- ▧ = Danger Zone

"Apparent Temperatures"

Relative Humidity (%)	70	75	80	85	90	95	100	105	110	115	120
100	72	80	91	108	132						
95	71	79	89	105	128						
90	71	79	88	102	122						
85	71	78	87	99	117	141					
80	71	78	86	97	113	136					
75	70	77	86	95	109	130					
70	70	77	85	93	106	124	144				
65	70	76	83	91	102	119	138				
60	70	76	82	90	100	114	132	149			
55	69	75	81	89	98	110	126	142			
50	69	75	81	88	96	107	120	135	150		
45	68	74	80	87	95	104	115	129	143		
40	68	74	79	86	93	101	110	123	137	151	
35	67	73	79	85	91	98	107	118	130	143	
30	67	73	78	84	90	96	104	113	123	135	148
25	66	72	77	83	88	94	101	109	117	127	139
20	66	72	77	82	87	93	99	105	112	120	130
15	65	71	76	81	86	91	97	102	108	115	123
10	65	70	75	80	85	90	95	100	105	111	116
5	64	69	74	79	84	88	93	97	102	107	111
0	64	69	73	78	83	87	91	95	99	103	107

Air Temperature (Degrees F)

Source: Data from the National Oceanic and Atmospheric Administration.

Chart 4.2	Physical Readiness for Sports or Vigorous Training

Answer the PAR-Q before using this chart. If you had one or more "yes" answers, follow the directions for the PAR-Q concerning consultation with a physician. If you had all "no" answers on the PAR-Q, answer the additional questions below before beginning intensive training particularly for sports.

Yes	No	
☒	☐	1. Do you plan to participate on an organized team that will play intense competitive sports (i.e., varsity team, professional team)?
☐	☒	2. If you plan to participate in a collision sport (even on a less organized basis), such as football, boxing, rugby, or ice hockey, have you been knocked unconscious more than one time?
☐	☒	3. Do you currently have pain from a previous muscle injury?
☐	☒	4. Do you currently have symptoms from a previous back injury, or do you experience back pain as a result of involvement in physical activity?
☐	☒	5. Do you have any other symptoms during physical activity that give you reason to be concerned about your health?

If your answer to any of these questions is "yes," then you should consult with your personal physician by telephone or in person to determine if you have a potential problem with vigorous involvement in physical activity.

CONCEPT

5

How Much Exercise is Enough?

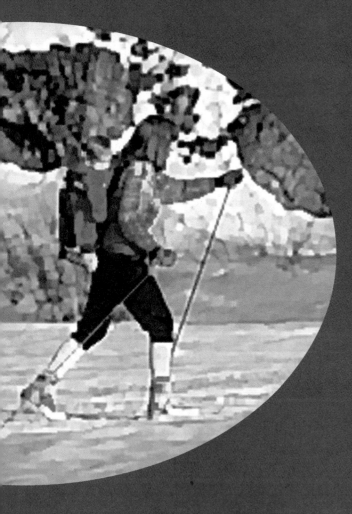

Concept 5

There is a minimal and an optimal amount of exercise necessary for developing each of the health-related aspects of physical fitness.

Introduction

Just as there is a correct dosage of medicine for treating an illness, there is a correct dosage of exercise for developing physical fitness. The minimum amount (dose) of exercise is called the threshold of training. The fitness target zone is the optimal amount of physical activity for developing physical fitness. New evidence indicates that the threshold for performance improvement differs from the threshold for achieving some health benefits of exercise.

Health Goals for the Year 2000

- Increase the proportion of people who do regular physical activity.
- Decrease the proportion of people who do no leisure-time physical activity.

Terms

FIT Formula

A formula used to describe the frequency, intensity, and length of time for exercise to produce fitness improvement.

Fitness Target Zone

Amounts of exercise that produce optimal improvements in physical fitness.

Health Benefit

A result of exercise that provides protection from hypokinetic disease or early death.

Overload Principle

A basic principle that specifies that you must perform exercise in greater than normal amounts (overload) to get an improvement in physical fitness.

Performance Benefit

A result of exercise that improves physical fitness and physical performance capabilities.

Principle of Progression

A corollary of the overload principle that indicates the need to gradually increase overload to achieve optimal benefits.

Principle of Specificity

A corollary of the overload principle that indicates a need for a specific type of exercise to improve each fitness component or fitness of a specific part of the body.

Threshold of Training

The minimum amount of exercise that will improve physical fitness.

The Facts

The **overload principle** is the basis for improving physical fitness.

In order for a muscle (including the heart muscle) to get stronger, it must be "overloaded," or worked against a load greater than normal. To increase flexibility, a muscle must be stretched longer than is normal. To increase muscular endurance, muscles must be exposed to sustained exercise for a longer than normal period. If overload is less than normal for a specific component of fitness, the result will be a decrease in that particular component of fitness. A normal amount of exercise will maintain the current fitness level.

There is no substitute for overload in developing physical fitness.

Many people do not overload enough to develop good fitness. Often the programs found in health clubs and in exercises described in popular books and magazines do not provide for adequate overload. Some people try exercise machines or quack devices that violate the overload principle and are therefore ineffective.

The **principle of specificity** is an important law of exercise that should be observed if optimal fitness is to be obtained.

The "principle of specificity" simply states that to develop a certain characteristic of fitness, you must overload specifically for that particular fitness component. For example, strength-building exercises may do little for developing cardiovascular fitness, and flexibility exercises may do little for altering body composition.

Overload is specific to each component of fitness and is also specific to each body part. If you exercise the legs, you build fitness of the legs. If you exercise the arms, you build fitness of the arms. For this reason, it is not unusual to see some people with disproportionate fitness development. Some gymnasts, for example, have good upper body development but poor leg development, whereas some soccer players have well-developed legs but lack upper body development.

Specificity is important in designing your warm-up, workout, and cool-down programs for specific activities. Training is most effective when it closely resembles the activity for which you are preparing. For example, if your goal is to improve your skill in putting the shot, it is not enough to overload the arm muscles. You should perform a training activity requiring overload while doing a putting motion that closely resembles what you use in the actual sport.

The **principle of progression** is an important corollary of the overload principle.

The progression concept indicates that overload should not be increased too slowly or too rapidly if fitness is to result. Obviously, the concepts of threshold of training and fitness target zones are based on the "progression principle." Beginners can exercise progressively by starting near threshold levels and gradually increasing in frequency, intensity, and time (duration) within the target zone. Exercise above the target zone is counterproductive and can be dangerous. For example, the weekend athlete who exercises vigorously only on weekends does not exercise often enough, and so violates the principle of progression. Many Americans, who consider themselves to be regular exercisers, violate the principle of progression by failing to exercise above threshold levels and in the exercise target zone. Clearly, it is possible to do too little and too much exercise to develop optimal fitness.

There is a **threshold of training** and a **fitness target zone** for each component of fitness.

The threshold of training is the minimum amount of exercise necessary to produce gains in fitness. What you normally do, or just a little more than your normal exercise, is not enough to cause improvements in fitness. Figure 5.1 shows the threshold of training and target zones for physical fitness improvement.

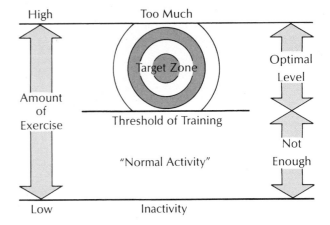

Figure 5.1
Exercise target zones.

The fitness target zone begins at the threshold of training and stops at the point where the benefits of exercise become counterproductive, as shown in figure 5.1. This is the optimal level of exercise.

Some people incorrectly associate the concepts of threshold of training and fitness target zones with only cardiovascular fitness. As the principle of specificity suggests, each component of fitness has its own threshold and target zone. Details for each of the health-related aspects of fitness are presented in Concepts 6–13.

The acronym FIT can help you remember the three important variables for determining threshold of training and fitness target zone levels.

For exercise to be effective, it must be done with enough Frequency and Intensity, and for a long enough Time. The first letter of these three words spells FIT and can be considered as the formula for fitness. **The FIT Formula** can help you remember these important factors.

F Frequency (how often)—Exercise must be performed regularly to be effective. The number of days a person exercises per week is used to determine frequency. Exercise frequency depends on the specific component to be developed. However, most fitness components require at least three days and up to six days of activity per week.

I Intensity (how hard)—Exercise must be hard enough to require more exertion than normal to produce gains in health-related fitness. The method for determining appropriate intensity varies with each aspect of fitness. For example, flexibility requires stretching muscles beyond normal length, cardiovascular fitness requires elevating the heart rate above normal, and strength requires increasing the resistance more than normal.

T Time (how long)—Exercise must be done for a significant length of time to be effective. Generally, an exercise period must be at least fifteen minutes in length to be effective, while longer times are recommended for optimal fitness gains. As the length of time increases, intensities of exercise may be decreased. Time of exercise involvement is also referred to as exercise duration.

Threshold levels and target zones change as your fitness level changes.

As you become more fit by doing correct exercises, your threshold of training and fitness target zones may change. Likewise, if you stop exercising for a period of time, they will also change. Your threshold of training and fitness target zones are based on your current physical fitness levels and your current exercise patterns.

It takes time for exercise to benefit health-related physical fitness.

Sometimes people just beginning an exercise program expect immediate results. They expect to see large losses in body fat in short periods, or great increases in muscle strength in just a few days. Evidence shows, however, that improvements in health-related physical fitness and the associated health benefits take several weeks to become apparent. Though some people report psychological benefits, such as "feeling better" and a "sense of personal accomplishment" almost immediately after beginning regular exercise, the physiological changes will take considerably longer to be realized. Proper preparation for exercise includes learning not to expect too much too soon, and not to do too much too soon. Attempts to overdo it and to try to get fit fast will probably be counterproductive, resulting in soreness and even injury. The key is to start slowly, stay with it, and enjoy the exercise. Benefits will come to those who persist.

The threshold of training necessary for producing noticeable improvements in health-related physical fitness differs from the threshold necessary for producing some of the health benefits of exercise.

The FIT formula as presented in this concept outlines the amount of exercise necessary to achieve what is called a **performance benefit.** A performance benefit results in a significant improvement in a specific component of health-related fitness. There is good evidence that adequate amounts of fitness are necessary for good health and, as noted in Concept 2, for improving performance in sports and physical activities.

New research has shown that some of the **health benefits** of exercise occur at levels less than those necessary for producing performance benefits. For example, reduced risk of heart disease can result from exercise that is less intense than the threshold of training illustrated in figure 5.1. Gardening, walking, and other activities of similar intensity have been shown to produce health benefits when done regularly and for a considerable duration. Whereas the performance and health benefits may occur within several weeks when exercise equals amounts prescribed by the FIT formula, the health benefits associated with less intense exercise are manifested only when regular exercise becomes a part of a permanent lifestyle. The lower threshold for sustained low intensity exercise is illustrated in figure 5.2.

Exercise in the target zone illustrated in figure 5.1 is recommended. However, less intense exercise should not be discounted as an important part of a healthy life-style.

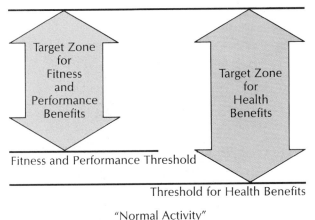

Figure 5.2

The threshold of training for health benefits of sustained low-intensity exercise.

Facts About Physical Fitness Testing

Periodic physical fitness testing can aid in determining if a person is exercising enough and is fit enough for health, performance, and quality living.

At some point, it is wise to have an expert test your fitness. This helps you get an accurate assessment of your current fitness level. *It is important, however, to learn to evaluate your own level of fitness.* Learning to evaluate your own fitness allows you to have a personal record of your fitness on a regular basis, keeps you from being dependent on others, and aids you in staying fit for a lifetime.

Comparison of physical fitness test results to health standards and improvement of your own fitness are more important than comparisons to other people.

In Western culture, we have a tendency to compare ourselves to others in almost all things we do. Rather than comparing your fitness scores to those of other people, you would be wise to concentrate on meeting good fitness standards and improving your personal fitness. Exceptionally high scores on fitness tests may improve performances in sports but probably are not necessary for good health. For example, a male having 10 to 15 percent body fat is considered to be more healthy than one having 25 to 30 percent body fat. However, having less than 10 percent of the body as fat is not necessarily more healthy than having 10 to 15 percent fat (though some people believe that low

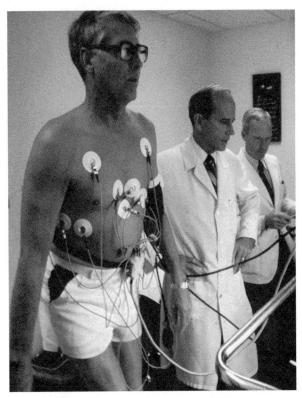

A fitness assessment by an expert can be useful.

levels of fatness may enhance performance in some sports). As you will learn later in this book, having too little body fat can be harmful to good health.

Heredity also plays an important role in the amount of physical fitness a person can attain. More than a few people have become discouraged after completing an exercise program only to find that they have scored lower on fitness tests than friends who are less active. Though it is clear that regular exercise is critical to optimal physical fitness, each person also has a hereditary predisposition to fitness. Although achieving good scores on fitness tests is a desirable goal, it is important to understand that hereditary predispositions to fitness limit one's potential for achieving exceptionally high scores. Meeting standards for good health and improving personal fitness are more important than comparisons to other people.

An assessment of all components of health-related fitness is important.

Because fitness has many different components, you will need to do many self-tests if you are going to get an accurate picture of your total fitness. It is recommended that each person do *several* tests of fitness for each component of health-related fitness. Several tests will give you a more complete and accurate picture of your total physical fitness.

An Important Note on Physical Fitness Testing

In this book we present many fitness tests. When possible, you should learn to give each test to yourself so that you can continue to reassess your fitness for a lifetime. Tests such as skin-fold measures are hard to administer to yourself, but you can learn to teach a friend or relative to measure you. You are encouraged to do as many tests as possible. For example, you may want to assess your cardiovascular fitness using all three tests described. You can use a summary of all tests to make accurate fitness assessments.

Finally, you should know how to use the Rating Scales in each concept to interpret your fitness results. Four rating categories are provided for you to rate each part of health-related fitness. These are illustrated and described in table 5.1. Your first goal should be to be sure that you do not rate low on any health-related fitness part. Ultimately you would like to achieve the "good fitness zone" for all parts of fitness. You may, for personal reasons, wish to achieve the high performance zone for some fitness components. The fitness ratings used in this book help you determine "how much fitness is enough" for your good health and wellness, but do not require you to compare yourself to others or set unrealistic standards.

Table 5.1
The Four Fitness Zones

High Performance Zone
The "high performance zone" is a good indicator of adequate fitness, but it is not necessary to reach this level to experience good health benefits. Achievement of high performance scores has more to do with performance on various physical tasks than it does with good health.

Good Fitness Zone
If you reach the "good fitness zone" you probably have enough of a specific fitness component to help reduce the risk of a specific hypokinetic condition, assuming that you maintain an active life-style. Even achievement in the good fitness zone may not result in optimal health benefits for inactive people.

Marginal Zone
"Marginal" scores indicate that some improvement is in order, but you are nearing minimal health standards set by experts.

Low Fit Zone
If you score "low" in fitness, you are probably less fit than you should be for your own good health and wellness.

Suggested Readings

American College of Sports Medicine. *Guidelines for Exercise Testing and Exercise Prescription.* 4th ed. Philadelphia: Lea & Febiger, 1991.

Paffenbarger, R., et al. "Physical Activity and Physical Fitness as Determinants of Health and Longevity." In Bouchard, C., et al. *Exercise, Fitness, and Health.* Champaign, IL: Human Kinetics Publishers, 1990.

SKELETAL SYSTEM

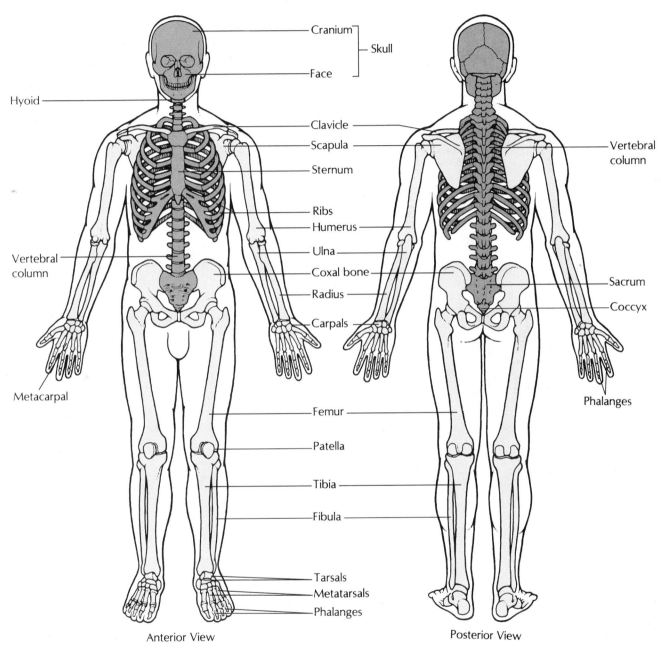

Cranium ⎤
          ⎬ Skull
Face ⎦

Hyoid

Clavicle
Scapula
Sternum

Ribs
Humerus
Ulna
Coxal bone
Radius

Carpals

Vertebral
column

Metacarpal

Femur

Patella

Tibia

Fibula

Tarsals
Metatarsals
Phalanges

Anterior View

Vertebral
column

Sacrum
Coccyx

Phalanges

Posterior View

THE MAJOR MUSCLE GROUPS

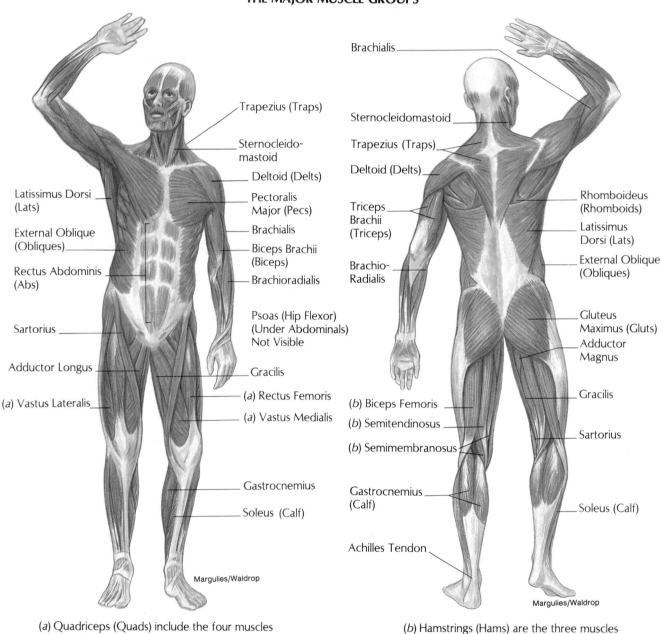

Brachialis

Trapezius (Traps)

Sternocleido-mastoid

Deltoid (Delts)

Pectoralis Major (Pecs)

Brachialis

Biceps Brachii (Biceps)

Brachioradialis

Psoas (Hip Flexor) (Under Abdominals) Not Visible

Gracilis

(a) Rectus Femoris

(a) Vastus Medialis

Gastrocnemius

Soleus (Calf)

Latissimus Dorsi (Lats)

External Oblique (Obliques)

Rectus Abdominis (Abs)

Sartorius

Adductor Longus

(a) Vastus Lateralis

Sternocleidomastoid

Trapezius (Traps)

Deltoid (Delts)

Triceps Brachii (Triceps)

Brachio-Radialis

(b) Biceps Femoris

(b) Semitendinosus

(b) Semimembranosus

Gastrocnemius (Calf)

Achilles Tendon

Rhomboideus (Rhomboids)

Latissimus Dorsi (Lats)

External Oblique (Obliques)

Gluteus Maximus (Gluts)

Adductor Magnus

Gracilis

Sartorius

Soleus (Calf)

Margulies/Waldrop

Margulies/Waldrop

(a) Quadriceps (Quads) include the four muscles identified by the letter (a) and the vastus intermedius (under the Rectus Femoris) not visible.

(b) Hamstrings (Hams) are the three muscles identified by the letter (b).

From Kent M. Van De Graaff and Stuart Ira Fox, *Concepts of Human Anatomy and Physiology*, 3d ed. Copyright © 1992 Wm. C. Brown Communications, Inc., Dubuque, Iowa. All Rights Reserved. Reprinted by permission.

MAJOR BLOOD VESSELS

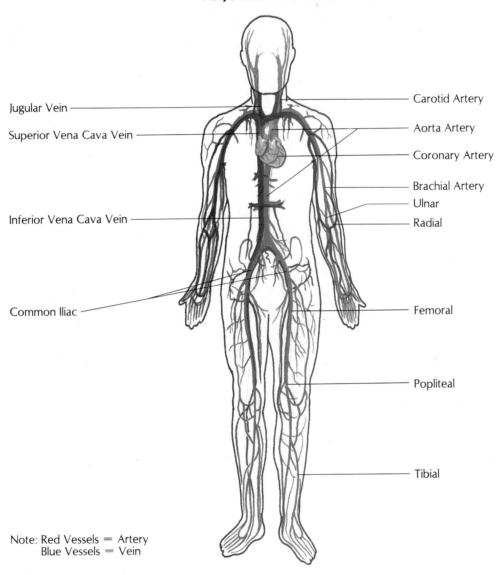

Jugular Vein

Superior Vena Cava Vein

Inferior Vena Cava Vein

Common Iliac

Carotid Artery

Aorta Artery

Coronary Artery

Brachial Artery

Ulnar

Radial

Femoral

Popliteal

Tibial

Note: Red Vessels = Artery
      Blue Vessels = Vein

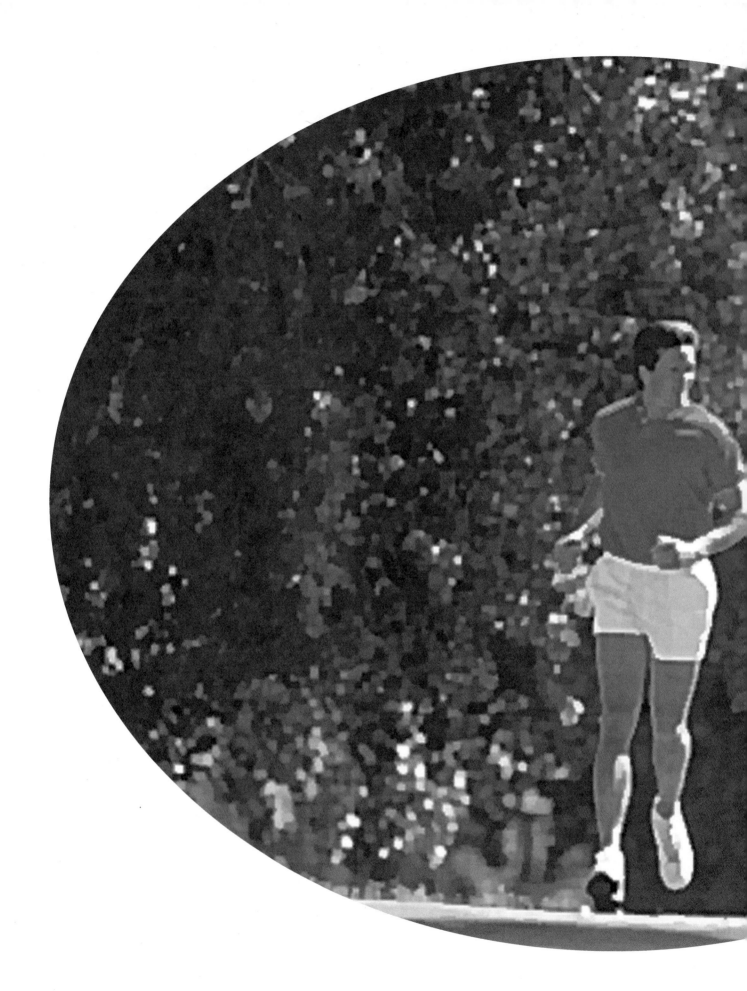

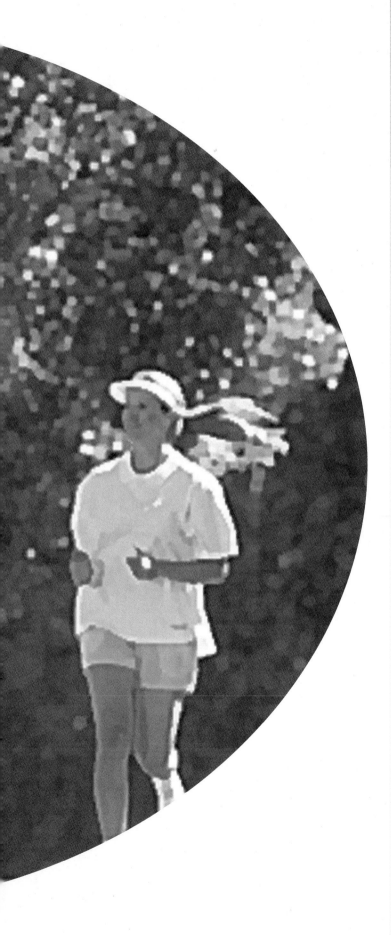

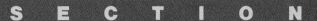

Health-Related Physical Fitness

6

Cardiovascular Fitness

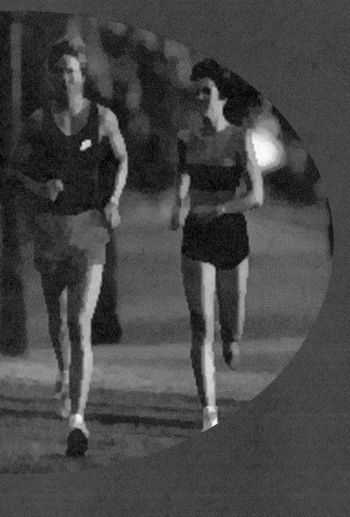

Concept 6

Cardiovascular fitness is probably the most important aspect of physical fitness because of its importance to good health and optimal physical performance.

Introduction

Cardiovascular fitness is frequently considered the most important aspect of physical fitness because those who possess it have a decreased risk of heart disease, the number-one killer in our society. Also, cardiovascular fitness is important to the effective performance of virtually all types of work and play activities.

Cardiovascular fitness is sometimes referred to as "cardiovascular endurance" because a person who possesses this type of fitness can persist in physical exercise for long periods of time without undue fatigue. It has been referred to as "cardio-respiratory fitness" because it requires delivery and utilization of oxygen, which is only possible if the circulatory and respiratory systems are capable of these functions.

The term *aerobic fitness* has also been used as a synonym for cardiovascular fitness because **aerobic capacity** is considered to be the best indicator of cardiovascular fitness and **aerobic exercise** is the preferred method for achieving it. Regardless of the words used to describe it, cardiovascular fitness is complex because it requires fitness of several body systems.

Health Goals for the Year 2000

- Reduce coronary heart disease deaths.
- Increase the proportion of people who engage in activity that promotes cardiovascular fitness.

Terms

Aerobic Capacity

Another term used for Maximal $\dot{V}O_2$.

Aerobic Exercise

Aerobic means "in the presence of oxygen." Aerobic exercise is activity for which the body is able to supply adequate oxygen to sustain performance for long periods of time.

Anaerobic Capacity

A measure of anaerobic fitness; the maximal work performed in a short burst of high intensity exercise.

Anaerobic Exercise

Anaerobic means "in the absence of oxygen." Anaerobic exercise is performed at an intensity so great that the body's demand for oxygen exceeds its ability to supply it.

Cardiovascular Fitness

The ability of the heart, blood vessels, blood, and respiratory system to supply fuel, especially oxygen, to the muscles and the ability of the muscles to utilize fuel to allow sustained exercise.

Fast-Twitch (FT) Muscle Fibers

The muscle fibers primarily used in anaerobic exercise or short, explosive exercise such as sprinting.

Health Benefit

In this concept, health benefit refers to reduced risk of heart disease associated with exercise.

Hemoglobin

Oxygen-carrying pigment of the red blood cells.

Lactic Acid

Substance that results from the process of supplying energy during anaerobic exercise; a cause of muscle fatigue.

Maximal Oxygen Uptake

A laboratory measure held to be the best measure of cardiovascular fitness. Commonly referred to as $\dot{V}O_2$ max or the volume ($\dot{V}$) of oxygen used when a person reaches his or her maximal (max) ability to supply it during exercise.

Performance Benefit

In this concept, performance benefit refers to an improved score on a cardiovascular fitness test or in performance of activities requiring cardiovascular fitness.

Ratings of Perceived Exertion (RPE)

The assessment of the intensity of exercise based on how the participant feels; a written questionnaire is used in assessment.

Slow-Twitch (ST) Muscle Fibers

Muscle fibers primarily used in aerobic or sustained, continuous exercise; also referred to as fatigue-resistant fibers.

Wingate Test

A laboratory measure of anaerobic capacity; a thirty-second, all-out stationary bicycle ride.

The Facts About Cardiovascular Fitness

Good cardiovascular fitness requires a fit heart muscle.

The heart is a muscle; to become stronger it must be exercised like any other muscle in the body. If the heart is exercised regularly, its strength increases; if not, it becomes weaker. Contrary to the belief that strenuous work harms the heart, research has found no evidence that regular, progressive exercise is bad for the normal heart. In fact, the heart muscle will increase in size and power when called upon to extend itself. The increase in size and power allows the heart to pump a greater volume of blood with fewer strokes per minute. For example, the average individual has a resting heart rate between seventy and eighty beats per minute, whereas it is not uncommon for a trained athlete's pulse to be in the low fifties or even in the forties.

The healthy heart is efficient in the work that it does.

The fit heart can convert about half of its fuel into energy. An automobile engine in good running condition converts about one-fourth of its fuel into energy. By comparison, the heart is an efficient engine.

The heart of a normal individual beats reflexively about 40 million times a year. During this time, over 4,000 gallons, or 10 tons, of blood are circulated each day, and every night the heart's workload is equivalent to a person carrying a thirty-pound pack to the top of the 102-story Empire State Building.

Good cardiovascular fitness requires a fit vascular system.

As illustrated in figure 6.1, blood containing a high concentration of oxygen is pumped by the left ventricle through the aorta (a major artery), where it is carried to the tissues. Blood flows through a sequence of arteries to capillaries and to veins. Veins carry the blood containing lesser amounts of oxygen back to the right side of the heart, first to the atrium and then to the ventricle. The right ventricle pumps the blood to the lungs. In the lungs, the blood picks up oxygen and carbon dioxide is removed. From the lungs, the oxygenated blood travels back to the heart, first to the left atrium and then to the left ventricle. The process then repeats itself.

Healthy arteries are elastic, free of obstruction, and expand to permit the flow of blood. Muscle layers line the arteries and control the size of the arterial opening on the impulse from nerve fibers. Unfit arteries may have a reduced internal diameter (atherosclerosis) because of deposits on the interior of their walls, or they may have hardened, nonelastic walls (arteriosclerosis).

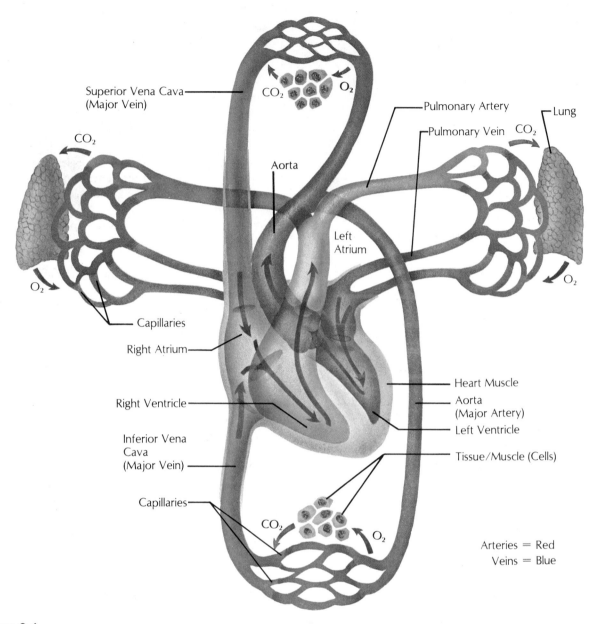

Figure 6.1

The cardiovascular system.

From John W. Hole, Jr., *Human Anatomy and Physiology*, 5th ed. Copyright © 1990 Wm. C. Brown Communications, Inc., Dubuque, Iowa. All Rights Reserved. Reprinted by permission.

Fit coronary arteries are especially important to good health. The blood in the four chambers of the heart does not directly nourish the heart. Rather, numerous small arteries within the heart muscle provide for coronary circulation (see figure 3.3, Concept 3). Poor coronary circulation precipitated by unhealthy arteries can be the cause of a heart attack (see figure 6.2).

Veins have thinner, less elastic walls than arteries as shown in figure 6.3. Also, veins contain small valves to prevent the backward flow of blood. Skeletal muscles assist the return of blood to the heart. The veins are intertwined in the muscle; therefore, when the muscle is contracted, the vein is squeezed, pushing the blood on its way back to the heart. A malfunction of the valves results in a failure to remove used blood at the proper rate. As a result, venous blood pools, especially in the legs, causing a condition known as varicose veins.

Capillaries are the transfer stations where oxygen and fuel are released and waste products, such as CO_2, are removed from the tissues. The veins receive the blood from the capillaries for the return trip to the heart.

Good cardiovascular fitness requires a fit respiratory system and fit blood.

The process of taking in oxygen (through the mouth and nose) and delivering it to the lungs, where it is picked up by the blood, is called external respiration. External res-

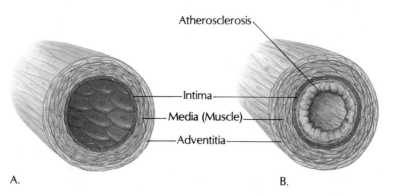

Figure 6.2

(*A*) Healthy, elastic artery, and (*B*) unhealthy artery.

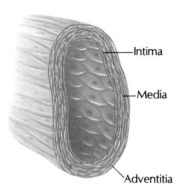

Figure 6.3

Healthy, nonelastic vein.

piration requires fit lungs as well as blood with adequate **hemoglobin** in the red blood cells (erythrocytes). Insufficient oxygen-carrying capacity of the blood is called anemia.

Delivering oxygen to the tissues from the blood is called internal respiration. Internal respiration requires an adequate number of healthy capillaries. In addition to delivering oxygen to the tissues, these systems remove CO_2. Good cardiovascular fitness requires fitness of both the external and internal respiratory systems.

Cardiovascular fitness requires fit muscle tissue capable of using oxygen.

Once the oxygen is delivered, the muscle tissues must be able to use oxygen to sustain physical performance. Cardiovascular fitness activities rely mostly on **slow-twitch (ST) muscle fibers.** These fibers, when trained, undergo changes that make them especially able to use oxygen. Outstanding distance runners often have high amounts of slow-twitch fibers and sprinters often have high amounts of **fast-twitch (FT) muscle fibers** (see Concept 10).

Facts About Exercise, Cardiovascular Fitness, and Heart Disease

---

Regular exercise reduces the risk of heart disease.

As documented in Concept 3, there is considerable evidence that regular exercise reduces the incidence of heart disease. Also, it reduces the chances of early death from heart disease. In fact, the benefits of exercise in preventing heart disease have been shown to be independent of other risk factors. Inactivity is now considered a primary risk factor for heart disease.

People with low cardiovascular fitness have increased risk of heart disease.

Although the benefits of regular exercise to good cardiovascular health have been well documented, the findings are less clear for cardiovascular fitness and reduced risk of heart disease. The best evidence indicates that people with low levels of cardiovascular fitness have a greater than normal risk of heart disease.

Threshold and Target Zones for Reducing Heart Disease Risk and Improving Cardiovascular Fitness

---

Aerobic exercise above the threshold of training and in the target zone will result in improved cardiovascular fitness.

Three factors must be considered in designing exercise programs for developing cardiovascular fitness: Frequency (number of days of exercise per week), Intensity (elevation of heart rate in exercise or amount of calories expended), and Time (length of each exercise period). Specific details are outlined in table 6.1.

Table 6.1
Threshold of Training and Target Zones for Aerobic Exercise

Performance and Health Benefit		Health Benefit
Frequency At least 3 and no more than 6 days a week. **Intensity** 60% to 80% of working heart rate range, or 70% to 85% of maximum heart rate, or exercise between 12 and 16 RPE. **Time** 20 to 60 minutes.	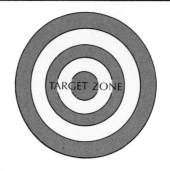	Better 2000 to 3500 calories expended per week. Good 1000 to 2000 calories expended per week.
Frequency 3 days a week. **Intensity** 60% of its working heart rate range or 70% of maximal heart rate or exercise at 12 RPE. **Time** 20 minutes.	THRESHOLD OF TRAINING	1000 calories expended per week in *regular* physical activity. or 1.35 calories per pound of body weight per day (3 calories per kg).

Calories can be counted to determine if a person is doing enough to receive cardiovascular benefits of exercise.

The threshold of training for producing many of the **health benefits** described in Concept 3 can be determined using a weekly calorie count. Scientific evidence suggests that people who regularly expend calories each week in activities such as walking, stair climbing, and sports reduce death rates considerably compared to those who do not exercise. As few as 500 to 1000 calories expended in exercise per week can reduce death rate, but most experts suggest that to insure a health benefit from exercise, a person should expend no less than 1.35 calories per pound of body weight each day. This amounts to 1000 to 2000 calories per week for most people if exercise is done daily.

For optimal health benefits an expenditure of 2000 to 3500 calories per week is recommended, because people doing this much exercise have 48 to 64 percent less risk of heart disease when compared to sedentary people. As the calories expended per week increase, the death rate decreases proportionally (see figure 6.4) up to 3500 calories. Because additional benefits do not occur for those expending more than 3500 calories per week, the target zone is 1000 to 3500 calories per week. For the health benefits to occur, calories must be expended in the target zone at least three days per week and over long periods of

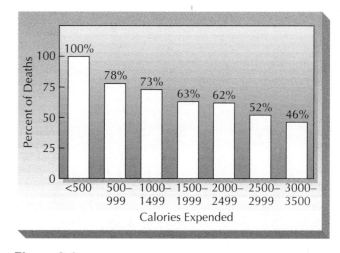

Figure 6.4
Deaths decrease as caloric expenditure increases. The baseline death rate was established for inactive people [< 500 calories].

Source: Data from R. Paffenbarger, et al., "Physical Activity and Physical Fitness as Determinants of Health and Longevity" in C. Bouchard, et al., *Exercise Fitness and Health*. Champaign, IL: Human Kinetics Publishers, 1990.

time. In other words, moderate exercise as described here must become *regular lifetime exercise* if optimal health benefits are to be obtained (see table 6.1). It should also be pointed out that some vigorous sports participation as part of the calories expended each week enhances the benefits of moderate regular calorie expenditure.

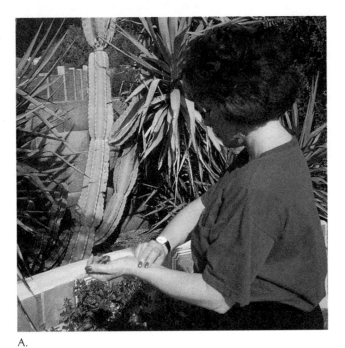

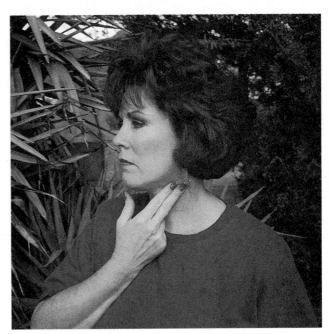

A.

B.

Figure 6.5
Counting your own pulse: (A) wrist (radial) and (B) neck (carotid).

Heart rate can provide the basis for determining if a person is doing enough exercise to improve cardiovascular fitness.

As noted in the previous section, expending a significant number of calories each week can result in reduced risk of cardiovascular disease and improved health. To achieve these benefits it is only necessary to do relatively low-level exercise for extended periods of time. For example, a 150-pound person could walk for an hour and a half five days a week at three miles per hour to expend 2000 calories a week. Both cardiovascular health and **performance benefits** (improved fitness test results) could be obtained in much shorter periods of time if exercise is done more intensely. For busy people this method is often preferred. To achieve fitness by using shorter duration exercise, your heart rate must be elevated to target zone intensity. (Details are presented in table 6.1 and subsequent sections of this concept.) In addition to producing cardiovascular health benefits, exercise that elevates the heart rate into the target zone has the added advantage of improved cardiovascular fitness test scores and improved performances in cardiovascular activities such as running, swimming, and cycling.

Learning to count heart rate properly is vital to determining intensity for aerobic exercise.

To determine the intensity of exercise for building cardiovascular fitness, it is important to know how to count your pulse. Each time the heart beats it pumps blood into the arteries. The surge of blood causes a pulse that can be felt by holding a finger against an artery. Major arteries that are easy to locate and are frequently used for pulse counts are the *carotid* taken on either side of the Adam's apple, and the *radial* taken just above the base of the thumb on the wrist (see figure 6.5). Heart rate (pulse) is important for determining the correct intensity of exercise for building cardiovascular fitness.

To count the pulse, simply place the fingertips (index and middle finger) over the artery at one of the previously mentioned locations. Move the fingers around until a strong pulse can be felt. Press gently so as not to cut off the blood flow through the artery. Counting the pulse with the thumb is not recommended because the thumb has a relatively strong pulse of its own and could be confusing when counting another person's pulse.

Counting the pulse at the carotid artery is the most popular procedure, probably because the carotid pulse is easy to locate. Some researchers suggest that caution should be used when taking carotid pulse counts because pressing on this artery can cause a reflex that slows the heart rate. This could result in incorrect heart rate counts. More recent research indicates that carotid palpations, when done properly, can be used safely to count heart rate for most people.

The radial pulse is a bit harder to find than the carotid pulse because of the many tendons near the wrist. Moving the fingers around to several locations just above the thumb on the wrist will help you locate this pulse. For older adults or those with known medical problems, this procedure is recommended.

Though less popular, the pulse can also be counted at the brachial artery. This is located on the inside of the upper arm just below the armpit.

Once the pulse is located, the heart rate can be determined in beats per minute. At rest, this is done simply by counting the number of beats in one minute. To determine exercise heart rate, it is best to count heart beats or pulses during exercise; however, during most activities this is difficult. Machines do exist that can count heartbeats during exercise, but they are not available to most people. The most practical method is to count the pulse *immediately* after exercise. During exercise, the heart rate increases; immediately after exercise, it begins to slow down or return to normal. In fact, the heart rate has already slowed considerably within one minute after exercise ceases. The key is to locate the pulse quickly and to count the rate for a short period of time. A full one-minute count after exercise does not give a good estimate of exercise heart rate, even if the pulse is quickly located, because the heart rate during the end of the count is much slower than it was during exercise. Keep moving while quickly locating the pulse, then stop and take a fifteen-second count. Multiply the number of pulses counted in a fifteen-second period by four to convert heart rate to beats per minute.

You can also count the pulse for ten seconds and multiply by six or count the pulse for six seconds and multiply by ten to estimate a one-minute heart rate. The latter method allows you to easily calculate heart rates by adding a zero to the six-second count. However, short duration pulse counts increase the chances of error because a miscount of one beat is multiplied by six or ten beats rather than by four beats.

The pulse rate should be counted after regular exercise, not after a sudden burst of activity. Some runners sprint the last few yards of their daily run and then count their pulse. Such a burst of exercise will elevate the heart rate considerably. This gives a false picture of the actual exercise heart rate. It would be wise for every person to learn to determine resting heart rate accurately and to estimate exercise heart rate by quickly and accurately making pulse counts after exercise.

In order to plan aerobic exercise for building cardiovascular fitness, it is important to know how to calculate heart rate threshold levels and target zones.

Two different procedures are commonly used to estimate threshold and target zone heart rates. The first involves calculating a percentage of your *working heart rate range,* also referred to by some as the maximum heart rate reserve. This method is considered by many to be the better of the two because it is more personal in that it uses your true resting heart rate in making the calculations. The second method, percentage of *maximal heart rate,* is easier to calculate but is less personalized. As noted in table 6.1,

the percentage of heart rate intensity necessary to get you in the target zone differs depending upon which method of heart rate calculation you use. In the following paragraphs, both methods of determining threshold and target zone heart rates are described.

Percentage of Working Heart Rate Range

To calculate your working heart rate range, you must know your resting and maximal heart rates.

The resting heart rate is easily determined by counting the pulse for one minute while sitting or lying. Ideally, this should be done early in the morning when you are rested, rather than late in the day when you have been involved in many activities.

Maximal heart rate is harder to determine. It could be measured by an electrocardiogram while exercising to exhaustion; however, for most people it is safer and better to estimate *maximal heart rate* by using a formula. This is done by subtracting your age from 220. Maximal heart rates are near 200 in young people but decrease with age. The formula for calculating your maximal heart rate and an example of the calculations for a twenty-two-year-old individual are shown in table 6.2.

The *working heart rate* is determined by subtracting the resting heart rate from the maximal heart rate. The heart always works in the range between the resting (the lowest) and the maximal (the highest) rate of your pulse. The formula for calculating the working heart rate and an example for the twenty-two-year-old with a resting heart rate of sixty-eight beats per minute are also shown in table 6.2.

The *threshold of training,* or *minimum heart rate,* for building cardiovascular fitness, is determined by calculating 60 percent of the working heart rate and then adding it to the resting heart rate. The upper limit of the target zone is 80 percent of the working heart rate added to the resting heart rate. The formula for determining threshold and the upper limit of the target heart rate zone, and examples for the hypothetical exerciser, are shown in table 6.2.

Percentage of Maximal Heart Rate

To use this method, first estimate your maximal heart rate just as you did for the previous method, then determine the threshold heart rate by calculating 70 percent of the maximal heart rate. The upper limit of the target zone is determined by calculating 85 percent of the maximal heart rate. Table 6.3 gives an example for a hypothetical twenty-two-year-old person.

This procedure, using a percentage of maximal heart rate, is deemed an acceptable alternative to the procedure using a percentage of working heart rate range because it provides target heart rates similar to those using 60–80 percent of the working heart rate range (see examples).

Table 6.2

Formula and Example for Calculating Target Heart Rates Using Percentage of Working Heart Rate Range (Example is for a twenty-two-year-old person with a resting heart rate of 68 bpm.)

Formula for Calculating Maximal Heart Rate	Example
220 − Age (in years) = Maximal Heart Rate	220 − 22 = 198 beats per minute
Formula for Calculating Working Heart Rate	**Example**
Maximal Heart Rate − Resting Heart Rate = Working Heart Rate	198 − 68 = 130
Formula for Calculating Threshold of Training Heart Rate	**Example**
Working Heart Rate × 60% + Resting Heart Rate = Threshold of Training Heart Rate	130 × .60 = 78 + 68 = 146
Formula for Calculating the Upper Limit of the Target Heart Rate Zone	**Example**
Working Heart Rate × 80% + Resting Heart Rate = Upper Limit for Target Heart Rate Zone	130 × .80 = 104 + 68 = 172

The target zone for this twenty-two-year-old is 146–172 bpm.

Table 6.3

Formula and Example for Calculating Target Heart Rates Using the Percentage of Maximal Heart Rate Procedure. (Example is for a twenty-two-year-old person.)

Formula for Calculating Maximal Heart Rate	Example
220 − Age (in years) = Maximal Heart Rate	220 − 22 = 198 beats per minute
Formula for Threshold Heart Rate	**Example**
Maximal Heart Rate × 70% Threshold of Training Heart Rate	198 × .70 = 138.6 (139)
Formula for Upper Limit Heart Rate	**Example**
Maximal Heart Rate × 85% Upper Limit for Target Heart Rate Zone	198 × .85 = 168.3 (168)

The target zone for this person is 139–168 bpm.

You should learn to calculate your threshold and target heart rate values using one of the two methods. Because the first method (percentage of working heart rate range) is a bit more difficult to calculate, a special chart (Chart 6A, p. 64) is presented in the Lab Resource Materials to assist you. Regardless of which method you use, you should exercise vigorously enough to bring your heart rate above threshold and into the target zone to get the cardiovascular performance benefits of exercise.

It should be noted that there are several possible sources of error in calculating threshold and target heart rates. First, the method of calculating maximal heart rate is an estimate based on typical values for typical people. Second, errors in counting are possible. Finally, it is possible that the count you make *after* exercise may not actually reflect your heart rate *during* exercise. For this reason, it is important that you make several estimates of your threshold and target heart rates, especially when you are first starting a cardiovascular fitness program.

> Ratings of perceived exertion during exercise can be useful as a guide to intensity of cardiovascular exercise.

The American College of Sports Medicine suggests that experienced exercisers can use **Ratings of Perceived Exertion (RPE)** to determine if they are exercising in the target zone. This prevents the need to stop and count heart rate during exercise. A rating of 12 (somewhat hard) is equal to threshold, and a rating of 16 (hard) is equal to the upper limit of the target zone. With practice, most people can learn to recognize when they are in the target zone using ratings of perceived exertion (see Lab 6C).

The Facts About Measuring Cardiovascular Fitness

> Though cardiovascular fitness can be measured in several ways, **maximal oxygen uptake** is considered the best method of evaluation.

A person's maximal oxygen uptake ($\dot{V}O_2$ max), also commonly referred to as *aerobic capacity,* is determined in a laboratory by measuring how much oxygen a person can use in one minute of maximal exercise. Great endurance

Cardiovascular Fitness **61**

athletes can extract five or six liters of oxygen per minute from the environment during an all-out treadmill run or bicycle ride. An average person extracts only two or three liters in a one-minute exercise session. $\dot{V}O_2$ max is often adjusted to account for a person's body size because bigger people may have higher scores due to their larger size. Scores are often reported as milliliters of oxygen per kilogram of body weight ($ml/O_2/kg$). This score is calculated by dividing your $\dot{V}O_2$ max value by your weight in kilograms.

Aerobic exercise is the most effective means of improving $\dot{V}O_2$ max.

As noted previously in this concept, good cardiovascular fitness requires a fit heart muscle, fit vascular and respiratory systems, fit blood, and fit muscles. Regular aerobic exercise improves these systems, which are essential for improved $\dot{V}O_2$ max.

$\dot{V}O_2$ max can be estimated using self-administered tests.

Several tests can be done with a minimum of equipment in or near your home. With proper instruction, you can learn to measure your own cardiovascular fitness using one of these methods. Commonly used tests are the step test, the twelve-minute run, the Astrand-Ryhming bicycle test, and the Rockport Walking Test (see pp. 64–67). Since these tests are not as accurate as a laboratory test of $\dot{V}O_2$ max, the use of more than one test is recommended to help you get a valid assessment of your cardiovascular fitness.

The Facts About Aerobic and Anaerobic Exercise

Aerobic exercise can be sustained for considerably longer periods than anaerobic exercise.

Regardless of the type of exercise you perform, you derive energy from high-energy fuel that must be available in muscle fibers. The breakdown of this high-energy fuel in the muscle cells allows you to perform all types of exercise. Unfortunately, the energy resulting from the breakdown of this fuel is used up in a matter of seconds. Carbohydrates stored in the cells can be broken down to replenish the high-energy fuel supply to allow performance to continue for an additional time (thirty to forty seconds for most people). The short-term, vigorous exercise performed in the absence of an adequate oxygen supply using these sources of energy is called **anaerobic exercise.**

Aerobic exercise, which means "in the presence of oxygen," is less vigorous and can be performed for much longer periods. Carbohydrates and fats available in the body can be used to rebuild the high-energy fuel necessary for doing regular exercises when oxygen is present.

Aerobic exercise produces cardiovascular fitness or aerobic capacity.

In accordance with the principle of specificity, regular aerobic exercise increases the body's ability to supply oxygen to the muscles as well as their ability to use it. Slow-twitch muscle fibers appear to benefit most from aerobic exercise.

Anaerobic exercise produces anaerobic capacity.

Anaerobic exercise produces **lactic acid** in the process of energy production. Muscle fatigue occurs when anaerobic energy supplies are depleted and lactic acid build-up occurs. Regular anaerobic exercise seems to allow the muscle to tolerate higher lactic acid levels before fatigue occurs. Also, anaerobic exercise improves anaerobic energy production capabilities, primarily in the fast-twitch fibers. These fibers appear to benefit most from anaerobic exercise. Anaerobic capacity is often measured in the laboratory using the **Wingate Test,** an all-out, thirty-second stationary bicycle ride at high resistance. The ability to perform a vigorous, short-term bout of exercise, and repeat it with a relatively short rest, will give you an indication of your anaerobic fitness.

Regular anaerobic exercise contributes to cardiovascular fitness development.

Though aerobic exercise is considered to be the preferred method of building cardiovascular fitness, anaerobic exercise can contribute to its development through increased heart rate and blood flow. Most experts agree that the primary contribution of anaerobic exercise to cardiovascular fitness is associated with improved delivery of oxygen in blood. Improvement of O_2 utilization within the cells seems to be specifically associated with aerobic exercise. Examples of anaerobic exercise, such as wind sprints or interval training, are presented in Concept 7.

Table 6.4

Threshold of Training and Target Zone for Anaerobic Exercise *

	Threshold of Training	Target Zone
Frequency **Intensity**	• 3 days a week	• 3–4 days a week.
	• Short Interval—100% of maximum speed running, swimming, or other exercise of short duration (10–30 seconds).	• Short Intervals—100% of maximum speed running, swimming, or other exercise of short duration (10–30 seconds).
	• Long Interval—90% of maximum speed running, swimming, or other exercise (30 seconds–2 minutes).	• Long Intervals—90–100% of maximum speed running, swimming, or other exercise (30 seconds–2 minutes).
Time	• Short Intervals—Exercise 10 seconds, rest 10 seconds. Repeat 20 times. or Exercise 20 seconds, rest 15 seconds. Repeat 10 times. or Exercise 30 seconds, rest 1–2 minutes. Repeat 8 times.	• Short Intervals—Same as threshold but repeat up to 30 times. or Same as threshold but repeat up to 20 times. or Same as threshold but repeat up to 18 times.
	• Long Intervals—Exercise 1 minute, rest 3–5 minutes. Repeat 5 times. or Exercise 2 minutes, rest 5–15 minutes. Repeat 4 times.	• Long Intervals—Same as threshold but repeat up to 15 times. or Same as threshold but repeat up to 10 times.

*The threshold of training and target zone values depicted in this table are for healthy young adults. For older people, or those who have not been active recently, aerobic training is recommended. Those with known medical problems should consult a physician to determine appropriate exercise amounts. This is only a sample of several formats for meeting anaerobic target zones.

Improved anaerobic capacity can contribute to performance in activities considered to be aerobic.

Many physical activities commonly considered to be aerobic—such as tennis, basketball, and racquetball—have an anaerobic component. These activities require periodic vigorous bursts of exercise. Regular anaerobic training will help you resist fatigue in these activities. Even participants in activities such as long-distance running may benefit from some anaerobic training, especially if performance times or winning races is important. A fast start may be anaerobic, a sprint past an opponent may be anaerobic, and a kick at the end will no doubt be anaerobic. Anaerobic training can help prepare a person for these circumstances.

There is a threshold and target zone for performing anaerobic exercise.

The frequency, intensity, and time for anaerobic exercise threshold and target zone are presented in table 6.4.

Suggested Readings

American College of Sports Medicine. *Guidelines for Exercise Testing and Exercise Prescription.* 4th ed. Philadelphia: Lea & Febiger, 1991.

American College of Sports Medicine. "The Recommended Quantity and Quality of Exercise for Developing and Maintaining Cardiorespiratory and Muscular Fitness in Healthy Adults." *Medicine and Science in Sports and Exercise* 22(1990):2.

Fletcher, G., et al. "American Heart Association: Statement on Exercise." *Circulation* 86(1992):2726.

LAB RESOURCE MATERIALS

(For use with Labs 6A, 6B, & 6C, pages L-11–L-16)

Chart 6A Threshold of Training and Target Zone Heart Rates
(Heart rates necessary to produce improved cardiovascular fitness) *

Resting Heart Rate		Age									
		Less than 25	25–29	30–34	35–39	40–44	45–49	50–54	55–59	60–64	Over 65
below 50	Threshold	136	133	130	127	124	121	118	115	112	109
	Target zone	136–166	133–164	130–160	127–156	124–152	121–148	118–144	115–140	112–136	109–134
50–54	Threshold	138	135	132	129	126	123	120	117	114	111
	Target zone	138–167	135–165	132–161	129–157	126–153	123–149	120–145	117–141	114–137	111–135
55–59	Threshold	140	137	134	131	128	125	122	119	116	113
	Target zone	140–168	137–166	134–162	131–158	128–154	125–150	122–146	119–142	116–138	113–136
60–64	Threshold	142	139	136	133	130	127	124	121	118	115
	Target zone	142–169	139–167	136–163	133–159	130–155	127–151	124–147	121–143	118–139	115–137
65–69	Threshold	144	141	138	135	132	129	126	123	120	117
	Target zone	144–170	141–168	138–164	135–160	132–156	129–152	126–148	123–144	120–140	117–138
70–74	Threshold	146	143	140	137	134	131	128	125	122	119
	Target zone	146–171	143–169	140–165	137–161	134–157	131–153	128–149	125–145	122–141	119–139
75–79	Threshold	148	145	142	139	136	133	130	127	124	121
	Target zone	148–172	145–170	142–166	139–162	136–158	133–154	130–150	127–146	124–142	121–140
80–85	Threshold	150	147	144	141	138	135	132	129	126	123
	Target zone	150–173	147–171	144–167	141–163	138–159	135–155	132–151	129–147	126–143	123–141
86 and over	Threshold	152	149	146	143	140	137	134	131	128	125
	Target zone	152–174	149–172	146–168	143–164	140–160	137–156	134–152	131–148	128–144	125–142

*Computed using 60 percent–80 percent of the working heart rate range.

Evaluating Cardiovascular Fitness

For an exercise program to be most effective, it should be based on personal needs. Some type of testing is necessary to determine your personal need for cardiovascular fitness. A treadmill test that includes continuous EKG monitoring or assessment of maximal oxygen uptake is the best test of cardiovascular fitness (see American College of Sports Medicine, 1986). However, there are some tests that do not require as much time and equipment and can give you a good estimate of cardiovascular fitness. The twelve-minute run, the step test, the Astrand-Ryhming bicycle test, and the Rockport Walking Test are some of these tests and are described here. Prior to performing any of these, be sure that you are physically and medically ready (Concept 4). Prepare yourself by doing some regular exercise for three to six weeks before actually taking the tests. If possible, take more than one test and use the summary of your test results to make a final assessment of your cardiovascular fitness.

The Twelve-Minute Run Test

- Locate an area where a specific distance is already marked, such as a school track or football field; or measure a specific distance using a bicycle or automobile odometer.
- Use a stopwatch or wristwatch to accurately time a twelve-minute period.
- For best results, warm up prior to the test, then run at a steady pace for the entire twelve minutes (cool down after the tests).
- Determine the distance you can run in twelve minutes in fractions of a mile. Depending upon your age, locate your score and rating on chart 6B.1.

The Step Test

- Warm up prior to exercise, and after finishing be sure to cool down.
- Step up and down on a twelve-inch bench for three minutes at a rate of twenty-four steps per minute. One

Chart 6B.1 Twelve-Minute Run Test (Scores in Miles)

Men (age)

Classification	17–26	27–39	40–49	50+
High performance zone	1.80+	1.60+	1.50+	1.40+
Good fitness zone	1.55–1.79	1.45–1.59	1.40–1.49	1.25–1.39
Marginal zone	1.35–1.54	1.30–1.44	1.25–1.39	1.10–1.24
Low zone	<1.35	<1.30	<1.25	<1.10

Women (age)

Classification	17–26	27–39	40–49	50+
High performance zone	1.45+	1.35+	1.25+	1.15+
Good fitness zone	1.25–1.44	1.20–1.34	1.15–1.24	1.05–1.14
Marginal zone	1.15–1.24	1.05–1.19	1.00–1.14	0.95–1.04
Low zone	<1.15	<1.05	<1.00	<.94

A chart showing the metric equivalents for this chart can be found in Appendix B.

step consists of four beats; that is, "up with the left foot, up with the right foot, down with the left foot, down with the right foot."

- Immediately after the exercise, sit down on the bench and relax. Don't talk.
- Locate your pulse or have another person locate it for you.
- Five seconds after the exercise ends, begin counting your pulse. Count the pulse for sixty seconds.
- Your score is your sixty-second heart rate. Locate your score and your rating on chart 6B.2.

Chart 6B.2 Step Test Rating Chart

Classification	Sixty-Second Heart Rate
High performance zone	84 or less
Good fitness zone	85–95
Marginal zone	96–119
Low zone	120 and above

As you grow older you will want to continue to score well on this rating chart. Because your maximal heart rate decreases as you age, you should be able to score well if you exercise regularly.

Source: Data from F. W. Kasch and J. L. Boyer, *Adult Fitness: Principles and Practices.* Copyright © 1968 Mayfield Publishing Company, Palo Alto, CA.

The Astrand-Ryhming Bicycle Test

- Ride a stationary bicycle ergometer for six minutes at a rate of fifty pedal cycles per minute (one push with each foot per cycle). Cool down after the test.

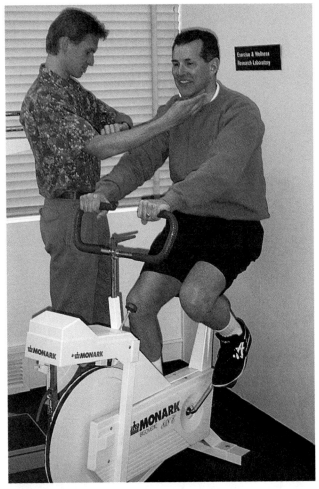

The bicycle test

- Set the bicycle at a work load between 300 and 1,200 kpm. For less fit or smaller people, a setting in the range of 300 to 600 is appropriate. Larger or fitter people will need to use a setting of 750 to 1,200. The work load should be enough to elevate the heart rate to at least 125 bpm but no more than 170 bpm during the ride.

- During the sixth minute of the ride (if the heart rate is in the correct range—see step 2), count the heart rate for the entire sixth minute. The carotid or radial pulse may be used.

- Use the nomogram to determine your predicted oxygen uptake score. Connect the point that represents your heart rate with the point on the right-hand scale that represents the workload you used in riding the bike (use the ♂ scale for men and the ♀ scale for women). Read your score at the point where a straight line connecting the two points crosses the $\dot{V}O_2$ max line. For example, the sample score for the woman represented by the dotted line is 2.55, or nearly 2.6. She had a heart rate of 150 and worked at a load of 600 kpm.

- Determine your score in terms of $\dot{V}O_2$ per kilogram of body weight by dividing your weight in kilograms into the score obtained from the nomogram. To compute your weight in kilograms, divide your weight in pounds by 2.2.

- To determine your cardiovascular fitness rating on the bicycle test, look up your $\dot{V}O_2$ per kilogram of body weight score on the nomogram.

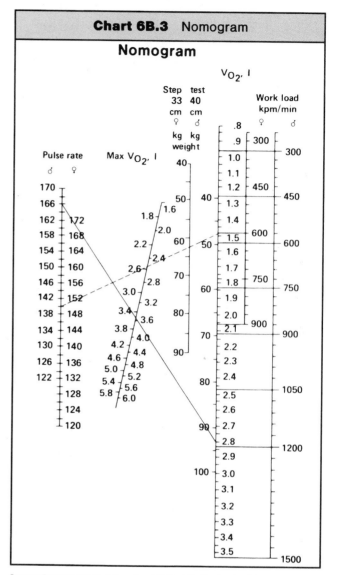

Chart 6B.3 Nomogram

Source: Data from P. O. Astrand and K. Rodahl, *Textbook of Work Physiology*, 1986.

Chart 6B.4 Bicycle Test *Rating Scale* (ml / O_2 / kg)

			Women		
Age	17–26	27–39	40–49	50–59	60–69
High performance zone	46+	40+	38+	35+	32+
Good fitness zone	36–45	33–39	30–37	28–34	24–31
Marginal zone	30–35	28–32	24–29	21–27	18–23
Low zone	<30	<28	<24	<21	<18
			Men		
Age	17–26	27–39	40–49	50–59	60–69
High performance zone	50+	46+	42+	39+	35+
Good fitness zone	43–49	35–45	32–41	29–38	26–34
Marginal zone	35–42	30–34	27–31	25–28	22–25
Low zone	<35	<30	<27	<25	<22

Source: Data from P. O. Astrand and K. Rodahl, *Textbook of Work Physiology*, 1986.

The Rockport Walking Test

- Warm up, then walk one mile as fast as you can. Record your time to the nearest second.

- Count your heart rate for 15 seconds immediately after the walk, then multiply by four to get a one-minute heart rate. Record your heart rate.

- Use your walking time and your post-exercise heart rate to determine your rating using Chart 6B.5 for males and 6B.6 for females.

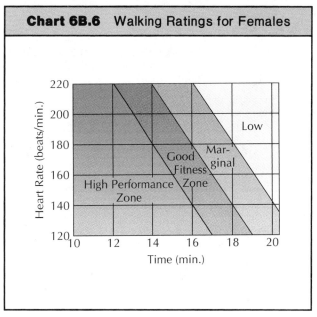

Chart 6B.6 Walking Ratings for Females

Adapted from the *One Mile Walk Test*, with permission of the author, James M. Rippe, M. D.

The ratings in chart 6B.6 are for ages 20–29. They provide reasonable ratings for people of all ages. For more specific ratings for different age groups the reader is referred to the original source (see reference list).

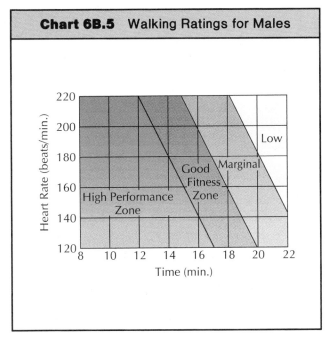

Chart 6B.5 Walking Ratings for Males

Adapted from the *One Mile Walk Test*, with permission of the author, James M. Rippe, M. D.

The ratings in chart 6B.5 are for ages 20–29. They provide reasonable ratings for people of all ages. For more specific ratings for different age groups the reader is referred to the original source (see reference list).

Chart 6.C	Ratings of Perceived Exertion (RPE)
Scale	**Verbal Rating**
6	
7	Very, very light
8	
9	Very light
10	
11	Fairly light
12	
13	Somewhat hard
14	
15	Hard
16	
17	Very hard
18	
19	Very, very hard
20	

From G. Borg, "Psychological Bases of Perceived Exertion" in *Medicine and Science in Sports and Exercise*, 14:377, 1982, © by the American College of Sports Medicine.

7

Aerobic and Anaerobic Exercise

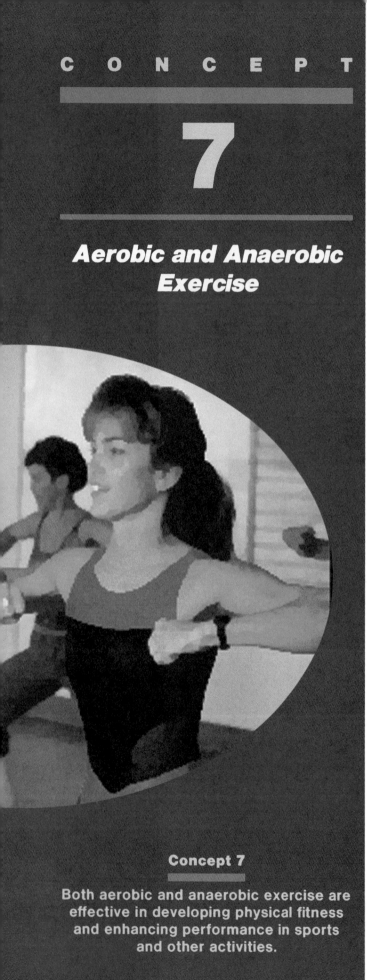

Concept 7

Both aerobic and anaerobic exercise are effective in developing physical fitness and enhancing performance in sports and other activities.

Introduction

Both **aerobic exercise** and **anaerobic exercise** enhance ability to perform many work and leisure activities. The various forms of aerobic exercise are particularly effective in building cardiovascular and other components of health-related fitness.

Health Goal for the Year 2000

▬ Increase proportion of people who engage in regular physical activity to improve cardiovascular fitness.

Terms

Aerobic Exercise

Aerobic means "in the presence of oxygen." Aerobic exercise is activity for which the body is able to supply adequate oxygen to sustain performance for long periods.

Anaerobic Exercise

Anaerobic means "in the absence of oxygen." Anaerobic exercise is performed at an intensity so great that the body's demand for oxygen exceeds its ability to supply it.

Continuous Aerobic Exercise

Exercise that is slow enough to be sustained for relatively long periods without frequent rest periods.

Intermittent Aerobic Exercise

Exercise that is alternated with frequent rest periods, often of relatively high intensity.

The Facts About Aerobic Exercise

Aerobic exercise is a good way to develop several components of health-related physical fitness.

When done in the cardiovascular fitness target zone, aerobic activities are excellent for building cardiovascular fitness. Because aerobic activities can be sustained for relatively long periods, they can result in considerable calorie expenditure and are very good for helping to control body fatness. Aerobic activities can also be of value in developing muscular endurance.

Aerobic exercise must be done at target levels to produce increases in cardiovascular fitness.

Some activities, such as slow walking, bowling, and golf, are technically considered to be aerobic because the body can meet the oxygen demands of these activities with little difficulty. Many people reserve the term *aerobic exercise* for activities that are done with enough frequency and intensity, and for a long enough time, to produce improvements in cardiovascular fitness (see Concept 6). Slow walking, golf, bowling, and even activities such as softball may not be effective in building cardiovascular fitness, depending on how they are performed.

Aerobic activities are exceptionally popular among adults.

Activities that have a strong anaerobic component, such as sprinting, football, baseball, and sprint swimming, are very popular among youth, whereas aerobic activities are more popular among adults. Adults report that they are most often involved in continuous swimming, jogging, cycling, walking, and calisthenics. All but vigorous calisthenics, sprint running, or sprint swimming are aerobic. When done at a slow or moderate pace, calisthenics are aerobic; when done continuously, they can be effective in producing the same benefits as jogging, swimming, and other aerobic activities.

To be effective in building all components of health-related physical fitness, aerobic exercise should be supplemented with other forms of exercise.

As already noted, aerobic exercise can be effective in aiding cardiovascular fitness, muscular endurance, and in reducing body fat. Except for some types of continuous calisthenics, aerobic exercise must be supplemented with exercises designed to build flexibility, strength, and, to a lesser extent, muscular endurance. If certain types of aerobic exercise, such as jogging, are done exclusively, they may actually reduce flexibility.

Aerobic exercise can be done either continuously or intermittently.

We generally think of aerobic exercise as being continuous in nature. Jogging, swimming, and cycling at a steady pace for long periods are classic examples of aerobic exercise. Experts have shown that aerobic exercise can be done intermittently as well as continuously. Both **continuous** and **intermittent aerobic exercise** can build cardiovascular fitness. For example, one recent study showed that

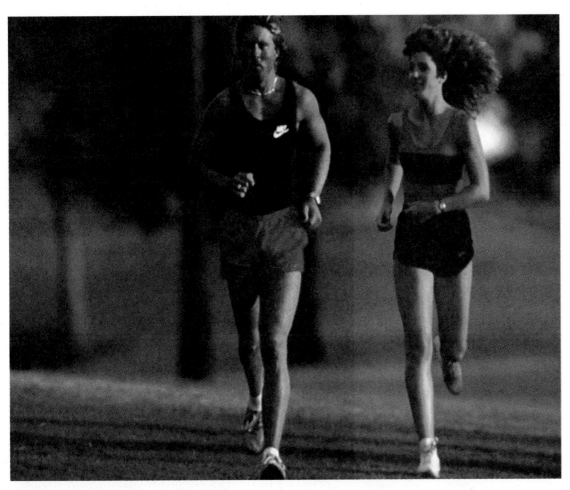

Jogging is a good example of aerobic exercise.

Table 7.1

Continuous versus Intermittent Exercise: Advantages and Disadvantages

Continuous	Intermittent
• Is done slowly and continuously, rather than in short, vigorous bursts; therefore, many people consider continuous exercise to be less demanding and more enjoyable.	• When done in the target zone, it has the same benefits as continuous exercise. If done intensely it can increase risk of soreness and injury for beginners.
• Is less intense and because of lower injury risk may be best for beginners, especially for those who are older and those who are just starting an exercise program after a long layoff.	• Three ten-minute or two fifteen-minute exercise sessions might be easier to schedule for busy people than one longer exercise period.
• Provides health benefits associated with cardiovascular fitness.	• May be more interesting to some people.
• May not provide optimal performance benefits for competitors.	• If done at relatively high intensity with alternating rest periods, it can be beneficial in preparing for competition.

three ten-minute exercise sessions in the target zone were as effective as one thirty-minute exercise session.

Aerobic interval training and interval dance exercise are examples of intermittent aerobic exercise. Sports such as basketball, tennis, and racquetball that are intermittent are often considered to be aerobic activities when they are performed for long periods without stopping. Though they are considered to be aerobic, they also involve periodic anaerobic exercise.

There are advantages and disadvantages of continuous and intermittent exercise.

The advantages and disadvantages of continuous and intermittent exercise are presented in table 7.1.

Not all aerobic exercise is equally safe.

Sports medicine experts indicate that certain types of aerobic exercise are more likely to result in injury than others. As shown in table 7.2, walking and low impact dance aerobics are among the least risky activities. Skating, an aerobic activity, is even more risky than most competitive sports. Among the most popular aerobic activities, running has the greatest risk, with cycling, high impact dance aerobics, and step aerobics having moderate risk of injury.

There Are Many Popular Forms of Aerobic Exercise

Some of the most popular forms of aerobic exercise are discussed briefly here.

Aerobic Exercise Machines

There are many kinds of aerobic exercise machines, including stairclimbers, cross-country ski machines, and stationary bicycles. Advantages of such machines are that they can be used in the home or in most fitness clubs and do not require excessive amounts of skill. There is some

evidence that use of these machines is fun and interesting initially, but that interest decreases with repeated use. Ski machines would seem to be most useful for people who ski on a regular basis, and bicycles would seem to be most interesting to those who do cycling. Aerobic exercise machines can be useful in developing cardiovascular fitness for those who use them to exercise in the target zone for fitness. The key to the effectiveness of the machines is persistent use over long periods of time.

Aerobic Interval Training

Interval training is one of the most common forms of intermittent exercise. Short bursts of energy, commonly referred to as *sprints,* are alternated with rest periods. For many years interval training was considered to be exclusively a form of anaerobic training, and as noted later in this concept, it is an excellent form of anaerobic training. However, athletes and coaches now feel that *aerobic interval training* may be quite important for competitors in sports such as swimming, running, and cycling. In aerobic interval training, repeated performances of relatively short exercise bouts are alternated with brief rest periods. The exercise bouts are performed at slower than race (for racers) pace and not so intensely as anaerobics. Proponents of aerobic interval training suggest that this procedure allows a greater volume of training in a shorter period. To date, the evidence supporting the superiority of this form of training for competitors is principally based on the testimony of coaches and athletes. Additional research is necessary.

An example of a schedule of aerobic interval training for a ten-km runner is illustrated in table 7.3. To use the schedule, locate your typical ten-km time in the left-hand column. Perform 400-meter runs at the time specified in the "pace" column. Repeat twenty times with intervals of ten to fifteen seconds between runs. Similar schedules can be developed with other activities such as swimming and cycling. This activity, however, is not recommended for those just beginning exercise (see table 7.1).

Table 7.2
Risk of Injury in Exercise

Activity	Injury per 1000 Hrs. of Activity
Skating	20
Basketball	18
Ave. competitive sports	16
Running/jogging	16
Racquetball	14
Ave. aerobic activity	10
Tennis	8
Cycling	6
High impact dance aerobics	6
Step aerobics	5
Aerobic exercise machines	3
Walking	2
Low impact dance aerobics	2

Source: Data from the Center for Sports Medicine at St. Francis Hospital, San Francisco, CA.

Table 7.3
Aerobic Interval Training Schedules for a Ten-Kilometer Runner

Best 10-km Time (Min:Sec)	Reps	Distance (Meters)	Rest (Sec)	Pace (Min:Sec)
46:00	20	400	10–15	2:00
43:00	20	400	10–15	1:52
40:00	20	400	10–15	1:45
37:00	20	400	10–15	1:37
34:00	20	400	10–15	1:30

From Jack H. Wilmore and David L. Costill, *Training for Sport and Activity*, 3d ed. Copyright © 1988 Wm. C. Brown Communications, Inc., Dubuque, Iowa. All Rights Reserved. Reprinted by permission.

Bicycling

Bicycling, when done continuously, is a form of aerobic exercise. This activity requires only a bicycle and some safety equipment, such as a helmet and a light and reflectors if done after dark. A tall flag is needed if biking in traffic. To be most effective in building physical fitness, you should pedal continuously, rather than coasting for long periods. Maintaining a steady pace is recommended. Riding a different course periodically can increase enjoyment of the activity.

Circuit Resistance Training (CRT)

Originally, circuit training was a type of physical training involving movement from one exercise station to another. A different type of exercise was performed at each station. In order to complete the circuit, you had to complete all the exercises at the different stations. Your goal was to perform the circuit in progressively shorter periods.

Recently, however, circuit training has been modified by some to include several strength overload stations. These stations may involve resistance exercises with free weights or exercise machines (see Concept 11 and Lab 11). There is some evidence that when CRT is done with high repetitions and moderate loads, it can make modest contributions to cardiovascular fitness. When aerobic exercise such as rides on stationary bicycles and running on treadmills is incorporated in the continuous exercise circuit, the contribution of this type of exercise to cardiovascular fitness increases. The key is continuous exercise. When repetitions of resistance training exercises are followed by relatively long rest periods (longer than the exercise time) they do little for cardiovascular fitness. One problem with this form of exercise, if cardiovascular fitness is the goal, is that the best of programs are ineffective if they cannot be performed properly. Some exercise clubs promote exercise circuits as a method of building both strength and cardiovascular fitness. Yet exercise stations are often crowded, and it is next to impossible to perform the circuit without long waiting periods. You may want to add aerobic exercise to your circuit during periods of waiting.

Cooper's Aerobics

Based on the needs of military personnel, Dr. Kenneth Cooper developed a physical fitness program that he called aerobics. In fact, he popularized the term. His program includes a variety of aerobic activities having point values for the different types of exercises involved. To develop fitness, especially cardiovascular fitness, a person is expected to earn thirty "aerobic points" per week. Aerobic points are part of Cooper's system for helping people to know when they are exercising frequently enough, intensely enough, and long enough. Many activities Cooper includes in his program are described in this concept. Table 7.4 charts some of the point values for various activities. (For more complete details on the Cooper aerobics program, refer to Cooper 1982, in the references.)

Continuous Calisthenics

Survey results repeatedly indicate that calisthenics are among the top two or three participant activities performed. Calisthenics, exercises such as the crunch and push-ups, are designed to build flexibility, strength, or muscular endurance in specific muscle groups. Even though most calisthenics are aerobic, they are often done intermittently. That is, calisthenic exercises are done a few at a time followed by a rest period. They may do little for cardiovascular fitness or fat control.

Table 7.4
Aerobic Points Chart

Points	Walking-Running (Time for 1 Mile)	Cycling (Speed for 2 Miles)	Swimming (300 yds.)	Handball, Basketball	Stationary Running for 5 Minutes	Stationary Running for 10 Minutes	Points
0	Over 20 min.	Less than 10 mph	Over 10 min.	Less than 10 min.	Less than 60 steps/min.	Less than 50 steps/min.	0
1	20:00–14:30 min.	10–15 mph	8:00–10:00 min.	10 min.	60–70 steps/min.	50–65 steps/min.	1
2	14:29–12:00 min.	16–20 mph	7:30–7:59 min.	20 min.	71–90 steps/min.	66–70 steps/min.	2
3	11:59–10:00 min.	Over 20 mph	6:00–7:29 min.	30 min.		71–80 steps/min.	3
4	9:59–8:00 min.			40 min.		81–90 steps/min.	4
5	7:59–6:30 min.			50 min.			5
6	Less than 6:30 min.			60 min.			6

Continuous calisthenics, or calisthenics that are done without stopping or with walking, jogging, rope jumping, or some other aerobic activity performed during the rest period, can develop virtually all health-related aspects of physical fitness. Fitness pioneer Dr. Thomas Cureton (1965) long advocated the use of continuous calisthenics, or what he referred to as "continuous rhythmical endurance exercise." Almost everyone can plan a continuous calisthenic program by selecting exercises for each fitness part that will elevate the heart rate to the optimal level and sustain this intensity an adequate length of time. As is the case with CRT, it is essential that resting between exercises be kept to a minimum. Continuous calisthenics can be done individually, but are also excellent for group use.

Cross-Country Skiing

In Europe, cross-country skiing is one of the most popular aerobic activities. Of course, this sport requires snow and a certain amount of specialized equipment. For those who can cross-country ski on a regular basis, studies show that it is one of the most effective types of cardiovascular fitness exercise.

Dance Aerobics

This activity was first popularized by Jackie Sorensen in the 1970s as "aerobic dance." Since then, other versions of the activity have been promoted as rhythmic aerobics,

jazzercise, and dancercize, to note but a few of the popular names. In most cases, dance aerobics consists of a preplanned or choreographed series of dance steps and exercises done to music. Most of the early programs were considered to be "high impact" because they included jumping, leaping, and hopping dance steps that resulted in stress on the feet and legs.

In an attempt to reduce the risk of injury or soreness, "low impact" dance aerobics were developed. In low impact dance aerobics, one foot stays on the floor at all times. Low impact dance aerobics are an especially wise choice for beginners and older exercisers. "Step aerobics," also known as "bench stepping," is another adaptation of dance aerobics. In this activity the performer steps up and down on a bench when performing the various dance steps. In most cases step aerobics is still considered to be low impact but higher in intensity than many forms of dance aerobics. Dance and step aerobics, when planned appropriately for individual participants, can be very effective in building cardiovascular fitness for both men and women. (See appendix E for a sample dance aerobics program.)

One problem with dance aerobics is that it is a preplanned exercise program; therefore, it requires all participants to do the same activity regardless of their fitness or activity levels. A vigorous routine could cause unfit people to overextend themselves, whereas an easy routine may not result in fitness gains for those who are already quite fit. Also, some dance aerobic routines have been

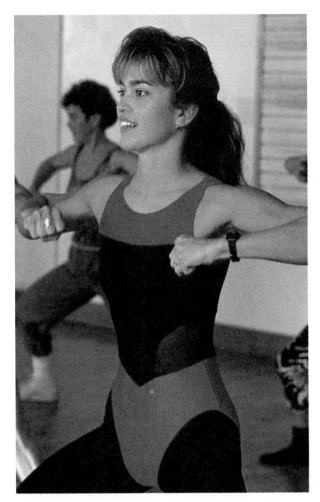
Dance aerobics is a popular form of exercise.

known to include contraindicated exercises. Good instructors encourage participants to adapt the steps and movements to meet their individual needs.

Hiking and Backpacking

Like walking and jogging, hiking is an excellent form of exercise. Hiking has the advantage of an out-of-doors setting, often in a very scenic environment. It does require some equipment, such as a rucksack and good hiking shoes, but highly specialized skills are not needed.

Backpacking is a form of hiking that usually covers longer distances and involves an overnight stay, often in the mountains. When done continuously, backpacking is excellent for building muscular endurance as well as cardiovascular fitness. Like other aerobic activities, it can be helpful in controlling body fatness. In recent years, it has become a popular activity; nearly eleven million American adults report regular involvement in backpacking.

Jogging/Running

The aerobic activity that has rapidly grown in popularity in recent years among both adult men and women is jogging or running. Though there is no official distinction between jogging and running, those who run more than a few miles per day, who participate in races, and who are concerned about improving the time in which they run a certain distance often prefer to be called runners rather than joggers. Fifteen to twenty million American adults report that they jog or run on a regular basis.

The major advantage of jogging/running is that it requires only a good pair of running shoes, some inexpensive exercise clothing, and very little skill. With effort, almost anyone can benefit from the activity and even improve performance if that is the goal.

There are some techniques that every jogger should be familiar with before starting a jogging program.

- *Foot Placement*—The heel of the foot hits the ground first in jogging. Your heel should strike before the rest of your foot (but not hard), then you should rock forward and push off with the ball of your foot. Contrary to some opinions, you should *not* jog on your toes. (A flat foot landing can be all right as long as you push off with the ball of your foot.) Your toes should point straight ahead. Your feet should stay under your knees and *not* swing out to the sides as you jog.
- *Length of Stride*—For efficiency, you should have a relatively long stride. Your stride should be several inches longer than your walking stride. If necessary, you may have to reach to lengthen your stride. Most older people find it more efficient to run with a shorter stride.
- *Arm Movement*—While you jog, you should swing your arms as well as your legs. The arms should be bent at about 90 degrees and should swing freely and alternately from front to back in the direction you are moving, not from side to side. Keep your arms and hands relaxed.
- *Body Position*—While jogging, you should hold your upper body nearly erect and your head and chest up. There should not be a conscious effort to lean forward as is the case in sprinting or fast running.

Rope Jumping

Rope jumping is aerobic if done at a slow or moderate pace, but is anaerobic if done vigorously. One study shows that typical exercisers jump very briskly, and for this reason cannot maintain the jumping continuously. Even those who are highly trained or who jump at a moderate pace find it difficult to continue this exercise long enough to build cardiovascular fitness because of leg fatigue, high heart rate, or loss of interest in the activity. To be most effective, a continuous routine involving several different jump steps should be used in combination with other forms of exercise. For example, rope jumping could be a part of a circuit-resistance training program or a dance aerobic routine.

Skating

Ice skating tends to be regional in its appeal, roller skating is often limited to roller rinks or amusement areas, and roller blades are most frequently used by young people. However, all three are examples of aerobic exercise that can be useful in promoting cardiovascular fitness when done regularly. Inline (roller-blades) skates, originally developed for training skiers in the off-season, have been improved through recent technology and are now a popular form of aerobic exercise. Because the risk of injury is greater for skating than for many other aerobic activities, special precautions should be taken when doing this activity, including wearing a helmet, as well as knee and elbow pads. Some degree of fitness and skill is necessary to perform skating safely and effectively.

Sports (Continuous)

As noted earlier in this concept, some activities at least partially anaerobic are considered aerobic if they are done at a continuous pace. Many sports have extended rest periods and do not allow for continuous involvement. Some sports considered to be good aerobic activities *when performed continuously* are basketball, handball, racquetball, and soccer. (For more information on sports, see Concept 15.)

Swimming and Water Exercises

The most recent exercise polls rank swimming as the first or second most popular form of regular exercise among adults. Most of those who swim for exercise swim laps or do water exercises. When done at a mild or moderate pace, both of these can be aerobic. When done continuously, these are excellent forms of cardiovascular exercise. Another popular but more structured program for this type of exercise is Aquadynamics, prepared by the President's Council for Physical Fitness and Sports (see references).

Walking

Approximately one-quarter of all adults report that they walk regularly for exercise. This exercise is probably so popular because it can be done easily by people of all ages and of all ability levels. In previous years the value of walking has been minimized. Because less than very brisk walking may not produce heart rates in the cardiovascular fitness target zone, it was sometimes considered to be a less than desirable form of exercise. Given the recent evidence indicating that regular calorie expenditure is most important in reducing the risk of heart disease, walking

Table 7.5

Walking Schedules for Expending 1000 Calories per Week

Days per Week	Pace	Time per Day (minutes)		
		*100 lb. (45 kg)	150 lb. (68 kg)	200 lb. (90 kg)
5	2 mph (3.2 kph)	96	62	46
	3 mph (4.8 kph)	44	48	38
	4 mph (6.4 kph)	48	36	24
6	2 mph	80	52	40
	3 mph	62	40	32
	4 mph	40	26	20
7	2 mph	68	44	34
	3 mph	54	36	26
	4 mph	34	24	18

*Body weight

is viewed in a different light. Walking is an excellent way to expend calories because it can be done for long periods. The calories expended also help in maintaining optimal body fatness. Since controlling fatness is associated with several health benefits, walking has a double benefit.

Table 7.5 illustrates the minutes per day and days per week necessary to accumulate an expenditure of 1000 calories per week at different rates of walking. Walkers could begin at lower levels (expending a minimum of 500 calories per week, for example), and gradually increase to the levels shown in Table 7.5—the amounts of walking that would produce a health benefit. Ideally, walkers would then continue to increase until they are regularly expending 2000 calories per week. Of course, walking can be combined with other more vigorous activities to expend greater amounts of calories in a shorter period of time.

If cardiovascular fitness benefits as evidenced by an increase in $\dot{V}O_2$ are desired, walking must be done intensely enough to elevate the heart rate to threshold levels. Walking is often most enjoyable when done with other people and when different walking routes are used to provide variety.

Different aerobic activities have different health-related benefits.

The health-related benefits of various aerobic activities are summarized in table 7.6.

The Facts About Anaerobic Exercise

Anaerobic exercise is useful for building cardiovascular and other aspects of physical fitness.

The types of health-related fitness that can be developed through anaerobic exercise programs are rated in table 7.7.

Table 7.6
Fitness Benefits Achieved through Aerobic Exercise

Program Type	Cardiovascular Fitness	Strength and Muscular Endurance	Flexibility	Body and Fat Control	Skill-Related Fitness Components	Enjoyment or Fun[1]
Aerobic exercise machines	***	**	*	***	—	—
Aerobic interval training	***	**	—	***	—	—
Bicycling	***	**	*	***	*	**
Circuit resistance training	*	***	*	**	*	**
Cooper's aerobics	***	*	*	***	*	**
Continuous calisthenics	***	**	***	***	*	**
Cross-country skiing	***	**	*	***	**	**
Dance aerobics	***	**	***	***	*	**
Hiking and backpacking	**	**	*	**	*	**
Jogging/running	***	*	*	***	—	**
Rope jumping	**	*	—	**	*	*
Skating	***	*	—	***	**	**
Swimming and water exercises	**	**	**	**	**	**
Walking	**	*	*	**	*	**

Key: *** = Very Good, ** = Good, * = Minimum, — = Low

[1]Enjoyment and fun are relative, and for this reason it is impossible to classify activities accurately. However, for the average person some activities seem to be more enjoyable than others. The above listed classifications reflect the opinions of the typical person. *Any of the activities listed above can be fun and enjoyable for a given person in the right circumstances.*

Table 7.7
Fitness Benefits Achieved through Anaerobic Exercise

Program Type	Cardiovascular Fitness	Strength and Muscular Endurance	Flexibility	Body and Fat Control	Skill-Related Fitness Components	Enjoyment or Fun[1]
Fartlek or "speed play"	**	**	—	***	**	*
Interval dance	**	**	—	***	*	*
Interval training (anaerobic)	**	**	—	***	***	*

Key: *** = Very Good, ** = Good, * = Minimum, — = Low

[1]Enjoyment and fun are relative, and for this reason it is impossible to classify activities accurately. However, for the average person some activities seem to be more enjoyable than others. The above listed classifications reflect the opinions of the typical person. *Any of the activities listed can be fun and enjoyable for a given person in the right circumstances.*

Popular Anaerobic Exercise Programs

Fartlek or "Speed Play"

Fartlek is a Swedish word for "speed play." This exercise was developed in Scandinavia where pinewood paths follow curves of lakes and up and down many hills, where the scenery takes your mind off the task at hand. The idea is to get away from the regimen of running on a track and to enjoy the woods, lakes, and mountains. Because of the terrain, the pace is never constant. The uphill path requires a slow pace, while a straight stretch or downhill trail allows for speed. In the "speed play" or fartlek system, you run easily for a time at a steady, hard speed, walk rapidly following that, alternate short sprints with walking, go full speed uphill, and perhaps at a fast pace for a while. You can plan your own speed play program using your own course, which may include both uphill and downhill running with other variations.

Interval Dance

Recently, *interval dance* exercise has become more popular. This is simply more intense dance exercise alternated with more frequent rest periods. In some cases, other forms of exercise, such as running, are alternated with dance exercise bouts. When properly planned, this form of exercise can be effective in producing cardiovascular fitness. Because it is a type of intermittent exercise, it has some advantages and disadvantages compared to traditional dance exercise (see table 7.1).

Interval Training Program (Anaerobic)

An anaerobic interval training program involves repeated fast anaerobic running or swimming for short periods of time, separated by measured intervals of slow recovery jogging or swimming. (Developed by Gerschler of Germany, the stress of anaerobic running raises the heart rate to near maximal from which it drops to a moderate level during recovery.) This program controls distance, pace, number of repetitions, and recovery interval, allowing for a wide variety of programs of various intensities. Guidelines for anaerobic exercise are presented in Concept 6 (see table 6.4).

Research suggests that short interval workouts should use maximum speed with rest intervals lasting from ten seconds to two minutes. These should be repeated eight to thirty times. Anaerobic interval training having long intervals uses 90 to 100 percent speed with rest intervals lasting from three to fifteen minutes. These should be repeated four to fifteen times. A sample short anaerobic interval program and a sample long interval running program are presented in table 7.8. Using the guidelines in Concept 6, you can plan your own anaerobic interval training program.

Table 7.8

Sample Anaerobic Interval Training Program (Moderate Intensity)

Short Intervals	Long Intervals
1. Do a flexibility and cardiovascular warm-up (see Concept 4).	1. Do a flexibility and cardiovascular warm-up (see Concept 4).
2. Run at 100% speed for 10 seconds (approximately 70 to 100 yards).	2. Run at 90% speed for one minute (approximately 300 to 500 yards).
3. Rest for 10 seconds by walking slowly.	3. Rest for 4 minutes by walking slowly.
4. Alternately repeat steps 2 and 3 until 20 runs have been completed.	4. Alternately repeat steps 2 and 3 until 5 runs have been completed.

Suggested Readings

Allsen, D. E., and P. Witbeck. *Raquetball.* 5th ed. Dubuque, Iowa: Wm. C. Brown Publishers, 1992.

Cheatum, B. A. *Golf.* 2d ed. Dubuque, Iowa: Wm. C. Brown Publishers, 1983.

Fisher, A. G., and P. E. Allsen. *Jogging.* 2d ed. Dubuque, Iowa: Wm. C. Brown Publishers, 1987.

Johnson, J. D. *Tennis.* 5th ed. Dubuque, Iowa: Wm. C. Brown Publishers, 1988.

McIntosh, M. *Lifetime Aerobics.* Dubuque, Iowa: Wm. C. Brown Publishers, 1990.

Rasch, P. J. *Weight Training.* 5th ed. Dubuque, Iowa: Wm. C. Brown Publishers, 1990.

Schunk, C. *Bowling.* 3d ed. Dubuque, Iowa: Wm. C. Brown Publishers, 1983.

Seiger, L. H., and J. Hesson. *Walking for Fitness.* Dubuque, Iowa: Wm. C. Brown Publishers, 1990.

Vickers, B. *Swimming.* 5th ed. Dubuque, Iowa: Wm. C. Brown Publishers, 1989.

8

Flexibility

Concept 8

Adequate flexibility permits freedom of movement and may contribute to ease and economy of muscular effort, success in certain activities, and less susceptibility to some types of injuries or musculoskeletal problems.

Introduction

Flexibility is a measure of the range of motion available at a joint or group of joints. It is determined by the shape of the bones and cartilage in the joint, and by the length and extensibility of muscles, tendons, ligaments, and fascia that cross the joint. Traditionally, flexibility has been the most neglected of the five health-related components of physical fitness. However, there has been a recent surge of interest in stretching exercises by athletes, fitness buffs, and researchers.

The range of movement at a joint may vary. It may be restricted so that the joint will not bend or straighten, and is said to be "tight" or "stiff," or to have "contractures." The deformed hand of an arthritic is an example of this extreme. At the other end of the spectrum is a high degree of flexibility referred to as "loose jointedness," **"hypermobility,"** or erroneously, as "double-jointedness." An example of this extreme is the contortionist seen at the circus. Each person, depending upon his or her individual needs, must have a reasonable amount of flexibility to perform efficiently and effectively in daily life.

Health Goals for the Year 2000

- Increase the proportion of people who engage in activity to enhance muscular strength, muscular endurance, and flexibility.

Terms

Active Stretch

Muscles are stretched by the active contraction of the opposing (antagonist) muscle. For example, when doing a calf stretch exercise, the muscles on the front of the shin contract to cause a stretch of the muscles on the back of the leg. (See figure 8.1A.)

Agonist Muscles

In this concept, agonist refers to the muscle group being stretched.

Antagonist Muscles

In this concept, antagonist refers to the muscle group opposing (on the opposite side of the limb from the agonist) the group being stretched.

Ballistic Stretch

Muscles are stretched by the force of momentum of a body part that is bounced, swung, or jerked, as in the calf stretch shown in figures 8.1D, E, and F. The foot is bounced forward either by antagonist muscle force or by an assist from another person, or gravity, or another body part.

77

Flexibility

Range of motion (ROM) in a joint or group of joints. Because muscle length is a major factor limiting the range of motion, those having long muscles that allow for good joint mobility are considered to have good flexibility.

Hamstrings

Three long muscles that cross both the back of the hip joint and the back of the knee joint, causing hip extension and knee flexion. They make up the bulk on the back of the thigh.

Hypermobility

Looseness or slackness in a normal plane of the muscles and ligaments (soft tissue) surrounding a joint.

Laxity

Motion in a joint outside the normal plane for that joint, due to loose ligaments (Steiner 1987).

Ligaments

Bands of tissue that connect bones.

Lumbar Muscles

Erector spinae and other muscles of the lower back (lumbar region of the spine); the muscles in the small of the back. These muscles are used to arch (hyperextend) the lower back.

Passive Stretch

Stretch imposed on a muscle by a force other than the opposing muscle, for example by another person (figure 8.1B), another body part (figure 8.1B), gravity (figure 8.1C), weights, or pulleys.

PNF Exercise (Proprioceptive Neuromuscular Facilitation)

Special exercise techniques to increase the contraction or the relaxation of muscles through reflex mechanisms (figure 8.1 G, H, and I).

Range of Motion (ROM)

The full motion possible in a joint.

Range of Motion Exercise

Exercises used to maintain existing joint mobility (to prevent loss of ROM).

Reciprocal Inhibition

Reflex relaxation in the muscle being stretched during the contraction of the antagonist.

Static Stretch

A muscle is slowly stretched and then held in that stretched position for several seconds.

Stiffness

Elasticity of the muscle–tendon unit.

Stretching (Flexibility) Exercise

Exercise used to increase the existing ROM at a joint by elongating muscles and other soft tissue.

Trigger Point

An especially irritable spot, usually a tight band or knot in a muscle or fascia. This often refers pain to another area of the body. For example, a trigger point in the shoulder might cause a headache. This condition is referred to as "myofascial pain syndrome" and is often caused by muscle tension, fatigue, or strain.

Some General Facts About Flexibility

There is no ideal standard for flexibility.

It is not known how much flexibility any one person should have in a joint. There are test norms available that list how hundreds of subjects of various ages, of both sexes, and in many walks of life have performed. But there is little scientific evidence to indicate that a person who can reach two inches past his or her toes on a sit-and-reach test is less fit than a person who can reach eight inches past the toes. Too much flexibility could be as detrimental as too little. The standards presented in chart 8.1 are based on the best available evidence.

Lack of use, injury, or disease can decrease joint mobility.

Arthritis and calcium deposits can damage a joint, and inflammation can cause pain that prevents movement. Failure to move a joint regularly through its full range of motion can lead to a shortening of muscles and **ligaments.** Static positions held for longer periods, such as in poor posture, working postures, and when a body part is immobilized by a cast, lead to shortened tissue and loss of mobility. Improper exercise that overdevelops one muscle group while neglecting the opposing group results in an imbalance that restricts flexibility.

Some people are unusually flexible because of a genetic trait that makes their joints "hypermobile."

In some families, the trait for loose joints is passed from generation to generation. This hypermobility is sometimes referred to as joint looseness. Studies show that those with this trait may be more prone to dislocated patellas. There is not much research evidence, but some experts believe that people with hypermobility or **laxity** may also be more susceptible to athletic or dance injuries, especially to the knee and ankle, and may be more apt to develop premature osteoarthritis. One recent study found that subjects who were "loose jointed" used more energy in walking and jogging than those who were medium or "tight jointed."

In the fifth century, Hippocrates noted the disadvantage of hyperextension of the elbow in archery. The hyperextended position for elbows and knees is not an efficient position from which to move because of a poor angle of muscle pull. For example, it is difficult to perform push-ups when the elbows lock into hyperextension because extra effort is required to unlock the joint. It may be advantageous for loose-jointed people to take extra care to strengthen muscles around the joints most used.

To maintain the *range of motion (ROM)* you presently have in your joints, you must regularly perform "range of motion exercises."

The adage: "If you don't use it, you'll lose it!" applies particularly to flexibility. Failure to use the joints regularly through their normal range results in loss of flexibility in a fairly short period. To maintain what you have, you should do "ROM exercises." Some athletes prefer to do this during the warm-up prior to a workout and save their stretching exercises until the end of the workout.

To increase the length of a muscle, you must stretch it (overload) more than its normal length.

There is much that is not known about flexibility, but the best evidence suggests that muscles should be stretched to about 10 percent beyond their normal length to bring about an improvement in flexibility. Exercises that do not cause an overload by stretching beyond normal will not increase flexibility.

Flexibility is specific to each joint of the body.

No one flexibility test will give an indication of your overall flexibility. For example, tight **hamstrings** and lumbar muscles might be revealed by a toe-touch test, but the range of motion in other joints may be quite different. The toe-touch test, done with both legs extended, does not distinguish between flexibility of the hamstrings and the lower back muscles, so it lacks specificity in its measurement.

Flexibility is influenced by several factors, including age, sex, and race.

As children grow older, their flexibility increases until adolescence when they become progressively less flexible. As a general rule, girls tend to be more flexible than boys.

This is probably due to anatomical differences in the joints, as well as to differences in the type and extent of activities the two sexes tend to choose. In adults, there is less difference between the sexes. Some races and ethnic groups have been reported to have specific joints that are hypermobile. For example, the thumb and finger joints of Middle Eastern people and East Indians tend to be more flexible.

Scores on flexibility tests may be influenced by several factors.

Your range of motion at any one time may be influenced by your motivation to exert maximum effort, your warm-up preparation, the presence of muscular soreness, your tolerance for pain, the room temperature, and your ability to relax. Recent studies have found a relationship between leg or trunk length and the scores made on the sit-and-reach test. For those of average build, this is not a factor, but for a small percentage of people it makes a significant difference unless the test specifically allows for differences in body build.

Studies of the influence of the temperature of the muscle on the effectiveness of a stretching exercise have produced contradictory results.

Some studies have shown that increasing the temperature of the muscle through warm-up exercises or the application of heat packs has resulted in improved scores on flexibility tests. Other studies have failed to find a difference between the flexibility of subjects who have warmed-up and those who did not warm-up.

Furthermore, some people believe that cooling the muscle with ice packs in the final phase of a stretch aids in lengthening the muscle, but a recent study has failed to confirm this (Lentell et al., 1992). Until scientists reach a consensus, it seems wise to continue the practice of the warm-up and cool-down with careful static stretching.

It is not necessary to sacrifice flexibility in order to develop strength.

A person with bulging muscles may become musclebound or have a restricted range of motion if strength training is done improperly. In any progressive resistance program, both agonists and antagonists should receive equal training, and all movements should be carried through the full range of motion. Properly conducted strength training does not cause a person to be musclebound. Furthermore, there is no evidence that a long muscle is any weaker than a short one. A good rule of thumb is: "Stretch what you strengthen and strengthen what you stretch."

Facts About the Benefits of Flexibility Exercises

Adequate flexibility may help prevent muscle strain and such orthopedic problems as backache.

Short, tight muscles are more apt to be injured by over-stretching than are long muscles. One common cause of backache is shortened **lumbar muscles** and hip flexor muscles. Short hamstrings are also associated with lower back problems. (See Concepts 16 and 17 for more discussion on back problems.) **Stretching (flexibility) exercises** may help prevent or alleviate some backaches, muscle cramps, and muscle strains.

Trigger points may sometimes be prevented or inactivated by static, or PNF stretching, of the muscles involved.

When body parts are held in static positions for long periods, or when muscles are chronically overloaded, fatigued, or chilled, myofascial trigger points may cause stiffness and local or referred pain. Often, the trigger point can be deactivated and the pain relieved by gentle but persistent stretching of the muscle, especially if accompanied or followed by the application of heat or cold.

Good flexibility may bring about improved athletic performance.

A hurdler must have good back and hip joint mobility to clear the hurdle. A swimmer requires shoulder and ankle flexibility for powerful strokes. A diver must be able to reach his or her toes in order to perform a good jackknife. Low back flexibility allows a runner to lengthen the stride. The fencer needs long hamstrings and hip adductors in order to lunge a long distance.

Even weight lifters have been shown to improve their performances by flexibility training. Those who trained were significantly better in the amount of weight they could bench press when it was performed with a "rebound" (no pause between the lowering and lifting phase) to take advantage of the elastic "snap-back" force. It has been hypothesized that the stretching exercises not only increase the length of the muscle, but can also decrease its **stiffness.** Other power athletes who use ballistic movements, such as baseball pitchers, high jumpers, shot putters, and so forth, might also benefit from this training.

It is widely believed that static muscle stretching is effective in relieving muscle spasms, muscle soreness, and shin splints.

One theory suggests that local muscle soreness may be caused by slight reflex contractions. It is believed that a **static stretch** of the affected muscle may relieve these slight

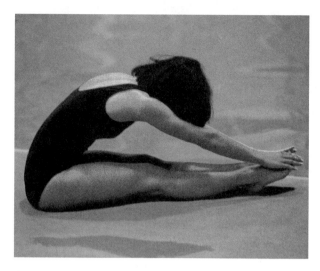

Athletic performance requires good flexibility.

contractions and thus relieve the pain. Even some cases of nonpathological shin splints may be relieved by such exercise.

Research studies to date do not support the conventional wisdom that stretching during a cool-down will *prevent* muscular soreness. In a recent controlled study, muscle soreness was deliberately induced in a group of subjects. When half of the group stretched immediately afterward and at intervals for 48 hours, they had no less soreness than the group who did not stretch (Buroker and Schwane 1989).

Stretching exercises are useful in preventing and remediating some cases of dysmenorrhea in women.

Painful menstruation (dysmenorrhea) of some types can be prevented or reduced by stretching the pelvic and hip joint fascia. Billig's exercise is an example of an effective exercise (see Concept 9, exercise 6).

Flexibility training has been shown to improve spinal mobility and the driving ability of older adults.

When older drivers performed stretching exercises, they improved their range of motion and were better able to look over their shoulders for blind spots, parallel parking, and backing into parking spaces ("Fitness Improves Driving," *Senior World* 1991).

It is normal for tissue to lose its elasticity with age, but a sedentary life-style is probably the greatest contributor to loss of flexibility with aging. Fortunately, the elderly do respond to training. Spinal mobility is important not only for driving, but also for daily activities such as tying one's shoes and reaching and twisting.

Facts About the Types of Stretching Exercises

There are several effective methods of exercising to develop flexibility.

Three commonly used types of stretching exercises are **static stretch, ballistic stretch,** and **PNF exercise (proprioceptive neuromuscular facilitation).** Each of these can be performed as an **active stretch** or as a **passive stretch.** All are effective in developing flexibility.

Static stretching is widely recommended because most experts believe it is less likely to cause injury.

Because static stretching is done slowly and held for a period, there is less probability of tearing the soft tissue, particularly if the force comes from your own muscles. Many believe static stretching is also less likely to cause delayed-onset muscle soreness, but one recent study found it caused greater soreness than ballistic stretching (Smith, et al., 1993).

Active-assisted stretch is safer and more effective than passive stretch.

When active stretch is used, the opposing muscles contract. This produces a reflex (**reciprocal inhibition**) relaxation in the muscles that you are trying to stretch. On the other hand, when a muscle is stretched passively by an outside force, there is no reflex relaxation. A muscle that is not relaxed cannot be stretched as far, and there is potential for injury.

There is one problem, however, with an active stretch. It is almost impossible to produce an overload by simply contracting the opposing muscles. Therefore, it is best to combine the active stretch with a passive assist. This gives the advantage of a relaxed muscle and a sufficient force to provide an overload to stretch it.

Ballistic stretching may be an important technique for active people.

A ballistic stretch uses momentum to produce the stretch. Momentum is produced by vigorous motion, such as flinging a body part or rocking it back and forth to create a bouncing movement. Because this may stretch the muscle farther than some other methods, there is the potential for injury. Some opponents argue that the sudden stretch of the ballistic motion elicits a myotatic reflex (stretch reflex), which then causes the muscle to contract and thus get shorter and stronger instead of longer. It is true that a myotatic reflex occurs (it also occurs in a static stretch), but the momentum is already spent so there is no overload on the muscle; therefore, *no* strength is developed. It should also be recognized that the active con-

traction of the **antagonist muscles** (opposite the muscle being stretched) causes a desirable reciprocal inhibition in the muscle being stretched.

Although not everyone agrees that the disadvantages of ballistic stretch outweigh the advantages, most experts do believe that static stretch is the preferred method for beginners, those with a history of muscle injury, and those who do not need exceptional levels of flexibility for athletic performances.

Since many athletic activities are ballistic in nature, sport-specific ballistic stretch is deemed appropriate for some athletes. The *principle of specificity* implies that one should train with the type of movements that are most likely to occur in the activity for which one is training. Since ballistic movement is very much a part of most athletic events (those requiring speed and power), it is appropriate to train using this type of movement. Even among athletes, however, static stretching is recommended prior to the use of ballistic stretching during a workout. Ballistic exercises are illustrated in figure 8.1D, E, and F. Examples of sport-specific ballistic stretches are shown on pages 95–96 in concept 9. Passive ballistic stretching is particularly risky and is not recommended for use outside of the clinic.

PNF (Proprioceptive Neuromuscular Facilitation) techniques have proven to be the most effective methods of improving flexibility.

PNF has been popular for rehabilitation since the 1960s. It consists of dozens of techniques to stimulate muscles to contract more strongly or to relax more fully so that they can be stretched. Three of the techniques that have become popular in fitness programs to improve the flexibility of healthy people are: contract-relax-antagonist-contract (CRAC), slow-reversal-hold-relax (SRHR), and contract-relax (CR).

The contract-relax-antagonist-contract technique involves three steps: (1) move the limb so the muscle to be stretched is elongated initially, then contract the **agonist muscles** isometrically against an immovable object or the resistance of a partner for three seconds; (2) relax the muscle two seconds; and (3) stretch the muscle immediately by contracting the antagonist for 10 to 15 seconds with an assist from a partner, gravity, or other body part (see fig. 8.1 G, H, I). Research shows that this and other types of PNF stretch are more effective than a simple static stretch. The SRHR procedure is the same as CRAC except that the agonist is passively stretched prior to step 1 (fig. 8.1G) and again after step 3 (fig. 8.1I).

A variation of this PNF procedure is contract-relax. This is the same procedure as the CRAC technique except that the static stretch is done passively. Following the isometric contraction, another body part, person, or gravity applies force to stretch the muscles. There is no contraction of the opposing muscles during the stretch. CRAC and SRHR are believed to be superior to CR in their effectiveness.

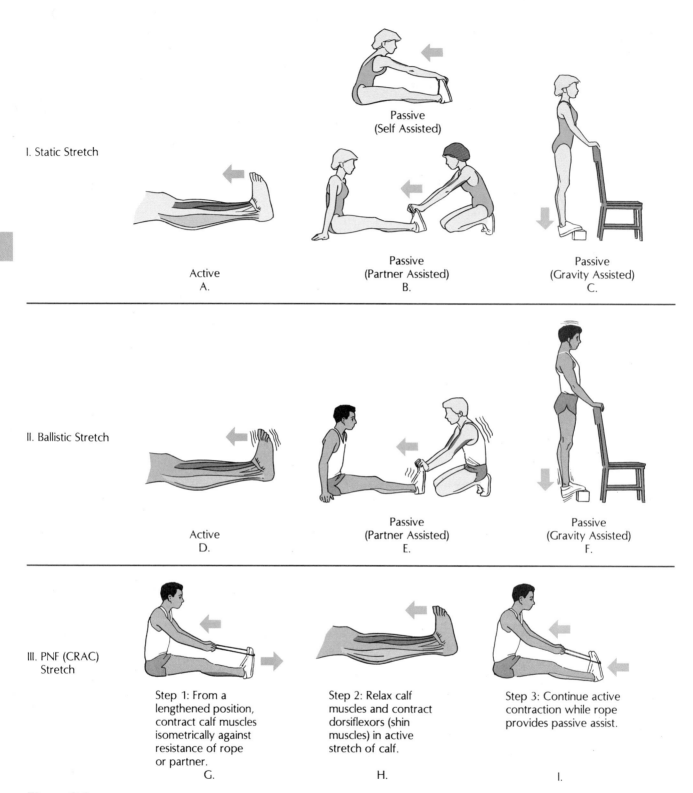

I. Static Stretch

Passive
(Self Assisted)

Active
A.

Passive
(Partner Assisted)
B.

Passive
(Gravity Assisted)
C.

II. Ballistic Stretch

Active
D.

Passive
(Partner Assisted)
E.

Passive
(Gravity Assisted)
F.

III. PNF (CRAC) Stretch

Step 1: From a lengthened position, contract calf muscles isometrically against resistance of rope or partner.
G.

Step 2: Relax calf muscles and contract dorsiflexors (shin muscles) in active stretch of calf.
H.

Step 3: Continue active contraction while rope provides passive assist.
I.

Figure 8.1

Examples of static, ballistic, PNF, active, and passive stretches of the calf muscles (gastrocnemius and soleus). Muscles shown in **dark red** are the muscles being contracted. Muscles shown in pink are those being stretched. *Note:* Bilateral toe touching is NOT recommended by the authors. It was chosen as a familiar exercise to illustrate the definitions.

Each form of flexibility exercise has its advantages and disadvantages.

The advantages and disadvantages of unassisted ballistic, static, and PNF exercises using active stretch with passive assist are summarized in table 8.1. The best method or methods for you may depend upon your physical condition, whether you wish to increase your range of motion or just maintain it, whether you have a partner to assist, and whether you are training for speed or power athletic events.

Facts About How to Increase Flexibility

For maximal effectiveness and minimal harm, there are guidelines that should be followed in performing flexibility exercises.

There is a correct and an incorrect way to exercise, and some exercises can even be harmful. Concept 9 presents guidelines for flexibility exercises and some samples of the exercises defined in this concept.

There is a minimum amount of exercise (threshold of training) and an optimal amount of exercise (target zone) necessary for developing flexibility.

The threshold of training and target zones for static, ballistic, and PNF stretching are presented in table 8.2. The time required to stretch tissue varies inversely with the force used. Low force requires more time, whereas high force requires less time.

Table 8.1

Comparison of Advantages and Disadvantages of Three Types of Flexibility Exercises

Advantages	Static-Active, Assisted	Ballistic-Active	PNF (CRAC), Assisted
	Rating*		
Less danger of overstretch	G–E	P–F	G–E
Useful to relieve muscle cramps or soreness	E	P	G
Strength may be developed	P	P	G
Utilizes reflexes to relax the stretched muscle	G	F	E
Specific to most athletics and daily activities such as speed and power skills	P	E	P
Convenient; less apt to need another person to assist	F	E	P–F
Efficient; requires less time	F	F	P
Effective in lengthening muscles	G	G	E

*Key: E = Excellent, G = Good, F = Fair, P = Poor

Table 8.2

Flexibility Threshold of Training and Fitness Target Zones *

	Threshold of Training			Target Zones		
	Static	**Ballistic**	**PNF (CRAC)**	**Static**	**Ballistic**	**PNF (CRAC)**
Frequency	• 3 days per week for all methods.			• 3 to 7 days per week for all methods.		
Intensity	• Stretch as far as you can go without pain; with slow movement, hold at the end of the range of motion.	• Stretch muscle beyond normal length with gentle bounce or swing, but do not exceed 10% of active-static range of motion.	• Same as static except use a maximum isometric contraction of the muscle prior to stretch.	• Add assist. • Avoid overstretch and pain for all methods.	• Same as threshold.	• Same as static. • Add assist.
Time	• Hold stretch 15 sec.; • 3 reps; rest 30 sec. between.	• Continuous reps for 30 sec. (this is 1 set).	• Hold isometric contraction 3 sec. • hold stretch 10–15 sec.; • 3 reps; • 30 sec. rest between reps.	• Hold 10–15 sec.; • 3 reps; 3 sets; • 30 sec. rest between reps; • 1 min. rest between sets.	• 1–3 sets; • rest 1 min. between sets.	• 1–3 reps of 3 sec. contraction and 10–15 sec. hold; • 30 sec. rest between reps; • 1 min. rest between sets.

Facts About Exercise Precautions

Overstretching may make a person more susceptible to injury or hamper performance.

Muscles and tendons have both extensibility and elasticity. Ligaments and the joint capsule are extensible but lack elasticity. When stretched, they remain in the lengthened state. If this occurs, the joint may lack stability and is susceptible to chronic dislocation or movement in an undesirable plane. This is particularly true of weight-bearing joints, such as the hip, knee, and ankle. Loose ligaments may allow the joint to twist abnormally, tearing the cartilage and other soft tissue. Remember these precautions:

- Don't force it to the point of pain.
- Elderly people or those with osteoporosis or arthritis should use special care.
- Avoid vigorous stretching after a body part has been immobilized (such as in a sling or cast) for a long period.

- Avoid stretching swollen joints.
- Avoid overstretching weak muscles.
- Use great care in applying passive stretch to a partner; go slowly and ask for feedback.
- Some (but not all) people with high blood pressure should avoid the PNF techniques because the isometric contractions may increase arterial blood pressure excessively.
- Beginners, should use static or PNF stretching rather than ballistic stretching.
- Athletes who use sport-specific ballistic stretching should precede this type of stretching with static stretching.

Suggested Readings

Alter, M. J. *The Science of Stretching.* Champaign, IL: Human Kinetics Publishers, 1988.

Alter, M. J. *Sports Stretch.* Champaign, IL: Human Kinetics Publishers, 1990.

Hardy, L., and D. Jones. "Dynamic Flexibility and Proprioceptive Neuromuscular Facilitation." *Research Quarterly for Exercise and Sport* 57(1986):150.

LAB RESOURCE MATERIALS

(For use with Lab 8, page L-21)

Flexibility Tests

Because it is impractical to test the flexibility of all joints, perform these tests for joints used frequently. Follow instructions carefully.

Test

1. *Modified Sit-and-Reach*
   (Flexibility Test of Hamstrings)
   a. Remove shoes and assume the position for the "backsaver toe touch" (fig. 4.2, p. 93), except place the sole of the foot of the extended leg flat against the box or bench seat, and place the head, back, and hips against a wall; 90 degree angle at the hips.

   b. Place one hand over the other and slowly reach forward as far as you can with arms fully extended; head and back remain in contact with the wall. A partner will slide the measuring stick on the bench until it touches the fingertips.

   c. With the measuring stick fixed in the new position, reach forward as far as possible, three times, holding the position on the third reach for at least two seconds while the partner reads the distance on the ruler. Keep the knee of the extended leg straight (see illustration).

   d. Repeat the test a second time and average the scores of the two trials.

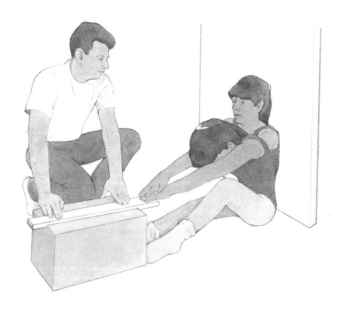

Test

2. *Shoulder Flexibility*

    a. Raise your right arm, bend your elbow, and reach down across your back as far as possible.

    b. At the same time, extend your left arm down and behind your back, bend your elbow up across your back, and try to cross your fingers over those of your right hand as shown in the accompanying illustration.

    c. Measure the distance to the nearest half-inch. If your fingers overlap, score as a plus; if they fail to meet, score as a minus; use a zero if your fingertips just touch.

    d. Repeat with your arms crossed in the opposite direction (left arm up). Most people will find that they are more flexible on one side than the other.

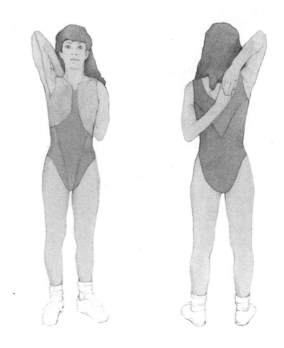

Test

3. *Hamstring and Hip Flexor Flexibility*

    a. Lie on your back on the floor beside a wall.

    b. Slowly lift one leg off the floor. Keep the other leg flat on the floor.

    c. Keep both legs straight.

    d. Continue to lift the leg until either leg begins to bend or the lower leg begins to lift off the floor.

    e. Place a yardstick against the wall and underneath the lifted leg.

    f. Hold the yardstick against the wall after the leg is lowered.

    g. Measure the angle created by the floor and the yardstick using a protractor. The greater the angle, the better your score.

    h. Repeat with the other leg.

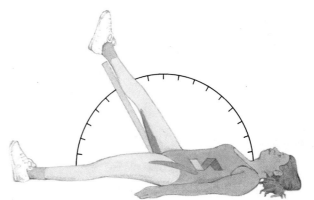

Note: For ease of testing, you may want to draw angles on a piece of posterboard as illustrated. If you have goniometers, you may be taught to use them instead.

Classification	Men				Women			
	Test 1	Test 2		Test 3	Test 1	Test 2		Test 3
		Right Up	Left Up			Right Up	Left up	
High performance zone	16+	5+	4+	111+	17+	6+	5+	111+
Good fitness zone	13–15	1–4	1–3	80–110	14–16	2–5	2–4	80–110
Marginal zone	10–12	0	0	60–79	11–13	1	1	60–79
Low zone	<9	<0	<0	<60	<10	<1	<1	<60

Chart 8.1 Flexibility *Rating Scale* for Tests 1, 2, 3*

*To convert to the metric system, see Appendix A.

9

Stretching Exercises

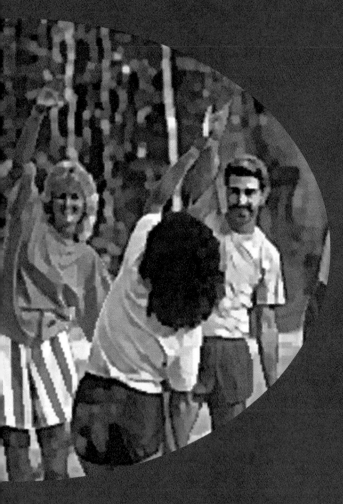

Concept 9

Stretching exercises are designed to maintain or increase flexibility by stretching the muscles and other soft tissue around the joints. This stretch may, in turn, prevent or alleviate some musculoskeletal problems.

Introduction

There are many ways to stretch muscles and improve flexibility through exercise (see Concept 8). The major types of muscle stretching exercises are static stretching, ballistic stretching, and PNF. These exercises can be done by yourself, using only your own muscles to stretch, gravity (body weight), or the assistance of other body parts or a partner. To increase flexibility, the muscles must be stretched beyond their normal range.

Health Goals for the Year 2000

- Increase the proportion of people who engage in activity to enhance muscular strength, muscular endurance, and flexibility.

Terms

- Detailed descriptions of important stretching and flexibility terms are presented in Concept 8.

The Facts

There is a correct way to perform stretching exercises.

Remember that stretching can *cause* muscle soreness, so "easy does it." Start below your threshold if you are unaccustomed to stretching a given muscle group, then work up to your target zone. The guidelines that follow will help you to gain the most benefit from your exercises.

- Warm the muscles *before you attempt to stretch them.*
- Exercises that do not cause a muscle to lengthen beyond normal may maintain, but will not increase, flexibility.
- To increase flexibility, the muscle must be overloaded (stretched beyond its normal length), but not to the point of pain. Remember, you want to stretch muscles, not joints!
- Exercises must be performed for each muscle group and at each joint where flexibility is desired.
- To protect adjacent joints, make certain the adjacent body parts are stabilized to prevent undesirable movement and are in good alignment to avoid strain.
- Stretch muscles of small joints in the extremities first, then progress toward the trunk with muscles of larger joints.
- Stretch muscles over joints one at a time before stretching at multiple joints simultaneously, for example, stretch muscles at the ankle, then the knee, then the ankle and knee simultaneously.
- If sport-specific ballistic stretching is used, precede it with static or PNF exercise.

- Avoid ballistic exercises on previously injured muscles or joints, especially the lower back muscles.
- Avoid *passive* ballistic stretches unless you are under the supervision of a registered or certified therapist or a trainer.
- If ballistic stretches are used, the bounces should be gentle and probably not exceed 10 percent of the normal static stretch range of motion. Avoid high-risk stretching exercises (see Concept 18).
- For static stretches, use the developmental stretch: stretch until you begin to feel pain, back off slightly and hold the position several seconds, then gradually try to stretch a little farther, back off, hold, etc. The stretch should feel slightly uncomfortable but should *not* be painful.
- For static stretches, increase the intensity of the stretch slowly, and also decrease it slowly after the hold.

There are certain areas of the body that especially need to be stretched for good health and fitness.

Areas of the body that are most likely to need stretching include:

- the muscles on the back of the legs (hamstrings) in order to prevent soreness, injury in sports, and referred back pain

- the muscles on the inside of the thigh in order to prevent back, leg, and foot strain.
- the calf muscles in order to prevent soreness and Achilles tendon injuries in jogging/running.
- the muscles on the front of the hip joint in order to prevent lordosis and backache
- the low back muscles in order to help prevent soreness and pain, as well as back injuries;
- the muscles on the front of the chest and shoulders in order to prevent rounded shoulders and limited range of movement in the shoulder joint.

The exercises pictured in this concept focus on these body areas.

Certain stretching exercises are good for therapeutic purposes, as well as for fitness.

Stretching exercises can be prescribed specifically to alleviate pain. Usually, the same exercise if done regularly can prevent the condition that originally caused the pain. Examples of therapeutic exercises include Exercise 1 (or some variation of it) to stretch the calf muscle. This will relieve muscle cramps in the lower leg. Exercise 6, Billig's exercise, can be used to relieve menstrual cramps (dysmenorrhea). The shin stretcher (Exercise 11) may relieve shin splints.

Sample Flexibility Exercises

These stretching exercises are intended primarily to develop flexibility. Exercises for different body parts are presented here. They include static and PNF type exercises. These exercises should be held for ten to sixty seconds. Muscles depicted in pink color are those primarily being stretched by the exercises.

1. Lower Leg Stretcher

Purpose

To stretch the calf muscles and Achilles tendon.

Position

Stand with the toes on a thick book or lower rung of a stall bar. Keep toes pointed straight ahead or slightly inward. Hold on to a support with the hands.

Movement

Rise up on toes (**contract**) as far as possible and hold for three seconds. **Relax** and lower heels to floor as far as possible; **hold.**

Note

Static stretch may alleviate spasms or cramps in calf muscles.

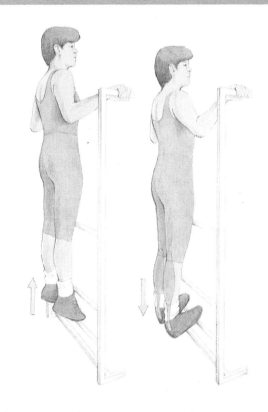

2. Sitting Stretcher

Purpose

To stretch muscles on inside of thighs.

Position

Sit with soles of feet together; place hands on knees or ankles and lean forearms against knees; resist (**contract**) by attempting to raise knees.

Movement

Hold three seconds; then **relax** and press the knees toward the floor as far as possible; **hold.**

Note

Useful for pregnant women and anyone whose thighs tend to rotate inward causing backache, knock-knees and flat feet.

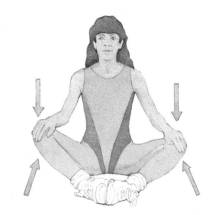

3. One-Leg Stretcher

Purpose

To stretch lower back and hamstring muscles.

Position

Stand with one foot on a bench, keeping both legs straight.

Movement

Contract hamstrings and gluteals by pressing down on bench with the heel for several seconds, then **relax** and bend the trunk forward, trying to touch the head to the knee. **Hold** for three seconds. Return to starting position and repeat with opposite leg. As flexibility improves, the arms can be used to pull the chest toward the legs. Do not allow either knee to lock.

Note

This is useful in relief of backache and correction of lordosis.

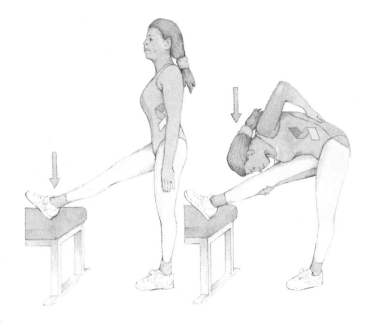

4. Leg Hug

Purpose

To stretch lower back and gluteals.

Position

Hook-lying position.

Movement

Contract gluteals and lumbar muscles. Lift hips. Hold for three seconds. **Relax** and pull knees to chest with arms as hard as possible; **hold.**

Note

Useful for backache and lordosis (also see Concept 17).

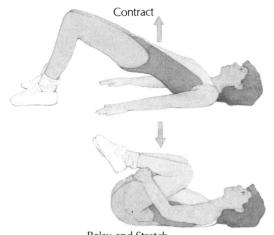

Contract

Relax and Stretch

5. Pectoral Stretch

Purpose

To stretch pectorals.

Position

Stand erect in doorway with arms raised 45°, elbows bent, and hands grasping doorjambs; feet in front stride position.

Movement

Press forward on door frame, **contracting** the arms maximally for three seconds. **Relax** and shift weight forward on legs so muscles on front of shoulder joint and chest are stretched; **hold.**
Repeat with arms raised 90°. Repeat with arms raised 135°.

Note

Useful to prevent or correct round shoulders and sunken chest.

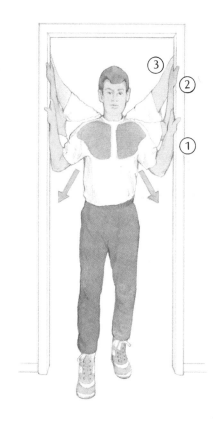

6. Billig's Exercise

Purpose

To stretch pelvic fascia, hip flexors, and inside of thigh.

Position

Stand with side to a wall and place the elbow and forearm against the wall at shoulder height. Tilt the pelvis backward, tightening the gluteal and abdominal muscles.

Movement

Place opposite hand on hip and push the hips toward the wall. Push forward and sideward (45°) with the hips. Do not twist the hips. **Hold.** Repeat on opposite side.

Note

Useful for preventing some cases of dysmenorrhea.

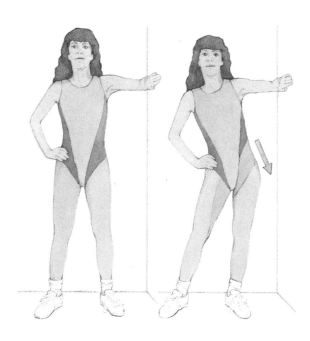

7. Lateral Trunk Stretcher

Purpose

To stretch trunk muscles.

Position

Sit on the floor.

Movement

Stretch left arm over head to right. Bend to right at waist, reaching as far to right as possible with left arm and as far as possible to the left with right arm; **hold.** Do not let trunk rotate. Repeat on opposite side. For less stretch, overhead arm may be bent at elbow.

Note

This exercise can be done in the standing position but is less effective.

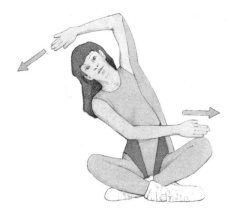

8. Hip and Thigh Stretcher

Purpose

To stretch iliopsoas and quadriceps.

Position

Place right knee directly above right ankle and **stretch** left leg backward so knee touches floor. If necessary, place hands on floor for balance.

Movement

Press pelvis forward and downward; **hold.** Repeat on opposite side. *Caution:* Do not bend front knee more than 90°.

Note

Useful for those who have lordosis or lower back problems.

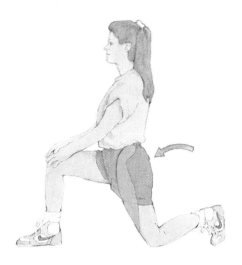

9. Arm Stretcher

Purpose

To stretch arm and chest muscles.

Position

Cross arms and turn palms of hands together. Raise arms overhead behind ears. Extend elbows.

Movement

Stretch as high as possible. **Hold.**

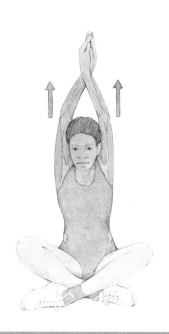

10. Shin Stretcher

Purpose

To relieve shin muscle soreness by stretching muscles on front of shin.

Position

Kneel on both knees, turn to right, and press down and **stretch** right ankle with right hand.

Movement

Move pelvis forward. **Hold.** Repeat on opposite side.

Note

Except when they are sore, most people need to strengthen rather than stretch these muscles.

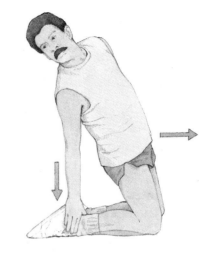

11. Hamstring Stretcher

Purpose

To stretch the muscles on the back of the hip, thigh, knee, and ankle.

Position

Start in a hook-lying position. Bring right knee to chest and grasp toes with right hand. Place left hand on back of right thigh.

Movement

(1) Pull knee toward chest; (2) push heel toward ceiling and pull toes toward shin; (3) attempt to straighten knee. Stretch and **hold.** Repeat on left side.

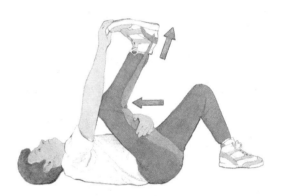

12. Trunk Twister

Purpose

To stretch the trunk muscles and muscles on the outside of hip.

Position

Sit with right leg extended, left leg bent and crossed over the right knee.

Movement

Place right arm on the left side of the left leg and push against that leg while turning the trunk as far as possible to the left; place left hand on floor behind buttocks. Stretch and **hold.** Reverse position and repeat on opposite side.

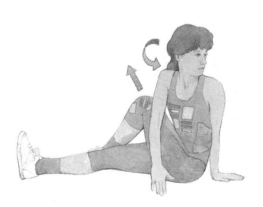

13. Rectus Femoris (Quadriceps) Stretch

Purpose

To stretch the rectus femoris (two-joint muscle on front of thigh).

Position

Sit in widest possible side-stride position. Lean to left on elbow and bend right knee 90°.

Movement

Place right hand on floor behind right calf and roll trunk backwards. Adjust until a pull is felt on the front of the right thigh, **not** on the inside of the right knee. **Hold.** Repeat on left leg.

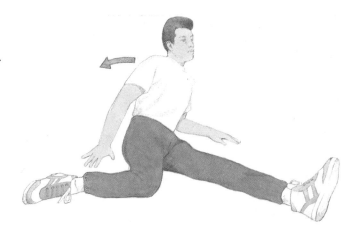

14. Lateral Thigh and Hip Stretch

Purpose

To stretch the iliotibial band and tensor fascia lata.

Position

Stand with left side to wall, left arm extended and palm of hand flat on wall for support. Cross left leg behind right and turn toes of both feet out slightly.

Movement

Bend left knee slightly and shift pelvis toward wall (left) as trunk bends toward right. Adjust until pull is felt down outside of left hip and thigh. **Hold.** Repeat on other side.

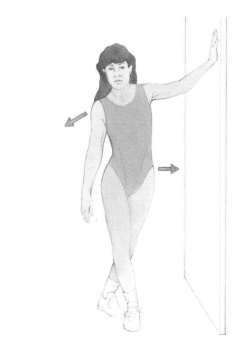

15. Arm Pretzel

Purpose

To stretch lateral rotators of the shoulder.

Position

Stand or sit with elbows flexed at right angles, palms up.

Movement

Cross right arm over left; grasp right thumb with left hand and pull gently downward, causing right arm to rotate laterally. Stretch and **hold.** Reverse arm position and repeat on left arm.

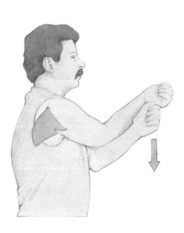

16. Spine Twist

Purpose

To stretch trunk rotators and lateral rotators of the thighs.

Position

Start in hook-lying position, arms extended at shoulder level.

Movement

Cross left knee over right; keep arms and shoulders on floor while touching knees to floor on left. Stretch and **hold.** Reverse leg position and lower knees to right.

17. Neck Rotation

Purpose

To stretch neck rotators.

See Exercise 5, p. 199.

18. Wand Exercise

Purpose

To stretch front of shoulder and chest.

See Exercise 2, p. 197.

19. Calf Stretcher

Purpose

To stretch the calf muscles and Achilles tendon.

See fig. 4.1, p. 37.

20. Back-saver Toe Touch

Purpose

To stretch the muscles on the back of the thigh (hamstrings).

See Exercise 6, p. 199.

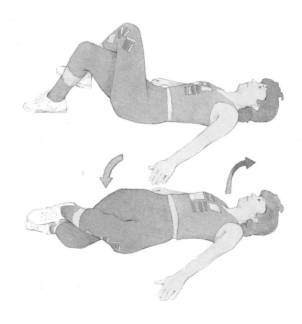

Purpose

To encourage flexibility and for fun and competition.

1. Two-Hand Ankle Wrap

Position

Stand with heels together.

Movement

Bend forward and place arms between knees; bend knees and wrap arms around legs, attempting to touch fingers in front of ankles. Hold ten seconds.

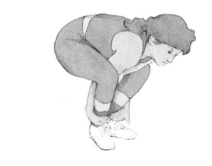

2. Wand Step-Through

Position

Stand; grasp wand with palms down, hands shoulder width apart.

Movement

(a) Bend forward and swing right leg around the outside of the right arm and over the wand (from front to back) into the "hole" made by the arms and wand. (b) Slide the wand around the back of the body by bringing the left arm over the head; then slide the wand under the hips and (c) step over the wand (from back to front) with the left foot, stepping out of the "hole."

Note

Arms finish in a palms-up position. Do not release the wand at any time.

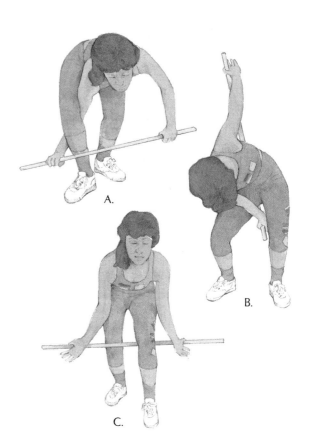

A.

B.

C.

3. Wring the Dishrag (with a partner)

Position

Partners stand facing each other, holding opposite hands.

Movement

Number one starts with the left leg and number two starts with the right leg. Each lifts the leg over the near arm and steps into the middle of the "hole" (formed by the arms); turn back to back while swinging the opposite arms overhead; step out of the hole with the opposite legs and end facing each other, hands still grasped.

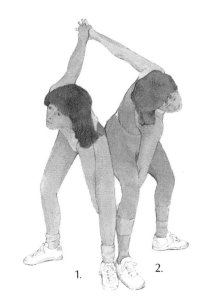

Sports-Specific Ballistic Stretches

Purpose

To aid one-handed throwing and striking skills (for example, racket sports forehand, backhand, and serve; baseball throw, or discus and shot put); and/or two-handed throwing or striking skills (for example, batting a softball or executing a golf drive or hammer throw).

1. Trunk Motions (with a partner):

Assume a position at the end of the backswing for any skill listed above. Partner grasps hand(s) and resists movement while the performer turns the trunk away from the partner, making a series of gentle bouncing movements, attempting to rotate the trunk as if performing the skill. Alternate roles with the partner.

Note

Avoid overstretching by too vigorous bouncing. If no partner is available, use a door frame for resistance or these sports actions can be practiced using elastic bands or inner tubes (attached to fixed objects) as resistance.

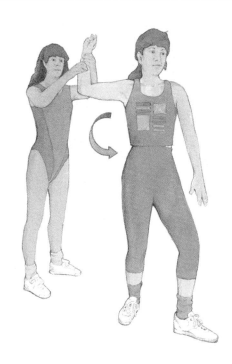

2. Arm and Trunk Motions

Stand and swing the racket, club, bat, or arm with or without a weight on the implement or on the wrist. Start by swinging backward and forward rhythmically and continuously. Gradually increase the speed and vigor of the swing to finally resemble the actual skill.

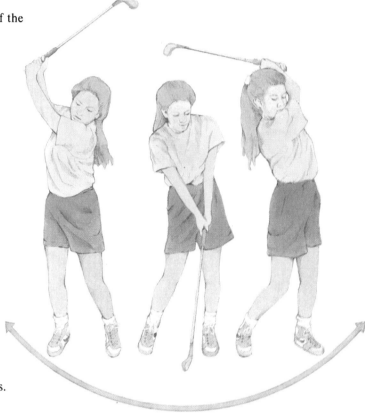

Note

If a weight is added, swing easily to avoid torn muscles.

Suggested Readings

Alter, M. J. *The Science of Stretching.* Champaign, Ill.: Human Kinetics Publishers, 1988.

Alter, M. J. *Sports Stretch.* Champaign, Ill.: Human Kinetics Publishers, 1990.

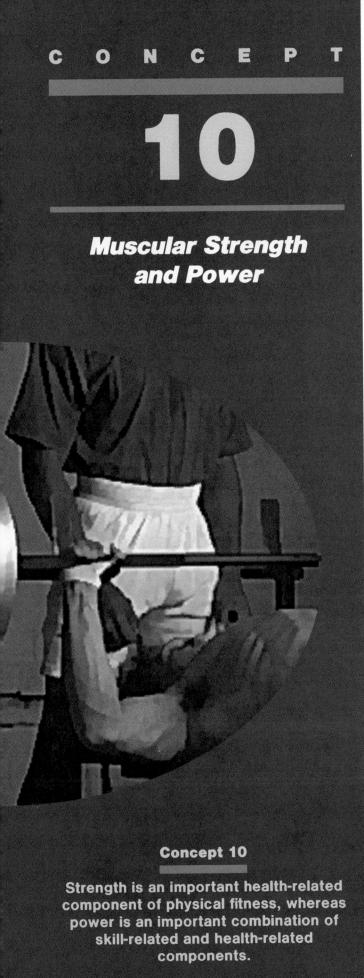

CONCEPT

10

Muscular Strength and Power

Concept 10

Strength is an important health-related component of physical fitness, whereas power is an important combination of skill-related and health-related components.

Introduction

Strength is measured by the amount of force you can produce with a single maximal effort. You need strength to increase work capacity; to decrease the chance of injury; to prevent low back pain, poor posture, and other hypokinetic diseases; to improve athletic performance; and perhaps to save life or property in an emergency. Strength training increases strength of bones, tendons, and ligaments, as well as muscles. It has been found to be therapeutic for patients with chronic pain.

Power training increases strength and endurance up to a point but is primarily useful in preparing you to perform activities that require power. Examples of activities requiring power are throwing, striking, and jumping skills in sports and dance or throwing heavy loads in farming and industry.

Health Goals for the Year 2000

- ▬ Increase the proportion of people who engage in activity to enhance muscular strength, muscular endurance, and flexibility.
- ▬ Reduce the proportion of male high school seniors who use anabolic steroids.

Terms

Absolute Strength

The maximum amount of force one can exert, e.g., maximum number of pounds or kilograms one can lift on one attempt. (See Relative Strength.)

Anabolic Steroid

A synthetic hormone similar to the male sex hormone testosterone. It functions androgenically to stimulate male characteristics and anabolically to increase muscle mass, weight, bone maturation, and virility.

Antagonistic Muscles

The muscles that have the opposite action from those that are contracting (agonists); normally, antagonists reflexly relax when agonists contract.

Concentric Contraction

An isotonic muscle contraction in which the muscle gets shorter as it contracts, such as when a joint is bent and two body parts move closer together. An example is the biceps muscle contraction that occurs when pulling up on a chinning bar.

"Definition" of Muscle

The detailed external appearance of a muscle.

Dynamic Contraction

A popular name for isotonic exercise.

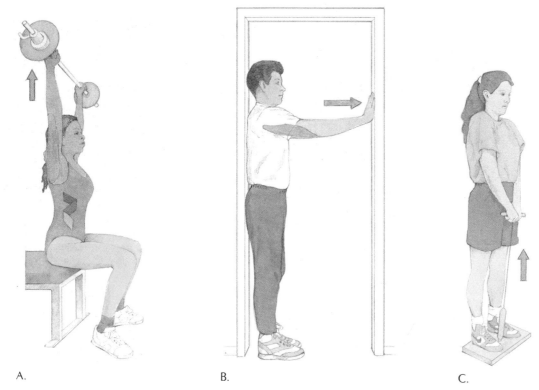

Figure 10.1

Examples of three strength exercises. (A) Isotonic, (B) isometric, (C) isokinetic.

Eccentric Contraction

"Negative exercise." An isotonic muscle contraction in which the muscle gets longer as it contracts; that is, when a weight is gradually lowered and the contracting muscle gets longer as it gives up tension. Lowering the body from a pullup on a chinning bar is an example of eccentric contraction of the biceps muscle.

Hypertrophy

Increase in the size of muscles as the result of strength training; increase in bulk.

Isokinetic

Isotonic concentric exercises done with a machine that regulates movement velocity and resistance (figure 10.1).

Isometric

A type of muscle contraction in which the muscle remains the same length. Isometric exercises are those in which no movement takes place while a force is exerted against an immovable object (also known as "static contraction") (figure 10.1).

Isotonic

Type of muscle contraction in which the muscle changes length, either shortening (concentrically) or lengthening (eccentrically). Isotonic exercises are those in which a resistance is raised and then lowered, as in weight training and calisthenics (also called "dynamic" or "phasic") (figure 10.1).

Plyometrics

An isometric or concentric isotonic muscle contraction performed after a prestretch or eccentric contraction of a muscle. A training technique used to develop explosive power. Referred to as "speed-strength training" in Eastern Europe and the Soviet Union, where it originated.

PRE

Progressive Resistance Exercise, such as those done with free weights or weight machines.

Relative Strength

Amount of force one can exert in relation to one's body weight or per unit of muscle cross-section; that is, if a 100-pound person lifts 250 pounds, he or she has lifted 2.5 pounds per pound of body weight, and thus has more relative strength than a

250-pound person who lifts 500 pounds, or 2 pounds per pound of body weight. The latter has more absolute strength.

RM (Repetitions Maximum)

The maximum amount of resistance one can move a given number of times; for example
1 RM = maximum weight lifted one time;
6 RM = maximum weight one can lift six times.

Sticking Point

The point in the range of motion where the weight cannot be lifted any farther without extreme effort or assistance; the weakest point in the movement.

The Basic Facts About Strength

There are three types of muscle tissue.

The three types of muscle tissue—smooth, cardiac, and skeletal—have different structures and functions. Smooth muscle tissue consists of long, spindle-shaped fibers; each fiber usually contains only one nucleus. The fibers are involuntary and are located in the walls of the esophagus, stomach, and intestines, where they function to move food and waste products through the digestive tract. Cardiac muscle tissue is also involuntary and, as its name implies, it is found only in the heart. Skeletal muscle tissues consist of long, cylindrical, multinucleated fibers. They provide the force needed to move the skeletal system and may be controlled voluntarily. Skeletal muscles are made up of slow- (red), intermediate-, and fast- (white) twitch fibers.

Some experts suggest that strength training using high resistance exercises tends to selectively develop fast-twitch muscle fibers.

Fast-twitch fibers generate greater tension than slow-twitch fibers, but they fatigue more quickly. They primarily use anaerobic metabolism. These fibers are particularly suited to fast, high-force activities such as explosive weight lifting movements, sprinting, and jumping.

An example of fast-twitch muscle fiber in animals is the white meat in the flying muscles of a chicken. The chicken is heavy and must exert a powerful force to fly a few feet up to a perch. A wild duck that flies for hundreds of miles has dark meat (slow-twitch fibers) in the flying muscles for better endurance.

The amount of force you can exert during a strength test depends upon the speed of contraction, muscle length, warm-up, and other muscle-related factors.

If you want to score high on a strength test, consider some of the secrets of success used by experienced lifters and proven by research. Generally, a muscle exerts the least

force as it becomes shorter (toward the end of a movement), and can exert more force during an isometric contraction than when it is shortening. The muscle exerts the most force when it is lengthening (lowering a weight). If a muscle is placed on a slight stretch immediately before it contracts, it can exert more force than it could if it started from a resting length.

Speed of contraction affects the amount of force that can be exerted. A slow contraction can lift a heavier weight than a fast contraction. If muscles are warmed up before lifting, more force can be exerted and heavier loads can be lifted.

Strength capacity differs with gender and age.

Women have less muscle mass than men and typically average 60 percent to 85 percent of the "absolute strength" of men. Women are as strong as men, however, in "relative strength." Maximum strength is usually reached in the twenties and declines with age. Regardless of age or gender, strength can be improved.

The Facts: Principles of Training

Strength is best developed by applying the "overload principle" so that exercise is done with a near maximum resistance with only a few repetitions.

In order to increase strength, the muscle must be contracted to at least 60 percent of its maximum. Strength training requires an overload in the amount of the resistance, while muscular endurance training (see Concept 11) requires an overload in the number of repetitions. Therefore, according to the law of specificity, when designing a program for strength development, high resistance and low repetitions at a moderately slow speed should be used for maximum effectiveness.

When you begin strength training, there will be marked improvements during the first couple of weeks. This is primarily due to motor learning factors rather than to muscle growth. Thereafter, improvements will be slow and the changes will be the result of hypertrophy of the muscle.

There is a threshold of training and a target zone for muscular strength development.

Experts generally agree that in **progressive resistance exercise (PRE)** using a maximum load (resistance) for three to eight repetitions in one to three sets three or four times per week will develop strength. Experts do *not* agree, however, on the ideal combination of repetitions, sets, and speed.

Table 10.1

Strength Threshold of Training and Fitness Target Zones for Beginners

	Threshold of Training			Target Zone		
	Isometrics	**Isotonics**	**Isokinetics**	**Isometrics**	**Isotonics**	**Isokinetics**
Frequency	• 2 days a week for each muscle group.			• Every other day for each muscle group.		
Intensity	• Use 65%–70% of maximum contraction (1 RM).	• Maximum resistance for every rep.	• 90% of 1 RM at set speed.	• Maximum contractions.	• Maximum resistance (for number of reps) on every set.	• Maximum effort at set speed.
Time	• 1 set; • 1 rep. held for 2–5 sec.; • Repeat once a day.	• 1 set; • 3–8 reps.	• 2 sets; • 3 reps lasting 3–4 sec. (30°–60° per sec.); • Rest 1 min. between sets.	• 1 set; • 6 rep., held 6–8 sec. (or 2 sets of 3 reps each); • Rest 30 sec. between reps.	• 3 sets; • 3–8 reps; • Rest 1 min. between sets.	• 3–5 sets; • 3–8 reps lasting 1–2 sec. (70°– 120° per sec.); • Rest 1 min. between sets.

Table 10.1 compares thresholds and target zones of **isometrics, isotonics,** and **isokinetics** that might be used by beginners who desire to improve pure strength. Note, however, if you are training for a specific skill these target zones may not be appropriate (refer to the following fact regarding the principle of specificity). If you are an advanced strength trainer, a body builder, or a competitive weight lifter, you will need special training programs to excel at these activities.

If the target zone is exceeded, an "overload syndrome" may result.

If the frequency, intensity, or time of your training program exceeds the optimum and you try to progress too fast, inflammatory changes in the muscles, tendons, or joints may occur. The ability of muscles to contract may decrease or loss of lean tissue may occur, so improvement stops and strength is actually lost.

Periodization of the athlete's training may help prevent "overtraining" or the "overload syndrome."

When an athlete trains for a single performance or perhaps several competitive events such as games or matches during a sport season, it requires careful planning to reach peak performance at the right time and to avoid overtraining and injuries. Periodization is a modern concept of manipulating repetition, resistance, and exercise selection so there are "peaks" and "valleys" (tapering-off) that are associated with the sports schedule. Training normally begins with high repetitions and low resistance. The resistance is gradually increased and the repetitions are decreased as each climax approaches (Stone 1990).

A strength training program should apply the "principle of specificity" by closely resembling the activity for which the strength is needed.

Specificity of training will enhance performance. If you want your arms to be stronger so you can *carry* heavy loads, or if you want finger strength to *grip* a heavy bowling ball, much of your strength exercise should be done isometrically, using the arm muscles the way you use them to carry loads or using the fingers the same way you hold a bowling ball. On the other hand, if the task for which you are training is performed *isotonically,* your strength program should be primarily isotonic use of the muscles involved in that skill.

If you are training for a particular skill that requires *explosive power,* such as in throwing, striking, kicking, or jumping, your strength exercises should be done with less resistance and greater speed. If you are training for a skill that uses both **concentric** and **eccentric contractions** or is **plyometric,** you should perform strength exercises using these characteristics.

If you are not training for a specific skill, but merely wish to develop pure strength, then consider the advantages and disadvantages of isometrics, isotonics, and isokinetics listed in table 10.2. You may wish to use a variety of methods to avoid boredom.

Training for cardiovascular endurance at the same time as strength training may prevent maximum results in both.

Studies have shown that simultaneously training for strength and cardiovascular endurance may not produce the same result as one could obtain while training for either one separately. Some people have interpreted this to mean

Table 10.2

Advantages and Disadvantages of Isometric, Isotonic, and Isokinetic Resistance Exercises*

	Isometrics (Statics)	Isotonics (Dynamics)	Isokinetics
In small space	E	F-G	F-G
No equipment or low-cost equipment	E	F-G	F-G
Provides feedback for motivation	P	E	F
Can rehabilitate immobilized joint	E	P	P
Builds strength through full range of motion	P	F-G	E
Less apt to cause soreness	E	F-G	E
Aids dynamic coordination	P	E	G
Safe for hypertensive	P	E	G-E
Amount of strength developed	F	E	E
Dynamic exercises and controlled testing	P	F-G	E
Hypertrophy	P	E	E
Power development	P	G	E
Rapid improvement in strength	E	F-G	F-G
Can accelerate to resemble sport skill	P	E	P

*Key: E = Excellent; G = Good; F = Fair; P = Poor

that they interfere with each other. The cause of this is not clear. It may be that the time spent on each one is less or that overtraining occurs rather than the fact that one inhibits the other. Whatever the cause, the differences are relatively minor and it should not prevent an individual from doing both concurrently.

Strength developed in one limb can be transferred to another unexercised limb.

When the right arm is trained with biceps curls until its strength increases, the unexercised left arm will also increase in strength, though not as much as the exercised arm. This phenomenon is called "transfer of training," "bilateral transfer," or "cross-education." The reason for this is not fully understood, but the phenomenon is sometimes applied to rehabilitation to prevent a limb from atrophying.

Progressive resistance exercise (PRE) is the most effective type of strength training program.

Muscles adapt only to the load placed upon them; therefore, in order to continue increasing strength, you must progressively increase the stress on the muscle as it adapts to each new load. Muscle groups differ in their strength potential, so each muscle group must have an individualized program (target zone). For example, the legs and trunk can usually lift greater loads than the arms.

The "double progressive system" is an effective variation of the PRE system.

The double progressive system of progression periodically adjusts both the resistance and the number of repetitions. For example, you may begin with three repetitions for the arms. Once a week, you add one repetition. When you have progressed to eight repetitions, increase the arm weight by five pounds. Decrease the repetitions to three and begin the progression again.

Facts About Types of Resistance Training

There are several good PRE programs for strength development, each having advantages and disadvantages.

Progressive resistance exercise can be performed in properly designed weight-training programs using free weights, constant resistance machines, variable (accommodating) resistance machines, isometrics, pulleys, calisthenics, springs, latex tubing, or isokinetic dynamometers. Machines may offer resistance by weight stacks, hydraulic or pneumatic pressure, or electrical resistance. Concept 12 describes some sample exercises and compares some of these programs. Weight training is considered the fastest and best method of improving strength. However, properly designed calisthenics are adequate for developing strength in most people.

The most popular form of strength exercise utilizes isotonic contractions of the muscles.

Isotonic (also called **dynamic**) exercise refers to such activities as weight training, calisthenics, and pulley weights, in which the muscles alternately shorten concentrically and lengthen eccentrically. Typically, the stress on the muscle in these types of exercises varies with speed, joint position, and muscle length. Thus, the muscle may work harder at the beginning of a lift than it does near the end of the range of motion or as the weight is lowered.

Isokinetics, plyometrics, and "negative" exercises are special forms of isotonic exercise. These are discussed later in this concept.

"Negative" exercise has no advantage over other types of exercise for strength development.

Contrary to the claims of some enthusiasts, there does not seem to be any difference between eccentric (negative) exercise and concentric (positive) exercise (see definitions) in terms of their effectiveness in developing strength. Eccentric exercise is performed more comfortably even though more weight can be handled. It is particularly useful in rehabilitation settings, but has a tendency to cause more muscle soreness. This type of exercise also requires the assistance of another person or the use of a special machine such as the Kin Com Biodex or Keiser dynamometers.

Eccentric contractions are combined with concentric contractions in most everyday activities and sports skills utilizing strength. For example, if you lift something you also lower it. Thus, to apply the law of specificity, some of the strength training for those activities should include both types of contractions.

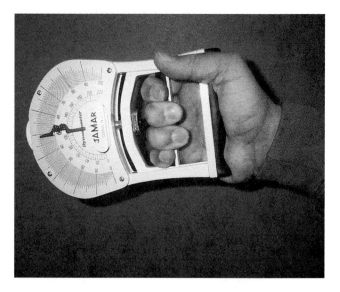

Isometric strength can be measured using a dynamometer.

Isometric strength exercises have advantages and disadvantages.

You can exert 15 percent to 20 percent more force with an isometric contraction than with a concentric one. Isometric exercises are effective for developing strength, require no equipment and only minimal space. They have been found to be quite useful for some athletes, such as wrestlers and gymnasts, and work especially well for people in the early stages of some rehabilitation programs. Research has shown that isotonic training can be enhanced significantly by using isometrics at the **sticking points** during isotonic lifts.

However, isometric exercises do not develop as much strength as isotonic and isokinetic exercises, nor do muscles hypertrophy as much. They work the muscle only at the angle of the joint used in the exercise. Isometrics may be dangerous for those with high blood pressure or cardiovascular disease. (See table 10.2 for a comparison with other types of exercise.)

Isokinetic exercises are effective for developing strength.

Isokinetic exercises are isotonic-concentric muscle contractions performed on devices such as the Apollo, Exer-Genie, Mini-Gym, Hydra-Fitness (hydraulic machine) or on electromechanical dynamometers, such as the Cybex II. These machines keep the velocity of the movement constant and match their resistance to the effort of the performer, permitting maximal tension to be exerted throughout the range of motion. For example, on the Cybex II, speeds may be preset from 0 to 300 degrees per second. This rate-limiting mechanism prevents the performer from moving faster no matter how much force is exerted.

Thus, isokinetic devices attempt to overcome the basic weakness of isotonics. On the other hand, these devices do not permit acceleration, so it is not possible to train specifically for sports skills, such as throwing or kicking, in which the limb is accelerated while applying maximum force and some of these devices permit only concentric contractions.

Isokinetic exercise has the advantage of being safer than most other forms of exercise and may be better for developing power (see Concept 11). It is not better for developing pure strength, however. More research is needed to determine the best training regimen for isokinetic exercise.

Variable resistance machines have some advantages over constant resistance machines and free weights.

Some machines, such as Nautilus and Universal, offer what is called "variable" or "accommodating resistance." The Nautilus, for example, uses a cam to adapt the resistance as the performer moves through the range of motion. The Universal Trainer uses a rolling pivot to do the same thing. These adaptations attempt to compensate for the weakness in isotonic constant resistance exercises, but they are only partially successful in adapting to the shape, sizes, and torque of individual human bodies. There is no evidence that variable resistance machines develop more strength than other devices, although they may strengthen a muscle through more of its range.

Free weights have some advantages and some disadvantages when compared to other methods of strength development.

Free weights include barbells and dumbbells, as well as homemade weights, such as sandbags or bottles filled with water. These are compared with weight machines (for example, Nautilus, Universal, Marcy, Hydra-Gym, Dynacam, and Paramount) in table 10.3. Both free weights and weight-stack machines are compared with other resistance machines in table 10.4.

Facts About Advanced Strength Training

Resistance training may be used as a competitive sport or as a recreational sport and as a means to improve fitness, especially muscular strength, endurance, and power.

There are three competitive sports associated with resistance training. Olympic weight lifting competitors use free weights and compete in two exercises: the snatch, and the

Table 10.3

Advantages and Disadvantages of Free Weights and Weight Machines

Free Weights	Weight Machines
• Requires balance and coordination; uses more muscles for stabilization.	• Other body parts are stabilized; easier to isolate particular muscle group.
• Truer to real-life situation, so skills transfer to daily life.	• Controlled path of weight not true to life.
• Creates more possibility of injury.	• Safer because weight cannot fall on participant.
• Requires spotters for safety.	• No spotters required.
• Takes more time to change weights.	• Easy and quick to change weights.
• Unlimited number of exercises possible.	• Restricted to range and angle of movement permitted by the machine.
• Less expensive.	• Expensive; need to go to club if cannot afford equipment; need more than one machine for variety.
• Loose equipment clutters area and may get lost or stolen.	• Machines are stationary but occupy large space.

clean and jerk. Power lifting competitors use free weights and compete in three lifts: the bench press, squat, and dead lift. Body building competitors use several forms of resistance training, and are judged on muscular hypertrophy and **definition of muscle.**

Advanced "lifters" use heavier resistance than most people during strength training; therefore, they use some techniques not recommended for the beginner.

The compressive force on the lumbar disks during a half-squat can be six to ten times the body weight. To reduce the spinal compression, prevent abdominal hernias, and aid in lifting more weight, advanced lifters are encouraged to use a belt with a rigid abdominal pad and a wide band across the lumbar spine. At the same time, they hold their breath until they get past the "sticking point" of a lift. The belt must be loosened between reps to breathe and to allow the blood to return to the heart. (Lander, et al. 1990). Holding the breath permits "trunk cavity pressurization" to relieve the load on the spine while the belt helps hold the abdominal contents in. Advanced lifting requires advanced training in proper techniques to avoid

Table 10.4
Comparison of Selected Resistance Training Devices*

	Free Weights	Weight-stack Machine	Compressed Air Machine	Hydraulic Machine	Isokinetic Machine
Concentric resistance	+	+	+	+	+
Eccentric resistance	+	+	+	−	+ −
Isometric resistance	+	+	+	+	−
Match resistance to effort through range of motion	−	+ −	+	+	+
Isolation of all major muscle groups	−	+ −	+	+	+
Safety features	−	+	+	+	+
Durability	+	+	+	+	+

From W. L. Wescott, "Strength Training" in *Sportcare & Fitness Magazine*, July/August 1988, p. 62. Copyright © 1988 Sportcare & Fitness, Wilmington, DE.

injury. Beginners should not attempt these lifts or hold the breath, but they may wish to use the belts if they have a history of back problems.

Training for bulk and "definition" may differ from strength training.

Most body builders use three to seven sets of ten to fifteen repetitions, rather than the three sets of three to eight repetitions recommended for most weight trainers. Body builders are more interested in **hypertrophy** (large muscles) than in strength. Sometimes, "definition" is difficult to obtain because it is obscured by fat. It should be noted that those with the largest looking muscles are not always the strongest.

Is There Strength in a Bottle?: The Facts

Taking anabolic steroids (A.S.) is not a safe and effective way for normal, healthy people to develop fitness.

Anabolic steroids are prescription drugs—a synthetic reproduction of the male hormone testosterone. Physicians use them to treat such conditions as muscle diseases, breast cancer, severe burns, rare types of anemia, and kidney disease. Because of their dangerous side effects, doctors use them in minimal doses. They are obtained on the black market or from unethical physicians, coaches, or trainers by some body builders, athletes, and an increasing number of nonathletes to enhance their strength or improve their

physique or appearance. Two million people are estimated to be using "roids." Steroids may be taken orally or injected. Usually they are taken in massive doses 20–100 times the normal therapeutic dose used for medical conditions. When combined with a resistance training program, they have been found to increase strength and muscle mass, but their adverse side effects far outweigh any benefits. In women, unlike men, some of these effects are irreversible (see table 10.5). As can be seen in the table, steroids (like all drugs) are dangerous. They can be addictive and produce more than seventy serious side effects, some of which may be fatal. Unfortunately, some studies show that many athletes who use anabolic steroids are familiar with the adverse effects, but say, "I don't care, I will use them anyway."

Injuries happen more easily and last longer in people who use steroids.

Even though steroids make muscles stronger, tendons and ligaments do not increase in strength proportionately. Therefore a strong muscle contraction can tear a tendon and/or a ligament. This is made more serious because steroids make the injury heal more slowly. When steroids increase muscle size, the extra muscle can grow around the bones and joints, causing them to break more easily (P. G. Peterson 1990).

The use of anabolic steroids can cause people to die.

The violent behavior sometimes seen in users often referred to as "roid rage" had led to the serious injury and death of other people. Many users have died from hepatitis or HIV/AIDS infections from shared needles, and

Table 10.5

Adverse Effects of Anabolic Steroids

Gender	Physical	Psychological
M/F	• Cancer of liver, testicles, or prostate	• Total personality changes
M/F	• Cardiac disease/early heart attacks	• Hostile and aggressive; violent behavior; sexual crimes
M/F	• Hypertension and increased risk of strokes	• Addiction (both psychological and physiological) to A.S.
M/S	• Edema (puffy face)	
M/F	• Scalp hair loss** (baldness in men)	• Inability to accept failure
M/F	• Nosebleeds	• Sleep disturbance (when cycled off drug)
M/F	• Premature closure of growth plates of long bones	• Depression
M/F	• Immune system may be suppressed	• Apathy
M/F	• Decreased HDL	• Wide mood swings
M/F	• Decreased aerobic capacity	• "Reverse anorexia" (eating compulsion)
M/F	• Altered glucose tolerance	
M/F	• Severe acne (face, chest, upper back and thighs)*	
M/F	• Oily skin*	
M/F	• Muscle or bone injuries	
M/F	• Injuries take longer to heal	
M/F	• Fever	
M/F	• Frequent headaches	
M/F	• Sterility	
M/F	• Death	
M	• Testicular atrophy	
M	• Prostate enlargement	
F	• Uterine atrophy	
M	• Decreased sperm count	
M	• Impotence	
M	• Feminine breast characteristics	
F	• Decreased breast size	
F	• Menstrual irregularities	
F	• Clitoral enlargement	
F	• Deepening voice**	
F	• Dark facial hair**	

Key: M = males; F = females

  * = In women, only partially reversible when drug is stopped

** = In women, irreversible when drug is stopped

others have died from the cancers and heart disease directly attributable to the use of steroids. Twenty-five Soviet athletes who competed in the 1980 Olympics died because of conditions attributed to steroid use, and the deaths of several American professional athletes have also been attributed to anabolic steroid use. Lyle Alzado's highly publicized death was one of those.

Human growth hormone (HGH) taken to increase strength may be even more dangerous than taking anabolic steroids.

HGH is produced by the pituitary gland but is made synthetically. Some athletes are taking it in addition to anabolic steroids or in place of anabolic steroids because it is difficult to detect in urine tests of competitors. It is believed to increase muscle mass and bone growth and hasten healing of tendons and cartilage; however, its adverse effects can be deforming and life threatening. They include the danger of irreversible acromegaly (gigantism) and gross deformities, cardiovascular disease, goiter, menstrual disorder, excessive sweating, lax muscles and ligaments, premature bone closure, decreased sexual desire, and impotence. In addition, the life span can be shortened by as much as twenty years.

Another hormone being used by some male athletes is human chorionic gonadotrophin (hCG), a substance found in the urine of pregnant women. It is being used to stimulate testosterone production before competition. The International Olympic Committee (IOC) has banned its use, but no test has been developed to detect it.

Some athletes have turned to dietary supplements and glandulars, which have been promoted as "safe substitutes" for anabolic steroids.

In an effort to avoid the undesirable side effects of anabolic steroids or the detection of its use by sports governing bodies who have banned it, some athletes or body builders are taking chemicals and supplements such as boron, chromium picolinate, gamma oryzanol and L-carnitine (see Concept 23). There is also a considerable market for "glandulars" such as ground-up bull testes, hypothalamus and pituitary glands, hearts, livers, spleens, and brains. These products have been advertised as "steroid alternatives." Dietitians, the F.D.A., and the National Council Against Health Fraud are alarmed at this practice and consider it potentially dangerous because these products have not been tested on humans or animals for safety and effectiveness. Very little is known about some of them. No research has been published to substantiate any claims for improved performance. A recent publication in *The Journal of the American Medical Association* cautions people concerning the use of "body building" supplements (Philen, et al. 1992).

The Facts About Proper Resistance Training Technique

There is a proper way to perform resistance training.

The following are some guidelines for safe and effective strength training for beginners.

- Make sure you are well prepared to begin. (See Concept 4 for details.)
- When beginning a weight program, start with weights that are too light so you can learn proper technique and avoid soreness and injury. Novices might, for example, start with one-fourth of their body weight for the military press; ten pounds less than the press for the curl; ten pounds more than the press for the bench press; and half of the body weight for back and leg exercises.
- Progress gradually. For example, use one set of three repetitions with a light weight to begin; add two repetitions when it gets easy, then another, until you reach eight repetitions; then drop back to three repetitions and add a second set. Repeat until you can do three sets. After this, the double progressive system (previously described) can be used, increasing the weight and the repetitions.
- Beginning weight trainers should probably train for endurance initially (see Concept 11). For example, a reasonable goal might be ten to fifteen repetitions at 50 percent to 70 percent of the maximum amount of weight they can lift for one repetition.
- Beginners should not attempt to use advanced techniques. After training for several months, you may wish to experiment with such things as supersets, split routines, and plateau systems used by advanced trainers.
- To ensure overall development, include all body parts and balance the strength of **antagonistic muscles.** For example, the ratio of quadriceps strength to hamstring strength should be 60:40. Exercise large muscles before small muscles.
- Athletes should train muscles the way they will be used in their skill, employing similar patterns, range of motion, and speed (the principle of specificity). This applies to anyone who knows the precise skill for which he or she is training.
- If you wish to develop a particular group of muscles, it is important to remember that it can be worked harder when it is *isolated* than when it is worked in combination with other muscle groups.

- Sports participants should include some eccentric training, such as plyometrics, to prevent injury to decelerating muscles during sports events and to develop power in accelerating muscles. Choose an exercise sequence that alternates muscle groups so muscles have a rest period before being used in another exercise.
- Make all movements through the full range of motion.
- Isometric training should be done at several joint angles.
- To avoid boredom, especially when you reach a plateau or sticking point, use such motivating techniques as music, record keeping, partners, competition, and variation in routine.
- To avoid overtraining, take a break by resting or choosing some other activity after eight to ten weeks. Also, try varying your training days so one is light (75 percent to 80 percent), one is medium (85 percent to 90 percent), and one is heavy (100 percent). It has been estimated that motivation can account for 10 percent to 15 percent of the score on a strength test. Varying the routine helps motivation.
- Lifters may reduce spinal and abdominal injury by using a belt which supports the back and abdomen.
- Unilateral training allows a muscle to exert more force than is possible when both sides of the body work simultaneously (bilaterally).

Most injuries can be prevented by using correct technique and proper care.

Refer to table 10.6 for some tips on injury prevention for the beginner.

The Facts: Common Misconceptions

There are many fallacies, myths, and superstitions associated with strength training.

Some common misconceptions about strength training have been refuted.

- It is *not* true that you will become musclebound and lose flexibility just because you do strength training. This could happen only if you train improperly. It has been found, however, that power lifters are less flexible than other weight lifters.

Table 10.6
How to Prevent Injury (for the Beginner)

- Warm up ten minutes before the workout and stay warm during the workout.
- Do not hold your breath while lifting. This may cause blackout or hernia.
- Avoid hyperventilation before lifting a weight.
- Avoid dangerous or high-risk exercises.
- Progress slowly.
- Use good shoes with good traction.
- Avoid arching your back. Keep the pelvis in normal alignment.
- Keep the weight close to the body.
- Do not lift from a stoop (bent-over with back rounded).
- Do not let the hips come up before your upper body when lifting from the floor.
- For bent-over rowing, put the head on a table and bend the knees or use one-arm rowing and support trunk with free hand.
- Stay in a squat as short a time as possible and do not do a full squat.
- Be sure collars are tight on free weights.
- Use a moderately slow, continuous, controlled movement and hold the final position a few seconds.
- Overload but don't overwhelm! A program that is too intense can cause injuries.
- Do not pause between repetitions.
- Try to keep a definite rhythm.
- Do not allow the weights to drop or bang.
- Do not train without medical supervision if you have a hernia, high blood pressure, fever, infection, recent surgery, heart disease or back problems.
- Use chalk or a towel to keep hands dry when handling weights.

- It is *not* true that women will become *masculine looking* if they develop strength. Contrary to popular belief, most women will not be able to develop as large and bulky muscles as men, nor will their muscles be as well defined. On a heavy resistance training program, women and men make about the same percentage change in strength and hypertrophy. The greater percentage of fat in most women prevents the muscle definition possible in men and camouflages the increase in bulk. (Until CAT scans were used in research studies, it was not evident that women achieved hypertrophy at the same rate as men.)

- Strength training does *not* make you move more slowly or make you more uncoordinated. Up to a point, increased strength may help to increase speed.
- The expression "*no pain, no gain*" is a fallacy. It may be helpful to strive for a burning sensation in the muscle, but this is not painful. If it hurts, you are probably harming yourself.
- Food supplements are not ergogenic aids and do *not* benefit muscle mass or strength building. You do need a balanced diet, however.
- Drugs do not make you fit. Anabolic steroids, growth hormones, diuretics, narcotics, and other drugs taken to enhance performance are extremely dangerous and ultimately produce an unhealthy person rather than a fit one.
- Strength training is *not* effective for cardiovascular fitness, flexibility, or weight loss. Muscles will get firmer, and desirable changes may occur in girth, but other aspects of fitness are specific and require specific training.
- It does *not* require two hours to complete a workout in weight training—unless you are a competitive lifter or body builder. If you are training for athletics, you will need forty-five to ninety minutes; the beginner or the person training for fitness or recreation can complete a circuit in thirty to forty-five minutes.

Facts About Power

Power is a combination of strength and speed, and is both health-related and skill-related.

Most experts classify power as a skill-related component of fitness (see Concept 2) because it is partially dependent on speed. On the other hand, power is also dependent on strength and can be classified as a health-related component to the extent that strength is involved. Thus, power falls somewhere in between the two distinct groups of fitness attributes. Certainly its use is not limited to sports and dance. We use power extensively in our daily activities every time we apply a force to move something quickly. Power is important in protective movements, such as a pedestrian jumping to dodge a car or a driver jerking the steering wheel to avoid a collision or jamming on the brakes to stop in an emergency. A worker heaves a heavy load from a truck to a dock, and a carpenter uses force to hammer a nail.

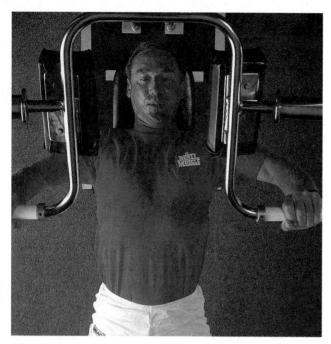
"No pain, no gain" is an exercise myth.

Power is usually neglected in fitness literature and often in fitness programs as well. Garnica (1986) called it the "most functional mode in which all human motion occurs." If this is true, all fitness programs should consider appropriate exercises that develop power.

The stronger person is not necessarily the more powerful.

Power is the amount of work per unit of time. To increase power, you must do more work in the same time or the same work in less time. If you extend your knee and move a 100-pound weight through a 90-degree arc in one second, you have twice as much power as a person who needs two seconds to complete the same movement. Power requires both strength and speed. Increasing one without the other limits power. Some "power athletes" (for example, football players) might benefit more by trying for less strength and more speed.

There is probably no one best training program for developing power, but the law of specificity applies.

If you need power for an activity in which you are required to move heavy weights, then you need to develop *strength-related power* by working against heavy resis-

tance at slower speeds. (See figure 10.2.) If you need to move light objects at great speed, such as in throwing a ball, you need to develop *speed-related power* by training at high speeds with relatively low resistance. There must be trade-offs between speed and power because the heavier the resistance, the slower the movement.

There is a target zone for optimum power.

Studies show that power is best developed when the force is between 30 and 60 percent of maximum. But the optimum is probably when the load and the speed are about one-third of maximum. (See figure 10.2.) Stamford (1985) uses the following illustration of the relationship between speed, strength, and power. If your maximum strength is represented by 2 and maximum speed by 2, then your power is $2 \times 2 = 4$. If you double your strength ($4 \times 2 = 8$), your power would be doubled. However, if your strength and speed were increased by only 50 percent, then even more power results ($3 \times 3 = 9$).

There are several effective techniques for developing power.

For specificity of training, as mentioned previously, much of an athlete's program should closely resemble the activity for which he or she is training, using similar speed, force, angle, range of motion, and so forth. However, if one is striving for all-round fitness or if an athlete is unable to perform the specific skill because of weather or injury or is seeking variety, then plyometrics, isokinetics, and weight training (especially with free weights or pulleys if simulating a sport skill) are effective means of developing power.

Plyometrics may be useful in athletic training for certain sports events requiring power.

A quick prestretch, or eccentric contraction of a muscle, immediately followed by an isometric or concentric contraction can produce more power. This has been called "preexertion countermovement," "wind up," or "plyometrics." Soviet Olympic coaches pioneered this area, developing drills for their athletes. Track and field athletes may, for example, perform a hopping drill for thirty to one hundred meters. This is called "depth jumping," "drop jumping," or "bounce loading." As the body lands, some of the major leg muscles lengthen in an eccentric contraction, then follow immediately with a strong concentric

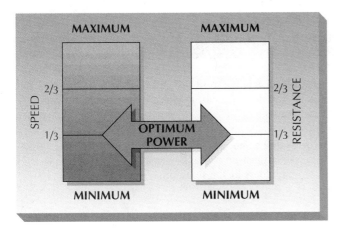

Figure 10.2
Optimum power is produced when the load and speed are each about one-third of maximum.

Table 10.7
Safety Guidelines for Plyometrics

- Adolescents whose bones are still growing should be limited to low-impact exercise (to avoid permanent growth-stunting damage to the growth plates).
- Progression should be gradual to avoid extreme muscle soreness.
- Adequate strength should be developed prior to plyometric training. (As a general rule, you should be able to do a "squat" with one and a half times your body weight.)
- Get a physician's approval prior to doing plyometrics if you have a history of injuries or if you are recovering from injury to the body part being trained.
- The landing surface should be semi-resilient, dry, and unobstructed.
- Shoes should have good lateral stability, be cushioned with an arch support, and have a nonslip sole.
- Obstacles used for jumping-over should be padded.
- The training should be preceded by a general and specific warm-up.
- The training sequence should:
  a. precede all other workouts (while you are fresh);
  b. include at least one spotter;
  c. be done no more than twice per week, with 48 hours rest between bouts;
  d. last about 30 minutes; and
  e. (for beginners) include 3 or 4 drills, with 2 or 3 sets per drill, 10–15 reps per set and 1–2 minutes rest between sets.

Source: Data from G. Brittenham, "Plyometric Exercise: A Word of Caution" in *Journal of Physical Education, Recreation, and Dance*, January 1992: 20–23. Reston, VA: American Alliance for Health, Physical Education, Recreation, and Dance.

contraction as the legs push off for the next jump or stride. The prestretch of the muscle during landing adds an elastic recoil that provides extra force to the push-off.

Plyometrics are used to apply the specificity principle to training for certain skills. Because eccentric exercise tends to result in more muscular soreness, it would be wise to proceed slowly with this type of training. It would also be important to have good flexibility before beginning a plyometrics program. Some guidelines are listed in table 10.7.

Power exercises can increase muscular endurance or strength.

Power exercises done at high speeds have been shown to increase muscular endurance. Likewise, power exercises that use heavy resistance at lower speeds will increase strength.

The principle of specificity should be applied to training programs for power events.

Athletes who need explosive power to perform their events should use training that closely resembles the event. Jumpers, for example, should jump as a part of their training programs in order to learn correct timing at the same time they are developing power. This also applies to Olympic weight lifters, shot-putters, jumpers, ballet dancers, and others. These athletes need both strength and endurance; however, studies show that too much of either

can have a negative effect on performance. If they use machines, it is better to use the leg press than a knee extension machine because the press more nearly resembles the leg action of the jump.

Suggested Readings

Philen, R., et al. "Survey of Advertising for Nutritional Supplements in Health and Body Building Magazines." *Journal of the American Medical Association* 268 (1992):1008.

Yesalis, C. *Anabolic Steroids in Sport and Exercise.* Champaign Ill.: Human Kinetics Publishers, 1993.

Lab Resource Materials

(For use with Lab 10, page L-25)

Directions: Within each group of exercises, start with the one that you believe is the most difficult one that you can perform. If you can pass it, try the next most difficult one. You receive points for the most difficult exercise that you can perform. Note: M = point values for males and F = point values for females.

Evaluating Isotonic Strength

I. **Push-Up:** Tests pectorals, triceps, abdominals, and other muscles.
(It is a failure if the hips pike or sag.)

Tests

1. One bent-knee push-up, keeping your body straight and rigid.

   Point values
   M = 0
   F = 3

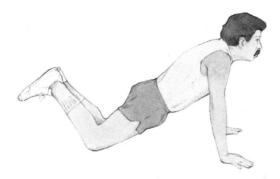

2. One straight-leg push-up, keeping your body rigid.

   Point values
   M = 3
   F = 6

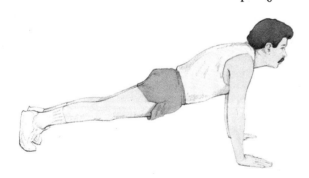

3. One straight-leg push-up, keeping your body rigid and your feet on the bench.

   Point values
   M = 6
   F = 8

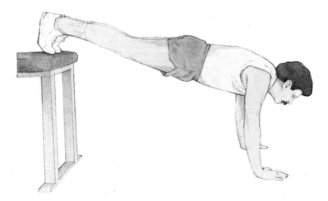

4. Same as no. 2, except have partner do a push-up on back of your shoulders at the same time.

   Point values
   M = 8
   F = 10

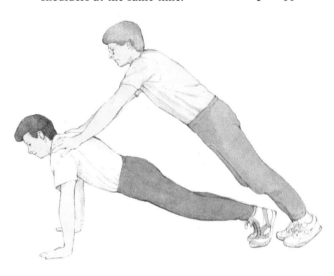

5. Same as no. 2, except use only one arm.

   Point values
   M = 10
   F = 12

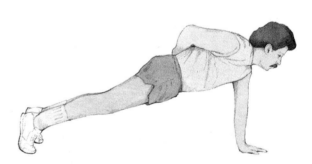

II. Pull-up: Tests biceps, latissimus, rhomboids, trapezius, and other muscles.

Tests

1. a. Hang from a bar placed at the height of the lower end of your sternum.
   b. Body should be inclined at a forty-five degree angle.
   c. Have partner brace your feet or brace against bench or wall.
   d. Pull up until your chin or chest touches the bar.

Point values
M = 1
F = 3

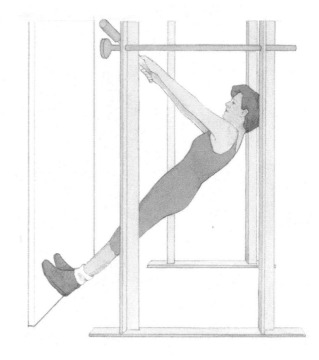

2. a. Stand on a chair and assume a position with palms facing body, elbows bent, and chin over bar.
   b. Remove chair.
   c. Slowly lower yourself, taking four seconds to extend the elbows.

Point values
M = 3
F = 6

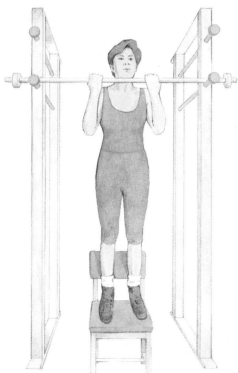

3. Perform one regulation chin-up (pull-up) from a hanging position with palms facing your body.

Point values
M = 6
F = 8

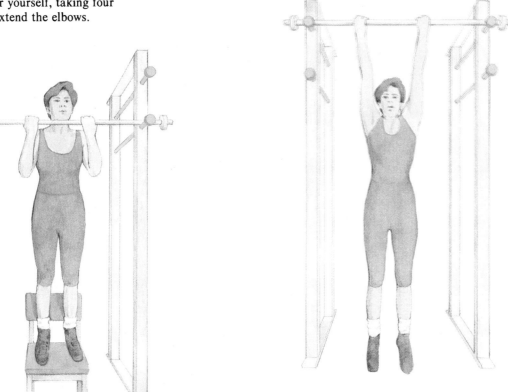

4. Same as no. 3, except pull up while two bleach bottles filled with water are suspended on the ends of a short rope across the back of your neck. (A towel may be used to pad the neck to prevent discomfort caused by the rope.)

Point values
M = 8
F = 10

5. Climb a rope to a height of ten feet above your head, using arms only (no leg use). *Caution:* Use a mat and spotters for safety.

Point values
M = 10
F = 12

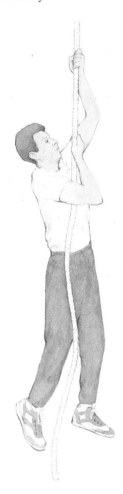

III. **One Leg Squat:** Tests hip and knee extensors (quadriceps, gluteals, hamstrings, etc).

Test

1. Squat on one leg and pick up a paper cup with one hand; return to a stand. Keep the back erect and maintain balance.
   a. Use one leg only.
   b. Use right leg only, then use left only.

Point values
M/F = 3
M/F = 6

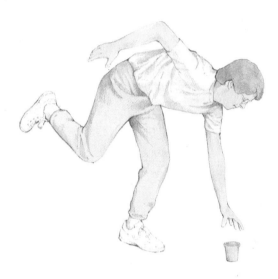

IV. **Trunk Lift:** Tests the strength of the upper back and neck muscles.

Test

1. Lie prone. Lift your upper trunk until the sternum leaves the floor (do not lift higher, causing an arch in the lower back). Keep your feet on the floor.
   a. Place the hands under the thighs.

Point values
M/F = 3

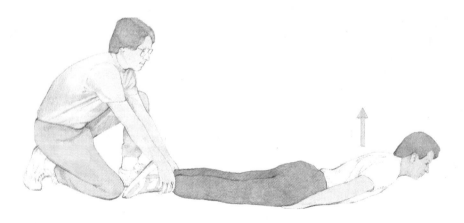

b. Same as "a," except clasp the hands behind the neck.

Point values
M/F = 6

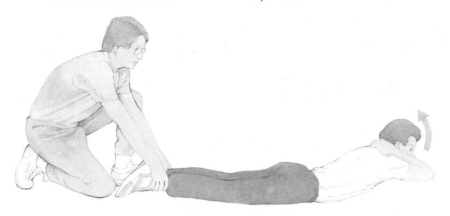

c. Same as "a," except extend both arms forward and clamp them against the ears.

Point values
M/F = 8

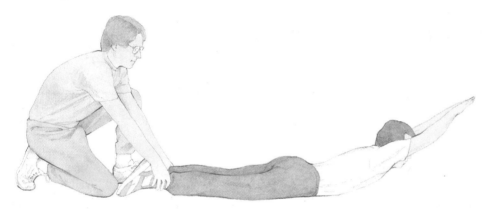

Evaluating Isometric Strength

Test

Grip Strength
Adjust a hand dynamometer to fit your hand size. Squeeze it as hard as possible. You may bend or straighten the arm, but do not touch the body with your hand, elbow, or arm. Perform with both right and left hands. (See photo p. 102.)
Note: When not being tested, perform the isometric strength exercises in Concept 12, or try to squeeze and indent a new tennis ball (*after* completing the dynamometer test).

Evaluating Leg Muscle Power

Test

Long Jump
Lie on a mat and have your partner mark your body length (height) from head to toe on the mat. Perform a standing long jump the distance of your body height if possible. Make two jumps and measure the better of the two.

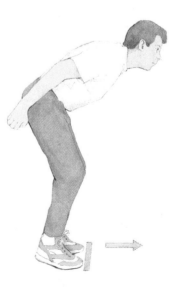

Chart 10.1 Isotonic Strength *Rating Scale* (Men and Women)

Classification	Age				
	17–26	27–39	40–49	50–59	60+
High performance zone	31+	28+	28+	26+	24+
Good fitness zone	24–30	22–27	22–27	20–25	19–23
Marginal zone	19–23	17–21	15–21	14–19	12–18
Low zone	<19	<17	<15	<14	<12

Chart 10.2 Isometric Strength *Rating Scale* for Men (Pounds)*

Classification	Left Grip	Right Grip	Total Score
High performance zone	125+	135+	260+
Good fitness zone	100–124	110–134	210–259
Marginal zone	90–99	95–109	185–209
Low zone	<90	<95	<185

Chart 10.3 Isometric Strength *Rating Scale* for Women (Pounds)*

Classification	Left Grip	Right Grip	Total Score
High performance zone	75+	85+	160+
Good fitness zone	60–74	70–84	130–159
Marginal zone	45–59	50–69	95–129
Low zone	<45	<50	<95

Charts 10.2 and 10.3 are suitable for use by young adults between 18 and 30 years of age. After 30, an adjustment of 0.5 of 1 percent per year is appropriate because some loss of muscle tissue typically occurs as you grow older.

*A chart showing the metric equivalents for charts 10.2 and 10.3 can be found in Appendix B.

Chart 10.4 Rating Scale of Leg Power (Men)					
Age	**17–26**	**27–39**	**40–49**	**50–59**	**60+**
Classification	Length of Jump (by height)				
High performance zone	ht.+	ht.+	¾ht.+	¾ht.+	½ht.+
Good performance zone*	¾ht.	¾ht.	½ht.	½ht.	½ht.
Marginal zone	½ht.	½ht.	⅓ht.	⅓ht.	⅓ht.
Low zone	<½ht.	<½ht.	<⅔ht.	<⅓ht.	<⅓ht.

*Because power is a skill-related fitness component and relates more to performance than to health, "good performance zone" is used rather than "good fitness zone."

Chart 10.5 Rating Scale of Leg Power (Women)					
Age	**17–26**	**27–39**	**40–49**	**50–59**	**60+**
Classification	Length of Jump (by height)				
Higher performance zone	¾ht.+	¾ht.+	¾ht.+	⅔ht.+	½ht.+
Good performance zone*	⅔ht.	⅔ht.	½ht.	½ht.	⅓ht.
Marginal zone	½ht.	½ht.	⅓ht	⅓ht.	¼ht.
Low zone	<½ht.	<½ht.	<⅓ht.	<⅓ht.	<¼ht.

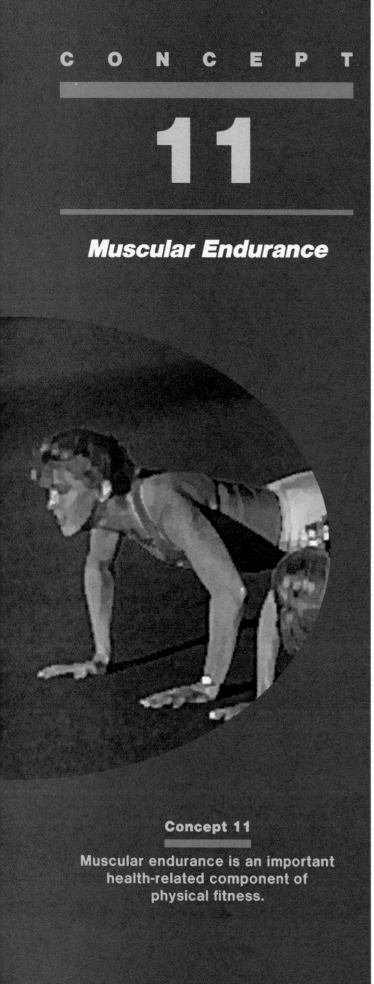

CONCEPT

11

Muscular Endurance

Concept 11

Muscular endurance is an important health-related component of physical fitness.

Introduction

When considering training programs, it is difficult to isolate **muscular endurance,** strength, and power from one another since a program designed specifically to develop one of these components would also tend to develop the other attributes to some degree. Muscular endurance is often neglected in discussions of fitness programs, and it is usually mentioned only in connection with strength, as if they were the same thing. Yet, experts agree that muscular endurance is a distinct and separate component of health-related fitness and that it requires a specific training program.

Health Goals for the Year 2000

- Increase the proportion of people who engage in activity to enhance muscular strength, muscular endurance, and flexibility.

Terms

- Also see Concept 10 terms.

Absolute Muscular Endurance (Dynamic type)

Endurance measured by the maximum number of repetitions (muscle contractions) one can perform against a given resistance; for example, the number of times you can lift 50 pounds in a bench press.

Dynamic Muscular Endurance

A muscle's ability to contract and relax repeatedly. This is usually measured by the number of times (repetitions) you can perform a body movement in a given time period. It is also called isotonic endurance.

Muscular Endurance

Fatigability of the skeletal muscles.

Relative Muscular Endurance (Dynamic type)

Endurance measured by the maximum number of repetitions one can perform against a resistance that is a given percentage of one's 1RM; for example, the number of times you can lift 50 percent of your 1RM.

Static Muscular Endurance

A muscle's ability to remain contracted for a long period. This is usually measured by the length of time you can hold a body position. It is also called isometric endurance.

Some Facts About Muscular Endurance

Benefits of Muscular Endurance

Muscular endurance is an important health-related component of physical fitness.

Muscular endurance is the capacity of a skeletal muscle or group of muscles to continue contracting over a long period. When you have good muscular endurance, you have the ability to resist fatigue and you can hold a position or carry something for a long period. You also have the ability to repeat a movement without getting tired.

When muscles become fatigued, they do not completely relax between contractions and are more susceptible to injury, and the rate of contraction slows, so less work is done. One's ability to withstand fatigue depends partly upon inheritance, partly upon the ability to tolerate pain and discomfort, and partly upon proper training. In the absence of fatigue, there is greater success and enjoyment in daily work activities and in athletic and recreational endeavors.

Good muscular endurance provides many other benefits.

In addition to providing resistance to fatigue, research has shown that a program (low load/high volume) of sufficient intensity can reduce cardiovascular disease risk by enhancing your blood lipid profile (increasing the HDL and decreasing cholesterol). Good muscular endurance also increases the static strength of bones, ligaments, and tendons. One study indicates it may be even more important than strength in the back muscles in terms of preventing back problems (Holmstrom et al. 1992).

It also increases the lean body mass, and produces small changes in body girth and skinfolds. (Noticeable changes in body weight and muscle hypertrophy, however, should *not* be expected.)

This is the type of training that beginning resistance trainers should engage in before using heavy resistance for strength; it is also believed to be safer for pregnant women, adolescents, and the elderly than high-load strength training.

Muscular endurance training tends to develop the slow-twitch fibers in your muscles.

As you train specifically for muscular endurance, the muscles adapt as a result of changes in slow-twitch fibers, including increased activity of aerobic enzymes in the muscle. Strength training, on the other hand, tends to produce changes in fast-twitch fibers, including increased activity of anaerobic enzymes.

Facts About Principles of Training

The overload principle applies to muscular endurance.

Though strength is developed by high resistance overload with low repetitions, **dynamic muscular endurance** requires just the opposite: higher repetitions and lower resistance. The ideal combination for maximum endurance is not known at this time. One study suggests that after progressing to twenty-five repetitions, it may be more effective to increase the resistance and keep the repetitions constant.

To develop **static muscular endurance,** the overload principle is applied by progressively increasing the length of time the muscles remain contracted against an immovable resistance and increasing the number of repetitions.

There is a threshold of training and a target zone for muscular endurance exercises.

There is a level of frequency, intensity, and time at which a training effect will begin to take place (threshold). There is also an optimal range, or target zone, where the most effective and efficient improvement will occur (see table 11.1). We do not know the exact range, but studies suggest that it has wide limits. The intensity, or resistance (load), is less important than the number of repetitions or the length of time a muscle contracts.

A muscular endurance training program should apply the principle of specificity by closely resembling the activity for which the endurance is needed.

Muscular endurance is specific to the muscles being used, the type of muscle contraction (static or dynamic), the speed or cadence of the movement, and the amount of resistance being moved.

For example, if you want endurance in the elbow flexor muscles (e.g., biceps), you must train those muscles. Performing muscular endurance exercise for the elbow extensor (e.g., triceps) or the leg muscles will not improve the muscular endurance of the biceps. Likewise, if you are trying to develop endurance for a dynamic task, you should do isotonic or isokinetic exercises. If you need endurance to hold you in a static position, do isometric exercises. If the activity requires a rapid movement, it is better to train with fast movements. There may be transfer from fast practice to slow movement in a skill, but the reverse it not necessarily true.

Garhammer (1986) believes that athletes wishing to develop muscular endurance for a particular sport may benefit more from performing the sport skill repeatedly than from doing special exercises such as resistance

Table 11.1

Muscular Endurance Threshold of Training and Fitness Target Zone

	Threshold of Training	Target Zone
Dynamic Endurance		
Frequency	• 2 days per week.	• Every other day.
Intensity	• Move 20%–30% of the maximum resistance you can lift.	• Move 40%–70% of the maximum resistance you can lift.
Time	• One set of 9 repetitions of each exercise.	• 2–5 sets of 9–25 repetitions. • Rest 15–60 sec. between sets.
Static Endurance		
Frequency	• 3 days per week.	• Every other day.
Intensity	• Hold a resistance 50%–100% of the weight you ultimately will need to hold in your work or leisure activity.	• Hold a resistance equal to and up to 50% greater than the amount you will need to hold in your work or leisure activity.
Time	• Hold for lengths of time 10%–50% shorter than the time you plan to do the activity. Repeat 10–20 times.	• Hold for lengths of time equal to and up to 20% greater than the time you plan to do the activity. For longer times, use fewer repetitions (5–10).
	• Rest 30 sec. between reps.	• Rest 30–60 sec. between reps.

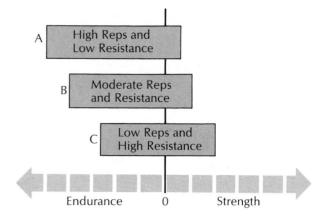

Figure 11.1

Comparison of absolute endurance and strength developed by different exercise regimens.

training. If injury or weather prevents practice of the sport, then resistance training for endurance would be an effective alternative.

Muscular endurance is slightly related to cardiovascular endurance, but it is not the same thing.

Cardiovascular endurance depends primarily upon the efficiency of the heart muscle, circulatory system, and respiratory system. It is developed with activities that stress these systems, such as running, cycling, and swimming. Muscular endurance depends upon the efficiency of the local skeletal muscles and the nerves that control them. You might train for cardiovascular endurance by running, but if the leg muscles lack the muscular endurance to continue contracting for more than five minutes, the cardiovascular system will not be stressed, even if it is in good condition.

Muscular endurance is related to strength, but is different.

Studies show that the person who is strength-trained will fatigue as much as four times faster than the person who is endurance-trained. However, there is a slight correlation between strength and endurance because the person who trains for strength will develop some endurance, and the person who trains for muscular endurance will develop some strength.

The graph in figure 11.1 illustrates the relationship between strength and **absolute muscular endurance.** In *A*, the training program calls for a high number of repetitions and light resistance. This results in a small gain in strength (the area of the bar to the right of the line), and a large increase in absolute endurance (the area of the bar to the left of the line). In *B*, the training program calls for a moderate number of repetitions (less than in *A*), and a moderate resistance (more than in *A*). This results in slightly less absolute endurance and slightly more strength than in program *A*. Program *C* results in the least gain in endurance and the most gain in strength because it uses high resistance and low repetitions. Thus, if you are primarily interested in muscular endurance, program *A* is your optimal choice.

Some endurance tests penalize the weaker person.

If you are tested on absolute endurance (the number of times you can move a designated number of pounds), a stronger person has an advantage. However, if you are tested on **relative muscular endurance** (the number of times you can move a designated percentage of your maximum strength), the stronger person does not have an advantage, and men and women can compete more evenly. In fact, on

Table 11.2
Absolute versus Relative Endurance: Percentage Change Due to Different Training Regimes.

	Absolute Endurance	Relative Endurance
Low resistance/high reps	5%	28%
Medium resistance/medium reps	8%	22%
High resistance/low reps	20%	7%

From T. Anderson and J. T. Kearney, "Effects of Three Resistance Training Programs on Muscular Strength and Absolute and Relative Endurance" in *Research Quarterly for Exercise and Sport*, 53:4. Copyright © 1982 American Alliance for Health, Physical Recreation, and Dance, Reston, VA. Reprinted by permission.

some tasks women have done as well or better than men on endurance. For example, the women at West Point Military Academy do as well as the men on sit-up tests.

Strength training will not help you improve your relative endurance.

This is illustrated in the research study on which the graph in figure 11.1 was based. When the relative endurance of the three training groups was calculated, it was discovered that although the Low Rep-High Resistance group had a 20 percent increase in absolute endurance (figure 11.1), it actually decreased 7 percent in relative endurance (table 11.2).

Muscular endurance and strength are part of the same continuum.

As mentioned previously, muscular strength and muscular endurance are similar but different. They are part of the same continuum (figure 11.2). This has led some writers to refer to muscular endurance as "strength-endurance." "Pure" strength is approached as one nears the end (right) of the continuum, where only one maximum contraction is made. As the number of repetitions increases and the force of the contractions decreases, one nears the other end (left) of the continuum and approaches "pure" endurance. In between the two extremes varying degrees of strength and endurance are combined. The activities listed along the continuum are examples that might represent points along the scale.

Facts About Training Programs

There are a variety of effective programs for developing muscular endurance.

All methods used in strength development are applicable to endurance development. Resistance training, calisthenics, isometrics, isokinetics, and such activities as running, swimming, circuit training, and aerobic dance can all be designed to increase muscular endurance. Even games, such as rope climbing, tug-of-war, Indian wrestling, and hopping races, can contribute to muscular endurance. Figure 11.3 illustrates an isokinetic endurance training device used by swimmers.

One popular method of training for muscular endurance is Circuit Resistance Training (CRT).

Circuit resistance training for muscular endurance consists of the performance of high repetitions of an exercise with low to moderate resistance, progressing from one station to another performing a different exercise at each station. The stations are usually placed in a circle. CRT typically employs about twenty to twenty-five reps against a resistance that is 30–40 percent of 1 RM for forty-five seconds. Fifteen seconds of rest is provided while changing stations. Approximately ten exercise stations are used, and the participant repeats the circuit two to three times (sets). A sample circuit is included in Lab 12B, page L-31.

Circuit training on weight or hydraulic machines has been found to be more effective than standard set weight training for caloric consumption during and after exercise and for improving cardiovascular endurance, although it is not as effective as aerobic exercises such as cycling or bench stepping.

High intensity endurance is best trained by multiple sets rather than by one set of repetitions to exhaustion.

There has been a long-running debate over which is more effective for developing muscular endurance: a single set of exercise to exhaustion, or the traditional method of multiple sets. Recent studies have shown that the traditional method is superior.

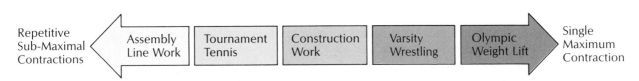

Repetitive Sub-Maximal Contractions ◁ Assembly Line Work | Tournament Tennis | Construction Work | Varsity Wrestling | Olympic Weight Lift ▷ Single Maximum Contraction

Figure 11.2
Muscular strength-endurance continuum.

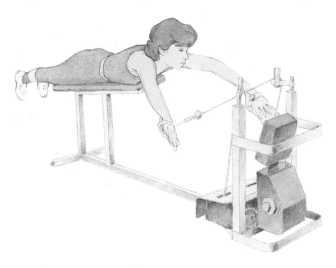

Figure 11.3
Isokinetic training device for swimmers.

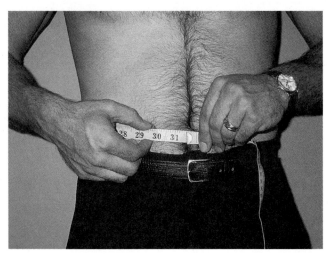

Exercise may help alter body measurements, but does not spot-reduce body fat.

Exercises to slim the figure/physique should be of the muscular endurance type.

Many men and women are interested in exercises designed to decrease girth measurements. High repetition, low resistance exercise is suitable for this because it usually brings about some strengthening and some decrease in skinfold and girth, which in turn, changes body contour. Exercises *do not* spot reduce fat (see Concept 24). Endurance exercises do speed up metabolism so more calories are burned, though if weight or fat reduction is desired, aerobic (cardiovascular) exercises are best. To increase girth, strength exercises such as those power lifters use for hypertrophy and/or a weight gain program are best (see Concept 10).

Endurance training may have a negative effect on strength and power.

Some studies have shown that for athletes who rely primarily on strength and power in their sports event, too much endurance training can cause a loss of strength and power because of modification of different muscle fibers. Strength and power athletes need some endurance training, but not too much, just as endurance athletes need some strength and power training, but not too much.

Some training methods can interfere with athletic performance.

Some research studies have shown that certain techniques used in training may actually cause a decrease in performance. For example, when distance runners were trained with weighted wristlets, anklets, and belts, they performed worse than runners who did not wear weights in training. In another study, people who were running and bicycling for aerobic endurance six days per week combined those exercises with a strength training program five days per week. The results yielded a decrease in strength development near the upper limits.

Guidelines for muscular endurance training programs are the same as those for strength development.

Performance guidelines for safety and effectiveness presented in Concept 10 should be reviewed before starting a program of exercise. It is particularly important that all muscle groups are exercised. For example, if your program for cardiovascular fitness stresses the muscles of the legs (front and back), then these might be omitted from your muscular endurance program and special attention given to the muscles on the inside and outside of the legs, and the muscles of the trunk and upper extremities.

Suggested Readings

Work, J. A. "Is Weight Training Safe during Pregnancy?" *Physician and SportsMedicine* 17(1989):257.
Yessis, M. "Latest Strength Techniques You Can Offer Your Clients." *Fitness Management* 5(1989):36.
Yessis, M. "Speaking of Strength." *Fitness Management* (1989):36.

Evaluating Muscular Endurance

1. Sitting Tucks (Dynamic)
Sit on the floor so that your back and feet are off the floor. Extend your arms forward for balance. Alternately draw your legs to your chest and extend them away from your body. Keep your feet and back off the floor. Repeat as many times as possible up to thirty-five.

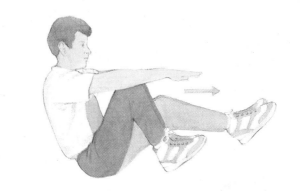

2. Ninety-Degree Push-Up (Dynamic)
Support the body in a push-up position from the toes. The hands should be under the shoulders, the back and legs straight, and the toes tucked under. Lower the body until the arms bend to 90 degrees and the upper arms are parallel to the floor. The rhythm should be approximately one push-up every three seconds. Repeat as many times as possible up to 35.

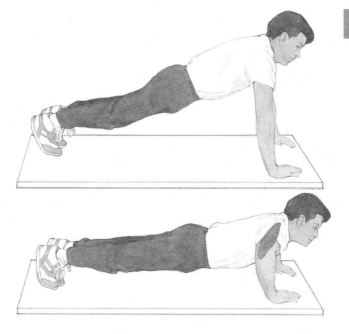

3. Flexed-Arm Support (Static)
Men: Support the body in a push-up position from the toes. The hands should be under the shoulders, the back and legs straight, and the toes tucked under. Lower the body until the arms bend to 90 degrees and the upper arms are parallel to the floor. *Women:* Use the same procedure as for men except support the push-up position from the knees instead of the toes. Hold the 90 degree position as long as possible.

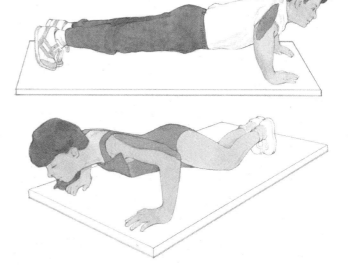

Chart 11.1 *Rating Scale* for Dynamic Muscular Endurance (Men)

Age	17–26		27–39		40–49		50–59		60+	
Classification	**Tucks**	**Push-Ups**	**Tucks**	**Push-Ups**	**Tucks**	**Push-Ups**	**Tucks**	**Push-Ups**	**Tucks**	**Push-Ups**
High performance zone	35+	29+	34+	27+	33+	26+	32+	24+	31+	22+
Good fitness zone	20–34	20–28	19–33	18–26	18–32	17–25	15–31	15–23	12–30	13–21
Marginal zone	15–19	16–19	13–18	15–17	12–17	14–16	10–14	12–14	8–11	10–12
Low zone	<15	<16	13	<15	<12	<14	<10	<12	<8	<10

Chart 11.2 *Rating Scale* for Dynamic Muscular Endurance (Women)

Age	17–26		27–39		40–49		50–59		60+	
Classification	**Tucks**	**Push-Ups**	**Tucks**	**Push-Ups**	**Tucks**	**Push-Ups**	**Tucks**	**Push-Ups**	**Tucks**	**Push-Ups**
High performance zone	25+	17+	24+	16+	23+	15+	22+	14+	21+	13+
Good fitness zone	20–24	12–16	19–23	11–15	18–22	10–14	17–21	9–13	10–20	8–12
Marginal zone	10–19	8–11	9–18	7–10	8–17	6–9	7–14	5–8	6–9	4–7
Low zone	<10	<8	<9	<7	<8	<6	<7	<5	<6	<4

Chart 11.3 *Rating-Scale* for Static Endurance (Flexed-Arm Support)

Classification	Score in Seconds
High performance zone	30>
Good fitness zone	20–29
Marginal zone	10–19
Low zone	<10

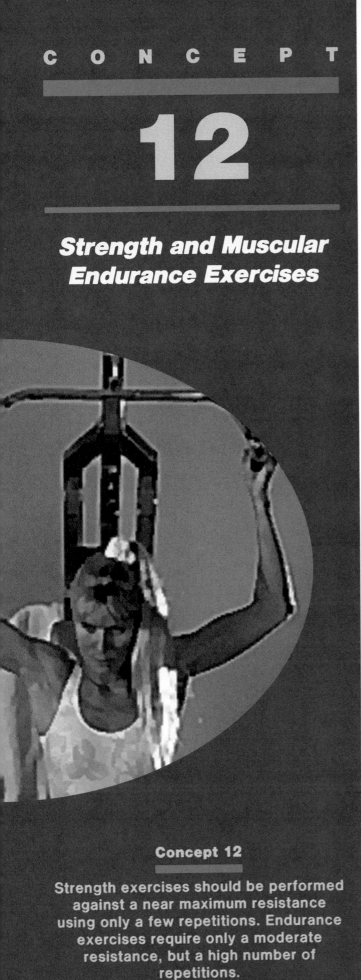

12

Strength and Muscular Endurance Exercises

Concept 12

Strength exercises should be performed against a near maximum resistance using only a few repetitions. Endurance exercises require only a moderate resistance, but a high number of repetitions.

Introduction

There are several kinds of strength and endurance exercises. Among the most popular are *isotonic calisthenics,* which require little or no special equipment; *isometric exercises,* which can be done in a small space; and *progressive resistance exercises (PRE),* which can be performed isotonically or isokinetically. The "Stations" mentioned in parentheses throughout this Concept refer to Universal stations pictured on page 137. The same muscles used in each exercise may be developed on the Universal machine. Other exercise machines can also be effective in developing strength and muscular endurance.

Health Goals for the Year 2000

- Increase the proportion of people who engage in activity to enhance muscular strength, muscular endurance, and flexibility.

Terms

- Detailed descriptions of important strength and muscular endurance terms are presented in Concept 10.

The Facts

Calisthenic exercises are among the most popular forms of exercise among adults.

Calisthenics, such as sit-ups and push-ups, are suitable for people of different ability levels, and can be used to improve both strength and muscular endurance. One disadvantage is that this type of exercise does little to increase strength unless more resistance is added. For example, doing a push-up will build strength to a point. However, once you can do several, adding more repetitions will only build muscular endurance but **not** strength. To develop additional strength, you can add more weights to increase the resistance or change the body position so there is a greater gravitational effect or more torque. For example, you can elevate your feet or wear a weighted vest while doing push-ups. Some calisthenics that you can do at home are illustrated on pages 124–128.

Resistance training with "free weights" is a popular form of isotonic progressive resistance exercise.

Free weights are weights that are not attached to a machine or exercise device. They can be put on a bar so that the weight can be adjusted as necessary for different exercises to provide optimal resistance. Weight training with free weights is very popular because it can be done in the home with inexpensive equipment. Homemade barbell weights can even be constructed from pieces of pipe and plastic bottles filled with water. Elastic tubes or bands may be substituted for the weights. These are available in varying strengths. Some exercises that are good for developing strength and muscular endurance are illustrated on pages 129–132.

Exercise with resistance training machines, pulley exercisers, and isokinetic machines have become more popular and more accessible in recent years.

Resistance training machines can be effective in developing strength and muscular endurance if used properly. They can save time because unlike free weights, the resistance can be changed easily and quickly. They are also safer because you are less likely to drop weights on machines. A disadvantage is that the kinds of exercises that can be done on these machines are more limited than those for free weights. Elastic bands or tubes may be substituted for the pulley device in these exercises. Some good exercises using resistance training machines and pulley exercisers are illustrated on pages 132–137. Isokinetic exercises are illustrated on page 145.

Isometric exercise is an effective and inexpensive way to build strength and muscular endurance.

Isometric exercise is an attractive form of exercise because it is effective in building strength and muscular endurance, and can be done in the home, office, or car, in a limited space and with no costly equipment. All that is necessary to do many isometric exercises are a piece of rope or a towel, and a doorway. It may be hard for some people to motivate themselves when performing isometrics because of the lack of movement involved. Also, isometric exercises may elevate blood pressure, and for that reason, those who have cardiovascular problems should be under the supervision of a physician when involved in them. Recent evidence indicates that for normal, healthy individuals, isometrics do not cause cardiovascular problems. Some good isometric exercises are illustrated on pages 138–144.

Sample Isotonic Exercises for Muscular Endurance and Mild Strengthening

The exercises suggested here should be performed as described until you are able to increase the repetitions to approximately twenty-five. Additional weight should then be added. Muscles depicted in color are those primarily involved in the exercises.

1. Full-Length Push-Ups

Purpose

Develop muscles of the arms, shoulders, and chest.

Position

Take front-leaning rest position, arms straight.

Movement

Lower chest to floor. Press to beginning position in same manner. Repeat. *Caution:* Do not arch back. (See stations 3, 7, and 9.) For a half push-up, press up until upper arm is parallel to floor.

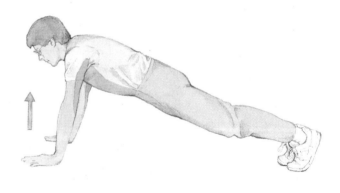

2. Bent-Knee Push-Ups

For those who cannot do full-length push-ups.

Purpose

Develop muscles of the arms, shoulders, and chest.

Position

Assume the push-up position, but rest the weight on the knees, not the feet.

Movement

Lower the body until the chest touches the floor; return to the starting position keeping the body straight. Repeat. *Caution:* Do not arch back. (See stations 2 and 9.) For a half push-up, see movement described in exercise 1, above.

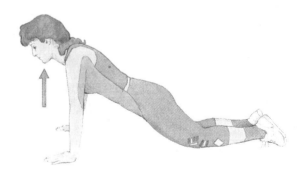

3. Bent-Knee Let-Downs

For those who cannot do bent-knee push-ups.

Purpose

Develop muscles of the arms, shoulders, and chest.

Position

Same as a bent-knee push-up position.

Movement

Slowly lower body to the floor, keeping the body line straight; return to the starting position in any manner. Repeat. *Caution:* Do not arch back. (See stations 2 and 9.)

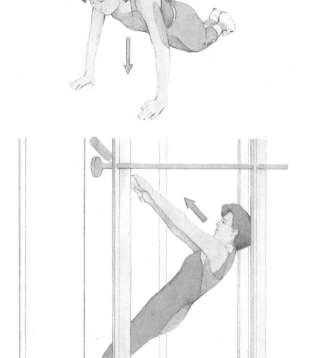

4. Modified Pull-Ups

Purpose

Develop muscles of the arms and shoulders.

Position

Hang (palms forward and shoulder width apart) from a low bar (may be placed across two chairs), heels on floor, with the body straight from feet to head.

Movement

Pull up keeping the body straight, touch the chest to the bar, then lower to the starting position. Stronger persons should perform exercise 5 (pull-up.) Repeat. (See stations 4, 6, and 12.)

5. Pull-Ups (Chinning)

Purpose

Develop muscles of the arms and shoulders.

Position

Hang from bar, palms forward, body and arms straight.

Movement

Pull up until chin is over bar. Repeat. (See station 6.)

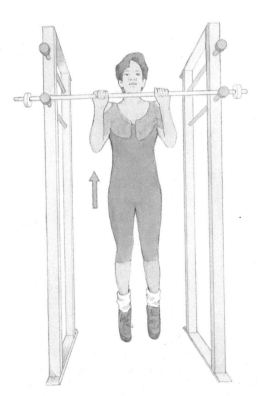

6. Reverse Curl

Purpose

Develop the lower abdominal muscles and correct abdominal ptosis.

Position

Lie on the floor. Bend the knees, place the feet flat on the floor, and place arms at sides.

Movement

Lift the knees to the chest, raising the hips off the floor; do not let the knees go past the shoulders. Return to the starting position. Repeat. (See stations 8 and 9.)

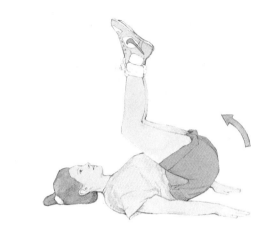

7. Crunch (Curl-Up)

Purpose

Develop the upper abdominal muscles and correct abdominal ptosis.

Position

Assume a hook-lying position with arms extended or crossed with hands on shoulders or palms on ears. If desired, legs may rest on bench to increase difficulty. For less resistance, place hands at side of body (do *not* put hands behind neck). For more resistance, move hands higher.

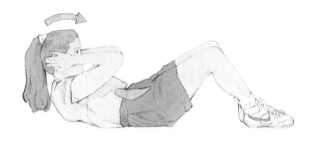

Movement

Curl up until shoulder blades leave floor, then roll down to the starting position. Repeat. (See station 9.) Note: Twisting the trunk on the curl-up develops the oblique abdominals.

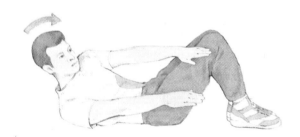

8. Leg Extension Exercise

Purpose

Develop muscles of the hips.

Position

Assume a knee-chest position, hands on floor with arms extended as far as possible.

Movement

Extend right leg upward in line with trunk, then lower, keeping it straight. Continue repetitions. Repeat with other leg. An ankle weight may be added to increase intensity. *Caution:* Do not allow back to arch, or leg to move higher than a line through the trunk. (See stations 5 and 16.)

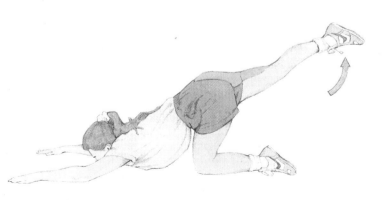

9. Upper Back Lift

Purpose

Develop muscles of the upper back. Correct kyphosis and round shoulders.

Position

Lie prone (face down) with hands clasped behind the neck.

Movement

Pull the shoulder blades together, raising the elbows off the floor. Slowly raise the head and chest off the floor by arching the upper back. Return to the starting position; repeat. For less resistance hands may be placed under thighs. *Caution:* Do not arch the lower back; lift only until the sternum (breast bone) clears the floor. (See station 11.)

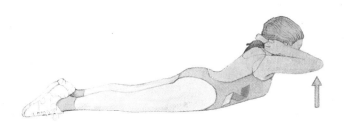

10. Side Leg Raises

Purpose

Develop muscles on the outside of thighs.

Position

Lie on the side. Point knees forward.

Movement

Raise the top leg 45 degrees, then return. Do the same number of repetitions with each leg. *Caution:* Keep knee and toes pointing forward.

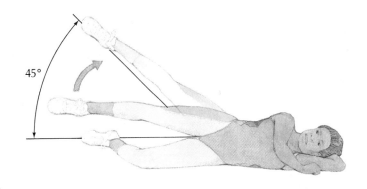

11. Lower Leg Lift

Purpose

Develop muscles on the inside of thighs.

Position

Lie on the side with the upper leg (foot) supported on a bench. Note: If no bench is available, bend top leg and cross it in front of bottom leg for support.

Movement

Raise the lower leg toward the ceiling; repeat. Roll to opposite side and repeat. Keep knees pointed forward.

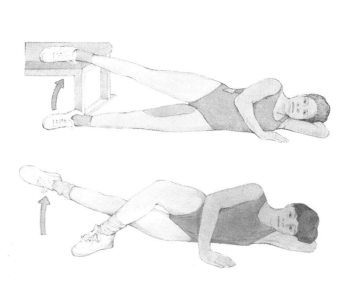

12. Alternate Leg Kneel

Purpose

Develop muscles of the legs and hips.

Position

Stand tall, feet together.

Movement

Take a step forward with the right foot, touching the left knee to the floor. The knees should be bent only to a 90-degree angle. Return to the starting position and step out with the other foot. Repeat, alternating right and left. (See stations 1, 10, and 16.)

13. Stationary Leg Change

Purpose

Develop muscles of the legs and hips.

Position

Crouch on the floor with weight on hands, left leg bent under the chest, right leg extended behind.

Movement

Alternate legs; bring right leg up while left leg goes back. Repeat. (See station 16.)

14. Knee-to-Nose Touch/Kneeling Leg Extensions

Purpose

Strength or endurance of lumbar and gluteal muscles; stretch low back.

Position

Kneel on all fours.

Movement

Pull knee toward nose, then extend leg horizontally (do not go higher). Repeat. Alternate legs. (See stations 1 and 16.)

Variations:

a. Keep knee extended as leg is raised and lowered.
b. Keep upper back straight and pull knee only to chest.

15. Lower Trunk Lift

Purpose

Develop lower back and hip strength.

See exercise 23 in Concept 18. (See station 11.)

16. Upper Trunk Lift

Purpose

Develop upper back strength.

See exercise 22 in Concept 18. (See station 11.)

These exercises may be used for strength or for muscular endurance. Muscles depicted in color are those primarily involved in the exercises. Before performing these exercises, review the resistance training guidelines in Concept 10. (Note: Elastic bands or tubes may be substituted for weights.)

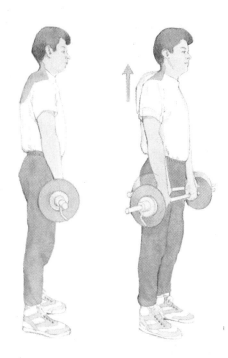

17. Shoulder Shrug

Purpose

Strengthen the muscles of the shoulder girdle.

Position

Stand with palms toward body, bar touching thighs, legs straight, and feet together.

Movement

Lift shoulders (try to touch ears) then roll shoulders smoothly backward, down, and forward. Repeat. (See stations 3 and 5.)

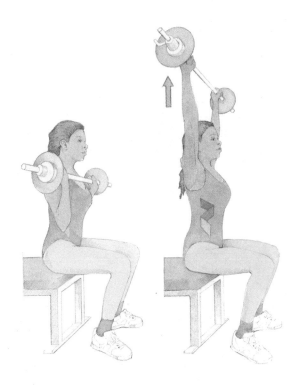

18. Military Press

Purpose

Strengthen the muscles of the shoulders and arms.

Position

Sit erect, bend elbows, palms facing forward at chest level, hands spread (slightly more than shoulder width). Have bar touching chest, spread feet (comfortable distance).

Movement

Move bar to overhead position (arms straight). Lower to chest position. Repeat. (See station 3.)

19. Half Squat

Purpose

Strengthen the muscles of the thighs and buttocks.

Position

Stand erect, feet turned out 45 degrees. Rest bar behind neck on shoulders. Spread hands in a comfortable position.

Movement

Squat slowly, keeping back straight, eyes ahead. Bend knees to 90 degrees; keep knees over feet. Pause, then stand. Repeat. (See stations 1, 10, and 16.)

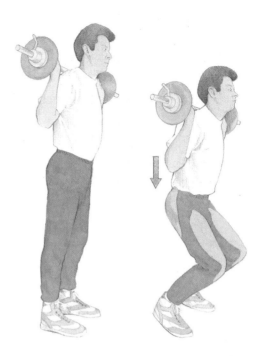

20. Biceps Curl

Purpose

Strengthen the muscles of the upper front part of the arms (biceps).

Position

Stand erect with back against a wall, palms forward; bar touching thighs. Spread feet in comfortable position.

Movement

Move bar to chin, keeping body straight and elbows near the sides. Lower to original position. Do not allow back to arch. Repeat. (See station 5.)

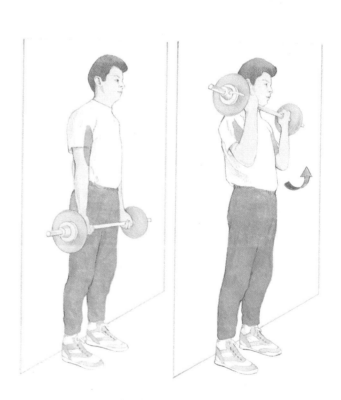

21. Triceps Curl

Purpose

Strengthen the muscles on the back of the upper arms (triceps).

Position

Sit erect, elbows and, palms facing up. Bar resting behind neck on shoulders, hands near center of bar, feet spread.

Movement

Keep upper arms stationary. Raise weight overhead, return bar to original position. Repeat. (See stations 6 and 7.)

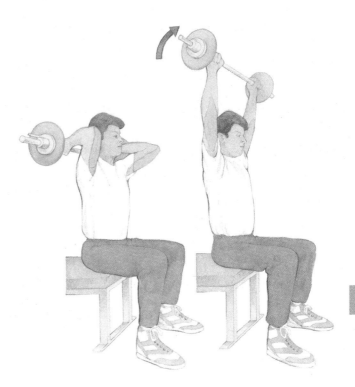

22. Toe Raise

Purpose

Strengthen muscles of the legs (calf).

Position

Stand erect with palms facing forward, hands wider than shoulder width apart, bar resting behind neck on shoulders. Rest balls of feet on two-inch block with heels on floor. Toes together, heels apart.

Movement

Rise on toes quickly, hold for one second. Lower heels to floor. Repeat. Keep toes in and heels out. (See stations 1 and 5.)

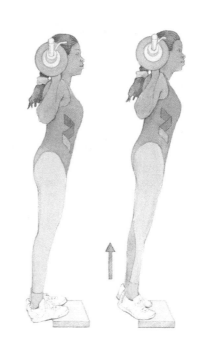

23. Upright Row

Purpose

Strengthen muscles of the shoulders and arms.

Position

Stand erect with palms facing body (loose), hands together at center of bar, bar touching thighs, feet spread, head erect, eyes straight ahead.

Movement

Pull bar to chin. Keep bar close to body and elbows well above bar. Lower to extended position. Repeat. Do not arch back. (See station 3.)

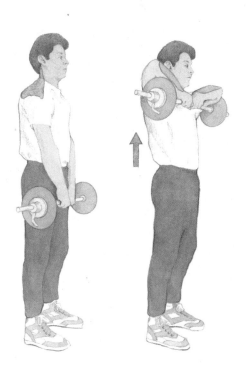

Sample Resistance Training Machine Pulley Exercises

These exercises may be used for strength or for muscular endurance. Before performing these exercises, review the resistance training guidelines in Concept 10. Muscles depicted in color are those primarily involved in the exercises.

24. Biceps Curl (Low Pulley)

Purpose

Strengthen the elbow flexor muscles on front of arm.

Position

Stand erect, arms at sides, palms up. Grasp bar.

Movement

Flex elbows, bringing bar to chest. Keep elbows pressed against sides. Lower; repeat; do not allow back to arch. (See station 12.)

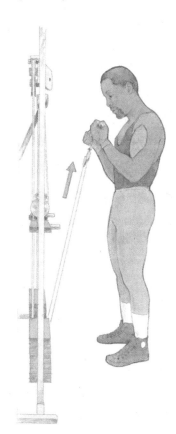

25. Seated Rowing (Low Pulley)

Purpose

Develop the upper arms and shoulders.

Position

Sit facing pulley, feet braced and knees slightly bent. Grasp bar, palms down with hands shoulder width apart.

Movement

Pull bar to chest, keeping elbows high and return; repeat. (See station 12.)

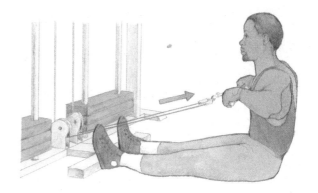

26. Leg Press

Purpose

Develop the thigh and hip muscles.

Position

Sit on chair with feet on pedals, knees bent to right angle. Grasp handles.

Movement

Extend legs and return; repeat. Do not lock knees when legs straighten. (See station 1.) Where two sets of pedals are available, the lower pedal emphasizes thigh muscles, the upper pedal emphasizes hip (gluteal) muscles.

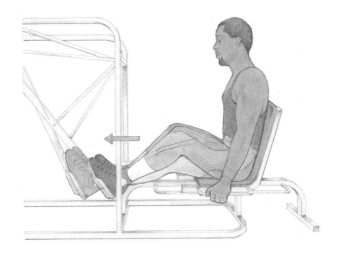

27. Lat Pull-down (High Pulley)

Purpose

Develop the latissimus ("lats"), biceps, and pectorals ("pecs").

Position

Tailor sit or kneel on both knees. Grasp bar with palms facing away from you, hands shoulder distance apart.

Movement

Pull bar down to chest and return; repeat.

Variations

Turn palms toward face or move hands out to ends of bar, or pull bar behind head. (See station 4.)

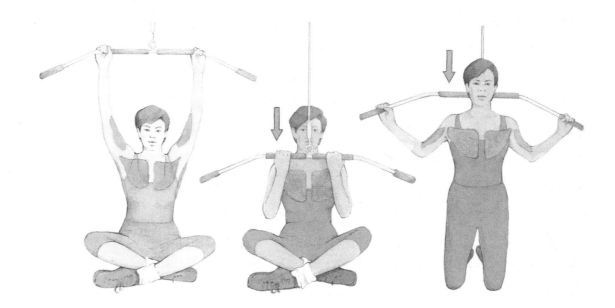

28. Triceps Curl

Purpose

Develop the triceps and other muscles on back of arm.

Position

Stand erect. Grasp bar near center, palms down.

Movement

With elbows clamped against sides, pull bar down to thighs and return to chest height without moving elbows; *Caution:* Do not lock knees or arch back; repeat. (See station 4.)

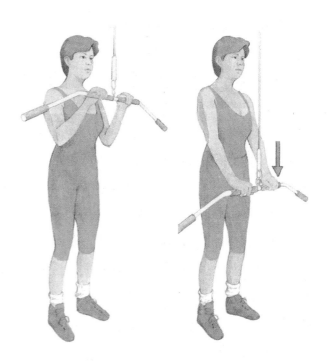

29. Bench Press

Purpose

Develop the chest (pectoral) and triceps muscles.

Position

Lie supine on bench with knees bent and feet flat on bench. Grasp handles at shoulder level.

Movement

Push bar up until arms are straight. Return; repeat; do not arch lower back. (See station 2.)

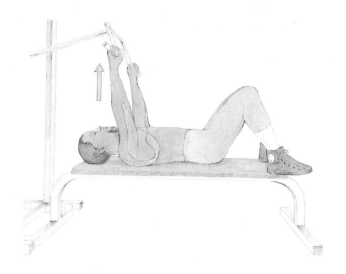

30. Ankle Press

Purpose

Develop the calf muscles.

Position

Sit at leg press station with legs straight. Grasp handles. Put ball of foot at lower edge of pedal.

Movement

Keeping knees straight, point toes by extending (plantar flexing) ankles. Return; repeat. (See station 1.)

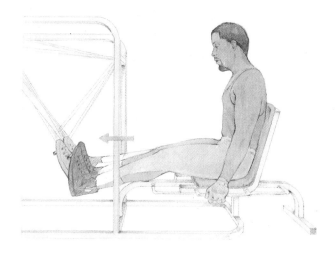

31. Knee Extension

Purpose

Develop the thigh (quadriceps) muscles.

Position

Sit on end of bench with ankles hooked under padded bar. Grasp edge of table.

Movement

Extend knees. Return; repeat. (See station 10.)

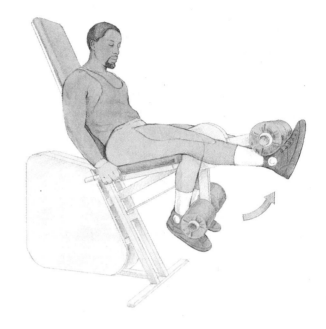

32. Hamstring Curl

Purpose

Develop the hamstrings (muscles on back of thigh) and other knee flexors.

Position

Lie prone on bench with ankles hooked under padded bar. Rest chin on hands or grasp bench.

Movement

Flex knees as far as possible without allowing hips to raise. Return; repeat. (See station 10.)

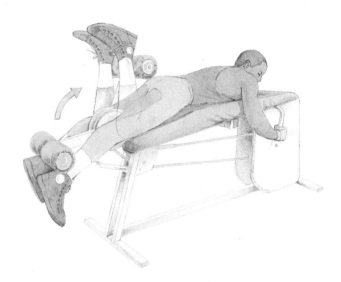

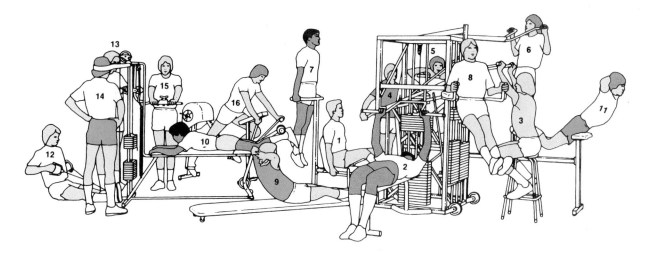

STATIONS

1. **Leg Press**—Push the pedal, extending the hips and knees; to strengthen the thigh (quadriceps) muscles.

*2. **Chest Press (Bench Press)**—Push upward on the handles, extending the elbows and bringing the upper arms toward the chest; to strengthen the chest muscles (pectorals) and the triceps on the back of the arms. Note: It is better if the feet are placed on the bench with knees and hips flexed and lower back flattened.

*3. **Shoulder Press (Military Press)**—Push upward on the handles, extending the elbows, bringing the arms toward the ears; to strengthen the shoulder (deltoids) and the back of the arm (triceps). Note: The stool should be closer to the machine than shown to prevent arching of the back.

4. **Lat Pull Down Bar or High Pulley**—Kneel or stand and pull the bar down behind the neck, alternating with a pull to the chest; to strengthen the biceps and the latissimus. To strengthen the triceps, perform a "triceps curl" by pulling the bar from chest height to waist or thigh level. Extend the elbows while keeping them hugged against your sides.

5. **Low Pulley and Dead Lift**—Perform "biceps curls" by standing and pulling your handle from thigh level to chest level, flexing the elbows while keeping elbows hugged close to the sides. Note: The Dead Lift is not recommended, but a sitting "Rowing" exercise (shown at station 12) may be substituted to strengthen the upper back muscles and biceps.

6. **Chinning**—Grasp handles and pull up until the chin is at hand level; to strengthen biceps, latissimus and upper back muscles.

7. **Dipping**—Support your weight on the handles, then lower the body by bending the elbows 90°, then push-up to a straight-arm position again; to strengthen triceps and upper pectorals (chest muscles).

*8. **Hip Flexors**—Support your weight on the forearms. Either with knees bent or knees straight, flex at the hip joint and lift one or both legs. Keep pelvis tilted backward and abdominals contracted; to strengthen hip flexors and lower abdominals. Note: This exercise may be hazardous to the back. Single and/or bent knee lifts are less hazardous than the exercise shown. Most people do not need to strengthen the hip flexors.

*9. **Abdominal (Tilt) Board**—Tilt the board at an angle appropriate for your ability. Perform sit-ups with knees bent (rather than as shown); to strengthen upper abdominals.

10. **Thigh and Knee**—"Hamstring Curl": lie prone with heels under pads and flex knees through a full range of motion; to strengthen the knee flexors (including hamstrings); "Knee Extensions": sit on end of bench with ankles under the lower set of pads. Extend the knees through a full range of motion to strengthen the knee extensors, including the quadriceps.

11. **Back Extension**—Adjust the apparatus so the feet can be braced while the pelvic bones rest on the pad. Let the trunk hang relaxed toward the floor. Extend the back until the trunk is parallel with the floor (Caution: do not arch the back); to strengthen the lower back muscles.

12. **Low Pulleys**—Sit with the feet braced, legs straight; grasp handles and keeping elbows out at chest level, pull handles to chest; to strengthen upper back muscles, including trapezius. To strengthen lower back muscles, lean the trunk backward at the hip joint during the pull.

13. **Wrist Conditioner**—Adjust the resistance, then grasp the handles, palm down, and rotate the handles by hyperextending the wrists; to strengthen the extensors. Reverse the direction of rotation to strengthen the wrist flexors.

14. **Neck Conditioner**—Place the strap around the forehead and flex the neck, or place the strap around the back or the side of the head and pull backward or sideward to strengthen the neck muscles. Caution: use only light resistance to avoid neck injury.

15. **Hand Gripper**—Adjust the resistance and grasp the handles, palm down. Alternate squeezing the right and the left; to improve grip strength.

16. **Real Runner**—Adjust the resistance; place the feet in the stirrups, the hands on the grips and the chest on the pad. Push and pull with the legs in a running motion; to strengthen the leg muscles.

Figure courtesy of Universal Gym Equipment, Inc., Cedar Rapids, IA.

Isometric exercises are intended primarily to develop muscular strength and endurance. Eighteen different exercises for different body parts are presented here. You should select exercises for your program (if you choose isometric exercise) that meet your own personal needs. All of the following exercises should be held for six to eight seconds and should be repeated several times a day. Muscles depicted in red are those primarily involved in the exercises. *Caution:* If you have high blood pressure, see your physician before doing these exercises. To make these exercises isotonic, elastic bands or tubes may be used for resistance.

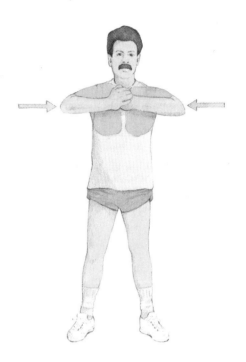

33. Chest Push

Purpose

Develop muscles of the chest and upper arms.

Position

Place left fist in palm of right hand. Keep hands close to chest, forearms parallel to floor.

Movement

Push hands together with maximum effort. (See station 2.)

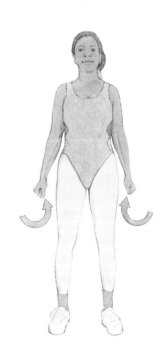

34. Fist Squeeze

Purpose

Develop muscles of the lower arm.

Position

Arms extended at side.

Movement

Clench fists as hard as possible. Repeat. (See stations 13 and 15.)

35. Shoulder Pull

Purpose

Develop muscles of the upper back and arms.

Position

Cup hands and interlock fingers or grasp opposite wrists. Keep hands close to chest, forearms parallel to floor.

Movement

Attempt to pull hands apart with maximum effort. (See station 12.)

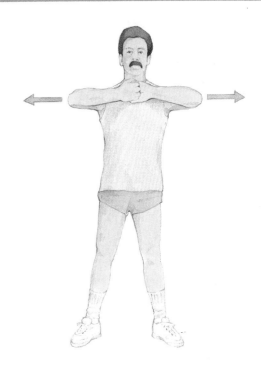

36. Neck Pull

Purpose

Develop muscles of the neck, upper back, and arms.

Position

Interlock fingers behind head, elbows pointing forward; head and neck erect.

Movement

Pull hands forward with maximum effort; resist with neck muscles. Keep chin down. (See station 14.)

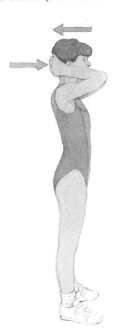

37. Leg Extension

Purpose

Develop muscles of the shoulders, legs, and hips.

Position

Loop rope under feet. Stand on rope (or towel), feet spread shoulder width. Keep back straight. Bend knees, grasp both ends of rope, back erect, arms straight, and buttocks low.

Movement

Try to straighten legs by lifting upward with maximum effort. (See stations 1 and 16.)

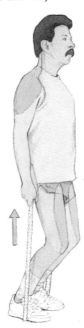

38. Overhead Pull

Purpose

Develop muscles of the arms.

Position

Fold rope in a double loop (or grasp towel). Grasp rope overhead, palms outward. Pull hands apart.

Movement

Push outward with maximum force. Repeat with palms turned in. (See stations 4, 6, and 12.)

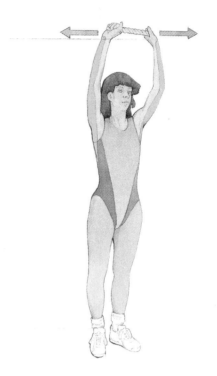

39. Curls

Purpose

Develop muscles on the front of the arms.

Position

Place rope (towel) loop behind thighs while standing in a half squat position. Grasp loop, palms up, shoulder width apart.

Movement

Lift upward with maximum effort. For reverse curls, repeat, gripping with palms down. (See stations 5 and 12.)

40. Foot Lift

Purpose

Develop muscles on back of legs.

Position

Stand on loop with left foot. Place loop around right ankle. Flex knee until taut.

Movement

Apply maximum force upward. Repeat forward and to side with each foot. (See station 10.)

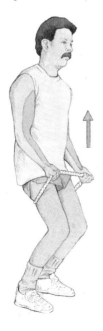

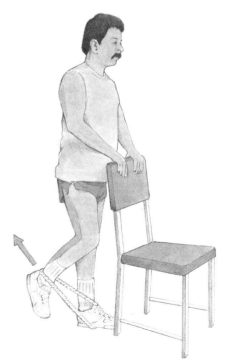

41. Military Press in Doorway

Purpose

Develop muscles of the arms and shoulders.

Position

Stand in doorway, face straight ahead, hands shoulder width apart, elbows bent.

Movement

Tighten leg, hip, and back muscles. Push upward as hard as possible. (See station 3.)

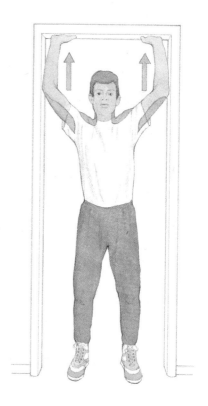

42. Arm Press in Doorway

Purpose

Develop tricep and pectoral muscles.

Position

Stand in doorway, back flat on one side of doorway, hands placed on other side.

Movement

Push with maximum force. (See stations 2 and 3.)

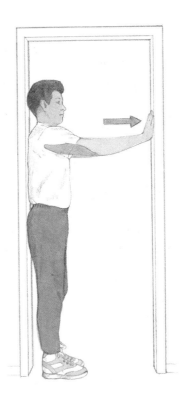

43. Leg Press in Doorway

Purpose

Develop muscles of the legs and hips.

Position

Sit in doorway facing side of door frame. Grasp molding behind head. Keep back flat on side of doorway, feet against other side.

Movement

Push legs with maximum force. (See stations 4 and 16.)

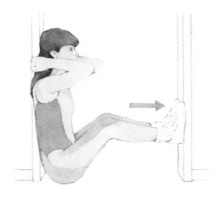

44. Wall Seat

Purpose

Develop muscles of the leg and hips.

Position

Assume half-sit position, back flat against wall, knees bent to 90 degrees.

Movement

Push back against wall with maximum force. (See stations 4 and 16.)

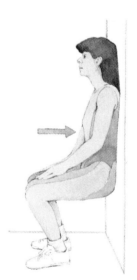

45. Triceps Curl

Purpose

Develop muscles on the back of the upper arm (triceps).

Position

Grasp towel (rope) at both ends. Hold left hand at small of back, right hand over shoulder.

Movement

Pull hands apart with maximum force; repeat exercise, reversing position of hands. (See stations 2, 3 and 7.)

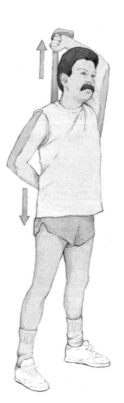

46. Knee Extension

Purpose

Develop muscles on the front of the thigh.

Position

Place towel (rope) around right ankle, knee bent to 90-degree angle.

Movement

Grasp towel with both hands behind back, extend leg downward with maximum force. Repeat exercise, changing legs. (See station 10.)

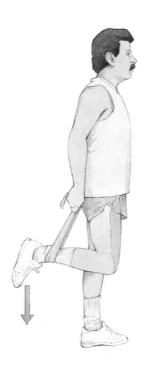

47. Waist Pull

Purpose

Develop muscles of the abdomen, chest, and arms.

Position

Grasp ends of towel (rope) palms in, towel around lower back, elbows flexed to right angle.

Movement

Pull forward on towel with maximum force while contracting abdomen and flattening back. (See stations 2 and 9.)

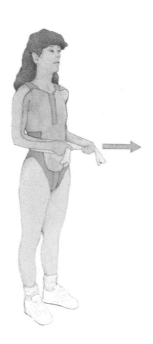

48. Bow Exercise

Purpose

Develop muscles of the shoulders and upper back.

Position

Take archer's position with bow (towel) drawn, left elbow partially extended, right hand at chin, right arm parallel to floor.

Movement

Grasp towel and pull arms away from each other. Exchange positions of hands and repeat. (See stations 7 and 12.)

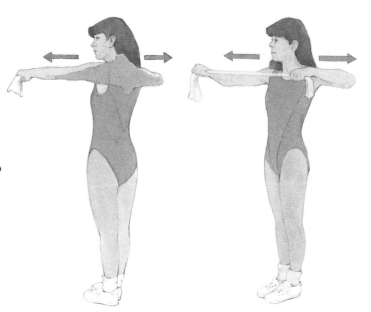

49. Gluteal Pinch

Purpose

Develop muscles of the buttocks.

Position

Lie prone, heels apart and big toes touching.

Movement

Squeeze the buttocks together. Hold several seconds. Slowly relax; repeat several times. (See station 1.)

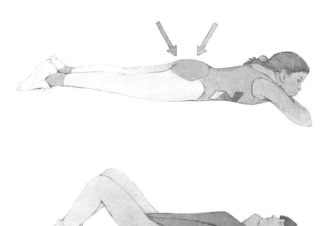

50. Pelvic Tilt

Purpose

Develop muscles of the abdomen and buttocks.

Position

Assume a supine position with the knees bent and slightly apart.

Movement

Press the spine down on the floor and hold for several seconds. Keep abdominals and gluteals tightened. (See stations 1 and 9.)

Exer-Genie Exercises

Examples of some of the isokinetic exercises that can be performed on the Exer-Genie are described below:

51. Back Extension

Keep the arms straight and bend the knees and hips until the handle can be grasped. Pull on the rope by extending knees, hips, and back, rolling the shoulders backward; strengthens hip, knee, and back extensors.

52. Straight-Leg Position

Stand erect and grasp handles with hands either palm-down or palm-up; perform "biceps curls" by hugging elbows to the sides while flexing elbows and pulling the handle to the chest; strengthens elbow flexors (biceps).

53. Curling and Abduction Position

Perform an "Upright Rowing" exercise by starting as in Position B with palms down, then pull the rope upward, bending the elbows out to the side and pulling the

shoulders back until the handle reaches chin level; strengthens elbow flexors (including biceps), shoulder rotators, deltoids, and upper back (including trapezius).

54. Press Overhead

Start with the handle at chin level, elbows bent and at the sides of the chest. Push the handle overhead by extending the elbows as in a "military press;" strengthens shoulders and arms (including deltoids and triceps).

55. Big Four

All of the muscle groups described above could be strengthened in one exercise by combining movements through the four positions into one continuous movement as shown in the illustration below.

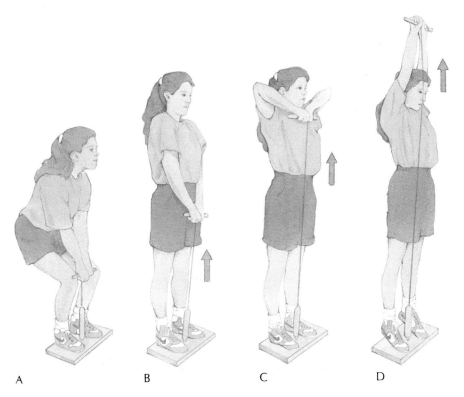

Figure 12.51
Big Four Exer-Genie. (*A*) Back-extension position; (*B*) straight-leg position; (*C*) curling and abduction position; (*D*) press overhead position.

LAB RESOURCE MATERIALS

(For use with Labs 12A and 12B, pages L-29–L-32)

Chart 12A.1 Sample Weight/Resistance Training Program					
Free Weight Exercise			**Machine Exercise**		
Name	**Number**	**Page**	**Name**	**Number**	**Page**
Shoulder shrug	17	129	Hamstring curl	32	136
Military press	18	129	Bench press	29	135
Half squat	19	130	Leg press	26	133
Biceps curl	20	130	Biceps curl	24	132
Triceps curl	21	131	Triceps curl	28	134
Toe raise	22	131	Ankle press	30	135
Upright row	23	132	Seated rowing	25	133

*See Appendix A to make metric conversions.

Chart 12A.2 Predicted 1 RM Based on Reps-to-Fatigue

Wt	\multicolumn{10}{c}{Repetitions}										Wt	\multicolumn{10}{c}{Repetitions}								

Wt	1	2	3	4	5	6	7	8	9	10	Wt	1	2	3	4	5	6	7	8	9	10
30	30	31	32	33	34	35	36	37	38	39	170	170	175	180	185	191	197	204	211	219	227
35	35	37	38	39	40	41	42	43	44	45	175	175	180	185	191	197	203	210	217	225	233
40	40	41	42	44	46	47	49	50	51	53	180	180	185	191	196	202	209	216	223	231	240
45	45	46	48	49	51	52	54	56	58	60	185	185	190	196	202	208	215	222	230	238	247
50	50	51	53	55	56	58	60	62	64	67	190	190	195	201	207	214	221	228	236	244	253
55	55	57	58	60	62	64	66	68	71	73	195	195	201	206	213	219	226	234	242	251	260
60	60	62	64	65	67	70	72	74	77	80	200	200	206	212	218	225	232	240	248	257	267
65	65	67	69	71	73	75	78	81	84	87	205	205	211	217	224	231	238	246	254	264	273
70	70	72	74	76	79	81	84	87	90	93	210	210	216	222	229	236	244	252	261	270	280
75	75	77	79	82	84	87	90	93	96	100	215	215	221	228	235	242	250	258	267	276	287
80	80	82	85	87	90	93	96	99	103	107	220	220	226	233	240	247	255	264	273	283	293
85	85	87	90	93	96	99	102	106	109	113	225	225	231	238	245	253	261	270	279	289	300
90	90	93	95	98	101	105	108	112	116	120	230	230	237	244	251	259	267	276	286	296	307
95	95	98	101	104	107	110	114	118	122	127	235	235	242	249	256	264	273	282	292	302	313
100	100	103	106	109	112	116	120	124	129	133	240	240	247	254	262	270	279	288	298	309	320
105	105	108	111	115	118	122	126	130	135	140	245	245	252	259	267	276	285	294	304	315	327
110	110	113	116	120	124	128	132	137	141	147	250	250	257	265	273	281	290	300	310	321	333
115	115	118	122	125	129	134	138	143	148	153	255	255	262	270	278	287	296	306	317	328	340
120	120	123	127	131	135	139	144	149	154	160	260	260	267	275	284	292	302	312	323	334	347
125	125	129	132	136	141	145	150	155	161	167	265	265	273	281	289	298	308	318	329	341	353
130	130	134	138	142	146	151	156	161	167	173	270	270	278	286	295	304	314	324	335	347	360
135	135	139	143	147	152	157	162	168	174	180	275	275	283	291	300	309	319	330	341	354	367
140	140	144	148	153	157	163	168	174	180	187	280	280	288	296	305	315	325	336	348	360	373
145	145	149	154	158	163	168	174	180	186	193	285	285	293	302	311	321	331	342	354	366	380
150	150	154	159	164	169	174	180	186	193	200	290	290	298	307	316	326	337	348	360	373	387
155	155	159	164	169	174	180	186	192	199	207	295	295	303	312	322	332	343	354	366	379	393
160	160	165	169	175	180	186	192	199	206	213	300	300	309	318	327	337	348	360	372	386	400
165	165	170	175	180	186	192	198	205	212	220	305	305	314	323	333	343	354	366	379	392	407

This chart is used as modified with permission from the *Journal of Physical Education, Recreation & Dance*, January, 1993, p. 89. *JOPERD* is a publication of the American Alliance for Health, Physical Education, Recreation and Dance, 1900 Association Drive, Reston, VA 22091.

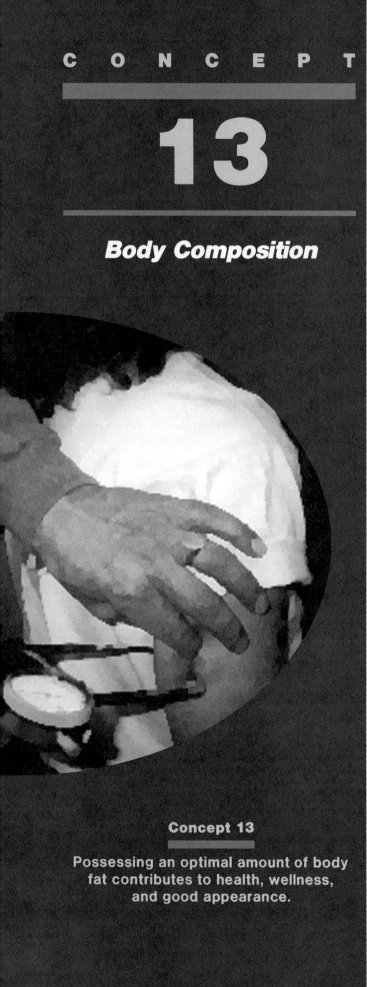

Concept 13

Possessing an optimal amount of body fat contributes to health, wellness, and good appearance.

Introduction

Body composition refers to the relative percentage of muscle, fat, bone, and other tissue of which the body is composed. Of primary concern, because of its association with various health problems, is body fatness. Being **overfat** or **underfat** can result in health concerns.

Some sources have suggested that the incidence of overfatness in our society is as high as 59 percent. Using body composition values associated with increased risk of various diseases, the Public Health Service estimates that 26 percent of adults in our society are overfat. National health goals have been established to reduce the fatness among people of all ages. Since eating disorders such as anorexia nervosa and bulimia are especially prevalent among teens, the national goal is to keep the percentage of overfat teens from increasing while at the same time reducing the incidence of those who have too little fat associated with eating disorders.

Health Goals for the Year 2000

- Reduce overfatness to no more than 20 percent of people aged 20 or more.
- Reduce overfatness to no more than 15 percent of people aged 12–19.
- Increase to 50 percent the proportion of overfat people who have adopted physical activity and sound nutrition to attain desirable body fatness.

Terms

Amenorrhea

Absence of or infrequent menstruation.

Calorie

A unit of energy supplied by food; the quantity of heat necessary to raise the temperature of a kilogram of water one degree centigrade (actually a kilocalorie but usually called a calorie for weight control purposes).

Caloric Balance

Consuming calories in amounts equal to the number of calories expended.

Diet

The usual food and drink for a person or animal.

Essential Fat

The minimum amount of fat in the body necessary to maintain healthful living.

MET

METs are multiples of the amount of energy expended at rest, or approximately 3.5 millimeters of oxygen per kilogram (2.2 pounds) of body weight per minute.

Nonessential Fat

Extra fat or fat reserves stored in the body.

Obesity

Extreme overfatness.

Overfat

Too much of the body weight composed of fat; for men, having more than 25 percent fat; for women, having more than 30 percent fat.

Overweight

Weight in excess of normal; not harmful unless it is accompanied by overfatness.

Percent Body Fat

The percentage of total body weight that is comprised of fat.

Somatotype

Inherent body build; ectomorph (thin), mesomorph (muscular), and endomorph (fat).

Underfat

Too little of the body weight composed of fat; for men, having less than 5 percent fat; for women, having less than 8 percent fat.

The Facts: The Meaning and Measurement of Fatness

There are standards that can be used to determine how much body fat an individual should possess.

Every person should possess at least a minimal amount of body fat for good health. This fat is called **essential fat** and is necessary for temperature regulation, shock absorption, and regulation of essential body nutrients, including vitamins A, D, E, and K. **Nonessential fat** accumulates when you take in more calories than you expend. When nonessential fat accumulates in excessive amounts, overfatness or even **obesity** can occur. For good health, an individual should not allow body fat levels to drop too low or to become too high. There is a desirable range of fatness for good health, different from the range suggested for those who have optimal performance in athletic events as a goal. Even for athletes, especially low levels

Table 13.1

Standards for Fatness (Percent Body Fat)

Classification	Men	Women
Essential fat	no less than 5%	no less than 8%
Desirable fatness for good performance	5%–13%	12%–22%
Desirable fatness for good health	10%–25%	18%–30%
Overfatness	more than 25%	more than 30%

From J. H. Wilmore, et al., "Body Composition: A Round Table" in *The Physician and Sportsmedicine*, 14:152, 1986. Copyright © 1986 *The Physician and Sportsmedicine*. Reproduced by permission of McGraw-Hill, Inc.

of body fatness are not desirable. Research has shown that attempts to attain and maintain too low a body fat level are associated with eating disorders such as anorexia nervosa and bulimia (see page 151). Also, there is evidence that excessive fat loss may result in **amenorrhea** in women. Table 13.1 provides standards of body fatness for both men and women.

When using height and weight to assess overweight, the body mass index (BMI) is considered to be a better measure than height-weight charts.

Individuals who are interested in controlling their weight often consult height-weight tables to determine their "desirable" weight. Being 20 percent or more above the recommended table weight is one commonly used indicator of obesity. The usefulness of these tables is limited because they reflect how an individual compares to "normal" people. They do not give an accurate estimate of the amount of fat a person has. A person who has a large muscle mass as a result of regular exercise could appear to be "overweight" using a height-weight table.

The Body Mass Index (BMI) is probably the best way to use height and weight to assess fatness. The BMI is calculated using a special formula and has a higher correlation with true body fatness than weights determined from height-weight tables. You may wish to calculate your BMI using Chart 13B.6 provided in the Lab Resource materials.

Overfat is more important than **overweight** in determining health and wellness.

Though height-weight tables and the BMI can provide guidelines for body fatness, neither is a true measure of body fatness. Because the amount of body fat, not the amount of weight, is the important factor in living a healthy life, it is better to determine the percentage of your body weight which is body fat (**percent body fat**).

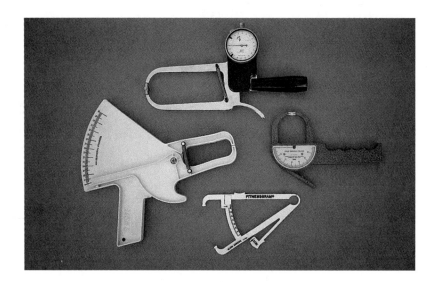

Figure 13.1
Skinfold calipers.

There are many ways to assess body fatness and leanness.

Underwater weighing, also referred to as "hydrostatic weighing," is considered the gold standard for assessing body fatness. In this laboratory procedure, a person is weighed underwater and out of the water. Corrections are made for the amount of air in the lungs when the underwater weight is measured. Using Archimedes principle, the body's density can be determined. Because the density of various body tissues is known, the amount of the total body fat can be determined. Body fatness is usually expressed in terms of a percentage of the total body weight. Because this procedure takes considerable time, equipment, and specialized training, it is not practical for use except in well-equipped laboratories. Other ways of measuring body fatness are X rays, ultrasound, impedence measurements, body girths, and skinfold measurements. Not all of these have been shown to be reliable and valid. Skinfold measurements are often used because they are relatively easy to do (see figure 13.1). This is not nearly as costly as underwater weighing or X rays. The better, more accurate calipers cost several hundred dollars. However, considerably less expensive calipers are now available. When used by a trained person, these calipers give a good estimate of fatness (see Lab Resource Materials on page 156). An expert's estimate of your body fatness determined by skinfold measurements is informative. It will also be useful for you to learn to use calipers correctly so that you can take your own measurements throughout your life.

Body fat is distributed throughout the body. About one-half of the body's fat is located around the various body organs and in the muscles. The other half of the body's fat is located just under the skin, or in skinfolds

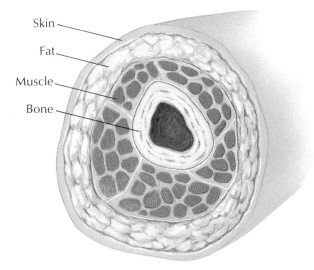

Figure 13.2
Location of body fat.

(figure 13.2). A skinfold is two thicknesses of skin and the amount of fat that lies just under the skin. At certain locations in the body, the thickness of the skinfolds can be used to obtain a good estimate of total body fatness (figure 13.3). In general, the more skinfolds measured, the more accurate the body fatness estimate. However, measurements with three skinfolds have been shown to be reasonably accurate and can be done in a relatively short period (see Lab Resource Materials).

Body girth measurements, especially those using only one or two body points, are less accurate than skinfolds but they are easy to do. As the sole measure of fatness, they should be used with caution. They can provide a useful second or third source of information about body fatness, however.

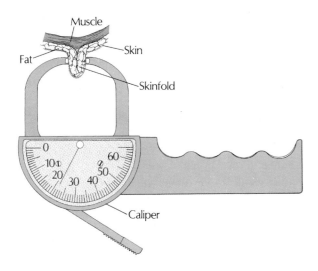

Figure 13.3
Measuring body fat.

The Facts About Body Composition and Health

Overfatness or obesity can contribute to degenerative diseases, health problems, and even shortened life.

Some diseases and health problems associated with overfatness and obesity are presented in Concept 3. In addition to the higher incidence of certain diseases and health problems, there is evidence that people who are moderately overfat have a 40 percent higher than normal risk of shortening their lifespan. More severe obesity results in a 70 percent higher than normal death rate. This is evidenced by the exorbitant life insurance premiums paid by obese individuals.

Recent statistics indicating that underweight people had a higher than normal risk of premature death are very deceptive. Many people included in the data were underweight because of terminal illnesses. Most experts agree that those people who are free from disease and who have lower than average amounts of body fat have a lower than average risk of premature death.

Excessive abdominal fat and excessive fatness of the upper body can increase the risk of various diseases.

Several research studies have shown that a relationship exists between the amount of abdominal fat and various health problems. For this reason it is important to keep both your total body fat and abdominal fat levels low, especially as you grow older. Other studies have shown that upper body fatness (from the waist up) produces a greater health risk than lower body fatness (from the waist down).

Skinfold measures of abdominal fatness could be used to help you monitor abdominal and upper body fatness. Another useful measurement that can be done at home is called the "waist-to-hip circumference ratio." This ratio is calculated using waist and hip circumference measurements. The technique for determining this ratio is described on page 162. A high ratio has been shown to be correlated with a high incidence of heart attack, stroke, chest pain, breast cancer, and death. Recent evidence indicates that people who exercise regularly accumulate less fat in the upper central regions of the body as they get older. This suggests that regular exercise throughout life will result in a smaller waist-to-hip ratio and a reduced risk of various life-style diseases.

Excessive desire to be thin or low in body fat can result in health problems.

In Western society the near obsession with thinness has been, at least in part, responsible for health conditions now referred to as eating disorders. Eating disorders, or altered eating habits, involve extreme restriction of food intake and/or regurgitation of food to avoid digestion. The most common disorders are anorexia nervosa, bulimia, and anorexia athletica. All of these disorders are most common among highly achievement-oriented girls and young women, although they effect virtually all segments of the population.

Anorexia nervosa is the most severe of the three disorders. In fact, if not treated, it is life threatening. Anorexics restrict food intake so severely that the body becomes emaciated. Among the many characteristics of the anorexic are fear of maturity and inaccurate body image. The anorexic starves herself/himself and may exercise compulsively or use laxatives to prevent the digestion of food in an attempt to attain excessive leanness. The anorexic's image of self is one of being "too fat" even when the person is too lean for good health. Assessing body fatness using procedures such as skinfolds and observation of the eating habits may help identify those with anorexia. Among anorexic girls and women, development of an adult figure is often feared. It is important that people with this disorder obtain medical and psychological help immediately, as the consequences are severe. Those with anorexia may also have some of the characteristics of the bulimic.

Bulimics may or may not be anorexic. It may not be possible to identify the bulimic with measures of body fatness, as they may be lean, normal, or excessively fat. The most common characteristics of bulimia are binging and purging. Binging means the periodic eating of large amounts of food at one time. A "binge" might occur after a relatively long period of dieting and often consists of junk foods containing empty calories. After a binge, the bulimic "purges" the body of the food by forced regurgitation. The bulimic may also use laxatives to purge. Another form of bulimia is binging on one day and starving on the next. The consequences of bulimia are not as severe as anorexia, but can result in serious mental and dental problems.

Anorexia athletica is a recently identified eating disorder that appears to be related to participation in sports and activities, such as ballet, that emphasize excessive body leanness. Studies show that participants in sports such as gymnastics, wrestling, body building, and activities such as ballet and cheerleading are most likely to develop anorexia athletica. This disorder has many of the symptoms of anorexia nervosa, but not of the same severity. In some cases, anorexia athletica can lead to anorexia nervosa.

Fear of obesity is a newly discovered condition that is not as severe as anorexia nervosa, but it can still have negative health consequences. This condition is most common among achievement-oriented teenagers who impose a self-restriction on caloric intake because they fear obesity. Consequences include stunting of growth, delayed puberty and sexual development, and decreased physical attractiveness. It is important to avoid excessive eating and inactivity to prevent the problems associated with overfatness and obesity; however, an overconcern for leanness can result in serious health problems, too.

Society can help reduce the incidence of eating disorders by changing its image of "attractiveness"—especially among young women. Many of the models and movie stars who convey the "ideal" image are anorexic or are exceptionally thin. Teachers and athletic coaches can help by educating people about these disorders, by not placing too much emphasis on leanness, and by screening students with procedures such as skinfolds and body mass index. Parents and friends can help by looking for excessive changes in body weight and lack of eating. Once an eating disorder is identified, it is important to help the individual obtain treatment for the problem.

The Facts About the Origin of Overfatness

Heredity plays a role in overfatness.

Some people have suggested that every individual is born with a set body weight. Advocates of this *set point theory* feel that it will be difficult for people to deviate from their "set point weight," which is predetermined by heredity. Though many experts question the validity of set point theory for humans, they agree that there is such a thing as a familial predisposition to obesity. For years, researchers have suggested that your body type, or **somatotype,** is inherited. Clearly, some people will have more difficulty than others controlling fatness because of their body types and because they come from families with a history of obesity. Scientists caution people from families

with a history of obesity *not to conclude that nothing can be done to prevent obesity*. It has been shown that weight reduction programs can be effective *among those with a predisposition to obesity*. Research also shows that regular exercise is especially effective in the control of genetically determined overfatness.

Glandular disorders can play a role in overfatness.

Glandular disorders can cause or contribute to overfatness. For example, thyroid problems can cause a low metabolic rate that results in fat gain. However, most experts suggest that only one to two percent of all overfatness is directly caused by problems of this type. Medical treatment is necessary for people suffering with these problems.

Fatness early in life leads to adult fatness.

Retention of baby fat is not a sign of good health. On the contrary, excess body fat in the early years is a health problem of considerable concern. As many as 25 percent of American schoolchildren are overfat. Of these children, four of five will become overfat adults. Twenty-eight of twenty-nine teenagers who are too fat will become overfat adults.

There is evidence that childhood overfatness results in hyperplasia, or an increased number of fat cells. People who have these extra fat cells are thought to have a greater tendency to become overfat. It was previously thought that only adult obesity was related to health problems. We now know that teens (ages 13–18) who are too fat are at greater risk of heart problems and cancer than their lean peers.

Changes in basal metabolic rate can be the cause of overfatness.

Basal metabolic rate (BMR) is highest during the growing years. The amount of food eaten increases to support this increased energy expenditure. When growing ceases, if eating does not decrease or activity level increase, fatness can result. Basal metabolism also decreases gradually as you grow older. One major reason for this is the loss of muscle mass associated with inactivity. Regular exercise throughout life helps keep the muscle mass higher, resulting in a higher BMR. Very recent evidence suggests that regular exercise can contribute in other ways to increased BMR. The higher BMR of active people helps them prevent overfatness, particularly in later life.

"Creeping obesity" is a problem as you grow older.

When people become less active and their BMR gradually decreases with age, even when eating habits remain the same, body fat increases. This is commonly referred to as "creeping obesity" because the increase in fatness is

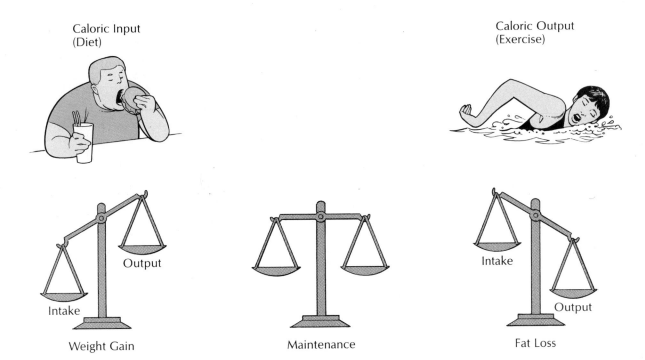

Caloric Input
(Diet)

Caloric Output
(Exercise)

Output

Intake

Weight Gain

Intake

Output

Fat Loss

Maintenance

Figure 13.4
Balancing calorie input and output.

gradual. For a typical person, creeping obesity could result in one-half to one pound of fat gain per year. People who stay active can keep muscle mass high and delay changes in BMR. For those who are not active, it is suggested that caloric intake decrease by three percent each decade after twenty-five so that by age sixty-five, caloric intake is at least ten percent less than it was at age twenty-five. The decrease in calorie intake for active people need not be as great.

The principal cause of most overfatness is the intake of more calories than are expended.

Though fatness may be associated with any of the factors mentioned previously, and overfatness is no doubt the result of multiple causes, excessive food (calorie) intake and/or lack of energy expenditure (exercise) are responsible for most overfatness. (See figure 13.4.) Threshold of training and target zones for body fat reduction, including information for both exercise and **diet** are presented in table 13.2.

Excess caloric intake or calorie expenditure results in an increase in fat cell size.

Overfatness can result in an increase in the number of fat cells among children. For adults, overfatness is a result of the increase in size of fat cells (*hypertrophy*). When fat cells become excessively large, they can cause dimples or lumps under the skin. Some people refer to these large fat cells as *cellulite*. Quacks try to create the impression that this type of fat is different from other types of fat and is removed from the body in different ways than regular fat. This is not true. All fatness among adults is a result of enlarged fat cells. All fat is lost as a result of reduction in fat cell size.

The Facts About Diet, Exercise, and Fatness

An overview of the role of diet and exercise in fat control is presented in this section. A more extensive discussion of practical methods for controlling body fatness is presented in Concept 14.

A combination of regular exercise and dietary restriction is the most effective means of losing body fat.

Studies indicate that exercise combined with dietary restriction is the *most* effective method of losing fat. One study of adult women indicated that diet alone resulted in loss of weight, but much of this loss was lean body tissue. Those studied who were dieting as well as exercising experienced similar weight losses, but this loss included more body fat. On the basis of this research, all weight loss programs should combine a lower caloric intake with a good physical exercise program.

Table 13.2
Threshold of Training and Target Zones for Body Fat Reduction

	Threshold of Training*		Target Zones*	
	Exercise	Diet	Exercise	Diet
Frequency	• To be effective, exercise must be regular, preferably daily, though fat can be lost over the long term with almost any frequency that results in increased caloric expenditure.	• It is best to reduce caloric intake consistently and daily. To restrict calories only on certain days is *not* best, though fat can be lost over a period of time by reducing caloric intake at any time.	• Daily moderate exercise is recommended. For those who do regular vigorous activity, 5 or 6 days per week may be best.	• It is best to diet consistently and daily.
Intensity	• To lose 1 pound of fat, you must expend 3,500 calories more than you normally expend.	• To lose 1 pound of fat, you must eat 3,500 calories fewer than you normally eat.	• Slow, low-intensity aerobic exercise that results in no more than 1–2 pounds of fat loss per week is best.	• Modest caloric restriction resulting in no more than 1–2 pounds of fat loss per week is best.
Time	• To be effective, exercise must be sustained long enough to expend a considerable number of calories. At least 15 minutes per exercise bout are necessary to result in consistent fat loss.	• Eating moderate meals is best. Do not skip meals.	• Exercise durations similar to those for achieving aerobic cardiovascular fitness seem best. An exercise duration of 30–60 minutes is recommended.	• Eating moderate meals is best. Skipping meals or fasting is *not* most effective.

*Note: It is best to combine exercise and diet to achieve the 3,500 caloric imbalance necessary to lose a pound of fat. Using both exercise and diet in the target zone is most effective.

Good exercise and diet habits can be useful in maintaining desirable body composition.

Table 13.2 illustrates how fat can be lost through regular exercise and proper dieting. However, not all people want to lose fat. For those who wish to maintain their current body composition, a **caloric balance** between intake and output is effective. For those who want to increase their lean body weight, increased caloric intake with increased exercise can result in the desired changes.

Exercise is one effective means of controlling body fat.

Though physical activity or exercise will not result in immediate and large decreases in body fat levels, there is increasing evidence that fat loss resulting from exercise may be more lasting than fat loss from dieting. Vigorous exercise can increase the resting energy expenditure up to thirteen times (13 **METs**).

Inactivity is more often the cause of childhood obesity than overeating. Many fat children eat less but are considerably less active than their nonfat peers. Excessive television watching may be one reason for inactivity among children. Studies show that adults who watch more than three hours of television per day are twice as likely to be obese as those who view television for less than one hour per day.

If you exercise moderately for an extra fifteen minutes a day, you will lose up to ten pounds in a year's time. Regular walking, jogging, swimming, or any type of sustained exercise can be effective in producing losses in body fat.

Exercise that can be sustained for relatively long periods is probably the most effective for losing body fat.

Table 13.3 shows the caloric expenditures for one hour of involvement in various recreational physical activities. The heavier the person, the more **calories** expended because more work is required to move larger bodies. Activities that are extremely vigorous can help in losing body fatness if done regularly. For many people, these may not be as effective as some less vigorous activities. For example, running at ten miles per hour (a six-minute mile) will cause a 150-pound person to expend 900 calories in one hour. Jogging about half as fast, or at five and one-half miles per hour (approximately an eleven-minute mile), will result in an expenditure of about 650 calories in the same amount of time. At first glance, the more vigorous exercise seems to be a better choice. But how many people can continue to run at a ten-mile-per-hour pace for a full hour? Each mile run at ten miles per hour results in an expenditure of 90 calories, while each mile run at five and one-half miles per hour results in an expenditure of 118 calories.

Table 13.3

Calories Expended per Hour in Various Physical Activities (Performed at a Recreational Level)*

Activity	Calories Used per Hour				
	100 lbs (146 kgs.)	120 lbs (55 kgs.)	150 lbs (68 kgs.)	180 lbs (82 kgs.)	200 lbs (91 kgs.)
Archery	180	204	240	276	300
Backpacking (40-lb. pack)	307	348	410	472	513
Badminton	255	289	340	391	425
Baseball	210	238	280	322	350
Basketball (half court)	225	255	300	345	375
Bicycling (normal speed)	157	178	210	242	263
Bowling	155	176	208	240	261
Canoeing (4 mph)	276	344	414	504	558
Circuit training	247	280	330	380	413
Dance, ballet (choreographed)	240	300	360	432	480
Dance, aerobics	315	357	420	483	525
Dance, modern (choreographed)	240	300	360	432	480
Dance, social	174	222	264	318	348
Fencing	225	255	300	345	375
Fitness calisthenics	232	263	310	357	388
Football	225	255	300	345	375
Golf (walking)	187	212	250	288	313
Gymnastics	232	263	310	357	388
Handball	450	510	600	690	750
Hiking	225	255	300	345	375
Horseback riding	180	204	240	276	300
Interval training	487	552	650	748	833
Jogging (5½ mph)	487	552	650	748	833
Judo/karate	232	263	310	357	388
Mountain climbing	450	510	600	690	750
Pool; billiards	97	110	130	150	163
Racquetball; paddleball	450	510	600	690	750
Rope jumping (continuous)	525	595	700	805	875
Rowing, crew	615	697	820	943	1025
Running (10 mph)	625	765	900	1035	1125
Sailing (pleasure)	135	153	180	207	225
Skating, ice	262	297	350	403	438
Skating, roller/inline	262	297	350	403	438
Skiing, cross-country	525	595	700	805	875
Skiing, downhill	450	510	600	690	750
Soccer	405	459	540	621	775
Softball (fast)	210	238	280	322	350
Softball (slow)	217	246	290	334	363
Surfing	416	467	550	633	684
Swimming (slow laps)	240	272	320	368	400
Swimming (fast laps)	420	530	630	768	846
Table tennis	180	204	240	276	300
Tennis	315	357	420	483	525
Volleyball	262	297	350	403	483
Walking	204	258	318	372	426
Waterskiing	306	390	468	564	636
Weight training	352	399	470	541	558

*Note: Locate your weight to determine the calories expended per hour in each of the activities shown in the table based on recreational involvement. More vigorous activity, as occurs in competitive athletics, may result in greater caloric expenditures.

From C. B. Corbin and R. Lindsey, *Fitness for Life*, 3d ed. Copyright © 1993 Scott, Foresman and Company. Reprinted by permission of Scott, Foresman and Company.

Per mile, you expend more calories in slow running. It takes longer to run a mile, but by the same token, you can also persist longer. The key is to expend as many calories as possible during each regular exercise period. Doing less vigorous activity for longer periods is better for fat control than doing very vigorous activities that can be done only for short periods.

Appetite is not necessarily increased through exercise.

The human animal was intended to be an active animal. For this reason, the human "appetite thermostat" (called the appestat by some) is set as if all people are active. Those who are inactive do not have a decreased appetite. Likewise, if a person is sedentary and then begins regular exercise, the appetite does not necessarily increase because this "appetite thermostat" expects activity. Very vigorous activity does not necessarily cause an appetite increase that is proportional to the calories expended in the vigorous exercise.

Suggested Readings

Avery, C. "Abdominal Obesity: Scaling Down This Deadly Risk." *Physician and Sportsmedicine* 19(1991):113.

Foreyt, J. "Factors Common to Successful Therapy for the Obese Patient." *Medicine and Science in Sports and Exercise* 23(1991):292.

Williams, M. H. *Nutrition for Fitness and Sport.* 3/e Dubuque, IA: Wm. C. Brown Publishers, 1992.

LAB RESOURCE MATERIALS

(For use with Labs 13A or 13B, pages L-33–L-36)

Evaluating Body Fatness

Skinfold Measurements

Skinfold measurements are made with skinfold calipers. Some of the more accurate and expensive calipers are the Harpenden, the Lange, and the Lafayette calipers. Some of the less expensive calipers include the Slimguide, the Fat-O-Meter, and the Adipometer. Regardless of the type employed, it is important to use a consistent procedure for "drawing up" or "pinching up" a skinfold and making the measurement with the caliper. The following procedures should be used for each skinfold site.

1. Lay the caliper down on a nearby table. Use the thumbs and index fingers of both hands to "draw up" a skinfold or layer of skin and fat. The fingers and thumbs of the two hands should be about one inch apart, or half an inch on either side of the location where the measurement is to be made.

2. The skinfolds are normally "drawn up" in a vertical line rather than a horizontal line. However, if the natural tendency of the skin aligns itself less than vertical, the measurement should be done on the natural line of the skinfold, rather than on the vertical.

3. Do not "pinch" the skinfold too hard. Draw it up so that your thumbs and fingers are not compressing the skinfold.

4. Once the skinfold is "drawn up," let go with your right hand and pick up the caliper. Open the jaws of the caliper and place them over the location of the skinfold to be measured and one-half inch from your left index finger and thumb. Allow the tips, or jaw faces, of the caliper to close on the skinfold at a level about where the skin would be normally.

5. Let the reading on the caliper "settle" for two or three seconds, then note the thickness of the skinfold in millimeters.

6. Three measurements should be taken at each location. Use the middle of the three values to determine your measurement. For example, if you had values of 10, 11, and 9, your measurement for that location would be 10. If the three measures vary by more than 3 millimeters from the lowest to the highest, you may want to take additional measurements.

Skinfold Locations for Women

A. *Triceps Skinfold*—Make a mark on the back of the right arm, one-half the distance between the tip of the shoulder and the tip of the elbow. Make the measurement at this location.

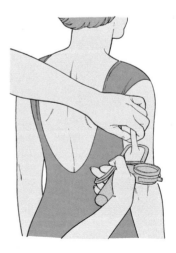

B. *Iliac Crest Skinfold*—Make a mark at the top front of the iliac crest. This skinfold is taken slightly diagonally because of the natural line of the skin.

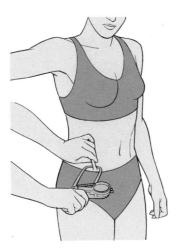

C. *Thigh Skinfold*—Make a mark on the front of the thigh midway between the hip and the knee. Make the measurement vertically at this location.

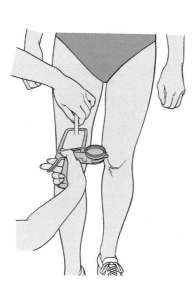

Skinfold Locations for Men

A. *Chest Skinfold*—Make a mark above and to the right of the right nipple (one-half the distance from the midline of the side and the nipple). The measurement at this location is often done on the diagonal because of the natural line of the skin.

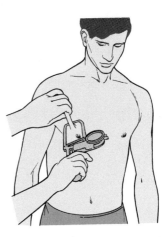

B. *Abdominal Skinfold*—Make a mark on the skin approximately one inch to the right of the navel. Make a vertical measurement at that location.

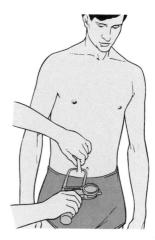

C. *Thigh Skinfold*—Make a mark on the front of the thigh midway between the hip and the knee. Make a vertical measurement at this location (same as for women).

Calculating Fatness from Skinfolds

1. Sum the three skinfolds (triceps, iliac crest, and thigh for women, chest, abdominal, and thigh for men).
2. Use the skinfold sum and your age to determine your percent fat using charts 13A.1 (men) and 13A.2 (women). Locate your sum of skinfolds in the left column and your age at the top of the chart. Your estimated body fat percentage is located where the values intersect.
3. Use chart 13A.3 to determine your fatness rating.

Sum of Skinfolds (mm)	Age to the Last Year								
	22 and Under	23 to 27	28 to 32	33 to 37	38 to 42	43 to 47	48 to 52	53 to 57	Over 58
8–10	1.3	1.8	2.3	2.9	3.4	3.9	4.5	5.0	5.5
11–13	2.2	2.8	3.3	3.9	4.4	4.9	5.5	6.0	6.5
14–16	3.2	3.8	4.3	4.8	5.4	5.9	6.4	7.0	7.5
17–19	4.2	4.7	5.3	5.8	6.3	6.9	7.4	8.0	8.5
20–22	5.1	5.7	6.2	6.8	7.3	7.9	8.4	8.9	9.5
23–25	6.1	6.6	7.2	7.7	8.3	8.8	9.4	9.9	10.5
26–28	7.0	7.6	8.1	8.7	9.2	9.8	10.3	10.9	11.4
29–31	8.0	8.5	9.1	9.6	10.2	10.7	11.3	11.8	12.4
32–34	8.9	9.4	10.0	10.5	11.1	11.6	12.2	12.8	13.3
35–37	9.8	10.4	10.9	11.5	12.0	12.6	13.1	13.7	14.3
38–40	10.7	11.3	11.8	12.4	12.9	13.5	14.1	14.6	15.2
41–43	11.6	12.2	12.7	13.3	13.8	14.4	15.0	15.5	16.1
44–46	12.5	13.1	13.6	14.2	14.7	15.3	15.9	16.4	17.0
47–49	13.4	13.9	14.5	15.1	15.6	16.2	16.8	17.3	17.9
50–52	14.3	14.8	15.4	15.9	16.5	17.1	17.6	18.1	18.8
53–55	15.1	15.7	16.2	16.8	17.4	17.9	18.5	18.2	19.7
56–58	16.0	16.5	17.1	17.7	18.2	18.8	19.4	20.0	20.5
59–61	16.9	17.4	17.9	18.5	19.1	19.7	20.2	20.8	21.4
62–64	17.6	18.2	18.8	19.4	19.9	20.5	21.1	21.7	22.2
65–67	18.5	19.0	19.6	20.2	20.8	21.3	21.9	22.5	23.1
68–70	19.3	19.9	20.4	21.0	21.6	22.2	22.7	23.3	23.9
71–73	20.1	20.7	21.2	21.8	22.4	23.0	23.6	24.1	24.7
74–76	20.9	21.5	22.0	22.6	23.2	23.8	24.4	25.0	25.5
77–79	21.7	22.2	22.8	23.4	24.0	24.6	25.2	25.8	26.3
80–82	22.4	23.0	23.6	24.2	24.8	25.4	25.9	26.5	27.1
83–85	23.2	23.8	24.4	25.0	25.5	26.1	26.7	27.3	27.9
86–88	24.0	24.5	25.1	25.5	26.3	26.9	27.5	28.1	28.7
89–91	24.7	25.3	25.9	25.7	27.1	27.6	28.2	28.8	29.4
92–94	25.4	26.0	26.6	27.2	27.8	28.4	29.0	29.6	30.2
95–97	26.1	26.7	27.3	27.9	28.5	29.1	29.7	30.3	30.9
98–100	26.9	27.4	28.0	28.6	29.2	29.8	30.4	31.0	31.6
101–103	27.5	28.1	28.7	29.3	29.9	30.5	31.1	31.7	32.3
104–106	28.2	28.8	29.4	30.0	30.6	31.2	31.8	32.4	33.0
107–109	28.9	29.5	30.1	30.7	31.3	31.9	32.5	33.1	33.7
110–112	29.6	30.2	30.8	31.4	32.0	32.6	33.2	33.8	34.4
113–115	30.2	30.8	31.4	32.0	32.6	33.2	33.8	34.5	35.1
116–118	30.9	31.5	32.1	32.7	33.3	33.9	34.5	35.1	35.7
119–121	31.5	32.1	32.7	33.3	33.9	34.5	35.1	35.7	36.4
122–124	32.1	32.7	33.3	33.9	34.5	35.1	35.8	36.4	37.0
125–127	32.7	33.3	33.9	34.5	35.1	35.8	36.4	37.0	37.6

*Percent fat calculated by the formula by Siri. Percent fat = $[(4.95/BD) - 4.5] \times 100$, where BD = body density.

From *Comprehensive Therapy*, 6(9):12–27, 1980. The Laux Company, Inc., P.O. Box 700, Ayer, MA 01432.

Chart 13A.2 Percent Fat Estimates for Women, Sum of Triceps, Iliac Crest, and Thigh Skinfolds*

Sum of Skinfolds (mm)	22 and Under	23 to 27	28 to 32	33 to 37	38 to 42	43 to 47	48 to 52	53 to 57	Over 58
23–25	9.7	9.9	10.2	10.4	10.7	10.9	11.2	11.4	11.7
26–28	11.0	11.2	11.5	11.7	12.0	12.3	12.5	12.7	13.0
29–31	12.3	12.5	12.8	13.0	13.3	13.5	13.8	14.0	14.3
32–34	13.6	13.8	14.0	14.3	14.5	14.8	15.0	15.3	15.5
35–37	14.8	15.0	15.3	15.5	15.8	16.0	16.3	16.5	16.8
38–40	16.0	16.3	16.5	16.7	17.0	17.2	17.5	17.7	18.0
41–43	17.2	17.4	17.7	17.9	18.2	18.4	18.7	18.9	19.2
44–46	18.3	18.6	18.8	19.1	19.3	19.6	19.8	20.1	20.3
47–49	19.5	19.7	20.0	20.2	20.5	20.7	21.0	21.2	21.5
50–52	20.6	20.8	21.1	21.3	21.6	21.8	22.1	22.3	22.6
53–55	21.7	21.9	22.1	22.4	22.6	22.9	23.1	23.4	23.6
56–58	22.7	23.0	23.2	23.4	23.7	23.9	24.2	24.4	24.7
59–61	23.7	24.0	24.2	24.5	24.7	25.0	25.2	25.5	25.7
62–64	24.7	25.0	25.2	25.5	35.7	26.0	26.7	26.4	26.7
65–67	25.7	25.9	26.2	26.4	26.7	26.9	27.2	27.4	27.7
68–70	26.6	26.9	27.1	27.4	27.6	27.9	28.1	28.4	28.6
71–73	27.5	27.8	28.0	28.3	28.5	28.8	28.0	29.3	29.5
74–76	28.4	28.7	28.9	29.2	29.4	29.7	29.9	30.2	30.4
77–79	29.3	29.5	29.8	30.0	30.3	30.5	30.8	31.0	31.3
80–82	30.1	30.4	30.6	30.9	31.1	31.4	31.6	31.9	32.1
83–85	30.9	31.2	31.4	31.7	31.9	32.2	32.4	32.7	32.9
86–88	31.7	32.0	32.2	32.5	32.7	32.9	33.2	33.4	33.7
89–91	32.5	32.7	33.0	33.2	33.5	33.7	33.9	34.2	34.4
92–94	33.2	33.4	33.7	33.9	34.2	34.4	34.7	34.9	35.2
95–97	33.9	34.1	34.4	34.6	34.9	35.1	35.4	35.6	35.9
98–100	34.6	34.8	35.1	35.3	35.5	35.8	36.0	36.3	36.5
101–103	35.3	35.4	35.7	35.9	36.2	36.4	36.7	36.9	37.2
104–106	35.8	36.1	36.3	36.6	36.8	37.1	37.3	37.5	37.8
107–109	36.4	36.7	36.9	37.1	37.4	37.6	37.9	38.1	38.4
110–112	37.0	37.2	37.5	37.7	38.0	38.2	38.5	38.7	38.9
113–115	37.5	37.8	38.0	38.2	38.5	38.7	39.0	39.2	39.5
116–118	38.0	38.3	38.5	38.8	39.0	39.3	39.5	39.7	40.0
119–121	38.5	38.7	39.0	39.2	39.5	39.7	40.0	40.2	40.5
122–124	39.0	39.2	39.4	39.7	39.9	40.2	40.4	40.7	40.9
125–127	39.4	39.6	39.9	40.1	40.4	40.6	40.9	41.1	41.4
128–130	39.8	40.0	40.3	40.5	40.8	41.0	41.3	41.5	41.8

*Percent fat calculated by the formula of Siri. Percent fat = [4.95/BD) − 4.5] × 100, where BD = body density.

From *Comprehensive Therapy*, 6(9):12–27, 1980. The Laux Company, Inc., P.O. Box 700, Ayer, MA 01432.

Chart 13A.3 Fatness *Rating Scale*

Classification	Men	Women
Excessively lean	Less than 5%	Less than 8%
High performance zone	5%–9%	12%–17%*
Good fitness zone	10%–20%	18%–25%
Marginal zone	21%–25%	26%–30%
Obese zone	> 25%	> 30%

It is recommended that these standards be maintained throughout life regardless of age.

*Experts believe that less than 12% is not desirable for females doing most types of athletic performance.

Determining the Waist-to-Hip Circumference Ratio

The Waist-to-Hip Circumference Ratio is recommended by experts (Van Stallie 1988) as the best available index for determining risk and disease associated with fat and weight distribution. As pointed out in Concept 13, disease and death risk are associated with abdominal and upper body fatness. When a person has both high fatness and a high waist-to-hip ratio, additional risks exist. The following steps should be taken in making measurements and calculating the waist-to-hip ratio.

1. Both measurements should be done with a nonelastic tape. Make the measurements while standing with the feet together and the arms at the sides, elevated only high enough to allow the measurements. Be sure that the tape is horizontal around the entire circumference.

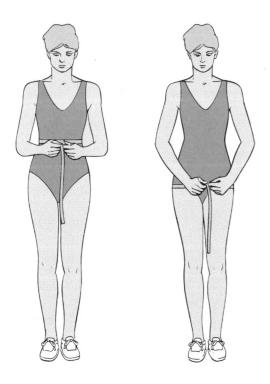

Chart 13A.4 Waist-to-Hip Ratio *Rating Scale*

Classification	Men	Women
High risk	> 1.0	> .85
Moderately high risk	.90–1.0	.80–.85
Lower risk	< .90	< .80

Source: Data from Van Stallie, 1988.

Record scores to the nearest millimeter or 1/16th of an inch. Use the same units of measure for both circumferences (millimeters or 1/16th of an inch). The tape should be pulled snugly but not to the point of causing an indentation in the skin.

2. *Waist Measurement.* Measure at the natural waist (smallest waist circumference). If there is no natural waist, the measurement should be made at the level of the umbilicus. Measure at the end of a normal inspiration.

3. *Hip Measurement.* Measure at the maximum circumference of the buttocks. It is recommended that the measurement be made in briefs that do not add significantly to the measurement.

4. Divide the hip measurement into the waist measurement to determine your waist-to-hip ratio.

5. Use chart 13A.4 to determine your rating for the waist-to-hip ratio.

Height-Weight Measurements

1. *Height.* Measure your height in inches or centimeters. Take the measurement without shoes, but add 2.5 centimeters or 1 inch to measurements, as the charts are based on heels of this height.

2. *Weight.* Measure your weight in pounds or kilograms without clothes. Add 3 pounds or 1.4 kilograms because charts are based on clothes of this weight. If weight must be taken with clothes on, wear indoor clothing of 3 pounds or 1.4 kilograms in weight.

3. Determine your frame size using the elbow breadth. The measurement is most accurate when done with a broad-faced sliding caliper. However, it can be done using a skinfold caliper or can be estimated with a metric ruler. The right arm is measured when it is elevated with the elbow bent at 90 degrees and the upper arm horizontal. The back of the hand should

face the person making the measurement. Using the caliper, measure the distance between the epicondyles of the humerus (inside and outside bony points of the elbow). Measure to the nearest millimeter (1/10 of a centimeter). If a caliper is not available, place the thumb and the index finger of the left hand on the epicondyles of the humerus and measure the distance between the fingers with a metric ruler. Use your height and elbow breadth in centimeters to determine your frame size using chart 13B.1. Once you have determined your frame size, you need not repeat this procedure each time you use a height-weight chart.

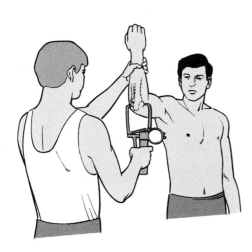

Chart 13B.2 Determination of "Desirable" Weight for Men

Height Feet	Inches	Small Frame	Medium Frame	Large Frame
5	2	128–134	131–141	138–150
5	3	130–136	133–143	140–153
5	4	132–138	135–145	142–156
5	5	134–140	137–148	144–160
5	6	136–142	139–151	146–164
5	7	138–145	142–154	149–168
5	8	140–148	145–157	152–172
5	9	142–151	148–160	155–176
5	10	144–154	151–163	158–180
5	11	146–157	154–166	161–184
6	0	149–160	157–170	164–188
6	1	152–164	160–174	168–192
6	2	155–168	164–178	172–197
6	3	158–172	167–182	176–202
6	4	162–176	171–187	181–207

Weights at ages 25–59 based on lowest mortality. Weight in pounds according to frame (in indoor clothing weighing 3 lbs., shoes with 1″ heels).

Courtesy of the Metropolitan Life Insurance Company.

To make a metric conversion, see Appendix A.

Chart 13B.1 Frame Size Determined from Height (ft. and in.) and Elbow Breadth (mm)

Height	Small	Frame Size Medium	Large
Males			
5′ 2½″ or less	< 64	64–72	> 72
5′ 3″–5′ 6½″	< 67	67–74	> 74
5′ 7″–5′ 10½″	< 69	69–76	> 76
5′ 11″–6′ 2½″	< 71	71–78	> 78
6′ 3″ or more	< 74	74–81	> 81
Females			
4′ 10½″ or less	< 56	56–64	> 64
4′ 11″–5′ 2½″	< 58	58–65	> 65
5′ 3″–5′ 6½″	< 59	59–66	> 66
5′ 7″–5′ 10½″	< 61	61–68	> 69
5′ 11″ or more	< 62	62–69	> 69

Height is given including one-inch heels.

Courtesy of the Metropolitan Life Insurance Company.

Chart 13B.3 Determination of "Desirable" Weight for Women

Height Feet	Inches	Small Frame	Medium Frame	Large Frame
4	10	102–111	109–121	118–131
4	11	103–113	111–123	120–134
5	0	104–115	113–126	122–137
5	1	106–118	115–129	125–140
5	2	108–121	118–132	128–143
5	3	111–124	121–135	131–147
5	4	114–127	124–138	134–151
5	5	117–130	127–141	137–155
5	6	120–133	130–144	140–159
5	7	123–136	133–147	143–163
5	8	126–139	136–150	146–167
5	9	129–142	139–153	149–170
5	10	132–145	142–156	152–173
5	11	135–148	145–159	155–176
6	0	138–151	148–162	158–179

Weights at ages 25–59 based on lowest mortality. Weight in pounds according to frame (in indoor clothing weighing 3 lbs., shoes with 1″ heels).

Courtesy of the Metropolitan Life Insurance Company.

To make a metric conversion, see Appendix A.

Chart 13B.4 Determination of Desirable Body Weight for Men (those above 16% fat)

16	18	20	22	24	**Estimated Percent Fat** 26	28	30	32	34	36	38	40
240	234	230	225	220	215	210	206	201	196	191	186	182
235	229	225	220	215	210	206	201	196	192	187	182	178
230	224	220	215	210	206	201	197	192	187	183	178	174
225	220	216	211	207	202	198	193	189	184	180	175	171
221	215	211	206	202	197	193	189	184	180	175	171	167
215	210	206	201	197	193	188	184	180	175	171	167	163
210	205	202	200	192	188	184	180	175	171	167	163	159
205	200	197	191	187	183	179	175	171	167	163	159	155
200	196	192	188	184	180	176	172	168	164	160	156	152
195	190	187	183	179	175	171	167	163	159	155	151	148
190	185	182	178	174	170	166	163	159	155	151	147	144
185	180	177	173	169	165	162	158	154	151	147	143	140
180	175	172	168	164	161	157	154	150	146	143	139	136
175	171	168	164	161	157	154	150	147	143	140	136	133
170	166	163	159	156	152	149	146	142	139	135	132	129
165	161	158	154	151	148	144	141	138	134	131	128	125
160	157	153	149	146	143	140	137	133	130	127	124	121
155	151	148	144	141	138	135	132	129	126	123	120	117
150	147	144	141	138	135	132	129	126	123	120	117	114
145	141	139	136	133	130	127	124	121	118	115	112	110
140	136	134	131	128	125	122	120	117	114	111	108	100
135	131	129	126	123	120	118	115	112	110	107	104	102
130	126	124	121	118	116	113	111	108	105	103	102	98
125	122	120	117	115	112	110	107	105	102	100	97	95
120	117	115	112	110	107	105	103	100	98	95	93	91

Along the side, locate your current body weight; across the top, locate your estimated percent fat. The intersection of the two entries is your desirable weight (fat-free body weight plus 16 percent fat). Example: 175 pounds is the desirable weight for a man who weighs 195 pounds and currently has a total body fat of 26 percent.

Note: This chart uses 16 percent as a "desirable" fat level for males. People who have less than 16 percent fat need NOT use it because they already possess a healthy body weight and level of body fat unless they have less than 5 percent body fat, in which case some gain in body fat is recommended. Sixteen percent was selected as a "desirable" level even though up to 20 percent fat is considered in the good fitness zone. For this reason it should be noted that this chart is designed to give you a general guideline for "desirable" weight and should NOT be used as an absolute standard, especially as you grow older.

To make a metric conversion, see Appendix A.

Body Mass Index (BMI)

The BMI is calculated using the following formula:

$$\frac{\text{body weight in kilograms}}{(\text{height in meters})^2}$$

Use the steps listed below to calculate your BMI.

1. Divide your weight in pounds by 2.2 to determine your weight in kilograms.

2. Multiply your height in inches by .0254 to determine your height in meters.

3. Square your height in meters (multiply your height in meters by your height in meters).

4. Divide the value you obtain in step 3 (square of height in meters) into the value you obtain in step 1 (weight in kilograms).

5. Use chart 13B.6 to obtain a rating for your BMI.

Chart 13B.5 Determination of Desirable Body Weight for Women (those above 20% fat)

	Estimated Percent Fat										
20	22	24	26	28	30	32	34	36	38	40
200	196	192	188	184	180	176	172	168	164	160
195	191	187	183	179	175	171	167	163	159	156
190	186	182	178	174	171	167	163	159	155	152
185	181	177	173	170	166	162	159	155	151	148
180	176	172	169	165	162	158	154	151	147	144
175	171	168	164	161	157	154	150	147	143	140
170	166	163	159	156	153	149	146	142	139	136
165	161	158	155	151	148	145	141	138	135	132
160	156	153	150	147	144	140	137	134	131	128
155	151	148	145	142	139	136	133	130	127	124
150	147	144	141	138	135	132	129	126	123	120
145	142	139	136	133	130	127	124	121	118	116
140	137	134	131	128	126	123	120	117	114	112
135	132	129	126	124	121	118	116	113	110	108
130	127	124	122	119	117	114	111	109	106	104
125	122	120	117	115	112	110	107	105	102	100
120	117	115	112	110	108	105	103	100	98	96
115	112	110	108	105	103	101	98	96	94	92
110	107	105	103	101	99	96	94	92	90	88
105	102	100	98	96	94	92	90	88	86	84
100	98	96	94	92	90	88	86	84	82	80
95	93	91	89	87	85	83	81	79	77	76
90	88	86	84	82	81	79	77	75	73	72

Along the side, locate your current body weight; across the top locate your estimated percent fat. The intersection of the two entries is your desirable weight (fat-free body weight plus 20 percent fat). Example: 150 pounds is the desirable weight for a woman who weighs 160 pounds and currently has a body fat amount of 26 percent.

Note: This chart uses 20 percent as a "desirable" fat level for females. People who have less than 20 percent need NOT use it because they already possess a healthy body weight and level of body fat unless they have less than 8 percent body fat, in which case some gain in body fat is recommended. Twenty percent was selected as a "desirable" level even though up to 25 percent fat is considered in the good fitness zone. For this reason, it should be noted that this chart is designed to give you a general guideline for "desirable" weight and should NOT be used as an absolute standard, especially as you grow older.

To make a metric conversion, see Appendix A.

Chart 13B.6 Rating Scale for Body Mass Index

Classification	Men	Women
High risk	27.8	27.3
Marginal	25.0–27.7	24.5–27.2
Good fitness zone	19.0–24.9	18.0–24.4
Low	17.9–18.9	15.0–17.9

Note: An excessively low BMI is not desirable. Low BMI values can be indicative of eating disorders and other health problems.

C O N C E P T

14

Controlling Body Fatness

Concept 14

There are various strategies for eating and exercising that can be useful in fat (weight) control.

Introduction

The benefits of maintaining desirable fat levels were discussed in Concepts 3 and 13. Estimates that 26 percent of adults are overfat is cause for concern. However, it is important to keep the concern about fat and weight control in perspective. A recent poll indicated that 96 percent of all adult males and 99 percent of all adult females would change something about their physical appearance. The leading concern was weight loss (see figure 14.1). Experts suggest that movies, television, and magazines have created an obsession with weight loss among many teens and adults. In many cases the concern is with losing weight rather than fat, and with appearance rather than good health. Caution is necessary so that we do not create more problems than we solve.

Because of the misplaced concern with weight loss among large numbers of people, the emphasis of this concept will be on fat loss for good health. When properly done, fat control can be safe and effective. This concept will make suggestions for losing, maintaining, and gaining body fat.

Health Goals for the Year 2000

- Reduce overfatness to no more than 20 percent of people aged 20 or more.
- Reduce overfatness to no more than 15 percent of people aged 12 to 19.
- Increase to 50 percent the proportion of overfat people who have adopted physical activity and sound nutrition to attain desirable body fatness.

Terms

Behavioral Goal

A statement of intent to perform a specific behavior (changing a life-style) for a specific period of time. An example would be, "I will reduce the fat in my diet to 30 percent or less of my total calories."

Empty Calories

Calories in foods considered to have little nutritional value.

Long Term Goal

A statement of intent to change behavior or achieve a specific outcome in a period of months or years.

Negative Self-Talk

Self-defeating discussions with yourself focusing on your failures rather than your successes.

Outcome Goal

A statement of intent to achieve a specific test score (attainment of a specific standard) associated with good health or wellness. An example would be, "I will lower my body fat level by three percent."

Positive Self-Talk

Telling yourself positive, encouraging things that help you succeed in accomplishing your goals.

Short Term Goal

A statement of intent to change a behavior or outcome in a period of days or weeks.

The Facts: Life-Styles and Fat Control

The first step in fat control is establishing realistic goals.

Too many teens and adults, both men and women, establish unrealistic goals for their physical appearance. Fat, weight, and body proportions are all factors that can be changed, but people often set standards for themselves that will be difficult, if not impossible, to achieve. It is important that goals be set for fat and weight control that can be accomplished for both the short and the long term. This necessitates developing an understanding of your own body proportions as well as your body fatness. Unrealistic goals may result in eating disorders (see Concept 13), failure to meet goals, or the failure to maintain fat loss over time. The measurement procedures used in Labs 13A and 13B should help you establish realistic goals.

Goals that emphasize the behavior of eating less and exercising more are more effective than those emphasizing a specific outcome such as weight or fat lost (or gained).

Researchers have shown that setting **outcome goals,** or goals that set a specific amount of weight or fat loss (gain), can be discouraging. If a behavioral goal of eating a reasonable number of calories per day and expending a reasonable number of calories in exercise is met, outcome goals will be achieved. Most experts believe that **behavioral goals** work better than weight or fat loss goals, especially in the short term.

People who have a large amount of fat to lose may do better setting short-term rather than long-term goals.

Losing 50 pounds (22.7 kilograms) may seem impossible. Losing 2 pounds (1 kilogram) in a week may seem more achievable. Because your weight can fluctuate with the

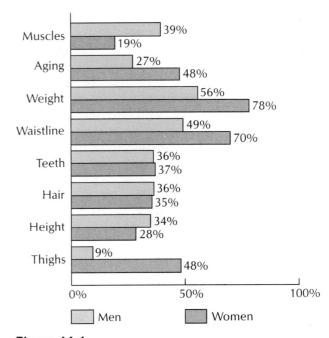

Figure 14.1

Physical appearance: what would people change?

From *Inside America* by Louis Harris. Copyright © 1985 by Louis Harris. Reprinted by permission of Random House, Inc.

amount of water lost or retained, daily monitoring of weight can also be discouraging. Weight may drop dramatically one day because of water loss and increase the next. Care must be taken not to worry too much about daily weight or fat losses or gains in the early stages of a program.

The best way to control body fatness is to establish a healthy life-style.

One way to ascertain whether fat control goals are realistic is to determine if they can be maintained for a lifetime. Diets that require severe caloric restriction or exercise programs that require exceptionally large caloric expenditure can be effective in fat loss over a short period, but are seldom maintained for a lifetime. Studies show that extreme programs for fat and weight control, designed to "take it off fast," result in long-term success rates of less than five percent. A healthy life-style includes a healthy diet and regular exercise. For some people it may be necessary to develop a daily habit of eating several hundred calories less than other people or maintaining an exercise schedule that expends more calories than the normal person if desirable body fat levels are to be maintained. These habits of "moderation" can realistically become part of your normal life-style.

Record keeping is important to meeting fat control goals and making moderation a part of your normal life-style.

Studies have shown that it is easy to fool yourself when determining the amount of food you have eaten or the amount of exercise you have done. Once fat control goals have been set, whether for weight loss, maintenance, or gain, it is important to keep records of your behavior. People often underestimate the amount of food they have eaten, particularly the number of calories consumed. They also tend to overestimate the amount of exercise they do. Keeping a diet log and an exercise log can help you monitor your behavior and maintain the life-style necessary to meet your goals. A log can also help you monitor changes in weight and body fatness. But remember, care should be taken to avoid too much emphasis on short-term weight changes. A sample log that can be used for record keeping is included in Lab 14 on page L-38.

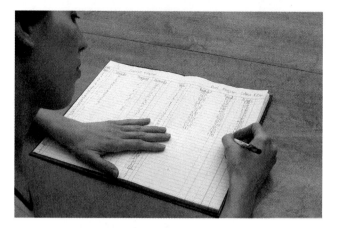

Keeping exercise and dietary records is important.

A basic knowledge of nutrition and exercise can help you in controlling fatness.

Many people are ignorant of the facts about foods and exercise. Information presented in this book should be helpful in separating fact from fiction. Concept 22 provides information about nutritional quackery, and Concept 24 provides information about exercise quackery, which should be useful in your attempts to control body fatness. Of course, much of this book deals with understanding the facts about fitness and exercise.

Some Facts About Eating and Fat Control

There are some general guidelines for eating that can help people interested in losing body fat.

- Restrict calories in moderate amounts per day rather than making large reductions in daily caloric intake.
- Choose foods from the lower portion of the food pyramid (see Concept 22).
- Eat less fat. Research shows that reduction in the fat in the diet not only results in fewer calories consumed (fats have more than twice the calories per gram as carbohydrates or proteins), but in greater body fat loss as well!
- Severely restrict **empty calories.** Foods with empty calories provide little nutrition and can account for an excessive amount of your daily caloric intake. Examples of these foods are candy (often high in simple sugar) and potato chips (often fried in saturated fat).
- Increase complex carbohydrates. Foods high in fiber, such as fresh fruits and vegetables, contain few calories for their volume. They are nutritious and filling, and are especially good foods for a fat loss program.
- Learn the difference between craving and hunger. Hunger is a physiological phenomenon that is a result of the body's need to supply energy to sustain life. A craving is simply a desire to eat

something; sometimes a food that is not particularly liked. When you feel the urge to eat, you may want to ask yourself: is this real hunger or a craving? Hunger is accompanied by growling of the stomach and is most likely to occur after long periods without food. If you have the urge to eat soon after a meal, it is probably from craving, not hunger.

There are some guidelines about shopping that can help people interested in fat control.

- Shop from a list. This helps you avoid the purchase of foods that contain empty calories and other foods that will tempt you to overeat.
- Shop with a friend. This is another way to help you avoid the purchase of unneeded foods. For this technique to work, the other person must be sensitive to your goals. In some cases, a friend can have a bad, rather than a good, influence.
- Shop on a full stomach to avoid the temptations of snacking on and buying junk food.
- Check the label for contents of foods. If the calories are not listed, be wary of buying them. Many so-called weight reduction foods have caloric contents equal to or in excess of normal foods.
- Consider foods that take some preparation time. If it takes time to prepare food, you may be less likely to eat it on the spur of the moment. It is acceptable to purchase foods prepackaged in small portions and that contain low caloric content, even if they require little preparation.

There are some guidelines about the way you eat that can be useful in fat loss.

- When you eat, do nothing else but eat. If you watch television, read, or do some other activity while you eat, you may be unaware of what you have eaten. Also, you should enjoy your eating, not share it with some other activity.

- Eat slowly. Taste your food. Pause between bites. Chew slowly. Don't take the next bite until you have swallowed what you have in your mouth. Periodically take a longer pause. Be the last one finished eating.
- Do not eat food you do not want. Some people do not want to waste food so they clean their plate even when they feel full.
- Follow an eating schedule. Eating at regular meal times can help you avoid snacking. If meals are spaced equally throughout the day, it can help reduce appetite.
- Do your eating in designated areas only. Designate areas such as the kitchen and dining room as eating areas.
- Eat meals of equal size. Some people try to restrict calories at one or two meals to save up for a big meal. Eating several *small* meals helps you to avoid hunger (fools the appetite) and helps you keep from losing control at one meal.
- Leave the table after eating and clear dishes early. Clearing the dishes and leaving the table help prevent you from taking extra unwanted bites and servings.
- Avoid second servings. Limit your intake to one moderate serving. If second servings are taken, make them one-half the size of first servings.
- Limit servings of salad dressings and condiments (catsup, etc.). These are often high in fat and calories, and can sometimes amount to greater calorie consumption than the food on which you put them.
- Limit servings of nonbasic parts of the meal. It is easy to consume large numbers of calories on alcohol, soft drinks, breads, and desserts. Limit these items.

There are some guidelines that are useful for controlling the home environment to aid in fat loss.

- Keep busy, especially at high-risk times or times when you are most likely to eat when you do not want to. If you have an urge to eat, exercise, talk to someone, go shopping, drink a glass of water, or find something active to do.
- Store food out of sight. Avoid containers that allow you to see food. It is especially important to limit the accessibility of foods that tempt you and foods with empty calories. "Foods that are out of sight, are out of mouth."
- Avoid serving food to others, especially between meals. Let them prepare their own snacks.
- If you snack, eat foods high in complex carbohydrates and low in fats, such as fresh fruits and carrot sticks.
- Freeze leftovers. Leftover foods are often tempting to eat. Freezing them so that it takes preparation to eat them will help you avoid temptation.

There are some guidelines for controlling the work environment to aid in fat loss.

- Take food from home rather than eating from vending machines or catering trucks. Even snacks should be brought from home, where they can be prepared based on guidelines listed above.
- Avoid snack machines. Most snacks from machines are high in calories and low in nutritional value. Fresh fruit from machines is an exception.
- If you eat out, plan your meal selection ahead of time. Write it down and know its calorie content. Be aware that many fast foods are high in caloric content and fat.
- Do not eat while working.
- Avoid sources of food provided by co-workers; for example, food in work rooms, such as birthday cakes, or candy in jars.
- Do something active during breaks. For example, take a walk.
- Have drinking water or low-calorie drinks available to substitute for snacks.

There are some guidelines about eating on special occasions that can be useful in fat loss.

- Practice ways to refuse food. Practice in front of a mirror or with friends. Know exactly what to say when you plan to refuse food. Do not let yourself be intimidated into eating something you do not want. For example, you might say something as simple as "No thank you." Be wary of persistent hosts. Do not let them make you feel guilty for not eating. Be polite but emphatic; give no indication that you might change your mind.
- In extreme cases, you may wish to avoid situations that create a high risk of overeating.
- Eat before you go out.
- When eating out, order à la carte.
- Do not stand near food sources.
- If you feel the urge to eat, talk to someone or find something else to occupy your thoughts.

Fad diets are not a satisfactory means to long-term weight reduction and may adversely affect your health.

There are hundreds of fad diets and diet books, but dietitians warn that there is no scientific basis for drastic juggling of food constituents. Such diets are usually unbalanced and may result in serious illness or even death, especially for the obese person who is already apt to be suffering from a number of health disorders. Fad diets cannot be maintained for long periods; therefore, the individual usually regains any lost weight. Less than five percent of those who lose weight maintain the loss for more than a year. Constant losing and gaining, known as the "yo-yo syndrome," may be as harmful as the original obese condition.

Total fasting is dangerous, as are crash (fast) diets. Crash diets that bring about weight loss by dehydration of only five percent in forty-eight hours have been shown to reduce the individual's working capacity by as much as forty percent. The practice of making weight in athletics, whether by dehydration, induced vomiting, or starvation diets, is dangerous to health and should be condemned. Much of the weight loss on such fad diets is valuable lean muscle mass.

Pill popping, hormone injections, and powder and liquid diets have little value in long-term weight control programs and present many health hazards. When in doubt, avoid diets that:

- Promise fast, easy solutions.
- Promise to help you achieve ideal weight without mental inspiration and perspiration.
- Favor one food as the answer to weight problems.
- Promise that your fat will melt away.

Many of the eating guidelines that are useful for fat loss are also valuable in maintaining desirable levels of body fat.

Once a person has achieved a desirable level of body fatness, it is important that this level be maintained throughout life. Many of the eating strategies for losing body fatness listed in the previous sections are also appropriate for maintaining body fat levels at desirable levels. If you follow them, you will develop new and healthier eating patterns that you will retain for the rest of your life.

Some people need to gain weight and can benefit from a change in their eating patterns.

Most people who want to gain weight want to gain lean body tissue. Only those who have body fat percentages less than what is considered to be essential for good health need to gain body fat (see Concept 13). Some eating guidelines for people interested in gaining weight are listed here.

- Increase the calories consumed. Increasing caloric intake by amounts of 500–1,000 calories a day will help most people gain weight over time.
- The majority of extra calories should come from complex carbohydrates. Breads, pasta, rice, fruits such as bananas, and potatoes are good sources. High-protein diets or diet supplements are not particularly effective if you maintain a normal diet. High-fat diets can result in weight gain but may not be best for good health, especially if they are high in saturated fat.

- If extra exercise results in extra calories expended, caloric intake will need to be adjusted to compensate. It may be difficult to eat when you are not hungry. Eating more than three meals per day may help.
- Drink lots of juice and milk. Grape and cranberry juices are good because they are high in calories.
- Eat snacks. Bananas, granola, nuts, and Grapenuts are high-calorie, healthy snacks.
- If weight gain does not occur over a period of weeks and months with extra caloric consumption, medical assistance may be necessary.

More calories are required to maintain weight during the growing years than in adulthood.

Typically, the people most likely to have difficulty in gaining weight are age ten to twenty. They have probably been told more than once that they will not have trouble gaining weight when they grow older. This is true for most people, but it is of little consolation to those who want to gain weight now. During adolescence, most people begin to gain weight, including muscle mass that can be enhanced with regular exercise. If they follow the guidelines just listed, they may have success in gaining weight. Excessive eating to gain weight (especially during adolescence) is not without its problems. The body requires more caloric intake during the teen years because the body is growing. A person who develops a habit of high caloric intake during this time may have a difficult time controlling fatness when the demands on the body are less.

Some Facts About Exercise and Fat Control

There are some guidelines for exercise that can be of value in losing or maintaining desirable body fat levels.

- Perform regular aerobic exercise. Since aerobic exercise can be maintained for a long period, it allows you to expend large numbers of calories. For this reason, it is the best type of exercise for fat loss and maintenance.
- Find a time, a place, and a type of exercise that will permit you to work out regularly. Regularity is the key. Exercise must be regular if it is to be of value. Consult Concept 19 for guidelines for adhering to regular exercise.
- Performing strength training can increase muscle mass and result in fat loss without loss in weight. If you follow the guidelines for strength training outlined in Concept 10, you can increase your muscle mass provided calorie intake is constant.

There are some guidelines for exercise that can be of value in gaining weight, including muscle mass.

- Performing strength training can aid in weight gain. It is the best form of exercise for people interested in gaining weight. Consult Concepts 10–12 for guidelines and specific strength training exercises. Of course, strength training is most effective in weight gain when accompanied by an increase in calorie intake.
- Excessive aerobic exercise may make it difficult to gain weight. Although some regular aerobic exercise is necessary for health and cardiovascular fitness, it may be necessary to limit aerobic exercise if weight gain is the goal. Studies have shown that extensive aerobic training can even cause a reduction in muscle mass. When training to gain weight, aerobic exercise expending no more than 3,500 calories per week is probably best. For a jogger, this would be approximately four to five miles a day. Aerobic exercise in moderate amounts can help some people relax and, therefore, expend less nervous energy.

Some Facts About Social and Psychological Strategies

The support of family and friends can be of great importance in fat control.

The importance of family and friends to successful exercise adherence can't be overemphasized (see Concept 19). Family and friends can also help you in changing and adhering to healthy eating practices. It is known that parents who overeat often have children who eat more than normal. In these cases, it is important for the entire family to participate in a program to control fatness. Family and friends should provide support for the person trying to gain or lose fat by helping them follow the guidelines presented in this Concept, rather than tempting the person to eat improperly. Unfortunately there is sometimes a danger of overemphasis on fat loss by a friend or family member. This can have the opposite effect of that intended if it is perceived as an attempt to control one's behavior. Studies have shown that the use of extrinsic rewards such as money or special gifts for achieving goals may be effective in the *short* term, but may result in resentment rather than adherence over the long term. Encouragement and support rather than control of behavior is the key!

Group support can be one of the best reinforcers of proper eating and exercise behavior.

Group support has been found to be beneficial to many individuals who are attempting to change their behavior.

In Concept 23, the importance of group support in reducing stress is discussed. Alcoholics have found that the support of others is critical to their rehabilitation (Alcoholics Anonymous grew as a result of this need). If you want to alter your body composition, especially to lose body fat, group support is important if you are to make permanent life-style changes in diet and exercise. Groups such as Overeaters Anonymous and Weight Watchers have been organized to help those who need the support of peers in attaining and maintaining desirable fat levels for a lifetime.

There are some psychological strategies that can be of assistance in eating and exercising to attain and maintain a desirable level of body fatness.

- Avoid food fantasies. Sometimes the thought of food is what causes overeating. Practice restructuring your thought process to something other than food fantasies. Use mental imagery to create a mind's eye view of something you enjoy other than food. When food fantasies occur, you may want to exercise or engage in some activity that refocuses your attention.
- Avoid weight fantasies. Sometimes the thought of being excessively thin or muscular occurs. By itself, this may not be bad. If, however, it causes you to become discouraged and makes your goals seem unattainable, it is bad. When weight fantasies occur, do some other activity to redirect your focus of attention or imagine something other than the weight fantasy. Altering mental fantasies takes practice.
- Avoid **negative self-talk.** One type of negative self-talk occurs when a person starts self-criticism for not meeting a goal. For example, if a person is determined not to eat more than one serving of food at a party, but fails to meet this goal, he or she might say "It's no use stopping now; I've already blown it." It is not too late. Failing to meet goals can happen to anyone. Negative self-talk makes it easy to fail in the future. A more appropriate response would involve **positive self-talk** such as "I'm not going to eat anything else tonight. I can do it."

Suggested Readings

Brownell, K., et al. "Matching Weight Control Programs to Individuals." *The Weight Control Digest* 1(1991):65.

Clark, N. "How to Gain Weight Healthfully." *Physician and Sportsmedicine* 19(1991):53.

Work, J. "Exercise for the Overweight Patient." *Physician and Sportsmedicine* 18(1990):113.

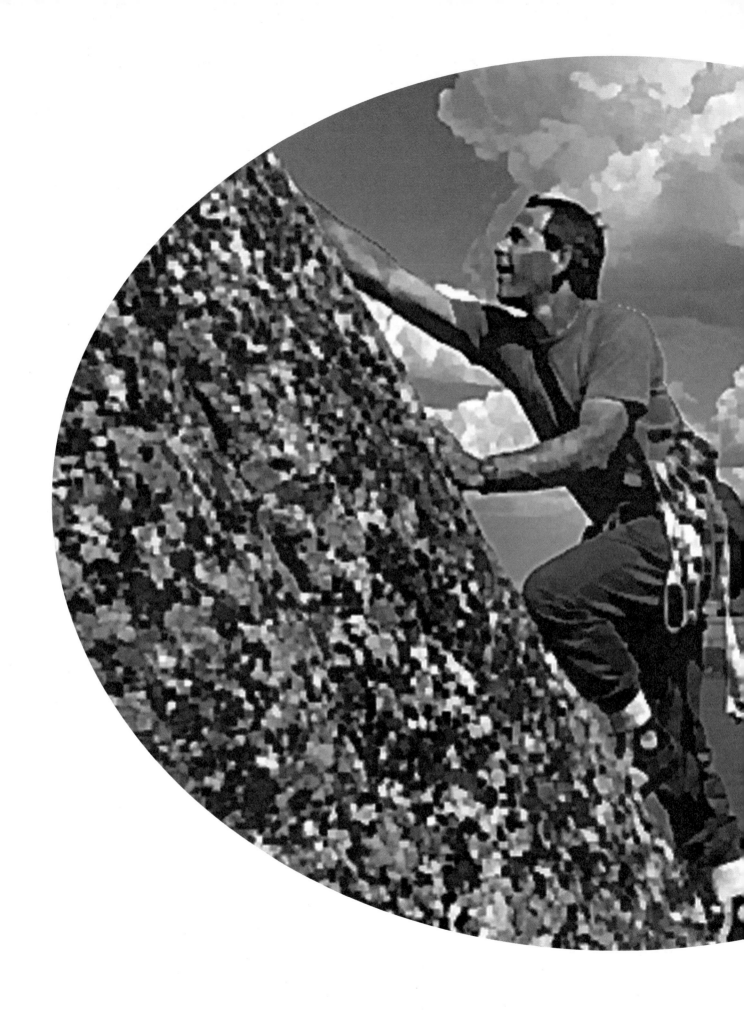

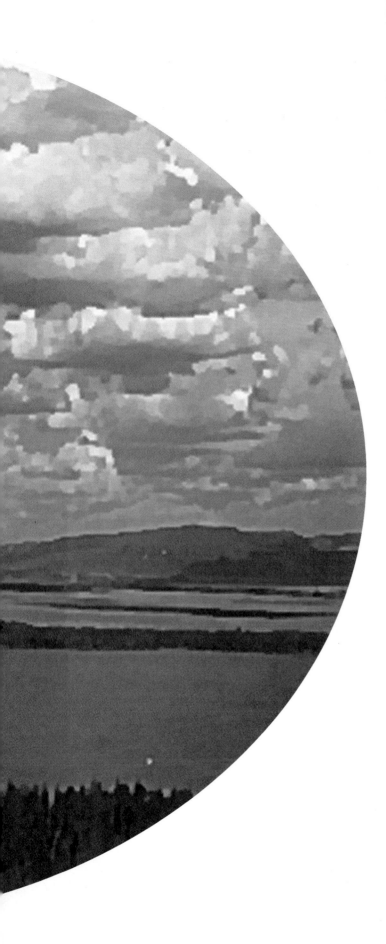

IV

Special Exercise Considerations

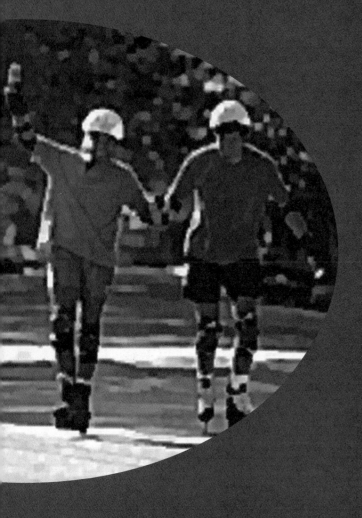

C O N C E P T

15

Sports, Physical Activity, and Skill-Related Physical Fitness

Concept 15

Everyone, regardless of physical ability, can find a sport or physical activity to enjoy for a lifetime.

Introduction

Sports are an important part of Western culture. Virtually all people are involved with sports, either as a spectator or as a participant. Sports can be used as recreational activities for enjoying free time or, if done as a participant, can be a significant part of a personal physical fitness program. Learning about your personal skill-related physical fitness (also called **motor fitness** or **sports fitness**), can help you select a sport that is well suited to your personal needs and interests. In addition to sports, there are other physical activities that are enjoyable as lifetime recreational pursuits.

Health Goals for the Year 2000

- Increase the proportion of people who engage in regular physical activity.
- Reduce the proportion of people who engage in no free-time physical activity.
- Increase worksite physical activity programs.

Terms

Fitness Activities

Fitness activities are physical activities that are particularly good for promoting physical fitness, such as aerobic and anaerobic exercises (Concept 7), stretching exercises (Concept 9), strength and muscular endurance exercises (Concept 12), and preplanned exercise programs. Some sports such as swimming, running, and cycling when not done competitively are also considered to be fitness and/or aerobic activities.

Lifetime Sport

A sport suitable for people of all ages; a sport that can be performed "from the cradle to the grave" (for a lifetime).

Motor Fitness

A term commonly used for skill-related fitness.

Preplanned Exercise Programs

Preplanned exercise programs are exercise regimes planned by someone other than the person doing the exercise. Often they are designed for a large group of people rather than for one individual.

Self-Promoting Activities

Physical activities in which the performer is not required to have a high level of skill to perform with some degree of success.

Sport

An activity that involves competition between teams or individuals in which the goal is to beat the opponent or win the game. Except in the case of ties, there is a winner and a loser. Activities such as swimming, cycling, jogging/running are classified as sports by some writers; however, in this text they are defined as aerobic activities rather than as sports because most adults do not perform these activities competitively.

Sports Fitness

A term commonly used for skill-related physical fitness.

The Facts About Sports

Sports can be a good form of leisure.

True leisure is a state of mind associated with a feeling of freedom and being able to enjoy yourself. Sports receive the highest ratings of all daily activities in terms of perceived feelings of freedom. Sport is rated as something "I want to do" more often than other work or free-time activities, such as cultural activities and home leisure.

The most popular participation sports are not the same as the most popular spectator sports.

Team sports are the most popular spectator sports, with football leading the list. Other popular spectator sports, as well as the most popular participation sports among adults, are listed in table 15.1. The sports that adults enjoy watching are not the same as the ones they enjoy playing.

The most popular sports share characteristics that contribute to their popularity.

The most popular sports are often considered to be **lifetime sports** because they can be done at any age. The characteristics that make these sports appropriate for lifelong participation probably contribute significantly to their popularity. Six of the top ten are individual sports that do not require a large group of people to play them. Often the popular sports are adapted so that people without exceptional skill can play them. For example, bowling uses a "handicap system" to allow people with a wide range of abilities to compete. Slow pitch softball is much more popular than fast pitch because it allows people of all abilities to play successfully.

Sports are most enjoyable when the challenge is optimal.

One of the primary reasons why sports participation is so popular is that sports provide a challenge. For the greatest enjoyment, the challenge of the activity should be balanced by the person's skill in the sport. If you choose to play against one of lesser skill, you will not be challenged.

Table 15.1
Popular Sports

Sport	Participation Rank	Spectator Rank
Bowling	1	9
Pool/billiards	2	*
Race cycling	3	*
Softball	4	*
Volleyball	5	*
Golf	6	6 (tie)
Basketball	7	3
Table tennis	8	*
Baseball	9	2
Tennis	10	5
Football	*	1
Ice hockey	*	4
Boxing	*	6 (tie)
Ice skating	*	6 (tie)
Wrestling	*	10

*Not in top ten sports.

Source: Data from the Gallup Poll.

On the other hand, if you lack skill or your opponent has considerably more skill, the activity will be frustrating. For optimal challenge and enjoyment the skills of a given sport should be learned before participation. Likewise, an opponent of similar skill level should be chosen.

Participation in sports can contribute to good health-related physical fitness.

The health-related fitness benefits of participation in the ten most popular sports are presented in table 15.2. Several of the top participation sports, such as softball and pool/billiards, are *not* particularly good activities for building health-related physical fitness. However, experts now agree that regular participation of some kind is better than no participation at all.

There are benefits to both watching and participating in sports.

Active involvement in sports can have many physical, social, and personal benefits. Though watching sports will not build physical fitness, it does have other benefits. According to recent research, watching sports "almost always" makes people feel happy when their team wins and gives them a feeling of accomplishment and pride, even though they did not participate. On the downside, when the favorite team loses, feelings of depression and lack of accomplishment may occur. In extreme cases, displays of poor sportsmanship and even violence have occurred.

Table 15.2

Achieving Fitness through Sports

Sport	Rank	Cardiovascular Fitness	Muscular Endurance	Strength	Flexibility	Fat Control
Bowling	1	*	*	–	–	*
Pool/billiards	2	–	–	–	–	–
Race cycling	3	***	***	**	*	***
Softball	4	*	*	–	–	*
Volleyball	5	**	**	*	*	**
Golf (walking)	6	**	**	*	*	**
Basketball	7	***	**	*	–	***
Table tennis	8	*	*	–	*	*
Baseball	9	*	*	–	–	*
Tennis	10	**	**	*	*	**

*** Very Good   ** Good   * Minimum   – Low

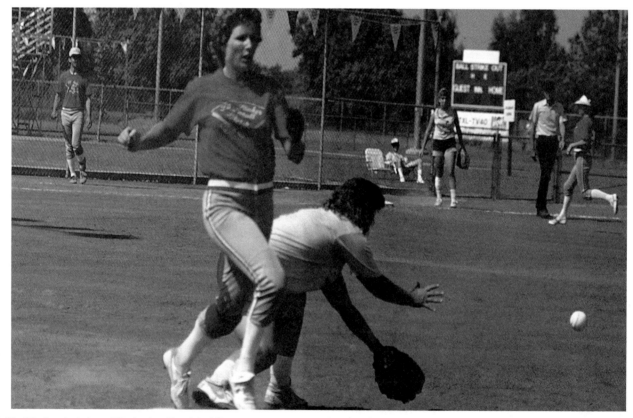

Softball is fun, but does little for health-related fitness components such as cardiovascular fitness.

In many cases, a person needs to exercise to get fit for sports rather than play sports to get fit.

Many sports require a considerable amount of fitness, especially those involving vigorous competition, yet the sport may do relatively little to develop fitness. For example, you need considerable strength, muscular endurance, and flexibility to play football. However, football is not a particularly good activity for developing these aspects of fitness.

> Though recreational sports skills are learned by most people early in life, lifetime sports skills can be learned at any age.

Research evidence suggests that most skills are learned early in life. In fact, one study indicates that as many as 85 percent of all recreational skills are learned by the age of twelve. This does not mean that "old dogs cannot learn new tricks," but it does suggest a need to teach skills to children at an early age.

> Sports are activities that can be enjoyed by virtually all people.

It is true that sports are most popular among younger people. Yet sports are enjoyed by people of all ages and abilities. The senior olympics and masters sports programs have expanded participation for people of all ages. In some locations, softball leagues for people age 75 and older have been formed.

Many people with physical disabilities now participate in a wide variety of sports, including wheelchair basketball and beep-beep softball for the blind. The Special Olympics, and other similar programs, have provided many sports opportunities for people with special physical needs and those with learning difficulties.

The Facts About Nonsport Activities

> Nonsport **fitness activities** are more popular for participation than most sports.

The most popular participation activities among adults are listed in table 15.3. Only three of the top lifetime activities are sports. Four are considered to be fitness activities, including swimming, bicycling, running/jogging, and weight training. These fitness activities, according to recent statistics, are not only among the most popular, they are also ones in which participants are most likely to perform on a regular basis throughout the year. The remaining three in the top ten are outdoor activities, one of which—hiking—has significant health-related fitness benefits. Note: swimming, bicycling, and running/jogging are not classified as sports because most participants in these activities do not compete on a regular basis. Race cycling as opposed to bicycling is classified as a sport.

> Many of the most popular participation activities are considered to be **self-promoting** activities.

Close scrutiny of the most popular lifetime fitness and outdoor activities indicates that they can be done, like

Table 15.3

Rankings of the Most Popular Lifetime Physical Activities

Activity	Rank	Activity	Rank
Swimming	1	Softball	11
Fishing	2	Volleyball	12
Bicycling	3	Motorboating	13
Bowling	4	Dance exercise	14
Camping	5	Golf	15
Hiking	6	Basketball	16
Pool/billiards	7	Table tennis	17
Running/jogging	8	Calisthenics	18
Weight training	9	Hunting	19
Race cycling	10	Baseball	20

Source: Data from the Gallup Poll.

popular lifetime sports, without the need for large groups of people, and they do not require a high degree of skill. Activities with these characteristics are considered to be self-promoting activities because they make the performer feel good. Some people avoid activities that require a high degree of skill because they often result in failure rather than success. Failure causes self-criticism rather than self-promotion. People who have had little previous success in organized sports should consider individualized skill instruction if they want to participate. An alternative would be to choose participation in self-promoting activities such as swimming, bicycling, jogging, weight training, or dance exercise.

> Self-promoting activities are especially good for people with special needs.

Because self-promoting activities allow you to set your own standards of success and can be done individually or in small groups, they are especially suited to people with special needs. Wheelchair distance events, weight training, and aquatics are a few examples of these activities.

> **Preplanned exercise programs** are a popular form of exercise.

Among the twenty most popular types of physical activities are weight training, dance exercise, and calisthenics. All of these are programs that are frequently done in the home. Programs of this type are often preplanned and published as a booklet or in video format. You may like preplanned programs because someone else directs your program.

There can be some problems in performing preplanned exercise programs.

Because preplanned exercise programs are planned by one person (or group) for individuals of many different levels of fitness, they may not be equally effective for all people who use them.

When selecting a preplanned exercise program, the following suggestions may be useful.

- Find out who wrote the program. Is the person(s) an expert? What makes the person an expert? Look for a program written by someone with a good educational background in physical education, exercise physiology, or sports medicine. Programs written by movie stars and television celebrities are rarely sound.
- Choose a program with more than one level of exercise. A good program will have exercises for beginning, intermediate, and advanced levels of fitness. This allows you to select a program appropriate to your needs. Be skeptical of programs that include one set of exercises for all people.
- Make certain that all exercises are "good" exercises. In Concept 18, some contraindicated or "questionable" exercises are described. Avoid programs that include these exercises.
- Choose a program that meets your needs. Because physical fitness has many components, you need a program that includes exercises and activities for the fitness areas in which you need improvement.
- Choose a program that you enjoy enough to continue on a regular basis. No matter how good a program is, if you don't do it, it won't work.
- Choose a program that can be adapted to your need as your fitness improves.

Preplanned programs that are not well designed but provide motivation to exercise can be adapted to make them safe and effective programs.

Some preplanned exercise programs, especially those prepared by celebrities with little exercise expertise, can be modified to improve them. Exercise programs on videotape and television can provide motivation to do regular exercise. Well-informed people can adapt these programs to make them safe and effective. You may want to use table 15.4 as a guide to making the necessary modifications.

There are different kinds of preplanned exercise programs.

Popular preplanned programs include those developed by governmental agencies, such as the Adult Fitness Program (developed by the President's Council on Physical

Table 15.4
Guidelines for Adapting Preplanned Exercise Programs

1. If the program contains contraindicated or "bad" exercises, don't do them or substitute safe exercises.
2. Determine if the program gets you to exercise in the target zone for all parts of fitness. If not, supplement it with appropriate exercises. Many programs emphasize one component of fitness while neglecting others.
3. If the program is too difficult, don't continue. Modify with easier exercises that are more suited to your needs. For cardiovascular exercises, you may slow the speed of the exercise or eliminate arm movements to make them easier. Don't feel that you need to keep up with the instructor.
4. If you experience pain, stop exercising or reduce the intensity of the exercise. The "no pain, no gain" idea is a misconception!
5. If the program is too easy, supplement it with additional exercises.
6. Rotate programs regularly to keep your interest level high.

Fitness and Sport) and the Royal Canadian XBX and 5BX exercises. Some are developed commercially, such as videotapes of home exercises, programs published in books and magazines, and those already discussed in Concept 7 (dance aerobics routines and aquadynamics).

The Facts About Skill-Related Fitness

There are several components of skill-related physical fitness.

The six components of skill-related physical fitness identified in this book were chosen because they are among the most important to sports performance and easiest to measure. There are probably other abilities that contribute to the ability to perform skills of all kinds. For example, many experts consider various perceptual abilities such as depth and distance perception (ability to judge depth and distances accurately) and visual tracking (ability to visually follow a moving object) to be skill-related parts of physical fitness.

There are sub-components of each part of skill-related physical fitness.

Most of the six parts of skill-related physical fitness have sub-components. For example, coordination includes foot-eye coordination and hand-eye coordination, which are measured quite differently. The tests in this Concept were chosen to measure some of the skill-related fitness aspects most important to sports performance.

Skills are specific in nature.

An individual might possess ability in one area and not in another. For this reason, "general motor ability" probably does not really exist. Individuals do not have one general capacity for performing skills. Rather, the ability to play games or sports is determined by combined abilities in each of the separate motor skill components of agility, coordination, balance, reaction time, speed, and power. It is, however, possible and even likely that some performers will be above average in many areas.

The potential for possessing outstanding skill-related fitness is based on hereditary predispositions, but all aspects of skill-related fitness can be improved through regular practice.

In order for a skill to be improved, it must be repeated. Some skill-related fitness components, such as power, agility, balance, and coordination, can be enhanced greatly with practice. Others, such as speed and reaction time, can be improved somewhat but are determined to a greater extent by heredity.

Exceptional athletes tend to be outstanding in more than one component of skill-related fitness.

Though people possess skill-related fitness in varying degrees, great athletes are likely to be above average in most, if not all, aspects. Indeed, exceptional athletes must be exceptional in many areas of skill-related fitness. Different sports require different skills, each of which requires varying degrees of the six components of skill-related fitness.

Excellence in one skill-related fitness component may compensate for a lack in another.

Each individual possesses a specific level of each skill-related fitness aspect. The performer should learn his or her other strengths and weaknesses in order to produce optimal performances. For example, a tennis player may use coordination to compensate for lack of speed.

Excellence in skill-related fitness may compensate for a lack of health-related fitness when playing sports and games.

As you grow older, health-related fitness potential declines much more rapidly than many components of skill-related fitness. You may use superior skill-related fitness to compensate. For example, a baseball pitcher who lacks the strength and power to dominate hitters may rely on a pitch such as a knuckleball, which is more dependent on coordination than on power.

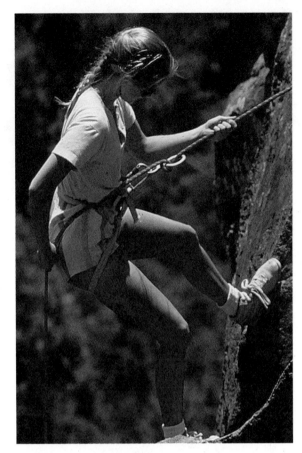

Different activities require different components of skill-related fitness.

Health-related fitness is important in playing sports and games.

Health-related fitness is not a substitute for skill-related fitness when it comes to performing successfully in sports. However, good health-related fitness is critical to exceptional performances of many kinds. For example, a gymnast with coordination, balance, and agility must have strength and flexibility to excel, and a football player with power and coordination must have cardiovascular fitness and muscular endurance to perform at optimal levels.

Skill-related fitness can be improved by performing activities that require the use of specific skill-related fitness components.

Skill-related fitness components are prerequisites to the successful performance of many sports skills. At the same time, the performance of sports skills, which require the use of different skill-related fitness components, will contribute to improvement in those fitness aspects. Table 15.5

Table 15.5
Skill-Related Benefits of Sports and Other Activities

Activity	Balance	Coordination	Reaction Time	Agility	Power	Speed
Archery	Good	Excellent	Poor	Poor	Poor	Poor
Backpacking	Fair	Fair	Poor	Fair	Fair	Poor
Badminton	Fair	Excellent	Good	Good	Fair	Good
Baseball	Good	Excellent	Excellent	Good	Excellent	Good
Basketball	Good	Excellent	Excellent	Excellent	Excellent	Good
Bicycling	Excellent	Fair	Fair	Poor	Poor	Fair
Bowling	Good	Excellent	Poor	Fair	Fair	Fair
Canoeing	Good	Good	Fair	Poor	Good	Poor
Circuit training	Fair	Fair	Poor	Fair	Good	Fair
Dance, aerobic	Fair	Excellent	Fair	Good	Poor	Poor
Dance, ballet	Excellent	Excellent	Fair	Excellent	Good	Poor
Dance, disco	Fair	Good	Fair	Excellent	Poor	Fair
Dance, modern	Excellent	Excellent	Fair	Excellent	Good	Poor
Dance, social	Fair	Good	Fair	Good	Poor	Fair
Fencing	Good	Excellent	Excellent	Good	Good	Excellent
Fitness calisthenics	Fair	Fair	Poor	Good	Fair	Poor
Football	Good	Good	Excellent	Excellent	Excellent	Excellent
Golf (walking)	Fair	Excellent	Poor	Fair	Good	Poor
Gymnastics	Excellent	Excellent	Good	Excellent	Excellent	Fair
Handball	Fair	Excellent	Good	Excellent	Good	Good
Hiking	Fair	Fair	Poor	Fair	Fair	Poor
Horseback riding	Good	Good	Fair	Good	Poor	Poor
Interval training	Fair	Fair	Poor	Poor	Poor	Fair
Jogging	Fair	Fair	Poor	Poor	Poor	Poor
Judo	Good	Excellent	Excellent	Excellent	Excellent	Excellent
Karate	Good	Excellent	Excellent	Excellent	Excellent	Excellent
Mountain climbing	Excellent	Excellent	Fair	Good	Good	Poor
Pool; billiards	Fair	Good	Poor	Fair	Fair	Poor
Racquetball; paddleball	Fair	Excellent	Good	Excellent	Fair	Good
Rope jumping	Fair	Good	Fair	Good	Fair	Poor
Rowing, crew	Fair	Excellent	Poor	Good	Excellent	Fair
Sailing	Good	Good	Good	Good	Fair	Poor
Skating, ice	Excellent	Good	Fair	Good	Fair	Good
Skating, roller	Excellent	Good	Poor	Good	Fair	Good
Skiing, cross-country	Fair	Excellent	Poor	Good	Excellent	Fair
Skiing, downhill	Excellent	Excellent	Good	Excellent	Good	Poor
Soccer	Fair	Excellent	Good	Excellent	Good	Good
Softball (fast)	Fair	Excellent	Excellent	Good	Good	Good
Softball (slow)	Fair	Excellent	Good	Fair	Good	Good
Surfing	Excellent	Excellent	Good	Excellent	Good	Poor
Swimming (laps)	Fair	Good	Poor	Good	Fair	Poor
Table tennis	Fair	Good	Good	Fair	Fair	Fair
Tennis	Fair	Excellent	Good	Good	Good	Good
Volleyball	Fair	Excellent	Good	Good	Fair	Fair
Walking	Fair	Fair	Poor	Poor	Poor	Poor
Waterskiing	Good	Good	Poor	Good	Fair	Poor
Weight training	Fair	Fair	Poor	Poor	Fair	Poor

From C. B. Corbin and R. Lindsey, *Fitness for Life*, 4th ed. Copyright © 1993 Scott, Foresman and Company. Reprinted by permission of Scott, Foresman and Company.

shows the activities that require each component of skill-related fitness. The table also gives you an idea about which activities tend to promote development of various skill-related fitness components. Though it is true that skill-related fitness is based on hereditary predispositions, all people can improve their skill-related fitness with participation in the appropriate activities.

Assessing your own skill-related fitness may help you choose a lifetime sport that best suits your abilities.

You can learn to assess your own skill-related fitness using some simple tests. Some of the tests are provided on pages 180–182. You may want to use the results of these tests and table 15.5 to help you choose a lifetime activity. Consider an activity that requires the parts of fitness on which you have your better scores.

Some Facts About Skill-Related Fitness and Wellness

Good skill-related fitness may help you achieve good health-related fitness.

Individuals who possess good skill-related fitness have the potential to succeed in sports and games. Regular participation in these activities can lead to improved health-related fitness throughout life. Research shows that people who make an effort to learn activities involving skill-related fitness are more likely to be active in sports and games for a lifetime.

Skill-related fitness may improve your ability to work efficiently.

In manual labor, skillful performance improves efficiency. For example, a ditchdigger with great ditchdigging skills uses less energy than one who has not mastered the skill. Seemingly simple skills are often quite complex and may require some proficiency in each of the skill-related fitness components.

Skill-related fitness may improve your ability to meet emergencies.

Good agility would enable you to dodge an oncoming car; good balance would lessen the likelihood of a fall; and good reaction time would decrease the chances of being hit by a flying object. Each aspect of skill-related fitness contributes in its own way to your ability to avoid injury and meet emergencies.

Good skill-related fitness is beneficial to carrying out the normal daily routine and enjoying your leisure time.

Walking, sitting, climbing, pushing, pulling, and other such tasks require varying degrees of skill-related fitness. Accordingly, improved fitness resulting from regular practice may improve efficiency in performing daily activities and in enjoying leisure or recreational time.

Suggested Readings

Magill, R. A. *Motor Learning: Concepts and Applications.* 4th ed. Dubuque, IA: Wm. C. Brown Communications, Inc., 1993.

LAB RESOURCE MATERIALS
(For use with Lab 15A, page L-39)

Important Note: Because skill-related physical fitness does not relate directly to good health, the rating charts used in this section differ from those used in earlier concepts. The rating charts that follow can be used to compare your scores to those of other people. You DO NOT need exceptional scores on skill-related fitness to be able to enjoy sports and other types of physical activity. After the age of thirty, you should adjust ratings by one percent per year.

Evaluating Skill-Related Physical Fitness

I. Evaluating agility: The Illinois agility run[1]
An agility course using four chairs ten feet apart, and a thirty-foot running area will be set up as depicted in this illustration. The test is performed as follows:
1. Lie prone with your hands by your shoulders and your head at the starting line. On the signal to begin, run the course as fast as possible.
2. Your score is the time required to complete the course.

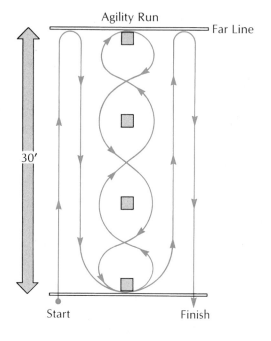

Agility Run

Far Line

30'

Start   Finish

II. Evaluating balance: The Bass test of dynamic balance[2]
Eleven circles (9½-inch) are drawn on the floor as shown in the illustration. The test is performed as follows:

1. Stand on the right foot in circle X. *Leap* forward to circle one, then circles two through ten, alternating feet with each leap.
2. The feet must leave the floor on each leap and the heel may not touch. Only the ball of the foot may land on the floor.
3. Remain in each circle for five seconds before leaping to the next circle. (A count of five will be made for you aloud.)
4. Practice trials are allowed.
5. The score is fifty, plus the number of seconds taken to complete the test, minus the number of errors.
6. For every error, deduct three points each. Errors include touching the heel, moving the supporting foot, touching outside a circle, or touching any body part to the floor other than the supporting foot.
7. Scores should be plotted on the appropriate rating scales.

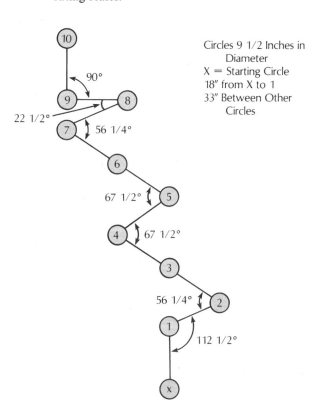

Circles 9 1/2 Inches in Diameter
X = Starting Circle
18" from X to 1
33" Between Other Circles

90°

22 1/2°

56 1/4°

67 1/2°

67 1/2°

56 1/4°

112 1/2°

Chart 15.1	Agility *Rating Scale*	
Classification	**Men**	**Women**
Excellent	15.8 or faster	17.4 or faster
Very good	16.7–15.9	18.6–17.5
Good	18.6–16.8	22.3–18.7
Fair	18.8–18.7	23.4–22.4
Poor	18.9 or slower	23.5 or slower

[1]Source: Data from Adams, et al., *Foundations of Physical Activity*, 1965, p. 111.

[2]Source: C. H. McCloy, *Tests and Measurements in Health and Physical Education*, Appleton-Century-Crofts, page 106, 1954.

Chart 15.2	Bass Test *Rating Scale*
Rating	**Score**
Excellent	90–100
Very good	80–89
Good	60–79
Fair	30–59
Poor	0–29

Chart 15.3	Coordination *Rating Scale*	
Classification	**Men**	**Women**
Excellent	14–15	13–15
Very good	11–13	10–12
Good	5–10	4–9
Fair	3–4	2–3
Poor	0–2	0–1

III. Evaluating coordination: The stick test of coordination

The stick test of coordination requires you to juggle three wooden wands. The wands are used to perform a one-half flip and a full flip as shown in the illustrations.

1. *One-Half Flip*—Hold two twenty-four-inch (one-half inch in diameter) dowel rods, one in each hand. Support a third rod of the same size across the other two. Toss the supported rod in the air so that it makes a half turn. Catch the thrown rod with the two held rods.
2. *Full Flip*—Perform the preceding task, letting the supported rod turn a full flip.

The test is performed as follows:

1. Practice the half-flip and the full flip several times before taking the test.
2. When you are ready, attempt a half-flip five times. Score one point for each successful attempt.
3. When you are ready, attempt the full flip five times. Score two points for each successful attempt.

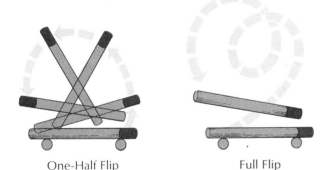

One-Half Flip   Full Flip

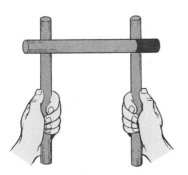

Hand Position

IV. Evaluating power: The vertical jump test

The test is performed as follows:

1. Hold a piece of chalk so its end is even with your fingertips.
2. Stand with both feet on the floor and your side to the wall and reach and mark as high as possible.
3. Jump upward with both feet as high as possible. Swing arms upward and make a chalk mark on a 5′ × 1′ wall chart marked off in half-inch horizontal lines placed six feet from the floor.
4. Measure the distance between the reaching height and the jumping height.
5. Your score is the best of three jumps.

Chart 15.4	Power *Rating Scale*	
Classification	**Men**	**Women**
Excellent	25½″ or more	23½″ or more
Very good	21″–25″	19″–23″
Good	16½″–20½″	14½″–18½″
Fair	12½″–16″	10½″–14″
Poor	12″ or less	10″ or less

Metric conversions for this chart appear in Appendix B.

V. Evaluating reaction time: The stick drop test

To perform the stick drop test of reaction time, you will need a yardstick, a table, a chair, and a partner to help with the test. To perform the test, follow these procedures:

1. Sit in the chair next to the table so that your elbow and lower arm rest on the table comfortably. The heel of your hand should rest on the table so that only your fingers and thumb extend beyond the edge of the table.
2. Your partner holds a yardstick at the very top, allowing it to dangle between your thumb and fingers.
3. The yardstick should be held so that the 24-inch-mark is even with your thumb and index finger. No part of your hand should touch the yardstick.
4. Without warning, your partner will drop the stick and you will catch it with your thumb and index finger.

5. Your score is the number of inches read on the yardstick just above the thumb and index finger after you catch the yardstick.
6. Try the test three times. Your partner should be careful not to drop the stick at predictable time intervals so that you cannot guess when it will be dropped. It is important that you react to the dropping of the stick only.
7. Use the middle of your three scores (example: if your scores are 21, 18, and 19, your middle score is 19). The higher your score, the faster your reaction time.

Chart 15.5 Reaction Time *Rating Scale*	
Classification	**Score in Inches**
Excellent	More than 21
Very good	19–21
Good	16–18¾
Fair	13–15¾
Poor	Below 13

Metric conversions for this chart appear in Appendix B.

VI. Evaluating speed: Running test of speed

To perform the running test of speed, it will be necessary to have a specially marked running course, a stopwatch, a whistle, and a partner to help you with the test. To perform the test, follow this procedure:

1. Mark a running course on a hard surface so that there is a starting line and a series of nine additional lines, each two yards apart, the first marked at a distance ten yards from the starting line.

2. From a distance one or two yards behind the starting line, begin to run as fast as you can. As you cross the starting line, your partner starts a stopwatch.
3. Run as fast as you can until you hear the whistle that your partner will blow exactly three seconds after the stopwatch was started. Your partner marks your location at the time when the whistle was blown.
4. Your score is the distance you were able to cover in three seconds. You may practice the test and take more than one trial if time allows. Use the better of your distances on the last two trials as your score.

Chart 15.6 Speed *Rating Scale*		
Classification	**Men**	**Women**
Excellent	24–26 yards	22–26 yards
Very good	22–23 yards	20–21 yards
Good	18–21 yards	16–19 yards
Fair	16–17 yards	14–15 yards
Poor	Less than 16 yards	Less than 14 yards

Metric conversions for this chart appear in Appendix B.

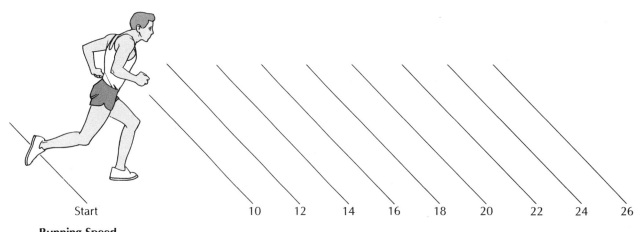

Start   10   12   14   16   18   20   22   24   26

Running Speed

CONCEPT

16

Body Mechanics: Posture and Care of the Back and Neck

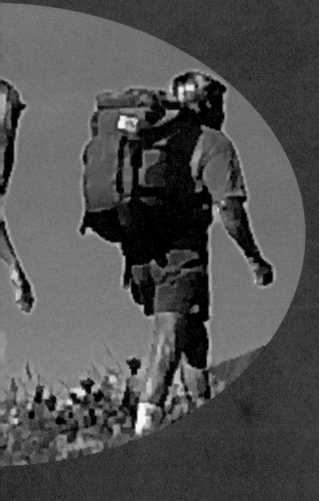

Concept 16

Because the human body is a system of weights and levers, its efficiency and effectiveness at rest or in motion can be improved by the application of sound mechanical and anatomical principles.

Introduction

"Body mechanics" is the application of physical laws to the human body. The bones of the body act as levers or simple machines, with the muscles supplying the force to move them. Therefore, mechanical laws can be applied to the body to aid in performing more and better work with less energy while avoiding strain or injury.

This concept focuses on three aspects of body mechanics. The first part of the concept discusses the mechanics of body alignment while sitting or standing (*static postures*). The second part of the concept emphasizes the *prevention of low back and neck pain* through proper body mechanics. The third section of the concept stresses *dynamic postures* for activities of daily living.

Health Goal for the Year 2000

- Reduce activity limitation due to chronic back conditions.

Terms

Center of Gravity

The center of the mass of an object.

Cervical Lordosis

Excessive hyperextension in the neck region ("swayback of the neck").

Effectiveness

The degree to which the purpose is accomplished.

Head Forward

The head is thrust forward in front of the gravity line; also called "poke neck."

Herniated Disk

The soft nucleus of the spinal disk protrudes through a small tear in the surrounding tissue; also called prolapse.

Hyperextended Knees

The knees are thrust backward in a locked position.

Intervertebral Disk

Spinal disk (disc); a cushion of cartilage between the bodies of the vertebrae. Each disk consists of a fibrous outer ring (annulus fibrosus) and a pulpy center (nucleus pulposus).

Kyphosis

Increased curvature (flexion) in the upper back; called "hump back" or "dorsal kyphosis." In the lower back it is called "flat back" or "lumbar kyphosis."

Linear Motion

Movement in a straight line.

Lumbar Lordosis

Increased curvature (hyperextension) in the lower back (lumbar region), with a forward pelvic tilt; commonly known as "swayback."

Posture

The relationship of body parts, whether standing, lying, sitting, or moving. Good posture is the relationship of body parts that allows you to function most effectively, with the least expenditure of energy and with a minimum amount of strain on muscles, tendons, ligaments, and joints.

Ptosis (Abdominal)

Sagging, protruding abdomen.

Referred Pain

Pain that appears to be located in one area, while in reality it originates in another area.

Round Shoulders

The tips of the shoulders are drawn forward in front of the line of gravity.

Sciatica

Pain radiating down the sciatic nerve in the back of the hip and leg.

Scoliosis

A lateral curvature with some rotation of the spine; the most serious and deforming of all postural deviations.

Trigger Points

See Concept 8.

The Facts About Static Postures

Good **posture** has aesthetic benefits.

The first impression one person makes on another is usually a visual one. Good posture can help convey an impression of alertness, confidence, and attractiveness.

There is probably no one best posture for all individuals, because body build affects the balance of body parts. In general, certain relationships are desirable, however.

In the standing position, the head should be centered over the trunk, the shoulders should be down and back, but relaxed, with the chest high and the abdomen flat. The spine

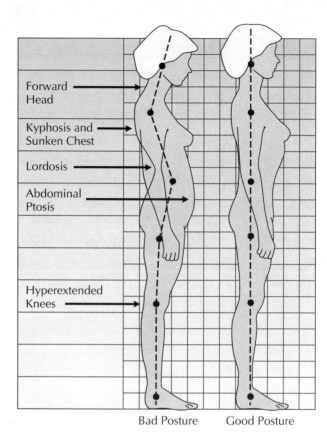

Forward Head

Kyphosis and Sunken Chest

Lordosis

Abdominal Ptosis

Hyperextended Knees

Bad Posture   Good Posture

Figure 16.1

Comparison of bad and good posture.

should have gentle curves when viewed from the side, but should be straight as seen from the back. When the pelvis is tilted properly, the pubis falls directly underneath the lower tip of the sternum. The knees should be relaxed, with the kneecaps pointed straight ahead. The feet should point straight ahead and the weight should be borne over the heel, on the outside border of the sole, and across the ball of the foot and toes.

Clinical evidence cited by physicians and opinions of educators indicate that poor posture can cause a number of health problems.

For example:

- Protruding abdomen and **lumbar lordosis** may contribute to painful menstruation, back injury, and low back syndrome.
- A forward position of the head can result in headache, dizziness, and neck, shoulder, and arm pain.
- **Rounded shoulders** may impair respiratory capacity.

- **Hyperextended knees** may predispose a person to knee injury and cause the pelvis to tilt forward, producing lumbar lordosis.
- Unbalanced postural lines can cause excessive tension in muscle groups, produce joint strain, stretch ligaments, damage joint cartilage leading to its degeneration, and become a factor in arthritic changes.
- Poor posture creates mechanical stresses that perpetuate myofascial **trigger points.**

> If one part of the body is out of line, other parts must move out of line to balance it, thus increasing the strain on muscles, ligaments, and joints.

The body is made in segments that are held balanced in a vertical column by muscles and ligaments. If gravity or a short muscle pulls one segment out of line, other portions of the body will move out of alignment to compensate, producing worse posture, more stress and strain, and possible deformity of the musculoskeletal system.

> Approximately 80 percent of the adult population suffers from acquired foot defects.

Most foot defects are acquired and are preventable. They are most often caused by improperly fitting shoes and socks; excessive hard use (such as in athletics); long standing or walking on hard surfaces; obesity or rapid weight gain (as in pregnancy); and improper bearing of weight through poor foot and leg alignment.

> There are many causes of poor posture, including hereditary, congenital, and disease conditions, as well as certain environmental factors.

Some environmental factors that may contribute to poor posture include ill-fitting clothing and shoes, chronic fatigue, improperly fitting furniture (including poor chairs, beds, and mattresses), emotional and personality problems, poor work habits, lack of physical fitness due to inactivity, and lack of knowledge relating to good posture. Some posture problems, especially **scoliosis,** may be congenital, hereditary, or acquired, but can often be corrected with exercise, braces, and/or other medical procedures. Early detection is critical in treating these problems.

> Lordosis usually results from weak abdominals and short hip flexor muscles.

As can be seen in figure 16.1, the lower part of the back normally has a slight inward curvature. If the lower back curve is too great, the muscles of the low back are more easily fatigued, more likely to suffer muscle spasms, and more prone to injury.

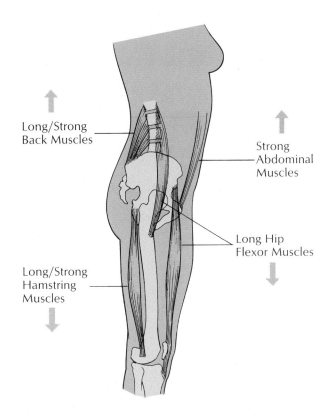

Figure 16.2
Balanced muscle strength and length permit good postural alignment.

The best way to prevent lordosis is to have strong abdominal muscles and long, but not too strong, hip flexor muscles. The strong abdominal muscles pull the bottom of the pelvis upward and help keep the top of the pelvis tipped backward, eliminating excessive back curve (fig. 16.2).

If the hip flexor muscles are too strong, or not long enough, they have the opposite effect of strong abdominal muscles; that is, they tip the top of the pelvis forward, causing excessive low back curve (lordosis). (See fig. 16.3.) This is why it is important to have long, but not too strong, hip flexor muscles. As a general rule, flexibility exercises to lengthen the hip flexor muscles, as well as strength and endurance exercises for the abdominal muscles, are recommended. For obvious reasons, exercises to increase the strength of the hip flexor muscles are not recommended for those with back pain.

> **Abdominal ptosis** can increase the risk of back pain.

If the abdomen sticks out too far over the belt line, problems with the back muscles can result. The extra weight of the protruding abdomen can cause lordosis by pulling the top of the pelvis forward. This can result in extra strain on the low back muscles and can precipitate muscle fatigue, soreness, or injury. Strengthening of the abdominal muscles and a loss of body fat, if you are overfat, are advised for this problem.

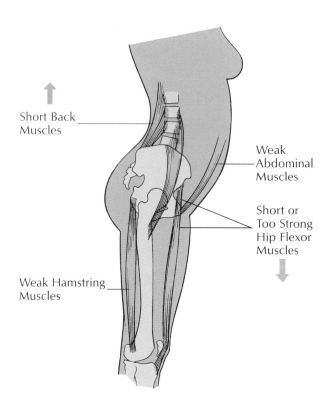

Short Back
Muscles

Weak
Abdominal
Muscles

Short or
Too Strong
Hip Flexor
Muscles

Weak Hamstring
Muscles

Figure 16.3
Unbalanced muscular development may cause poor posture or back problems.

Poor posture, especially lordosis, can cause back strain and pain and can make the back more susceptible to injury.

The forward tilt of the pelvis may cause the sacral bone or one of the lumbar vertebrae to press on nerve roots with consequent low back pain and **sciatica.** To be on the safe side, some authorities advise those who have lordosis and weak abdominals to eliminate all exercises that hyperextend the spine. Incidence of lordosis is about the same for men as it is for women, except that women experience an added back strain during pregnancy.

Some people have a "flat back" (lumbar **kyphosis**) in the lower back region that can lead to backaches.

There is an increased interest among therapists in patients who lack a normal lordotic curve in the lumbar spine. Robin McKenzie's theories and exercises (1980, 1981, 1983) have become increasingly popular in the treatment of people who sit for long periods with the back flat and pelvis tilted backward or those who engage in prolonged bending, heavy lifting, and long standing with flat back postures.

These people may need to regain a normal lordotic curve and probably need to perform relaxed static stretches with the back in hyperextension, such as the Press-Up Exercise shown in Concept 17, page 204. They may also benefit from the use of lumbar support (rolls or pillows) during sitting.

The Facts About Backaches and Neckaches

Backache has been called "a twentieth-century epidemic," "the nemesis of medicine," and "the albatross of industry" (Zamula 1989), because most people (sixty to eighty percent of all Americans) will see a physician about a backache during their lifetimes.

Backache is second only to headaches as a common medical complaint. An estimated 30–70 percent of Americans have recurring back problems, and two million cannot hold jobs as a result. It is the most frequent cause of inactivity in individuals under the age of forty-five. It most often affects people between the ages of 25 and 60. Even teenagers have backaches. (One study indicated that 26 percent of teenagers have backaches.) Athletes also have backaches, but the condition is more common in people who are not highly fit.

The causes of backache are varied, but it is rarely a dramatic event such as trauma in a diving or an automobile accident.

Incorrect postures when standing, sitting, lying, or working are responsible for many back problems. Compounding this are weak muscles and muscular imbalance. Other causes of low back pain include improper exercises (Concept 18); incorrect techniques in sports; repetitive, forced hyperextension of the back; and other preventable causes. Some of these are reflected in the list of risk factors in table 16.1. (The list excludes known causes such as trauma, tumors, and congenital abnormalities.) What you may not know is that in 80 percent of the cases, physicians are unable to pinpoint the exact cause.

The overwhelming majority of backaches and neckaches are avoidable. A common cause of backache is muscular strain, frequently precipitated by poor body mechanics in daily activities or during exercise.

When lifting improperly, there is great pressure on the lumbar disks and severe stress on the lumbar muscles and ligaments. Many popular exercises place great strain on the back (see Concept 18). Sleeping flat on the back or abdomen on a soft mattress can also cause lower back strain.

Table 16.1
Backache Risk Factors: Activities or Characteristics That Predispose People to Suffer Back Pain

• Overweight	• Trunk muscle imbalance
• Frequent bending over	• Previous back problems
• Frequent lifting of heavy loads	• Participation in gymnastics, javelin throw, diving, weight lifting, skiing, football, rowing, and swimming butterfly
• Regular exposure to vibration	• Repetitive and large range or rapid acceleration or decelleration of spine
• Lack of lumbar flexibility	• Increased age
• Lack of hamstring flexibility	• Osteoporosis
• Weak trunk extensor muscles	

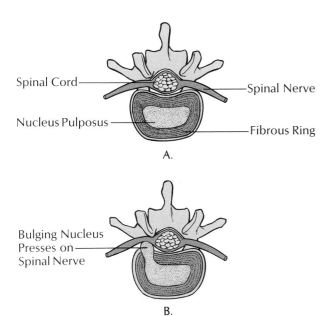

Figure 16.4
Normal disk (*A*) and herniated disk (*B*).

There is no such thing as a slipped disk.

Disk problems are frequently misunderstood. **Intervertebral disks** may herniate or rupture, but they do not slip (figure 16.4). Material from the pulpy center part of the disk (the nucleus pulposus) may bulge outward and press on spinal nerves, causing pain, and a protective reflex (muscle spasm) may occur to protect it. This causes a lack of circulation to the muscle and more pain, and more muscles tense up to prevent movement. Stiffness results and the muscles become weaker; chronic back pain may set in unless this vicious pain cycle can be stopped (figure 16.5). If it persists, bones may develop spurs, disks may degenerate, the patient may go to bed and worry and tense up, and the cycle may go on indefinitely.

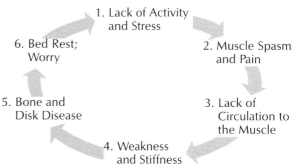

Figure 16.5
The vicious cycle of back pain.

The disks in the lumbar area are subjected to greater compression and torque because they are at the bottom of the spine. They are, therefore, more apt to be damaged. Sudden twisting and flexion or extension movements, such as suddenly reaching for a ball in tennis or racquetball, may precipitate a **herniated disk.** It is more apt to happen when the disk is degenerated from overuse (figure 16.6). It is more common in men than women and in people who do heavy manual labor. Degenerated disks are normal with aging, but not uncommon in athletes. One study shows gymnasts' disks were comparable to the disks of 65-year-old men. However, in spite of what popular literature and certain unethical "back doctors" may tell you, studies show that a herniated disk is rarely the cause of back pain—occurring in only five to ten percent of the cases.

The neck is probably strained more frequently than the lower back.

The neck is constructed with the same curve and has the same mechanical problems as the lower back. The postural fault of **head forward** places a chronic strain on the

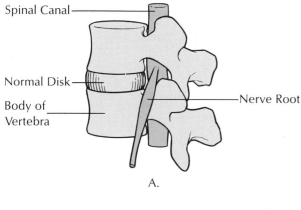

A.

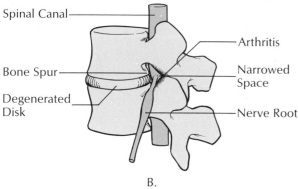

B.

Figure 16.6
Normal disk (*A*) and degenerated disk with nerve impingement and arthritic changes (*B*).

posterior neck muscles. Tension in these muscles can lead to myofascial trigger points, causing headache or **referred pain** in the face, scalp, shoulder, arm, and chest.

Kyphosis is a contributing factor in neck pain.

The more the upper back is flexed, the greater the compensating curve (**cervical lordosis**) in the neck. The sharpest angle is between the fourth and sixth cervical vertebrae, creating wear and tear (microtrauma) that accelerates disk degeneration and arthritic changes, which can ultimately result in nerve and artery impingement.

The causes of chronic neck pain are many, and they have a complex interaction that varies with the individual and makes it difficult to diagnose and prevent or treat.

Some of the causes of chronic neck pain (and the often accompanying shoulder pain) includes workplace design, posture, work habits, physical fitness, and stress. The risk factors that predispose a person to suffering from neck pain are listed in table 16.2.

Table 16.2
Some Risk Factors for Chronic Neck (and Shoulder) Pain

- Poor posture (especially cervical lordosis and kyphosis)
- In women, large breasts
- Weak neck muscles (especially flexors and rotators)
- Stress
- Job dissatisfaction
- Job monotony (repetitive motion or position)
- Degenerated disks
- Desk or chair too low or high
- Wearing bifocals (to read computer screen)
- Arthritis
- Previous neck injury
- Hold/carry loads for long periods (e.g., purse, briefcase, baby)

Facts About Prevention and Intervention

Practicing good body mechanics and posture can help prevent back problems.

Several practical suggestions for modifying everyday activities are listed here.

- To relieve back stress due to a swayback during prolonged standing, try to keep the lower back flat by propping one foot on a stool or rail; alternate feet occasionally. Dentists, hair dressers, barbers, and store clerks are particularly susceptible to back problems because they must stand while working.
- If your back arches excessively when sitting, use a hard chair with a straight back and armrests, placing the spine against it; keep one or both knees higher than the hips by crossing the legs (alternate sides) or by using a foot rest and keeping the knees bent. If your back flattens when you sit, use a lumbar roll behind your lower back. (See fig. 16.7.)
- When driving a car, to avoid a swayback position place a hard seat and backrest combination over the seat of the automobile; pull the seat forward so the legs are bent when operating the pedals. If your back flattens when you drive, use a lumbar support pillow.
- When lying, keep the knees and hips bent; avoid lying on the abdomen. When lying on the back, a pillow or lift should be placed under the knees.
- Avoid improper lifting and carrying. Especially avoid bending over or straightening the spine while twisting. (This can be more damaging from a sitting position than from a standing position.)

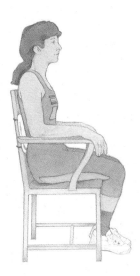

Figure 16.7
A proper chair and good posture can prevent back problems from prolonged sitting.

- Do exercises to strengthen abdominal and hip extensors, and to stretch the hip flexors and lumbar muscles if they are tight.
- Avoid hazardous exercises (see Concept 18).
- General exercises involving the entire body, such as walking, jogging, swimming, and bicycling are important in preventing weak or tight muscles.
- Warm up before engaging in strenuous activity.
- Get adequate rest and sleep. Avoid pushing yourself mentally or physically to the point of exhaustion.
- Vary the working position by changing from one task to another before feeling fatigued. When working at a desk, get up and stretch occasionally to relieve tension.
- Sleep on a firm mattress or place a three-fourths-inch-thick plywood board under the mattress.
- Avoid sudden, jerky back movements, especially twisting.
- The smaller the waistline, the lesser the strain on the lower back. Avoid obesity.

Practicing good body mechanics and posture can prevent or alleviate neck pain.

Some modifications of your daily activities are suggested here.

- Use appropriate back and seat supports when sitting for longer periods.
- Use proper tools and equipment to reduce neck strain; for example, use a paint roller with an extension to reach overhead, thus reducing the need to hold the arms overhead and to hyperextend the neck.
- Maintain good posture when carrying heavy loads; don't lean forward, sideways, or backward.

- When sleeping, use a good pillow that supports your head in a neutral position—not too high or too low.
- Adjust sports equipment to permit good posture; for example, adjust bicycle seat and handle bars to permit good body alignment.
- When you have a neckache,
  a. lie down;
  b. apply heat or ice;
  c. massage the neck and shoulders; and
  d. stretch the neck muscles.
- Avoid long periods of desk sitting or driving; take frequent breaks and adjust the seat and headrest for maximum support.
- To avoid injury, use safe sports equipment and techniques, e.g., proper helmet and cervical collar (if indicated); look before you dive in water.
- When shaving, don't tilt the head backward.
- Wash your hair in the shower rather than in the sink.
- Try to work at eye level; for example, when typing put the copy on a vertical typist's stand; when working above head level, get on a stool or ladder to avoid tipping the head back.
- Do not sit in front row theater seats so you don't have to tip your head back.

The Facts About Dynamic Postures: Lifting and Carrying

The best method for lifting or carrying a given object depends upon its size, weight, shape, and position in space. However, here are some general principles that are applicable to lifting with both hands, including the weight lifting squats.

- *Stand close to the object and assume a wide base.* Stand in a forward-backward stride position with the object at the side of the body, or assume a side-stride position with the object between the knees. The purpose of lifting from this position is to allow you to lift straight upward from a stable position, utilizing the most efficient leverage.
- *Keep the head up and the back fairly erect with the normal lordotic curve maintained, and bend at the hips and knees. Squat, do not bend, regardless of how light the object may be.* The back was never meant to be used as a lever for lifting. Avoid leaning forward to pick up objects without bending the knees because of the strain placed on the muscles and joints of the spine. This kind of back strain can occur when improperly making a bed or when lifting a child out of a crib.
- *Lower your body only as far as necessary, directly downward.* Squatting lower than is necessary is a waste of energy, but more importantly perhaps, deep knee bends can damage the structures of the knee joints.

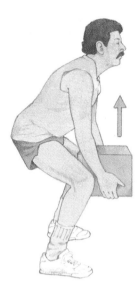

Figure 16.8

Maintain a normal curve in the back when lifting an object with both hands.

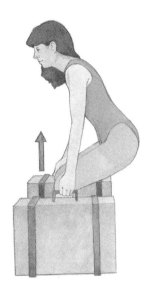

Figure 16.9

Divide a heavy load.

• *Grasp the object, tighten the lower back muscles, then lift with your leg muscles, keeping the object close to the body's center of gravity.* (See figure 16.8.) The leg muscles are the strongest in the body. If the back is kept erect, use of the legs for lifting allows a maximal force to be applied to the load without wasting energy. Do not twist during the lift. If the object is heavy, hold your breath on the lift (this produces "trunk cavity pressurization," which helps to reduce the load on the spine). A lumbar belt may also help protect the spine.

• *Carry the object close to the body's center of gravity and no higher than waist level (except when carrying on the shoulder, head, or back).* When objects are carried in front of the body above the level of the waist, you must lean backward to balance the load, producing an undesirable arch in the lower back. Carrying loads at the midline of the body, such as in a knapsack or on the head or shoulders, is **effective** in reducing the stress on the skeletal system.

• *Push or pull heavy objects, if this can be done efficiently, rather than lifting them.* Theoretically, it takes about thirty-four times more force to lift than to slide an object across the floor. The size, shape, and friction of the object determine whether or not it is feasible to push or pull it.

• *Divide the load if possible, carrying half in each arm. If the load cannot be divided, alternate it from one side of the body to the other.* (See figure 16.9.) When walking with the weight carried on one side of the body, the force on the opposite hip is much greater than when the load is distributed on both sides. This is true even when the bilateral load is twice as great as the unilateral load. If the weight must be carried on only one side, the opposite arm should be raised to counterbalance the load and to help keep the center of gravity over the base.

• *Avoid hyperextending the neck and the back when lifting and lowering an object from overhead. Any lift above waist level is inefficient.* Occasionally, you must reach overhead to lift an object from a high shelf. To avoid back and neck strain, climb a ladder or stand on a stool so you don't have to raise your arms overhead. If this is not practical, reach for the object with your weight on the forward foot, and then step backward on the rear foot as the object is lowered.

• *Do not try to lift or carry loads too heavy for you.* The most economical load for the average adult is about thirty-five percent of the body weight. Obviously, with strength training, you can safely lift a greater load.

One-handed lifts are executed with the same body mechanics as a two-handed lift, except for the use of one arm to support the trunk.

Some guidelines for one-handed lifting are included below (Boyce and Jackson 1991). (Remember to use the same squat technique as described for the two-handed lifts, above).

A. *When lifting from the floor, follow these four steps:*

 1. Squat and support the weight of the trunk by putting the left hand on the floor while grasping the weight with the right.

 2. Remain in this position and lift the weight to the right thigh.

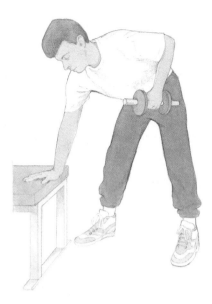

Figure 16.10
When lifting with one hand (as in upright rowing), support the trunk with the other hand.

3. Shift your upper body weight toward the right while the left hand moves from the floor to the left thigh.
4. Push with the left hand on the thigh to help raise the trunk as the legs extend.

Reverse these steps to return the weight to the floor.

B. *For one-arm upright rowing or for lifting loads from awkward, bent-over positions such as a car trunk or a baby's crib:*

Use a technique similar to the one-arm lift from the floor. Support the trunk with your free arm by leaning on something for support while lifting with the other arm. This saves the back muscles from having to do the work (see figure 16.10).

The Facts About Dynamic Postures: Pushing and Pulling

The choice to push or to pull a load depends upon the nature of the task.

When deciding whether to push or pull an object, you must consider such factors as desired direction, type of movement, distance to be moved, and friction. If a downward force is desired, pushing would be best. If an upward force is desirable, pulling is probably better. Pushing tends to increase friction because of the downward force, but may offer better control because the object is closer to the person. Pulling decreases friction if there is an upward component to the force.

Pushing and pulling are forms of lifting; therefore, the same mechanical principles may be applied.

When pushing or pulling, the back should be kept as erect as possible, a wide stance should be used, and the leg muscles should do the work rather than the back or arms. You may alternate the working muscles by changing positions occasionally; that is, face forward, then backward, then sideward.

Force should be applied as nearly as possible in the desired line of direction.

If **linear motion** is desired, you should apply force at the center of the object's gravity and push or pull in the desired direction by leaning from the hips in that direction. To move an object horizontally, the upward and downward components of the push or pull should be reduced to a minimum. When pulling, increasing the length of the handle reduces the vertical component.

If there is a great deal of friction, the force should be applied below the object's center of gravity. Sufficient force should be applied continuously to keep the load moving, because it takes more force to start an object moving (overcoming inertia) than to keep it going.

When rotary motion is desired, apply force away from the center of gravity of the object.

Objects that are too heavy or too awkward to be moved as a whole, such as a refrigerator or couch, can be moved by applying force alternately at one end and then the other, so that a pivoting or "walking" action is employed to rotate the object.

The Facts About Dynamic Postures: Saving Energy During Work

When working with the arms in front of the body, a pulling motion is easier than a pushing motion.

The pulling motion uses the stronger flexor muscles, whereas a pushing motion employs the seldom-used extensors that are usually weaker. Thus, counterclockwise circular movements are easier for the right hand, and clockwise circular movements easier for the left hand.

Organize work to avoid stooping or unnatural positions that cause strain.

• Sideward flexion of the trunk is more strenuous than forward trunk flexion.

- Avoid constant arm extension, whether forward or sideward.
- Whenever possible, sit while working but stand occasionally.
- The arms should move either together or in opposite directions. When the conditions allow, use both hands in opposite and symmetrical motions while working.
- Tools most often used should be the closest to reach.
- When working with the hands, the workbench or kitchen cabinet should be about 2 to 4 inches below the waist. The office desk should be about 29 to 30 inches high for the average man and about 27 to 29 inches high for the average woman.

Some types of arm movements are more accurate than others.

Horizontal movements are more precise than vertical ones. Circular movements are better than zigzag ones. Movements toward the body are easier to control than those away from the body. Rhythmic movements are more accurate and less tiring than abrupt movements.

Suggested Readings

Field, R. "How Humans Sit." *The American Way* (April 15, 1988):pp. 28–29.

Zamula, E. "Back Talk: Advice for Suffering Spines." *FDA Consumer* 23(1989):28.

LAB RESOURCE MATERIALS

(For use with Lab 16A, page L-43)

Chart 16.1 Posture Evaluation			
Side View	**Points**	**Back View**	**Points**
Head forward	_____	Tilted head	_____
Sunken chest	_____	Protruding scapulae	_____
Round shoulders	_____	Symptoms of scoliosis: Shoulders uneven	_____
Kyphosis	_____	Hips uneven	_____
Lordosis	_____	Lateral curvature of spine (Adams' position)	_____
Abdominal ptosis	_____	One side of back high (Adams' position)	_____
Hyperextended knees Body lean	_____		
		Total score_____	

Chart 16.2 Posture *Rating Scale*	
Classification	**Total Score**
Excellent	0–2
Very good	3–4
Good	5–7
Fair	8–11
Poor	12 or more

LAB RESOURCE MATERIALS

(For use with Labs 16B–16C, pages L-45 and L-47)

Chart 16.3 Healthy Back Tests

These tests are among the ones used by physicians and therapists to make differential diagnoses of back problems. You and your partner can use them to determine if you have muscle tightness that may make you "at risk" for back problems. Discontinue any of these tests if they produce pain or numbness, or tingling sensations in the back, hips, or legs. Experiencing any of these sensations may be an indication that you have a low back problem that requires diagnosis by your physician. Partners should use *great caution* in applying force. Be gentle and listen to your partner's feedback.

	Pass	Fail

Test 1—Back to Wall

Stand with your back against a wall, with head, heels, shoulders, and calves of legs touching the wall as shown in the diagram. Try to flatten your neck and the hollow of your back by pressing your buttocks down against the wall. Your partner should just be able to place a hand in the space between the wall and the small of your back. If this space is greater than the thickness of his/her hand, you probably have lordosis with shortened lumbar and hip flexor muscles.

Test 2—Straight Leg-Lift

Lie on your back with hands behind your neck. The partner on your left should stabilize your right leg by placing his/her right hand on the knee. With the left hand, your partner should grasp the left ankle and raise your left leg as near to a right angle as possible. In this position (as shown in the diagram), your lower back should be in contact with the floor. Your right leg should remain straight and on the floor throughout the test. If your left leg bends at the knee, short hamstring muscles are indicated. If your back arches and/or your right leg does not remain flat on the floor, short lumbar muscles or hip flexor muscles (or both) are indicated. Repeat the test on the opposite side. (Both sides must pass in order to pass the test.)

Test 3—Thomas Test

Lie on your back on a table or bench with your right leg extended beyond the edge of the table (approximately one-third of the thigh off the table). Bring your left knee to your chest and pull the thigh down tightly with your hands. Your lower back should remain flat against the table as shown in the diagram. Your right thigh should remain on the table. If your right thigh lifts off the table while the left knee is hugged to chest, a tight hip flexor (iliopsoas) on that side is indicated. Repeat on the opposite side. (Both sides must pass in order to pass the test.)

Test 4—Ely's Test

Lie prone; flex right knee. Partner *gently* pushes right heel toward the buttocks. Stop when resistance is felt or when partner expresses discomfort. Pelvis should remain on floor with no flexion at hip. Knee should bend freely 135 degrees, or heel should touch buttocks if there is no tightness in the quadriceps muscles. Repeat on the other side. (You must pass on both sides to pass the test.)

Chart 16.3 *Continued*

	Pass	Fail

Test 5—Ober's Test ☐ ☐

Lie on left side with left leg flexed 90 degrees at the hip and 90 degrees at the knee. Partner places right hip in neutral position (no flexion) and right knee in 90-degree flexion; partner then allows the weight of the leg to lower it toward the floor. If there is no tightness in the iliotibial band (fascia and muscles on lateral side of leg), the knee touches the floor without pain and the test is passed. Repeat on the other side. (Both sides must pass in order to pass the test.)

Test 6—Press-Up (Straight Arm) ☐ ☐

Perform the press-up as described in exercise no. 13. If you can press to a straight arm position, keeping your pubis in contact with the floor, and if your partner determines that the arch in your back is a continuous curve (not just a sharp angle at the lumbosacral joint), then there is adequate flexibility in spinal extension.

Test 7—Knee Roll ☐ ☐

Lie supine with both knees and hips flexed 90 degrees, arms extended to the sides at shoulder level. Keep the knees and hips in that position and lower them to the floor on the right and then on the left. If you can accomplish this and still keep your shoulders in contact with the floor, then you have adequate rotation in the spine, especially at the lumbar and thoracic junction. (You must pass both sides in order to pass the test.)

Chart 16.4 Healthy Back Test Ratings	
	Number of Tests Passed
Excellent	7
Very good	6
Good	5
Fair	4
Poor	1–3

Chart 16.5 Backache Risk Assessment

Check "yes" if the statement applies to you; check "no" if it does not apply. Total the number of "yes" answers.

	Yes	No
1. I often have a backache at the end of the day.	☐	☐
2. I usually don't think of my back when I lift and carry things.	☐	☐
3. I often move heavy loads without getting help.	☐	☐
4. I'm not sure I use good body mechanics when I work.	☐	☐
5. I frequently push and pull things.	☐	☐
6. I do a lot of bending over.	☐	☐
7. I do a lot of reaching in work or exercise and sports.	☐	☐
8. I do a lot of twisting in work or exercise and sports.	☐	☐
9. I do a lot of lifting and carrying.	☐	☐
10. I don't do strength exercises for my back and abdomen regularly.	☐	☐
11. I don't do stretching exercises for my trunk, hips, and legs regularly.	☐	☐
12. I sit for long periods without a break.	☐	☐
13. I spend a lot of time leaning over my work.	☐	☐
14. I do exercises that are considered "questionable."	☐	☐

Total _____

Chart 16.6 Back Risk Rating

	Number of Yes Answers
Extremely high risk	10–14
High risk	7–9
Moderate risk	4–6
Some risk	1–3
Low risk	0

17

Exercises for Good Posture and Care of the Neck and Back

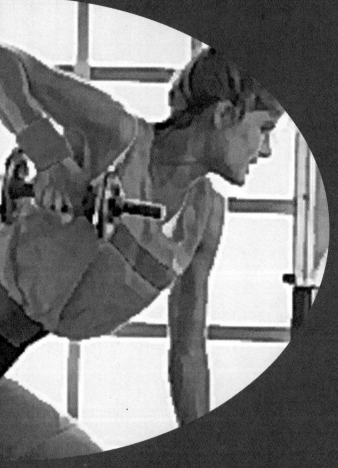

Concept 17

Exercise plays an important role in the prevention and correction of neck and backaches and poor posture.

Introduction

Exercises included in previous concepts were presented with health-related fitness in mind. The exercises included in this concept are not really so different. They are either flexibility or strength exercises for specific muscle groups; however, each is selected specifically to help correct a postural problem or to remove the cause of neck and back pain. To that extent these exercises may be classified as "therapeutic." These same exercises may be called "preventative" because they can be used to prevent postural or spine problems.

Whether therapeutic or preventative, the exercises will not be effective unless they are done faithfully and with the "FIT Formula" applied. Those who have back and neck pain should seek the advice of a physician to make certain that it is safe for them to perform the exercises.

Health Goal for the Year 2000

▬ Reduce activity limitations due to chronic back conditions.

Terms

▬ See Concept 16.

Exercise is one of the most frequently prescribed treatments for painful spines.

Treatments range from surgical removal of a disk or fusion, to more conservative measures such as injections, electrical stimulation, muscle relaxants, antiinflammatory drugs, vapo-coolant spray, bracing, traction, bed rest, heat, cryotherapy, massage, and therapeutic exercise. Regardless of the treatment used, 70 to 85 percent of back patients recover spontaneously. Of those, 70 percent will have no symptoms by the end of three weeks and 90 percent will recover in two months (Tietz 1985). The various treatment modalities may simply make patients more comfortable or they may hasten the recovery.

Exercise has been found to be helpful in treating all kinds of chronic pain. (Resistance exercises and aerobic exercises have been particularly helpful in pain clinics.) Aerobic exercise is also known to help nourish the spinal disks.

Exercise can serve to prevent or correct some of the underlying causes of back and neck pain by strengthening weak muscles and stretching short ones. In the process of creating muscle balance, it improves postural alignment and body mechanics and relaxes muscle spasms.

Exercises for the correction of postural deviations are generally based on this assumption: if the problem is a functional deformity, regardless of the factors causing it, muscular imbalance will be present.

If the muscles on one side of a joint are stronger than the muscles on the opposite side of that joint, the body part is pulled in the direction of the stronger muscles. Corrective exercises are usually designed to strengthen the long, weak muscles and to stretch the short, strong ones in order to have equal pull in both directions. For example, those with lumbar lordosis may need to strengthen the abdominals and hamstrings, and stretch the lower back and hip flexor muscles.

Some people are unable to lift loads safely because tight and/or weak muscles may prevent them from using proper body mechanics.

Some people have backaches because they lift improperly. In many instances the poor technique is caused by muscle imbalance, such as hamstrings or gluteals too tight to permit the lower back to retain its normal curve during the squat and lift; or calf muscles too tight to allow the heels to remain on the floor during the squat; or abdominals too weak to support the back and quadriceps and gluteals too weak to lift the weight of the body and the load. Proper exercise could remediate these problems.

Exercises for Good Posture and Care of the Neck and Back

The exercises suggested here should be performed as described until you are able to increase repetitions. Most people need to do all of these exercises regularly, but some may need to perform only selected exercises to meet their specific needs. Muscles depicted in color are those primarily involved in the exercise.

1. Wand Exercise

Purpose

To help prevent and correct round shoulders and kyphosis by stretching the muscles on the anterior side of the shoulder joint.

Position

Sit with wand grasped at ends. Raise wand overhead. Be certain that the head does not slide forward into a "poke neck" position. Keep the chin tucked and neck straight.

Movement

Bring wand down behind shoulder blades. Keep spine erect. Hold. Hands may be moved closer together to increase stretch on chest muscles.

Note

If this is an easy exercise for you, try straightening the elbows and bringing the wand to waist level in back of you.

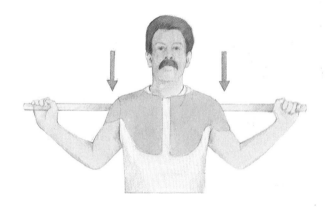

2. Pectoral Stretch

Purpose

To stretch pectorals and prevent or correct kyphosis and round shoulders.

See exercise 5, p. 89.

3. Side Bender

Purpose

To stretch trunk lateral flexors and help prevent and correct backaches by maintaining flexibility in the spine.

Position

Stand with feet shoulder width apart.

Movement

Stretch left arm overhead to right. Bend to right at waist reaching as far to right as possible with left arm; reach as far as possible to the left with right arm; hold. Do not let trunk rotate or lower back arch. Repeat on opposite side.

Note

This exercise is made more effective if a weight is held in the hand opposite the side being stretched. More stretch occurs also if the hip on the stretched side is dropped and most of the weight is borne by the opposite foot.

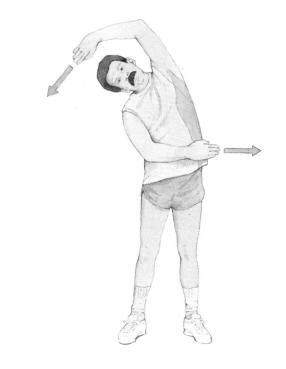

4. Isometric Neck Exercises

Purpose

To strengthen the neck muscles and prevent or correct forward head and cervical lordosis, as well as upper back and neck trigger points and pain.

Position

Assume good head and neck posture by tucking the chin, flattening the neck, and pushing the crown of the head up (axial extension). Sit; place one or both hands on the head as shown.

Movement

Apply resistance sideward, backward, and forward. Contract the neck muscles to prevent the head and neck from moving. Hold six seconds; repeat up to six times.

Note

For neck muscles, it is probably best to use less than a maximal contraction, especially in the presence of arthritis, degenerated disks, or injury.

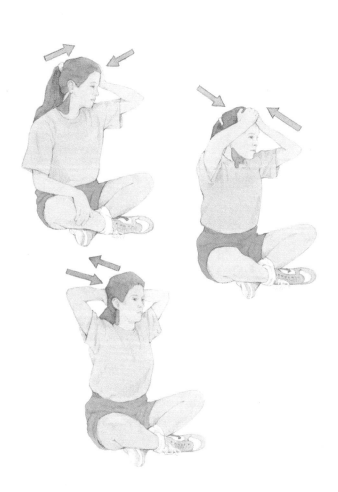

5. Neck Rotation Exercise

Purpose

This PNF exercise strengthens and stretches the neck rotators. It should always be done with the head and neck in axial extension (good alignment). It is particularly useful for relieving trigger point pain and stiffness.

Position

Place palm of left hand against left cheek; point fingers toward ear and point elbow forward.

Movement

Try to turn head and neck left while resisting with left hand. Hold six seconds. Relax and turn head to right as far as possible; hold ten seconds. Repeat four times; then repeat on opposite side.

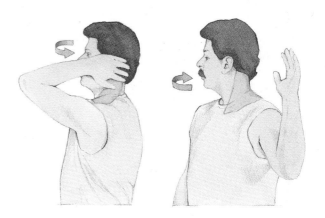

6. Back-Saver Hamstring Stretch

Purpose

To stretch hamstrings and calf muscles, and help prevent or correct backache caused in part by short hamstrings.

Position

Sit on the floor with the feet against the wall or an immovable object. Bend left knee and bring foot close to buttocks. Clasp hands behind back.

Movement

Bend forward from hips, keeping lower back as straight as possible. Let bent knee rotate outward so trunk can move forward. Lean forward keeping back flat; hold and repeat on each leg.

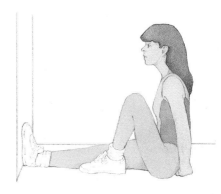

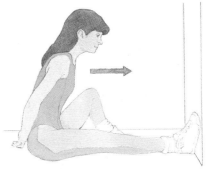

7. Hip and Thigh Stretcher

Purpose

To stretch hip flexor muscles, and help prevent or correct forward pelvic tilt, lumbar lordosis, and backache.

See exercise 8, p. 90.

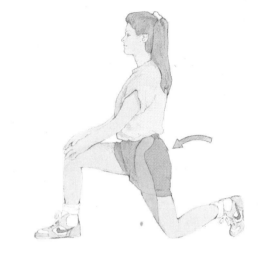

8. Low Back Stretcher

Purpose

To stretch hip flexors, gluteals, and lumbar muscles, and help prevent or correct lumbar lordosis and backache.

Position

Supine position.

Movement

Draw one knee up to the chest and pull thigh down tightly with the hands, then slowly return to the original position. Repeat with other knee. Do not grasp knee; grasp thigh. If a partner or a weight stabilizes the extended leg, the hip flexor muscles on that leg will also be stretched.

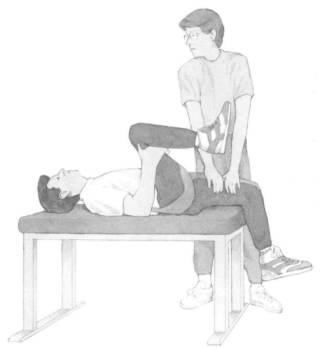

9. Single Knee-to-Chest

Purpose

To stretch lower back, gluteals, and hamstring muscles and help prevent or correct lordosis and backache.

Position

Supine with knees bent.

Movement

Use hands on back of thigh to draw one knee to the chest, then extend the knee and point the foot toward the ceiling; hold. Return to the starting position by drawing the knee back to the chest before sliding the foot to the floor. Repeat with other leg.

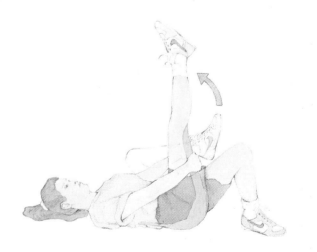

10. Double Knee-to-Chest

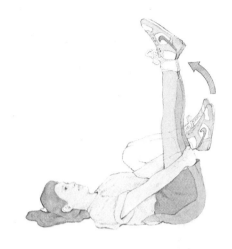

Purpose

To stretch lower back, gluteals, and hamstring muscles, and help prevent or correct lordosis and backache (advanced exercise).

Same as Single Knee-to-Chest, except use both legs simultaneously.

Note

If you are a back patient, this is more advanced than the preceding exercises and it should not be attempted until the others have been performed for three to four weeks.

11. Calf Stretcher

Purpose

To stretch the calf muscles (gastronemius and soleus) to enable you to squat correctly when performing lifts.

See fig. 4.1, p. 37.

12. Lower Leg Stretcher

Purpose

Same as calf stretcher except it is a more advanced exercise.

See exercise #1, p. 87.

13. Half-Squat with Weights

Purpose

To strengthen hip and knee extensors; to train specifically for squatting and lifting.

See exercise #19, p. 130.

14. Pelvic Tilt

Purpose

To strengthen abdominals and help prevent or correct lumbar lordosis, abdominal ptosis, and backache.

Position

Supine with knees bent.

Movement

Tighten the abdominal muscles and tilt the pelvis backward; try to flatten the lower back against the floor. At the same time, tighten the hip and thigh muscles. Hold, then relax. Breathe normally during the contraction, do not hold the breath.

15. Reverse Curl

Purpose

To strengthen lower abdominals and to correct or prevent abdominal ptosis and backache. (This is more advanced than the pelvic tilt.)

See exercise #6, p. 126.

16. Crunch (Curl-Up)

Purpose

To strengthen upper abdominals; to correct or prevent abdominal ptosis, lordosis, or backache.

See fig. 18.16, p. 213.

17. Crunch with Twist (on Bench)

Purpose

To strengthen the oblique abdominals and help prevent or correct lumbar lordosis, abdominal ptosis, and backache.

Position

Lie supine with feet on bench, knees bent 90 degrees. Arms may be extended or on shoulders or hands on ears (the most difficult).

Movement

Flatten the lower back and curl the head, neck, and shoulders until the shoulder blades leave the floor, twisting the upper trunk so the right shoulder is higher than the left. Reach toward the right knee with the left elbow. Hold; return and repeat to the opposite side.

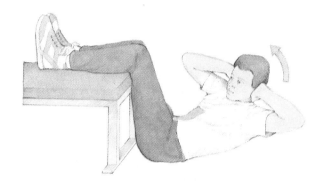

18. Sitting Tucks

Purpose

To strengthen the lower abdominals and increase their endurance; improve posture and prevent backache. (This is an advanced exercise.)

See Test #1 on p. 121 in the Lab Resource Material for Concept 11.

19. Standing Crunch

Purpose

To strengthen abdominals, prevent or correct lordosis, abdominal ptosis, and backaches.

Position

Stand erect, holding ends of elastic resistance (tubes or bands) in each hand at shoulder level. Contract abdominals and tilt pelvis backward, flattening the lower back.

Movement

Pull on the elastic resistance by curling the chest toward the pubis, keeping the pelvis tilted backward.

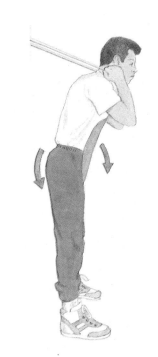

20. Arm Lift

Purpose

To strengthen scapular adductors and help prevent or correct round shoulders and kyphosis.

Position

a. Least difficult: lie prone with arms in reverse-T; forehead resting on floor.

b. More advanced—same as "a" except extend arms overhead and hold against the ears.

Movement

Maintain the arm position and contract the muscles between the shoulder blades, lifting the arms as high as possible without raising head and trunk. Hold; relax and repeat.

Note

If the arms are first pressed against the floor before lifting, this becomes a PNF exercise and range of motion may be greater.

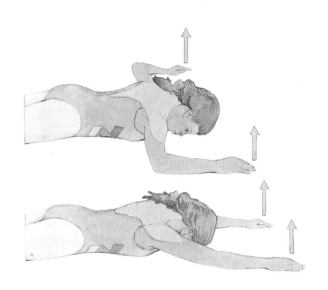

21. Seated Rowing

Purpose

To strengthen the scapular adductors (rhomboid and trapezius) and to prevent or correct kyphosis, round shoulders, head forward or cervical lordosis, and neck pain. See exercise #25, p. 133.

22. Upper Trunk Lift

Purpose

Develop upper back strength.

Position

Lie on a table or bench with the upper half of the body hanging over the edge.

Movement

Have a partner stabilize the feet while the trunk is raised parallel to the floor, then lower the trunk to the starting position. Place hands behind neck. Do not raise past the horizontal or arch the back.

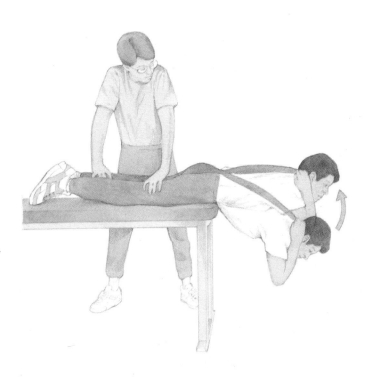

23. Lower Trunk Lift

Purpose

Develop low back and hip strength.

Position

Lie prone on bench or table with legs hanging over the edge.

Movement

Have a partner stabilize the upper back or grasp the edges of the table with hands. Raise the legs parallel to the floor and lower them. Do not raise past the horizontal or arch the back. Suggested progression: (1) Begin by alternating legs; when you can do 25 reps, (2) add ankle weights; when you can do 25 reps, (3) lift both legs simultaneously (no weights).

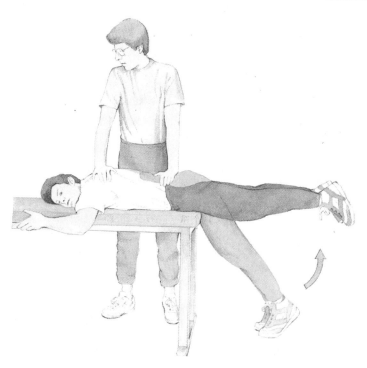

24. Press-Up (McKenzie Extension Exercise)

Purpose

To increase flexibility of lumbar spine, reduce tension on posterior disks and longitudinal ligaments, and restore normal lordotic curve, especially for those with a flat lumbar spine.

Position

Prone with hands under the face.

Movement

Slowly press up to a rest position on forearms; keep pelvis on floor. Relax and *hold* ten seconds. Repeat once; do several times a day. Progress to gradually straightening the elbows while keeping the pubic bone on the floor. *Caution:* Do *not* perform if you have lordosis or if it produces any pain or discomfort in the back or legs.

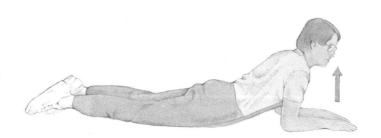

Note

A prone press-up will feel good as a stretch after doing abdominal strength or endurance exercises. This relaxed lordotic position can be performed while standing. Place the hands in the small of the back and gently arch the back and hold. This should feel good after sitting for a long period with the back flat.

25. Bridging

Purpose

To strengthen hip extensors, especially gluteal muscles and help prevent and correct lordosis and forward pelvic tilt.

Position

Supine with knees bent and feet close to buttocks.

Movement

Contract gluteals, lifting buttocks and lower back off floor. Hold; relax; repeat. Do not allow the lower back to arch.

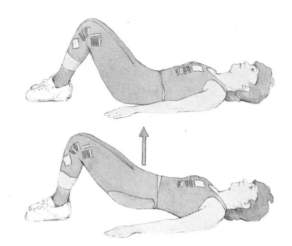

26. Wall Slide

Purpose

To help prevent or correct poor spinal alignment by teaching the feel of flattening the neck and back, and tilting the pelvis.

Position

Stand with heels 4 to 6 inches from wall, arms at sides.

Movement

Flatten neck and lumbar region to wall by flexing knees and sliding down wall until spine can be forced against it. Slide up wall, maintaining flat spine. Walk away from wall, keeping curves flat. Return to wall and check alignment. Repeat with hands behind neck and elbows touching wall. Repeat with arms at sides and sandbag on head. Repeated flexion and extension of the knees can develop strength in the quadriceps muscles on the front of the thigh.

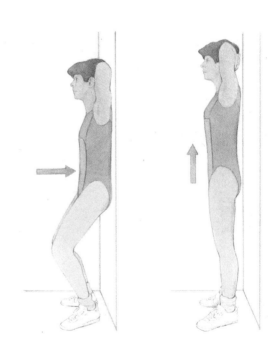

27. Supine Trunk Twist

Purpose

To increase flexibility of spine and stretch rotator muscles.

Position

Lie supine, arms extended at shoulder level; left foot on right patella.

Movement

Twist the lower body by lowering left knee to touch floor on right. Turn head to left; try to keep shoulders and arms on floor.

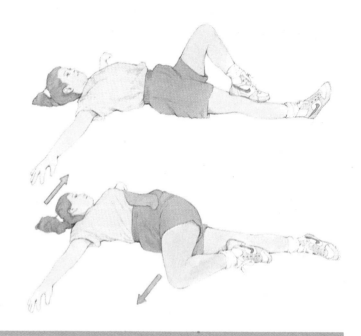

Suggested Readings

Field, R. "How Humans Sit." *The American Way* (April 15, 1988):pp. 28–29.

Zamula, E. "Back Talk: Advice for Suffering Spines." *FDA Consumer* 23(1989):28.

18

Exercise Cautions

Concept 18

Some exercises should be used with caution or not used at all because they are "high risk" exercises or because they may cause more harm than good.

Introduction

There are literally thousands of exercises from which one can choose, but they must be chosen carefully because *all* exercises are not good for *all* people. Some exercises should be avoided because there is some risk of injury. We term these exercises "questionable" or "hazardous." Some of these exercises so drastically violate the mechanics of the human frame that they are dangerous and should probably never be used by anyone.

Studies indicate that many commercial enterprises do not employ properly trained instructors. Those who are qualified to advise you about exercise have college degrees and four to eight years of study in such courses as anatomy, physiology, kinesiology, preventive and therapeutic exercise, and physiology of exercise. These qualified individuals are physical educators, kinesiotherapists, and physical therapists. On-the-job training, a good physique or figure, and good dancing ability are not sufficient qualifications for teaching or advising about exercise.

If you have had knowledgeable instructors, you may recognize some of these exercises, but others listed here may set off a protest such as: "I've been doing that all my life and it never has hurt me!"

This Concept explains the difference between individually prescribed exercise and mass prescription; what is good for you may not be good for me. The difference between microtrauma and acute injury, and the significance of the number of repetitions will also be discussed. Exercises that are believed to be potentially hazardous for most people are presented with the reasons for classifying them as such. Alternative exercises that may be safer are then suggested. The old saying "when in doubt, don't do it" is a good philosophy when choosing exercises, because there are always safe, effective alternative exercises for any specific muscle group.

Health Goal for the Year 2000

- Increase the proportion of people who engage in appropriate physical activity for promoting health-related physical fitness.

Terms

Bursa

Small sac filled with fluid and situated between muscles, or between muscles and bones, to prevent friction.

Hyperflexion

Bending (flexing) a joint more than normal; excessive bending.

Hyperventilation

"Overbreathing"; forced, rapid, or deep breathing.

Microtrauma

Injury so small it is not detected at the time it occurs.

Pyriformis Syndrome

Muscle spasm and nerve entrapment in the pyriformis muscle of the buttocks region causing pain in the buttock and referred pain down the leg (sciatica).

Sciatica

Pain along the sciatic nerve in the buttock and leg.

Spondylolysis

A stress fracture of a vertebra at the pars interarticularis.

Spondylolisthesis

Forward displacement of a vertebra, usually the fourth or fifth lumbar.

Torque

A twisting or rotating force.

Valsalva Maneuver

Exerting force with the epiglottis closed, thus increasing pressure in the thorax and raising arterial pressure. When released, arterial pressure drops rapidly, blood vessels expand and are then filled, causing a lag in blood flow to the left ventricle. When this occurs, the subject may become dizzy or feel faint. May be caused by holding the breath while exerting force.

The Facts: Rationale

There is a difference between exercises that are good when prescribed for a particular individual and those that are good for everyone (mass prescription).

Individual Prescription

An example of an exercise program in which the exercise is individually prescribed is the clinical setting. A therapist works with one patient and takes a case history, administers tests and measurements to determine which muscles are weak or strong, or short or long. A determination of existing limitations that might make any given exercise indicated or contraindicated is made, and then exercises are prescribed for that person. The patient is supervised in the correct execution of the movements.

For example, in a back care program for an individual with lumbar lordosis or lumbar degenerative disk disease and arthritis, back hyperextension exercises might be contraindicated. However, another client might have a flat lumbar spine with limited range of motion, in which

case, a set of back hyperextension exercises (McKenzie 1981) would be indicated. Thus, the classification of exercises in this Concept does not necessarily apply to the setting where individual prescription is done by a qualified professional. A qualified professional is one who is expert in applied anatomy, kinesiology, therapeutic exercise, and functional tests as well as being knowledgeable about pathomechanics and other acute and chronic conditions. Typically this includes physical therapists, kinesiotherapists, and physical educators with graduate specialization in corrective/remedial/therapeutic physical education.

Mass Prescription

When a physical educator, aerobics instructor, or coach leads a group of people in exercises, or a book or magazine describes a great exercise to "slim and trim" and all participants in the group or all readers perform the same exercise, this is a *mass prescription*. There is little if any consideration for individual differences except perhaps some allowance made in the number of repetitions or in the amount of weight (resistance) used.

Some of the exercises that would be appropriate for an individual would not be appropriate for all individuals in the group. Since it is not practical to prescribe individually for everyone, it is necessary to consider what the needs of the majority may be and choose the least harmful (but most effective exercises) for the group.

Some exercises can produce microtrauma, and some may cause acute injuries.

Microtrauma refers to "a silent injury"; that is, an injury that results from chronic, repetitive motions such as the ones we use in calisthenics or sports. Other terms which appear frequently in the scientific literature include *Repetitive Motion Syndrome, Cumulative Trauma Disorder,* and *Overuse Syndrome.* They all refer to injury caused by repetitive movement. We may violate the integrity of our joints by performing, for example, forty backward arm circles with the palms down (see fig. 18.29) three days per week for ten or twenty years. The "wear and tear" is usually not noticed by the participant until the friction over time wears down the tendon, ligament, and/or bone, resulting in tendonitis, bursitis, and arthritis, perhaps between ages forty to fifty. Chances are, when the injury reaches an acute stage in later life, the cause of the injury is never really identified and it will be attributed to "old age." Because the injury is unseen and unfelt, the participant views the exercise as harmless. [**Note:** Many of the changes in the musculoskeletal system normally attributed to aging are found in *young* athletes. Degenerated disks are not an uncommon finding.]

The term acute injury as used here refers to the stress, strain, or sprain that produces pain at the time it occurs or within a few hours of performing the exercise.

For example, violating the integrity of the knee joint by placing torque on it during a toe touch or knee bend can tear the ligament and cartilage on the inside of the knee so the participant knows immediately that an injury occurred during that exercise. Some of the exercises termed "questionable" in this Concept are capable of producing this kind of injury, whereas others in the list are more apt to produce the "silent" microtrauma. Some exercises can produce both types of injury.

Some exercises may be reasonably safe for most people when performed only once, but become hazardous when done repetitively.

An acute exercise injury in any hazardous activity may occur the first time you place yourself at risk, or it may never happen. The odds of performing a hazardous activity safely decrease as the number of repetitions increase. It is like playing Russian Roulette! You may have performed bilateral straight leg raises for years and never had a backache but, as the saying goes "you are living on borrowed time." Microtrauma, on the other hand, occurs with each repetition of an exercise that violates physiologic movements or normal joint mechanics. It is true that we cannot avoid all wear and tear on the body, and it is true that we must "use it or lose it," but we can *reduce* wear and tear by eliminating hazardous activities because *if we do not use it **correctly**, then we will also lose it!* Some of the exercises that are considered questionable because of microtrauma can probably be performed safely when the number of repetitions is very small and they are rarely used. For example, if it feels comfortable, hyperextending the back in the Press-Up (McKenzie's) exercise (page 204) is probably safe when done once as a static stretch after a series of abdominal strengthening exercises, but repetitive hyperextension exercises even if comfortable are hazardous.

The Facts: Questionable Exercises and Safer Alternatives

Common exercises when misused or abused are potentially harmful.

Unless a qualified person evaluates the individual participant and determines one of these exercises to be indicated for that individual, it is prudent to choose a safer exercise to accomplish the same purpose. This concept does not include every possible "questionable" exercise, and space does not permit the inclusion of all good alternative exercises.

Questionable Exercises

1. *Repetitive hyperextension of the lower back* has several objections. First, it stretches the abdominals. These muscles are too long and weak in most people and should not be further lengthened. Second, it can be harmful to the back, causing an impingement on the nerve, compression and even herniation of the disk, myofascial "trigger points" and **spondylolysis.** Examples of exercises in which this occurs include *cobras, back bends, straight leglifts, straight leg sit-ups, prone back lifts, donkey kicks, fire hydrants, prone swans, backward trunk circling, weight lifting with the back arched, and landing from a jump with the back arched.* One of the back hyperextension exercises commonly seen is the *swan* shown in figure 18.1, used to strengthen the back muscles.

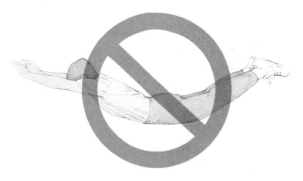

Figure 18.1
Swan.

ALTERNATIVE. Lie prone over a roll of blankets or pillows and extend the back to a neutral position (figure 18.2). Or substitute exercise 9 in Concept 12 and exercises 22 and 23 in Concept 17.

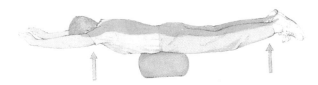

Figure 18.2
Back extension.

2. The same hazards are present in the *back-arching abdominal stretch* exercise shown in figure 18.3. This exercise can stretch the hip flexors, quadriceps, and shoulder flexors (such as the pectorals) as well as the abdominals, but it has the additional problem of possibly **hyperflexing** the knee joint, because of the arm pull (see discussion

of knee, exercise 11). If your goal is stretching the hip flexors and quadriceps, try substituting the *hip and thigh stretcher* (see figure 18.22). If used for the shoulders, substitute the PNF *pectoral stretch* (see figure 18.4).

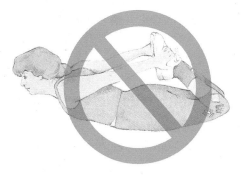

Figure 18.3
Back-arching abdominal stretch.

ALTERNATIVE. Stand erect in doorway with arms raised 45 degrees, elbows bent, and hands grasping doorjambs; feet in front-stride position. Press forward on door frame, contracting the arms maximally for several seconds. Relax and shift weight on legs so muscles on front of shoulder joint and chest are stretched; hold. Repeat with arms at 90 degrees and 135 degrees (figure 18.4).

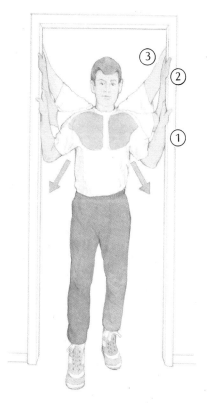

Figure 18.4
Pectoral stretch.

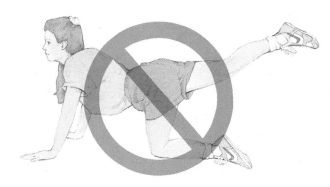

Figure 18.5
Donkey kick.

3. The *donkey kick* exercise (figure 18.5) is performed for the purpose of developing strength and/or endurance of the buttocks muscles (hip extensors). It may involve touching the nose with the knee, followed by a ballistic backward kick, a lifting of the head (*neck hyperextension*), and *hyperextension of the lower back*. As discussed earlier, hyperextension of the back is generally undesirable in exercises for the "masses." The same is true for the neck (see exercise 6 for a discussion of the neck). This exercise should be modified as shown in the *knee-to-nose touch* (figure 18.6), so the leg does not lift higher than the hips, and the neck and lower back are not allowed to hyperextend.
    ALTERNATIVE. Kneel on "all fours." Pull knee to nose, then extend leg and head to horizontal (do not go higher). Repeat. Then change legs.

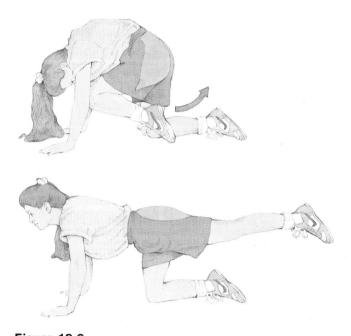

Figure 18.6
Knee-to-nose touch.

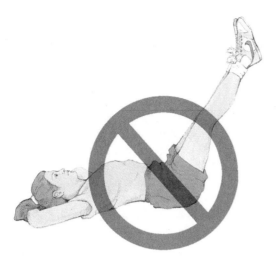

Figure 18.7
Double leg lift.

4. The *double leg lift* (figure 18.7) is usually used with the intent of strengthening the lower abdominals, when in fact it is primarily a hip-flexor (iliopsoas) strengthening exercise. The iliopsoas attaches to the lower back and tilts the pelvis forward, arching the back. Most people have overdeveloped the hip flexors and do not need to further strengthen those muscles. Even if the abdominals are strong enough to contract isometrically to prevent hyperextension of the lower back, the exercise produces excess compression on the disks. The same criticism is true of *straight-leg sit-ups*. These can displace the fifth lumbar vertebra (spondylolisthesis). A *bent-knee sit-up*, which is usually used to strengthen the upper abdominals, creates less shearing force on the spine, but some recent studies have shown it produces greater compression on the lumbar disks than the straight-leg sit-up. (**Note:** A complete discussion of these and other abdominal exercises is found in Sharpe, Liehmohn, and Snodgrass 1988.) An example of a safer and better exercise to strengthen the lower abdominals is the *reverse curl* (figure 18.8).

ALTERNATIVE. Lie supine, knees bent, feet flat on floor (hook-lying), arms at side. Lift knees to chest, raising hips off floor. Do not let knees go past the shoulders. Return to starting position and repeat.

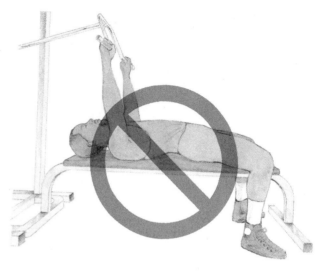

Figure 18.9
Bench press, back arched.

5. The *bench press* or similar exercises lying on a bench can be hazardous when the back is arched during lifting on a weight machine (figure 18.9). ALTERNATIVE. To prevent *lumbar hyperextension* and possible strain on the lower back, bend the knees and place the feet on the bench in a "hook-lying" position as shown in figure 18.10. If the bench is too short, substitute a longer one or place a chair at the end of the bench.

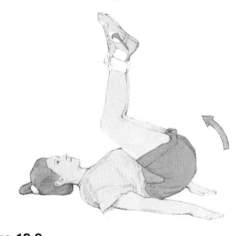

Figure 18.8
Reverse curl.

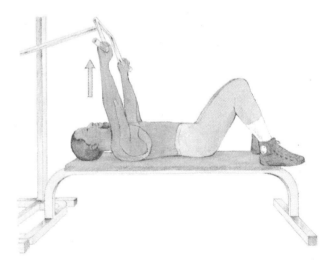

Figure 18.10
Bench press, knees bent.

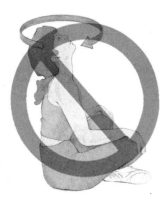

Figure 18.11
Neck circling.

6. As a general rule, exercises that *hyperextend the neck* should be avoided. Tipping the head backward during an exercise, such as is done in *neck circling* (figure 18.11), can pinch arteries and nerves in the neck and at the base of the skull, grind down the disks, and produce dizziness or myofascial trigger points. It also aggravates arthritis and degenerated disks. (**Note:** figures 18.1, 18.3, and 18.5 also show improper neck positions.) Another hazardous neck exercise is *bridging* on the head. This places extreme pressure on the cervical disks. If the purpose of the exercise is relaxation of the neck, substitute the *Head Clock* in figure 18.12. If your purpose in doing the exercise is strengthening, try some isometrics keeping your head in good alignment, using your hands as the resistance, or use contract-relax *PNF neck rotation* (page 199).

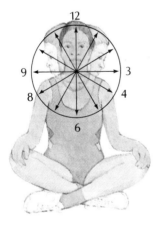

Figure 18.12
Head clock.

ALTERNATIVE. Pretend your neck is a clock face with the chin at 12:00 when you assume good posture. Flex the neck and point the chin at 6:00, hold, return to 12:00; repeat pointing at 4:00 and 8:00, then turn the head to 3:00 and 9:00.

7. As a general rule, exercises that force the *neck and upper back into hyperflexion* should not be used. It has been estimated that 80 percent of the population has forward head and kyphosis (hump back) with accompanying weak muscles. *Hyperflexion of the neck* can be as harmful as hyperextension by causing excessive stretch on the ligaments and nerves. It can also aggravate preexisting thin disks and arthritic conditions. Examples of exercises that tend to promote these conditions include *shoulder stand bicycling* (figure 18.13) and the Yoga positions called the *plough* and the *plough shear* (not shown).

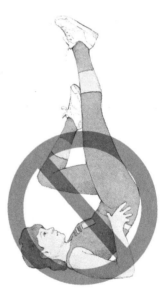

Figure 18.13
Shoulder stand bicycle.

If the purpose for these exercises is to reduce gravitational effects on the circulatory system or internal organs, try lying on a tilt board with the feet elevated. If the purpose is to warm up the muscles in the legs, try a *stationary leg change* (exercise 13, page 128). If the purpose for doing the exercise is to stretch the lower back, try the *leg hug* (figure 18.14) or *single knee-to-chest* exercise (see figure 18.28).

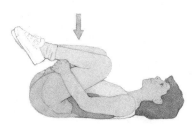

Figure 18.14
Leg hug.

ALTERNATIVE. From a hook-lying position, bring both knees to the chest and wrap the arms around the back of the knees. Pull knees to chest and hold.

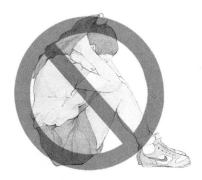

Figure 18.15
Hands-behind-the-head sit-up.

8. Placing the *hands behind the neck or head during the sit-up* (figure 18.15) and *crunch* allows the arms to pull the *head and neck into hyperflexion,* stretching the posterior ligaments, as described in exercise 7. If the hands are not placed at the sides or across the chest, then the hands should be placed so the *palms or fists cover the ears* (see figure 18.16) to prevent pulling on the neck. Another alternative is to *cross the hands behind the upper back by reaching* down the spine as far as possible (about the third or fourth thoracic vertebra) and holding this position while *resting the weight of the head on the arms.*

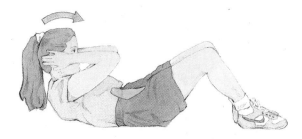

Figure 18.16
Crunch (hands on ears).

ALTERNATIVE. Assume a hook-lying position, with palms of hands lightly covering ears. Curl up until scapulae leave the floor, then roll down to starting position and repeat.

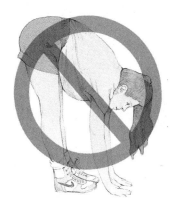

Figure 18.17
Standing toe touch.

9. *The knee joint should not be hyperextended.* This action stretches the ligaments and joint capsule of the knee. Bending the back while the legs are straight may cause back strain, particularly if the movement is done ballistically as in the *standing toe touch* (figure 18.17). Repetitive *bilateral straight-leg toe touches,* whether standing or sitting, may stretch the lower back excessively if the hamstrings are very tight. This can lead to backache and **spondylolisthesis.** If performed only on rare occasions as a test, there is less chance of injury than if incorporated into a regular exercise program. *Standing hamstring stretches with the back flat* have also been condemned (especially when done ballistically) because they can produce degenerative changes at the lumbosacral joint. Safer stretches of the lower back include the *leg hug* (see figure 18.14), and *single knee-to-chest*

(see figure 18.28). To stretch the hamstrings, substitute a sitting or lying stretch such as the *back-saver stretch* (figure 18.18) or the *hamstring stretcher* (see figure 18.26).

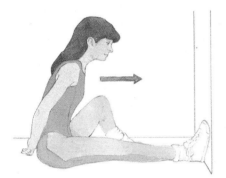

Figure 18.18
Back-saver hamstring stretch.

ALTERNATIVE. Sit with one foot against the wall, one knee bent, foot close to buttocks. Clasp hands behind back and bend forward, keeping lower back as straight as possible. Allow bent knee to move laterally so trunk can move forward. Stretch and hold.

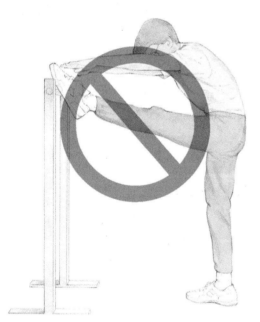

Figure 18.19
Bar stretch.

10. *Leg stretches at the ballet bar* (figure 18.19) may be potentially harmful. Some experts have found that where the extended leg is raised 90 degrees or more and the trunk is bent over the leg, it may lead to **sciatica** and **pyriformis syndrome,** especially in the person who has limited flexibility. Substitute some of the back and hamstring stretching exercises suggested in figures 18.8, 18.26, and 18.28.

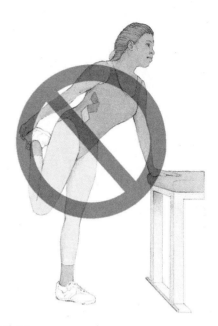

Figure 18.20
Shin and quadriceps stretch.

11. When the *knee is hyperflexed* 120 degrees or more, the ligaments and joint capsule are apt to be stretched and the cartilage may be damaged. Among the many exercises that place this type of stress on the knee joint are certain so-called "*quadriceps*" stretching exercises. (Note: one of the quadriceps, the rectus femoris, is not stretched by this exercise.) Figure 18.20 illustrates this position and also shows the *shin muscle being stretched*. It is usually not necessary to stretch the shin muscles, since they tend to be weak and elongated; however, if you need to stretch the shin muscles to relieve muscle soreness, try the *shin stretcher* (figure 18.21). To avoid injuring the knee when stretching the quadriceps substitute the *hip and thigh stretcher* (figure 18.22).

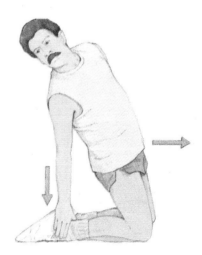

Figure 18.21
Shin stretch.

ALTERNATIVE. Kneel on both knees, turn to right, and press down on right ankle with right hand and hold. Keep hips thrust forward to avoid hyperflexing knees. Do not sit on heels. Repeat on left side.

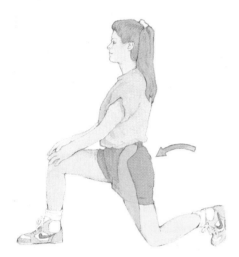

Figure 18.22
Hip and thigh stretcher.

ALTERNATIVE. Kneel with right knee directly above right ankle and stretch left leg backward so knee touches floor. If necessary, place hands on floor for balance. Press pelvis forward and downward and hold stretch for several seconds. Repeat on right side. Do not bend front knee more than 90 degrees. This stretches the rectus femoris and more importantly, the hip flexors (iliopsoas).

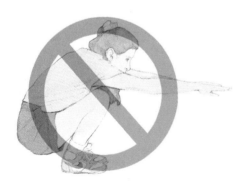

Figure 18.23
Deep knee bends.

12. *Deep squatting exercises* (figure 18.23), with or without weights, placing the knee joint in hyperflexion tends to "wedge it open," stretching the ligaments, irritating the synovial membrane, and possibly damaging the cartilage. There is even greater stress on the joint when the lower leg and foot are not in straight alignment with the knee. If you are performing squats to strengthen the knee and hip extensors, then try substituting the

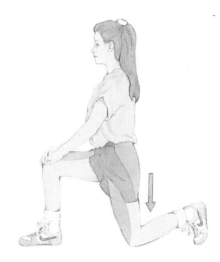

Figure 18.24
Alternate leg kneel (lunge).

forward lunge (figure 18.24) or *half squat* (also called parallel squat) (knees at right angle) with free weight or knee extensions and leg presses on a resistance machine.

ALTERNATIVE. From a standing position, with or without a free weight, take a step forward with right foot, touching left knee to floor. The front knee should be bent only to a 90-degree angle. Return to start and lunge forward with other foot. Repeat, alternating right and left.

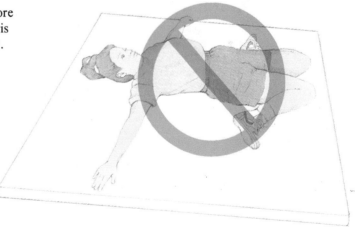

Figure 18.25
The hero.

13. The *hero* places the knee in a rotated position with **torque** on the flexed knee, which is apt to stretch the ligaments and capsule, and damage the cartilage. It may also cause strain in the groin muscles and the lower back. If the exercise is used to stretch the quadriceps, refer to exercise 11 regarding quadriceps stretching. The *hurdler's stretch* (not shown) is a sitting toe-touch exercise with one leg turned out rather than two, as shown in the hero (figure 18.25). It produces the same

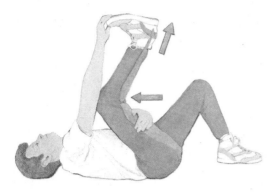

Figure 18.26
Hamstring stretcher.

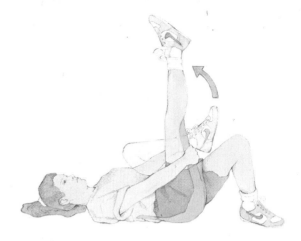

Figure 18.28
Single knee-to-chest.

kind of stress on the knee joint. Try substituting the *hamstring stretch* (figure 18.26) or *backsaver hamstring stretch* (figure 18.18).
ALTERNATIVE. Lie supine in a hook-lying position. Raise left leg and grasp toes with left hand while pulling on back of thigh with right hand. Push heel toward ceiling and hold. Repeat on other leg. (You may pull on a rope placed around the ankle of the extended leg, rather than pulling on the toe and thigh.)

ALTERNATIVE. From the hook-lying position, draw one knee to the chest by pulling on the thigh with the hands, then extend the knee toward the ceiling; hold. Pull to chest again and return to starting position. Repeat with other leg.

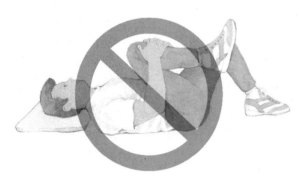

Figure 18.27
Knee pull-down.

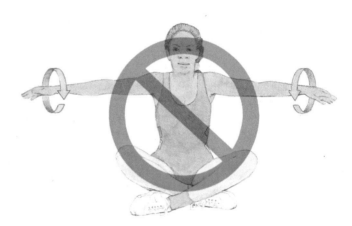

Figure 18.29
Forward arm circles (palms down).

14. *Hyperflexing the knee* by pulling it to the body with the arms or hands placed on top of the shin places undue stress on the knee joint. The *knee pull-down* exercise is one example (figure 18.27). (This position of the knee is also seen in figures 18.20–23). In this case, the exercise is intended to stretch the lower back. The hand position should be changed to hug the thigh rather than the shin to make this a good exercise. Try *single knee-to-chest* (figure 18.28) or *leg hug* (figure 18.14).

15. *Arm circles with the palms down* (circumduction with the arms straight out to the sides) figure 18.29) may cause the bony knob near the head of the humerus to impinge upon a shoulder ligament or the lip of the socket, and squeeze some of the muscles and the **bursa** in the shoulder every time the arm is lifted. In addition, if these are done in a forward direction (top of the circle is forward), there is a tendency to emphasize the use of the stronger chest muscles (pectorals) rather than to

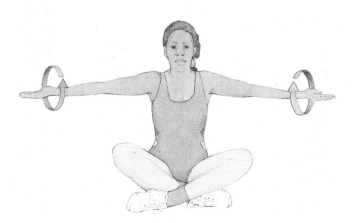

Figure 18.30
Backward arm circles (palms up).

stretch those muscles and emphasize the weaker upper back muscles. Finally, if they are done while standing, there is a tendency for the head to protrude forward and the low back to arch. This exercise is best done as modified in figure 18.30. To strengthen the upper back muscles, try *arm lifts* (page 203) or *seated rowing* (page 133). To stretch the pectorals try *pectoral stretch* (page 89).

ALTERNATIVE. Sit, turn palms up and pull in chin, contract abdominals. Circle arms backward.

Some Guidelines for Avoiding Hazardous Exercises

Most hazardous exercises can be avoided.

Follow these general guidelines, except where a physician or qualified professional has prescribed otherwise for you.

- Do not hyperflex the knee or neck.
- Do not hyperextend the knee, neck, or lower back.
- Do not apply a twisting or lateral force to the knee.
- Avoid holding your breath during exercise (heavy resistance training is an exception).
- Avoid stretching already long/weak muscles and avoid shortening already short/strong muscles.
  a. Most people should especially avoid aggravation of common postural faults: head forward, "hump back," protruding abdomen, inward rotation of the thigh, and pronation of the foot (see Concept 17).
  b. Most people need to stretch the chest muscles, hip flexors, calf, hamstrings, lower back, and medial thigh rotators.

  c. Most people need to strengthen the abdominals, the muscles between the shoulder blades, upper and lower back extensors, the lateral hip rotators, and the shin muscles.
- Avoid overstretching any joint so that ligaments and joint capsules are stretched.
- Be especially careful when using passive stretches by another person (unless it is a therapist). Avoid passive neck stretches and any ballistic passive stretches.
- Avoid movements that place acute compressional forces on spinal disks, such as extending and rotating the spine simultaneously, trunk and neck circling, and double leg lifts. (See Concept 17 for specific neck and back cautions.)
- Avoid movements that cause joint impingements or cartilage damage, such as arm circles in palm-down position. (See discussion under microtrauma.)
- If the nature of your sport regularly requires the violation of good mechanics (such as the need for a baseball catcher to assume a deep squat position or a gymnast to perform double leg raises), make certain that the muscles and joints are as fit as possible to endure the stress.
- Avoid fast, forceful hyperextension and flexion of the spine.

Other Important Facts

Manual stretching of the shoulders as done by some competitive swimmers has been found to create instability in the shoulder joint.

The practice of some athletes of using the passive assistance of a partner can cause excessive stretch. Examples of such exercises are pulling the arms backward at shoulder level until they cross each other behind the back; or pulling the bent elbows together making them touch while the hands are on the back of the head. Competitive swimmers sometimes begin such practices while they are in children's swimming programs and continue them through their competitive years. Such overstretching has resulted in painful shoulders and disability.

Repeatedly rising on the toes and heels may weaken the long arches of the feet.

Tiptoeing exercises will develop the calf muscles, but at the same time, they will stretch the muscles and ligaments that help support the long arch of the foot. "Heel walking" may have the same effect; that is, it may develop strong shin muscles while further weakening the arch. The potential harm is lessened if these exercises are performed with the toes turned in slightly.

Isometric exercises may be harmful to some people.

Isometric exercises have advantages (see Concept 10), but they may be more dangerous to heart patients than isotonic exercises, because they cause a marked rise in blood pressure and may produce irregular heartbeats. People with high blood pressure or heart trouble should not perform isometrics. Isometric exercise (as well as heavy weight training) for adolescents is also questionable because the bones of adolescents have not matured and growth may be affected.

Jogging and aerobic dance exercises are excellent for cardiovascular conditioning, weight control, and improvement of a variety of conditions; however, reasonable caution should be observed.

Jogging has been used successfully in rehabilitating cardiac patients and those with pulmonary emphysema; in weight reduction of diabetics; in relaxing insomniacs, the emotionally disturbed, and migraine patients; and in reducing the discomfort accompanying arthritis in the legs and back. Like many other exercises, jogging should not be done without a physician's approval for those with arthritis, osteoporosis, and heart and circulatory diseases. It is *not* harmful to women, although some women may need to wear a special bra as a comfort measure. Jogging can cause shin splints, blisters, and foot, ankle, knee, and hip problems. Using the proper footwear and learning how to jog correctly will minimize these hazards. If you have poor leg or foot alignment, you would be wise to jog only three or four days per week because studies show that the risk of injury is greatest for those who jog every day. Or you should choose another activity such as cycling or swimming. The same fitness levels will result with less risk of injury.

Aerobic dance exercise has some of the same hazards as jogging; these include the overstress syndromes from too many hours of high impact landings on the floor. The most common problems are shin splints, Achilles tendon injuries, arch strains, and pain under the knee cap. Most of these problems can be prevented by warming up and stretching properly before exercising, by using low impact movements, and by avoiding hazardous exercises such as those described in this concept. More recently there have been increasing reports of dizziness, hearing loss, and impaired balance—in pupils and in teachers. Loud music can cause hearing loss, and high-impact landings may cause inner ear damage, but the causes are not now understood (JOPERD 1990). A qualified physical education teacher will be more apt to teach/lead safe classes than a person with no qualifications other than being a good dancer and looking good in a leotard or being a celebrity.

Equipment that can be hazardous for some people is the "gravity inversion boot" and similar devices designed to allow a person to hang upside down.

These devices are supposed to be effective for the treatment of backache. However, studies have shown that during hanging (inactively or while oscillating), significant increases occur in systemic blood pressure; intraocular and retinal arterial pressure (in the eye) doubles; and pulse and other heart irregularities occur. Therefore, this type of equipment is potentially dangerous to the elderly and medically compromised, and to people with high blood pressure, glaucoma, diabetes, and heart abnormalities.

Exercise can alter the effect of drugs in the body, as well as the effect of certain disorders.

The effect of drugs used to treat thyroid disease may be altered by exercise. Likewise, patients taking certain medicine for asthma and collagen diseases may not be able to perform exercises that require moderate or heavy exertion in a normal fashion. Exercise alters the effect of nonsteroidal analgesics and anti-inflammatory drugs (like aspirin). During exercise, these drugs can cause increased oxygen consumption and increased carbon dioxide production, as well as promote sweating and dehydration. Muscle relaxants may cause depression and hinder coordination. (See Concept 10 for a discussion of steroids and growth hormone.)

The valsalva maneuver should be avoided when exerting great force in weight lifting, calisthenics, and isometrics.

Dizziness, blackouts, and inguinal hernias may result from the valsalva maneuver. This can be prevented in heavy weight lifting by avoiding **hyperventilation,** squatting as briefly as possible, and raising the weight as rapidly as possible to a position where it can be supported while breathing normally. In all other activities, breathe normally! Do *not* hold your breath during exercise.

Suggested Readings

Liemohn, W. S., et al. "Unresolved Controversies in Back Management." *Journal of Orthopaedic and Sports Physical Therapy* 9(1988):239.

Lindsey, R., and C. Corbin. "Questionable Exercise—Some Alternatives." *Journal of Physical Education, Recreation and Dance* 60(1989):26.

Luttgens, K., et al. *Kinesiology: Scientific Basis of Human Motion.* 8th/e. Dubuque, IA: Wm. C. Brown Publishers, 1992.

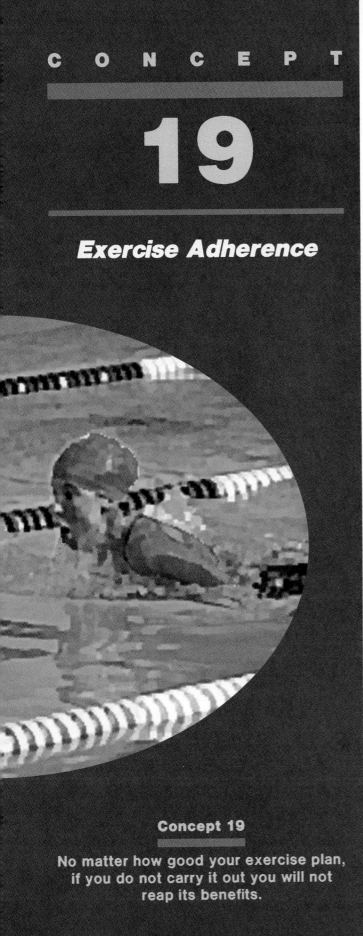

C O N C E P T

19

Exercise Adherence

Concept 19

No matter how good your exercise plan, if you do not carry it out you will not reap its benefits.

Introduction

You have read about the benefits of exercise and the amount of exercise necessary for developing each of the physical components of fitness. Now the challenge is to make exercise a permanent part of your life-style. **Exercise adherence** is the term used in this concept to describe staying with exercise for a lifetime. The purpose of this concept is to help you become a person who adheres to a program of regular exercise.

There are three types of factors that aid you in exercise adherence: **predisposing factors, enabling factors, and reinforcing factors.** Many of these factors will be outlined in this concept.

Health Goal for the Year 2000

- Increase the proportion of people who do lifetime physical activity.

Terms

Enabling Factor

Anything that helps you to carry out your exercise plan.

Exercise Adherence

Adopting regular exercise as part of your life-style.

Mental Practice

Imagining yourself going through the performance of a skill without actually physically performing it.

Overlearning

To practice a skill repeatedly in an attempt to make the skill a habit.

Paralysis by Analysis

Overanalysis of skill behavior. This occurs when more information is supplied than the performer can really use or when concentration on too many details of skill results in interference with performance.

Positive Addiction

Exceptional adherence; the formation of a habit that is exceptionally difficult to break but that has positive rather than negative consequences.

Predisposing Factor

Anything that makes you more likely to decide that you should make exercise a regular part of your life-style.

Reinforcing Factor

Anything that provides encouragement to maintain regular exercise for a lifetime.

Self-confidence

The belief that you can be successful at something; in this case, the belief that you can be successful in sports and physical activities, and can improve your physical fitness.

Self-criticism

Punishing yourself or getting angry with yourself because you did not perform as well as you think you should; negative "self-talk."

Self-monitoring

The ability to set your own goals and to keep records to accurately determine (without the help of others) if your goals are being met.

Self-motivation

The internal desire to start or continue a behavior; in this case, regular exercise. Sometimes referred to as "intrinsic motivation."

Skill Analysis

Breaking the performance of a skill into component parts and critically evaluating each phase of the performance.

The Facts About Predisposing Factors

Knowledge of exercise and fitness predisposes you to exercise adherence.

Many people have misconceptions about exercise. Dispelling these misconceptions and providing people with knowledge can help them know the value of exercise, how to perform it without injury, and how to get the most from their efforts. By itself, knowledge does not guarantee that people will start an exercise program. However, a sound fitness and exercise education is one predisposing factor to lifetime exercise.

Holding beliefs that exercise and fitness are important predisposes you to exercise adherence.

A belief is something that you think is true. It may or may not be based on fact. If you believe that exercise is important, you are more likely to be a regular exerciser than if you do not believe it is important. For example, if you believe that exercise helps you sleep better, you may do regular exercise even if there is little scientific evidence that the belief is true. Some experts think that believing

in the importance of exercise is more important than real knowledge about it. Unfortunately, the reverse may also be true. If you believe exercise is of no value, even though it is, you may be less likely to do regular exercise. Sound beliefs based on knowledge are most likely to lead to exercise adherence.

Enjoyment of exercise predisposes you to exercise adherence.

Enjoyment is a subjective feeling. It is hard to explain why some people enjoy exercise and others do not. What is clear is that many people who enjoy exercise would probably choose to do it even if it did not contribute to optimal health and well-being. In fact, some people would probably do it even if it had negative consequences. This is evidenced by the fact that some people participate in sports when they are injured or ill. Some experts believe that knowledge and beliefs can improve one's attitude or positive feelings about exercise. It may also be true that people who enjoy exercise are motivated to learn more about it and are more likely to believe that it is good for them. Since all people do not enjoy the same activities, it is important that you identify the form of exercise that you most enjoy if you are to adhere to exercise.

Feeling comfortable about the way you look predisposes you to exercise adherence.

People who are self-conscious about the way they look may avoid exercise because they feel that people might make fun of them. The feeling of self-consciousness is probably more important than actual appearance. Some people who are very fit and attractive feel uncomfortable in exercise clothes and in formal exercise classes or facilities. Being too fat, quite lean, or unfit does not always lead to feelings of self-consciousness. Some things you can do to reduce self-consciousness include: wearing exercise clothes that cover your body, avoiding exercise in highly visible places, exercising with supportive friends, listening to music, or finding other ways to keep you from thinking about what other people think about you. In reality, they may be admiring your dedication!

Self-confidence predisposes you to exercise adherence.

People who have self-confidence are more likely to engage in exercise and physical activity than those who lack self-confidence. Lack of confidence can result from lack of experience, pressure from others, comparisons to other people or unrealistic standards, lack of skill, and many other factors. Perhaps the most important reason for low self-confidence is **self-criticism.** If an activity makes you angry with yourself, it undermines your confidence. Improving your skills may reduce self-criticism. Selecting an activity that requires less skill may also help. Jogging/running, walking, cycling, swimming, and home calisthenics are quite popular because they do not produce self-criticism. Also, since self-criticism is often based on comparisons to other people, it is important to remember that most people are far more critical of themselves than of other people. The most competent people do not always have the most confidence. Some people with good skills lack confidence, and some with lesser skills exhibit high confidence.

Self-motivation predisposes you to exercise adherence.

People with self-motivation do things for personal or internal reasons. They do not rely on external incentives such as money, awards, or even recognition as a source of motivation. The reasons why some people have self-motivation is not entirely clear. However, we do know that people who start exercise early in life and who have not depended on external rewards to enjoy their exercise are most likely to have self-motivation. Reliance on external rewards such as trophies, money, and other material rewards has been shown to undermine self-motivation. This is evidenced by the fact that some athletes perceive performance in their sport as work rather than play. Self-motivation is highest when you are not threatened by failure and when the activity is one that you typically enjoy.

People with a previous history of involvement in physical activity are more likely to adhere to exercise than those who have not participated regularly.

You **can** teach an old dog new tricks! It is possible to get a habitual nonexerciser to become active. However, the people most likely to become active in the future are those who have been active in the past. Of course, people who have a history of participating in activity are also likely to enjoy it, to be self-confident, and to be self-motivated. If you are not a person who has a history of regular exercise, there is nothing you can do about it. However, there are things you can do to change your knowledge, beliefs, attitudes, self-confidence, and self-motivation.

The Facts About Enabling Factors

Possessing skill in a variety of physical activities enables you to adhere to exercise.

You do NOT have to be a great performer to enjoy sports and physical activity. However, having some skill enables you to be more active.

It is advisable to practice and perhaps seek instruction to enhance enjoyment of a lifetime activity, especially if you are unskilled. People with greater skill are more likely to get involved because they are more likely to be successful. However, there is another way to increase satisfaction from sports participation. Research suggests that you must be 65 to 75 percent as good as your partner if either of you is to enjoy the activity. For this reason, it is not only advisable to improve your skills, but you should find a playing partner or group of similar ability.

There are certain guidelines that can be followed to help you learn and enjoy lifetime sports and physical activities.

- *When learning a new activity, concentrate on the general idea of the skill first; worry about details later.* For example, a diver who concentrates on pointing the toes and keeping the legs straight at the end of a flip may land flat on his/her back. To make it all the way over, he/she should concentrate on merely doing the flip. When the general idea is *mastered*, then concentrate on details.

- *The beginner should be careful not to emphasize too many details at one time.* After the general idea of the skill is learned, the learner can begin to focus on the details, one or two at a time. Concentration on too many details at one time may result in **paralysis by analysis.** For example, a golfer who is told to keep the head down, the left arm straight, and the knees bent, cannot possibly concentrate on all of these details at once. As a result, neither the details nor the general idea of the golf swing are performed properly.

- *Once the general idea of a skill is learned, a skill analysis of the performance may be helpful.* Be careful not to overanalyze; it may be helpful to have a knowledgeable person help you locate strengths and weaknesses. Movies and videotapes of performances have been known to be of help to learners.

- *In the early stages of learning a lifetime sport or physical activity, it is not wise to engage in competition.* Beginners who compete are likely to concentrate on beating their opponent rather than on learning a skill properly. For example, in bowling, the beginner may abandon the newly learned hook ball in favor of the "sure thing" straight ball. This may make the person more successful immediately, but is not likely to improve the person's bowling skills for the future.

- *To be performed well, lifetime sports skills must be overlearned.* Oftentimes, when you learn a new activity, you begin to play the game immediately. The best way to learn a skill is to overlearn it, or practice it until it becomes habit. Frequently, games do not allow you to overlearn skills. For example, during a game is not a good time to

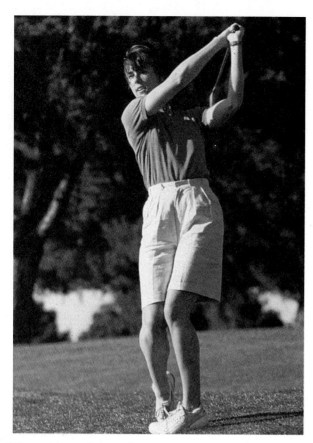
Skills enable you to be active.

learn the tennis serve because there may be only a few opportunities to serve. For the beginner, it would be much more productive to hit many services (overlearn) with a friend until the general idea of the serve is well learned. Further, the beginner *should not* sacrifice speed to concentrate on serving for accuracy. Accuracy will come with practice of a properly performed skill.

- *When unlearning an old (incorrect) skill and learning a new (correct) skill, a person's performance may get worse before it gets better.* For example, a golfer with a baseball swing may want to learn the correct golf swing. It is important for the learner to understand that the score may worsen during the relearning stage. As the new skill is overlearned, skill will improve as will the golf score.
- **Mental practice** *may aid skill learning.* Mental practice may benefit performance of motor skills, especially if the performer has had previous experience in performing the skill. Mental practice can be especially useful in sports when the performer cannot participate regularly because of weather, business, or lack of time.

- *For beginners, practicing in front of other people may be detrimental to learning a skill.* Research indicates that an audience may inhibit the beginner's learning of a new sports skill. This is especially true if the learner feels that his or her performance is being evaluated by someone in the audience.

Possessing good physical fitness enables you to adhere to exercise.

Some people feel that they are unable to exercise because they might get injured. Possessing health-related fitness can reduce the risk of injury and fatigue. Both injury and fatigue are sources of inactivity. Skill-related fitness also aids in the performance of various physical activities, though it is not a requirement for enjoying them. Some people do not exercise because they lack fitness, and this leads to further lack of fitness. The best solution to breaking the inactivity cycle is to begin your program with a modest amount of exercise in an activity that you enjoy. Gradually take advantage of more rigorous activities when your fitness improves.

Accessibility to facilities and equipment enables you to adhere to exercise.

Repeatedly, people indicate that they are unable to exercise because the facilities are too far from home, the weather is bad, or the cost of using facilities is too great. These reasons may be merely excuses for not doing regular exercise. On the other hand, the easier it is to adhere, the more likely you are to do it. It is important that you find a place to exercise near or in the home, that you find a place to exercise when the weather is bad, and that you find a way to exercise that is within your budget. There are many forms of exercise that can be done at home at little or no cost. If you do not enjoy these, you should investigate public recreation opportunities. You may need to be creative. Some people who walk regularly go to nearby covered shopping malls to walk when the weather is bad. Others use old bicycle inner tubes as a substitute for resistance machines or milk bottles as a substitute for weights.

Selecting a type of exercise that is not too difficult enables you to adhere.

Corporate fitness programs have higher dropout rates when the exercise provided is exceptionally vigorous. Beginners are especially likely to adhere to programs that are moderate. More vigorous exercise may lead to injury and is more likely to be perceived as too difficult. Beginners should start gradually. Also, they might want to make ratings of perceived exertion (see Lab 6C) to learn to avoid exercise that seems too difficult.

Self-monitoring means being able to set your own exercise and fitness goals, and to keep records of your own progress. People who have clear, realistic exercise and fitness goals are more likely to adhere to exercise. Participants who keep records of their exercise and fitness progress are most likely to meet their exercise and fitness goals. Guidelines for goal setting and record keeping are presented in Concept 25 for your use in program planning.

The Facts About Reinforcing Factors

When family members support your exercise behavior, you are likely to continue it. However, exercise may take time away from family activities. If family members, especially one's spouse, feel that exercise is interfering with family obligations, regular exercise may diminish. It is important to involve family members in planning for regular exercise.

People who live in communities where regular exercise is typical are reinforced to continue exercise. Exercising with friends helps one adhere. Finding friends with similar interests and abilities is also important. An exercise leader who is encouraging and supportive can also reinforce exercise adherence. People who especially enjoy the social aspects of exercise should consider joining a sports or exercise group and/or choose sports and activities with a social component.

Some people avoid exercise because they see it as a source of failure. If done properly, anyone can succeed in exercise. As already noted, practice and becoming skilled in an activity can enhance your chances of success. Some other suggestions are listed here.

- *Do not equate success with winning.* Sports psychologists agree that one problem experienced by many adults is that they cannot enjoy competitive activities unless they win. Though most people enjoy winning, it must be realized

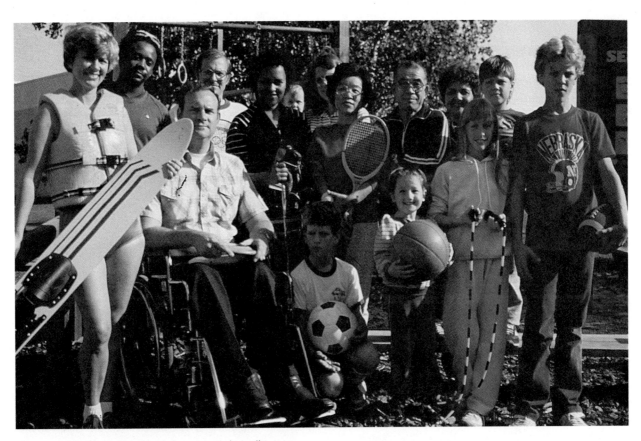

Support from friends and family reinforces exercise adherence.

that only 50 percent of the participants in most activities can win. Playing well and enjoying the sport also makes you a "winner."

- *Avoid comparing yourself and your accomplishments to those of other people.*
- *Consider long-term improvement as a successful accomplishment.*
- *Try using a handicap system when competing with those of unequal skill.* Such systems as those used in golf and bowling can be adapted for other activities to help "even up" the competition.
- *Competition may or may not make exercise fun.* Some people especially enjoy competition. Others, however, avoid competitive activities because they have not had success in competitive games. Whatever the benefits of regular physical activity, none should be exaggerated to the point of detracting from a fuller life. Overemphasis on sports can cause anxiety and even neurosis. In fact, some people create stress for themselves by being excessively competitive and increase their chances of getting stress-related diseases.

Support from medical and other experts reinforces exercise adherence.

A doctor's advice is the reason most often mentioned for doing regular exercise. Too often, the doctor's advice is given after a health problem already exists. When medical doctors, insurance companies, and employers place a priority on healthy lifestyles and preventing health problems, it sends a signal that regular exercise is a priority. You may wish to consider insurance companies that provide for regular preventive exams and other healthy life-styles. Also, if you have a choice you may wish to seek a place of employment that provides opportunities to exercise.

The popular media can provide reinforcement for exercise adherence.

In 1960 very few adults performed regular exercise in their free time. The number of exercisers has increased dramatically since then. Exercise has become popular. This is reflected in the advertisements on television, in newspapers, and in magazines. The trend toward regular exercise as the "normal" thing to do is reinforcing to exercise adherence.

The Facts About Positive Addiction to Exercise

Exercise adherence means regular lifetime exercise. **Positive addiction** is another term commonly used to describe this healthy life-style. The implication is that exercise is addicting, but unlike addictions such as drugs and smoking, the consequences of the addiction are positive. Experts have not established that exercise can be addicting, though it is generally agreed that some people develop very strong exercise habits (exceptional adherence) even to the point of activity neurosis (see Concept 3). Habitual exercisers regularly indicate that they have positive feelings, even feelings of euphoria, when they do regular, sustained exercise.

Morgan and O'Conner (1988) have suggested several possible explanations for the positive feelings associated with exercise. They refer to these positive feelings as "positive mood states." One theory is that the increase in body heat that accompanies exercise could result in reduction in muscle tension. Another theory is that involvement in exercise provides a "time out," or a period of time free from distractions. A regular exerciser gets away from the sources of stress and tension. This distraction may account for positive mood states. Researchers find little support for the "endorphin theory" popularized in many jogging books and magazines. This explanation suggests that regular exercise elevates endorphins, or substances in the brain, thought to be responsible for the positive feeling runners have referred to as the "runner's high."

Facts About Stages of Change

People who are nonexercisers do not become regular lifetime adherers overnight, nor do regular exercisers become sedentary all at once. Rather, people progress forward and backward through several stages of change.

The goal for all people should be to get to the stage of maintenance. People at the maintenance stage are true exercise adherers, they have the "exercise habit." At the other extreme are sedentary people who do no exercise at all. These people are at the precontemplation stage. Not only do they *not* do exercise, they are not even considering doing it.

Rather than trying to get sedentary people to move from the precontemplation stage directly to the maintenance stage, it is probably more effective to help them move through several more gradual stages. First, it is important to get people to contemplate exercise, to start thinking about it. Helping people with predisposing factors will help in this change. Next, it is useful to help people who are contemplating change to begin planning for exercise. In the next Concept you will learn how to plan or prepare for exercise. Writing down your plans is an important step toward taking action. Planning to improve enabling factors will help move you to the action stage.

People at the action stage are doing some type of exercise, but it is sporadic and often is not enough to produce all the benefits associated with the "exercise habit."

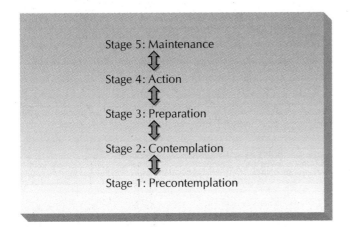

Figure 19.1

The stages of change for exercise adherence.

Source: Data from B. H. Marcus et al., 1992.

A large number of adults are currently at this stage. Both enabling and reinforcing factors are important at this stage. These factors can help you meet the goal of moving on to the maintenance stage and becoming a true lifetime exercise adherer.

Suggested Readings

Dishman, R. K. (ed.). *Exercise Adherence*. Champaign, Ill.: Human Kinetics Publishers, 1988.

King, A., et al. "Determinants of Physical Activity and Interventions in Adults." *Medicine and Science in Sports and Exercise* 24(1992):S221 (Supplement).

Sallis, J., et al. "Determinants of Exercise Behavior." *Exercise and Sport Sciences Reviews* 18(1990):307.

Sallis, J., et al. "Determinants of Physical Activity and Interventions in Youth." *Medicine and Science in Sports and Exercise* 24(1992):S248 (Supplement).

LAB RESOURCE MATERIALS

(For use with Lab 19, page L-53)

Chart 19.1 Exercise Adherence Questionnaire

The factors that predispose, enable, and reinforce exercise adherence are listed below. Read each statement. Check the box under the most appropriate response for you.

	Very True	Somewhat True	Not True
Predisposing Factors			
1. I am very knowledgeable about fitness and exercise.	☐	☐	☐
2. I have a strong belief that exercise is good for me.	☐	☐	☐
3. I enjoy doing regular exercise and physical activity.	☐	☐	☐
4. I am confident of my abilities in sports, exercise, and other physical activities.	☐	☐	☐
5. I am motivated to do physical activity without having to be encouraged by others or without receiving external rewards.	☐	☐	☐
6. I have been a regular exerciser most of my life.	☐	☐	☐
7. I like the way I look.	☐	☐	☐
			Subtotal _____
Enabling Factors			
8. I possess good sports skills.	☐	☐	☐
9. I possess good general physical fitness.	☐	☐	☐
10. I have a place to exercise and equipment that I can use in or near my home.	☐	☐	☐
11. I am capable of setting my own exercise goals and keeping track of my progress.	☐	☐	☐
			Subtotal _____
Reinforcing Factors			
12. I have the support of my family, especially my spouse (if married), for doing my regular exercise.	☐	☐	☐
13. I have many friends who enjoy the same kinds of exercise that I do.	☐	☐	☐
14. I am successful in most physical activities that I try.	☐	☐	☐
15. I have a doctor and/or employer who encourages me to exercise.	☐	☐	☐
			Subtotal _____
			Total _____

Score the Exercise Adherence Questionnaire as follows:

1. Give 2 points for every Very True answer, 1 point for each Somewhat True answer, and 0 points for each Not True answer.

2. Calculate your Predisposing Factors score by adding your points for items 1 through 7. This score indicates your general predisposition to start an exercise program.

3. Calculate your Enabling Factors score by adding your points for items 8 through 11. This score indicates the extent to which you have the qualities necessary to continue an exercise program once you have started one.

4. Calculate your Reinforcing Factors score by adding your points for items 12 through 15. This score indicates the encouragement and support you have for continuing your regular exercise.

5. Calculate your Total Score by adding the three subtotals. This score gives you a general idea of your tendency to adhere to exercise.

6. Use chart 19.2 to determine your ratings.

Chart 19.2 Exercise Adherence *Rating Scale*				
Classification	Predisposing Score	Enabling Score	Reinforcing Score	Total Score
Excellent	12–14	7–8	7–8	26–30
Very Good	10–11	6	6	22–25
Good	7–9	4–5	4–5	15–21
Fair	5–6	3	3	11–14
Poor	<5	<3	<3	<11

C O N C E P T

20

Planning for Physically Active Living

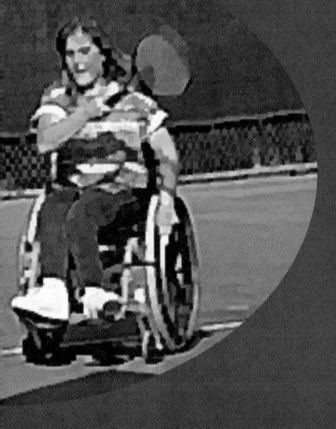

Concept 20

Planning for physically active living is essential to optimal physical fitness, health, and wellness.

Introduction

There is no single exercise program best suited for all people, nor is there one best life-style for health and wellness. When planning a program of exercise, it is important to consider your own unique needs and interests.

Health Goals for the Year 2000

- Increase the proportion of people who do daily exercise.
- Increase the proportion of people who engage in activity to promote cardiovascular fitness.
- Reduce the proportion of people who do no leisure-time physical activity.
- Increase the proportion of people who engage in activity to enhance muscular strength, muscular endurance, and flexibility.
- Increase proportion of overfat people who use sound dietary practices and regular exercise to attain appropriate body weight.

Terms

Behavioral Goal

A statement of intent to perform a specific behavior (changing a life-style) for a specific period of time. An example would be, "I will walk for fifteen minutes each morning before work."

Exercise Goals

An exercise or physical activity goal is a behavioral goal with exercise as the intended behavior.

Fitness Goals

A fitness goal is an outcome goal with a specific fitness score as the intended outcome.

Long Term Goal

A statement of intent to change behavior or achieve a specific outcome in a period of months or years.

Outcome Goal

A statement of intent to achieve a specific test score (attainment of a specific standard) associated with good health or wellness. An example would be, "I will lower my body fat level by three percent."

Short Term Goal

A statement of intent to change a behavior or outcome in a period of days or weeks.

Steps in Program Planning

There are several steps for planning an effective exercise program.

Step 1—Clarify your reasons for starting your exercise program.

Clarifying your purposes for starting an exercise program may help you to select activities that you will enjoy and continue for a lifetime. In Concept 2 you read about the reasons why people do or do not exercise regularly, and in Concept 19 you read about the factors that help people adhere to regular exercise. At this time it would be useful to review those concepts.

Step 2—Identify your fitness needs.

If you have no medical problems, the second step in program planning is to test your physical fitness on each of the health-related components.

Step 3—Establish your short term and long term goals.

Having established both your reasons (step 1) and your needs (step 2), it is now possible to develop your **exercise goals** and **fitness goals**. Some guidelines follow:

- **Be realistic.** The biggest problem with goal setting is that you may fail to meet your goals if they are too difficult to achieve. Failure to meet goals is discouraging. You should set goals that you have a realistic chance of achieving. This is especially true for short-term goals.
- **Focus on short term goals first. Short term goals** are easier to accomplish than long term goals. Realistic short term goals make you successful. One success leads to another. When you meet short term goals, establish new ones.
- **Short term goals should be exercise or *behavioral goals*.** If you exercise regularly, fitness will improve. Beginners who establish short term exercise goals and stick with them will be successful. Because fitness goals take more time to reach, they make poor short term goals. Exercise is a behavior that any one can do—it takes only effort. You can easily monitor a behavior to tell that you have met your goal. Outcomes such as fitness can be monitored, but when changes do not occur immediately you may get the feeling you have failed. **Outcome goals** or fitness goals are more appropriate **long term goals.**
- **Long term fitness goals should consider your heredity.** Your heredity limits your fitness. When establishing long term fitness goals, be careful not to base them on what other people can do. You may be setting yourself up for failure. Be sure

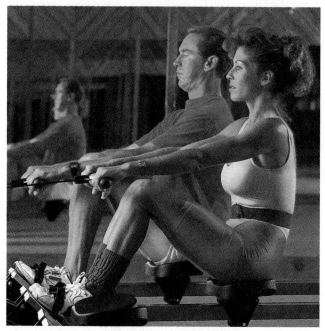

Select activities that you enjoy and that are best for meeting your own personal goals.

that the fitness outcomes you expect are based on health standards or scores slightly above what you can currently perform, rather than on performance scores of other people.

- **Consider maintenance goals as well as improvement goals.** There is a limit to the amount of fitness any person can achieve. You cannot improve forever. At some point it is reasonable to set "maintenance goals." Maintenance means staying active and fit when improvement goals have already been met.
- **Set goals that call for a life-style that you can maintain.** Exercise and fitness for a lifetime mean maintaining your program forever. If you set exercise or fitness goals that are excessive, you may burn out and quit exercising entirely. Consider the long term in setting your goals.
- **Put your goals in writing.** It is easy to forget your goals if they are not in writing. Writing them helps establish a commitment to yourself and clearly establishes your goals. You can revise them if necessary. Written goals are not cast in concrete.

Step 4—Select activities that are best for meeting your goals.

In reading this text, you have learned about the benefits of different types of physical activities. Use this information to select activities to include in your program. The activities should adhere to the FIT formula for the various components of fitness. They should be safe and meet your personal needs and interests. Include activities you have enjoyed in the past, ones that you feel will meet your future goals, and those in which you are likely to persist for a lifetime.

Table 20.1

Weekly Exercise Program (Sample)

Daily Schedules
(List the activities and times of day for each activity.)

Monday	Tuesday	Wednesday
7:00 a.m. "Special exercises" 5:30 p.m. Warm-up racquetball	7:00 a.m. "Special exercises" 12:30 p.m. Walk after lunch 5:30 p.m. Weight training (30 minutes)	7:00 a.m. "Special exercises" 5:30 p.m. Warm-up racquetball
Thursday	**Friday**	**Saturday**
7:00 a.m. "Special exercises" 12:30 p.m. Walk after lunch 5:30 p.m. Weight training (30 minutes)	7:00 a.m. "Special exercises" 12:30 p.m. Walk after lunch	afternoon - walk or swim Weight training (30 minutes)

Sunday	**Warm-Up and Cool-Down Activities**	**Program Evaluation** (Fill in after trying out your program.)
"Special exercises" when I get up. Other exercise if I have no other plans Tennis if I can find a partner & may take lessons.	Calf stretcher toe touch leg hug side stretch two-minute walk	This seems to be working pretty well. I find I usually walk rather than swim because it is inconvenient to go to the pool. I am taking tennis lessons.
	Special Exercises	
	sit-ups (bend knee) pectoral stretch Billigs' exercise contract-relax routine before bed when I am tense	

Step 5—Write a weekly plan and do it!

You are more likely to perform your program if you put it down in writing. To get you started, a sample **Weekly Exercise Program** is provided (see table 20.1). A blank weekly plan is provided in Lab 20 for you to write out your personal plan. Now do it! If you are going to adhere to this program, you must be able to manage your time. Time management is one of the keys to success. A hit-or-miss program may turn into no program at all. From the beginning, set aside a specific time and place for your activity. Place a high priority on your exercise time. Don't allow anything to interrupt your exercise schedule. Build exercise into your daily routine; make it as much a habit as taking a bath or eating regular meals. Some form of exercise should be done at least three days per week and as many as five to six days a week.

Step 6—Keep monthly records of exercise and fitness.

Record keeping can help you stick with your exercise program and can help you attain your fitness goals. Use a one-month calendar to keep track of your regular exercise and fitness changes. Steps in using the calendar are described in Lab 20.

Step 7—Periodically reevaluate and modify your program.

The weekly program you write in step 5 may be an excellent one. However, as time goes by your needs, interests, and goals change. For this reason, you should periodically reevaluate and revise your personal program. If you become bored with certain activities, you may wish to drop them and add other new and interesting activities. Changes in the weather, the availability of facilities, and personal schedules may all require program changes. Each time you change your program, follow steps 1 through 6. It is not necessary to do the same program forever; the key is to have a program that meets your current needs, interests, and goals.

Suggested Readings

American College of Sports Medicine. *Guidelines for Exercise Testing and Prescription.* 4th ed. Philadelphia: Lea & Febiger, 1991.

American College of Sports Medicine. "The Recommended Quantity and Quality of Exercise for Developing and Maintaining Cardiorespiratory and Muscular Fitness in Healthy Adults." *Medicine and Science in Sports and Exercise* 22(1990):2.

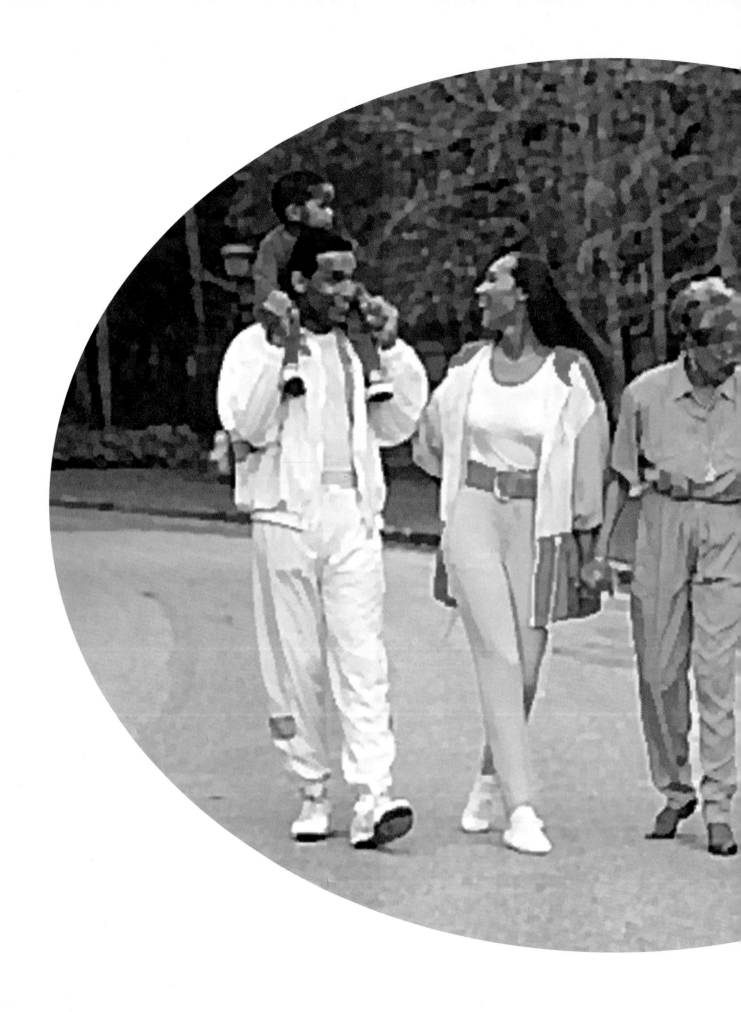

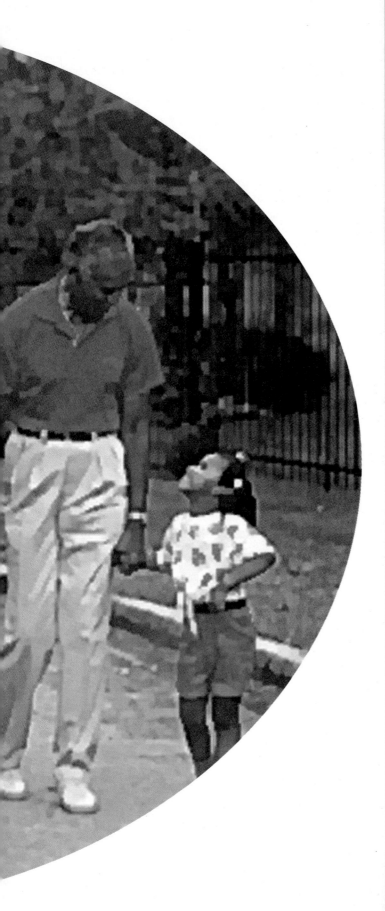

V

Healthy Life-Styles

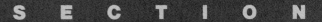

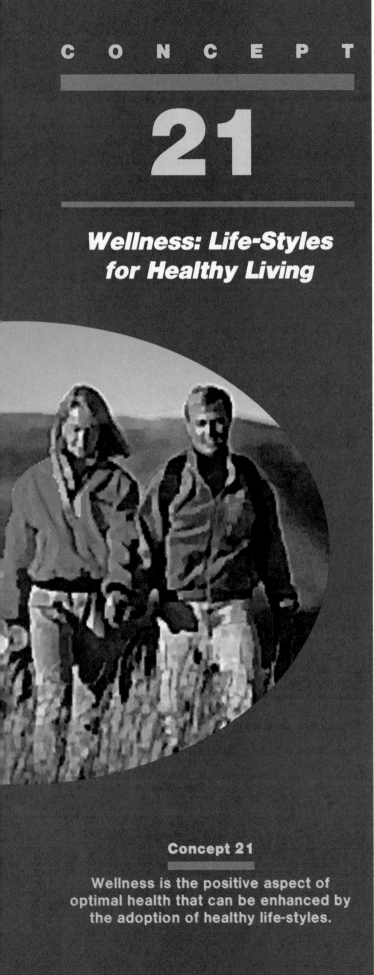

CONCEPT

21

Wellness: Life-Styles for Healthy Living

Concept 21

Wellness is the positive aspect of optimal health that can be enhanced by the adoption of healthy life-styles.

Introduction

Goals for the nation's optimal **health** have been established in a comprehensive document entitled *Healthy People 2000*. The intent of the document was to establish reasonable goals that, with a conscientious effort, could be achieved by the year 2000. "The challenge of *Healthy People 2000* is to use the combined strength of scientific knowledge, professional skill, individual commitment, community support, and political will to enable people to achieve their potential to live full, active lives. It means preventing premature death and preventing disability, preserving a physical environment that supports human life, cultivating family and community support, enhancing each individual's inherent abilities to respond and to act, and assuring that all Americans achieve and maintain a maximum level of functioning" (Public Health Service 1991, p. 6). Clearly the goals for the nation emphasize all of the components of optimal health, including **wellness,** as evidenced by a positive sense of well-being and quality living.

Health Goal for the Year 2000

■ Increase the span of optimally healthy life.

Terms

Emotional Wellness

A person's ability to cope with daily circumstances and to deal with personal feelings in a positive, optimistic, and constructive manner.

Health

Health is optimal well-being that contributes to quality of life. It is more than freedom from disease and illness, though freedom from disease is important to good health. Optimal health includes high-level emotional, intellectual, physical, social and spiritual wellness.

Intellectual Wellness

A person's ability to learn and to use information to enhance the quality of daily living and optimal functioning.

Mental Wellness

The goals for the nation's health refer to mental rather than emotional health and wellness. In this book mental wellness is considered to be the same as emotional wellness (see above).

Physical Wellness

A person's ability to function effectively in meeting the demands of the day's work and ability to use free time effectively. Physical wellness includes good physical fitness and the possession of useful motor skills.

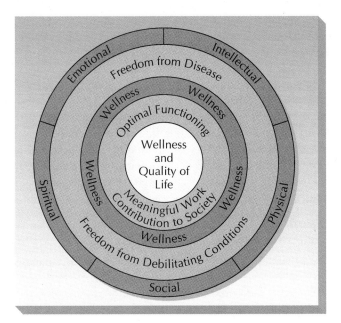

Figure 21.1
A model of optimal health and wellness.

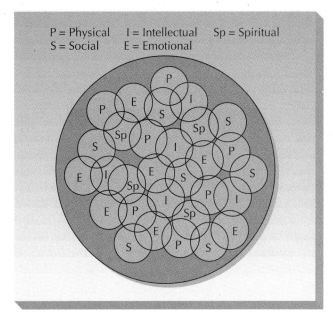

Figure 21.2
The integration of wellness dimensions.

Social Wellness

A person's ability to successfully interact with others and to establish meaningful relationships that enhance the quality of life for all people involved in the interaction (including self).

Spiritual Wellness

A person's ability to establish a values system and act on the system of beliefs as well as to establish and carry out meaningful and constructive life's goals. Spiritual wellness is often based on a belief in a force greater than the individual that helps one contribute to an improved quality of life of all people.

Wellness

Wellness is the integration of many dimensions, including emotional, intellectual, physical, spiritual, and social, that expands one's potential to live and work effectively and to make a significant contribution to society. Wellness is considered to be the positive component of good health. It reflects how one feels (a sense of well-being) about life as well as one's ability to function effectively.

The Facts About Wellness

Wellness is the positive component of optimal health.

Death, disease, illness, and debilitating conditions are the negative components of health. Death is the ultimate op-

posite of optimal health. Disease, illness, and debilitating conditions obviously detract from optimal health. Wellness has been recognized as the positive component of optimal health as evidenced by a sense of well-being reflected in optimal functioning, a quality of life, meaningful work, and a contribution to society (see figure 21.1).

Wellness is the integration of all parts of health that expands one's potential to live and work effectively and to make a significant contribution to society.

Wellness is the integration of many dimensions, including **emotional (mental), intellectual, physical, social, and spiritual.** Each of the five sections of figure 21.1 is meant to illustrate the importance of each dimension to total wellness.

Throughout this book references will be made to the various wellness dimensions to help the reader understand the importance of each dimension to integrated total wellness. Wellness is, however, an integrated state of being that is better depicted as many threads that can be woven together to produce a larger, integrated cord. Each specific dimension relates to each of the others and overlaps all others. The overlap is so frequent and so great that the specific contribution of each thread is almost indistinguishable when looking at the total (figure 21.2).

Wellness reflects how one feels about life as well as one's ability to function effectively.

As noted in table 21.1, a positive total outlook on life is essential to wellness. A total positive outlook is impacted by each of the wellness dimensions. A well person is one

Table 21.1

The Dimensions of Wellness

−	Wellness Dimensions	+
Depressed	Emotional-Mental	Happy
Ignorant	Intellectual	Informed
Unfit	Physical	Fit
Lonely	Social	Involved
Unfulfilled	Spiritual	Fulfilled
Negative	Total Outlook	Positive

who is satisfied in his/her work, who is spiritually fulfilled, enjoys leisure time, is physically fit, is socially involved, and has a positive emotional-mental outlook. This person is likely to have a positive total outlook on life. This person is happy and fulfilled. Many experts believe that a positive total outlook is a key to wellness.

The way one perceives each of the dimensions of wellness affects total outlook. Researchers have used the term self-perceptions to describe the feelings people have about their competence in each area of wellness. Many believe that self-perceptions are more important than actual performance when it comes to various wellness dimensions. For example, a person who has an important job may find less meaning and job satisfaction than another person with a much less important job.

Apparently one of the important factors for a person who has achieved high-level wellness and a positive life's outlook is the ability to reward himself/herself. A good self-reward system allows a person to feel good about self. Some people seem unable to give themselves credit for their life's experiences. The development of a system that allows a person to positively perceive the self is important. Of course, the adoption of positive life-styles that encourage improved self-perceptions is also important. The questionnaire at the end of this concept will help you assess your self-perceptions of the various wellness dimensions. For optimal wellness it would be important to find positive feelings about each dimension.

Feelings of wellness are important for people with disease and disability.

All people can benefit from enhanced wellness. Wellness, an improved quality of life, is possible for everyone, regardless of disabilities or disease states. Evidence is accumulating to indicate that people with a positive outlook are better able to resist the progress of disease and illness. Thinking positive thoughts has been associated with enhanced results from various medical treatments and better results from surgical procedures.

Because self-perceptions are important to wellness, positive perceptions of self are especially important to the wellness of people with disease, illness, and disability. The

concepts of wellness and optimal health must be considered in light of one's heredity and personal disabilities and disease states.

Wellness is a useful term that may be used by quacks as well as experts.

Health People 2000 recognizes that optimal health comes from an improved quality of life and ". . . is best measured by citizens' sense of well-being" (Public Health Service 1991, p. 6). Experts support the importance of wellness to optimal health.

Unfortunately, some individuals and groups have tried to identify wellness with products and services that promise benefits that cannot be documented. Because "well-being" is a subjective feeling that is hard to document, it is easy for quacks to make claims of improved wellness for their product or service without facts to back them up.

"Holistic health" is a term that is similarly abused. Optimal health includes many areas (see figure 21.2), thus the term holistic (total) is appropriate. In fact the word "health" originates from a root word meaning *wholeness*. Nevertheless, care should be used when considering services and products that make claims of wellness and/or holistic health to be sure that they are legitimate.

The Facts About Healthy Life-Styles

Three strategies are commonly employed in efforts designed to achieve optimal health for all people.

Disease and illness treatment, disease and illness prevention, and health and wellness promotion are three different strategies used to achieve optimal health. Disease and illness treatment includes efforts to treat and cure common diseases and illness that threaten society and are likely to result in pain, suffering, hospitalization, and/or premature death. Much of the burden for this strategy falls to those in the medical and health professions.

Disease and illness prevention includes efforts to prevent diseases and illnesses that threaten society and are likely to result in pain, suffering, hospitalization, and/or premature death. Though medical and public health agencies have a considerable responsibility in this area, much of the burden for implementing this strategy rests with communities and individuals within these communities.

Health and wellness promotion includes efforts to alter personal life-styles to enhance the quality of life that ". . . enables people to achieve their potential to live full, active lives" (Public Health Service 1991, p. 6). Whereas the treatment and prevention strategies focus on death, disease, and illness, promotion strategies focus on wellness.

> The principal path to wellness is health promotion associated with altering life-styles.

Just as physical fitness is a state of being that is altered by regular physical activity, wellness is a state of being (see figures 21.1 and 21.2) that is altered by one's behaviors. Life-styles are behaviors that are partially or totally in your own control. Some of the healthy life-styles considered to be very important to optimal wellness are presented in table 21.2.

Exercising Regularly

As noted throughout this book and particularly in Concept 3, regular exercise is associated with the reduced risk of many diseases. Regular physical activity is a positive addiction. It is habit-forming, but the result of the habit is positive, not negative. Regular exercise can be fun and can improve the quality of life. It is interesting to note that people who exercise regularly are likely to adopt other healthy life-styles. For example, regular exercisers are more likely than sedentary individuals to visit a physician for preventive examinations, practice preventive dentistry, and wear seat belts.

Eating Properly (Good Nutrition)

Good eating habits can help you feel and look your best. Failure to eat properly can result in many health problems. It has been shown that six of the ten leading causes of death in North America are linked to improper nutrition. The fact that millions of teenagers and adults regularly modify their diet suggests that they want to assume control of the way they look and of their health as it relates to nutrition. Unfortunately, many dietary modifica-

Table 21.2
Healthy Life-Styles

- Exercising regularly
- Eating properly
- Managing stress
- Avoiding destructive habits
- Practicing safe sex
- Adopting good safety habits
- Learning first aid
- Adopting good personal health behaviors
- Seeking and complying with medical advice
- Being an informed consumer
- Protecting the environment
- Managing time effectively

tions may have a negative rather than positive impact on health. Making *appropriate* changes in eating patterns is the key. Eating properly is a goal that is achievable.

Managing Stress

Nearly 30 million professionals and executives who rank among the highest in annual earnings indicate that they would like to find a way to get away from their ". . . steady diet of stress and tension" (Harris and Associates 1987). Reducing distress in your life and learning to cope with stress are associated with feelings of well-being and an improved quality of life. Stress reduction is possible for most people with alterations in life-style, though some people may need the help of an expert.

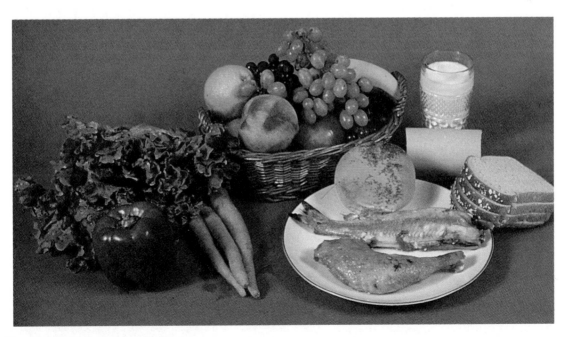

A healthy life-style includes eating healthy foods.

Table 21.3
Facts About Destructive Habits

Effects of the Tobacco Habit

- Smokers have five times the risk of heart attack as nonsmokers.
- Smoking tobacco is directly related to cancer (lung, oral, throat), emphysema, and other respiratory diseases.
- Use of smokeless tobacco is associated with heart disease and cancer.
- Pregnant women who smoke increase the risk of health problems for their unborn babies.
- Second-hand smoke (smoke created by smokers) can cause health problems for people who breathe it.

Facts About the Abuse of Alcohol

- Alcohol abuse is a known cause of traffic accidents, violent crimes, allergic reactions, and child and spouse abuse.
- Alcohol abuse is associated with diseases of the liver, cardiovascular system, digestive system, and nervous system, to name but a few.
- Alcohol use by pregnant women can result in medical problems for the unborn child.

Facts About the Abuse of Drugs

- Illegal or illicit drug use is associated with violent crimes, traffic accidents, the increased risk of diseases such as AIDS, suicide, absenteeism, and decreased work production, among other problems.
- Legal drugs taken in improper amounts, too frequently, or in combination with other drugs are associated with many of the same health problems as illegal drugs and alcohol.
- Anabolic steroid use has health risks and has been shown to be related to use of other illegal or illicit drugs.

Avoiding Destructive Habits

Among the most destructive of habits are the use of tobacco and alcohol, and the abuse of drugs. (See table 21.3.) These are life-style or health behaviors over which you have personal control, but once they are adopted they are exceptionally difficult to eliminate.

Smoking cigarettes, cigars, and pipes as well as the use of smokeless tobacco products, such as chewing tobacco and snuff, increase the risk of many diseases. Though it is best not to start using these products, stopping the use of tobacco after years of use is beneficial to health. Unfortunately, it is very difficult to stop smoking.

Addiction to alcohol is another disease that is difficult to conquer. Seventy percent of all American adults consume alcohol. Alcohol is a depressant to the central nervous system and can have other negative effects on the body, mind, and society.

Abuse of drugs is a destructive health habit that can result from abuse of legal or illegal drugs. Among the legal drugs most often abused are caffeine and various over-the-counter drugs. Caffeine is a stimulant found in many drinks including coffee, tea, and soft drinks. In 1980 it was classified as an addicting drug. Many adults also abuse over-the-counter drugs and prescription drugs with the intent of reducing health problems. Tranquilizers and sedatives (depressants), analgesics (pain relievers), antidepressants, and amphetamines (stimulants) are among the legal drugs that are most often abused.

Illicit drugs such as cocaine (coke and crack), marijuana, the opiates (heroin, morphine, codeine, and others), the psychedelics (LSD, mescaline, designer drugs), the deliriants (PCP and others), and inhalants are addicting drugs abused by a large number of Americans. As many as forty percent of young adults try drugs, and many become addicted. One in ten of those who do not use illicit drugs are affected each day by people who abuse these drugs.

Most people use drugs as medications at some time to treat medical conditions or to reduce disease symptoms. These drugs are often prescribed by a physician or are purchased over the counter. Drugs such as caffeine are in drinks consumed by huge numbers of children and adults each day. Good health and wellness would dictate avoidance of illegal drugs, responsible use of medication, and limited use of legal drugs such as over-the-counter drugs and those found in foods or drinks.

Practicing Safe Sex

Though sexually transmitted diseases (STD) are not currently among the leading killers, they are the source of much pain and suffering. The Human Immunodeficiency Virus (HIV) that causes Acquired Immunodeficiency Syndrome (AIDS) is now a major health problem. HIV/AIDS is a worldwide health problem that has reached epidemic proportion. Many STDs can be cured but others, such as HIV/AIDS, have no cure. Healthy life-styles are the key to prevention of the most common STDs, including chlamydia, genital herpes and warts, gonorrhea, hepatitis B, HIV/AIDS, and syphilis (see table 21.4).

Adopting Good Safety Habits

Accidents are a major cause of death in North America, accounting for more than six percent of all deaths in the United States. In addition, they result in many disabilities and problems that can detract from good health and wellness. All accidents cannot be prevented, but it is possible to adopt habits that greatly reduce the risk of accidents. Deaths from automobile accidents can be greatly reduced by regular use of seat belts. The proper maintenance of play and work equipment can greatly reduce injury and death rates. Many children die each year from water-related accidents that can be prevented by proper supervision, the use of proper safety devices such as life jackets, and knowledge of cardiopulmonary resuscitation. Proper

Table 21.4
Factors Associated with Reduced Risk of STDs.

- Abstaining from sexual activity.
- Limiting sexual activity to a noninfected partner. A lifetime partner who never has sex with other people or never uses illegal injection drugs is the only "safe" partner.
- Avoiding sexual activity or other activity that puts you in contact with semen, vaginal fluids, or blood.
- Using a new condom (latex) every time you have sex, especially with a partner who is not known to be "safe."
- Using a water-based lubricant with condoms (petroleum-based lubricants increase risk of condom failure).
- Not injecting illegal drugs.
- Never sharing a needle or drug paraphernalia.

storage of guns, use of smoke alarms, proper use of ladders, and proper maintenance of cars, motorcycles, and bicycles can also reduce accident risk.

Learning First Aid

Many deaths could be prevented if persons at the site of emergencies were able to administer first aid. Because they can prevent death, all people should be familiar with cardiopulmonary resuscitation (CPR) and the Heimlich Maneuver for assisting a person who is choking (fig. 21.3). Many agencies give extensive classes in first aid taught by qualified experts. It is best to learn these procedures in such a class. First aid for minor injuries and poisoning and for control of bleeding are other important procedures.

Adopting Good Personal Health Behaviors

Many of the healthy life-styles already discussed are good personal health habits. There are other simple personal health behaviors that are important to optimal health. These behaviors may be considered elementary because they are often taught in school and at home at a very young age. Still, there are many adults who fail to adopt these behaviors on a regular basis. Examples include regular brushing and flossing of the teeth; care of ears, eyes, and skin; proper sleep habits; proper innoculations for disease prevention and good posture (see Concepts 16 and 17). Health behaviors that prevent sexually transmitted diseases are also important.

Seeking and Complying with Medical Advice

Some people purposely avoid seeking the advice of a physician because they fear that something may be wrong. This occurs in spite of the evidence that delay in treatment greatly increases the risk of death for many diseases that can be cured or controlled. In addition to medical readiness exams for those beginning exercise (see Concept 4), regular preventive medical exams are important.

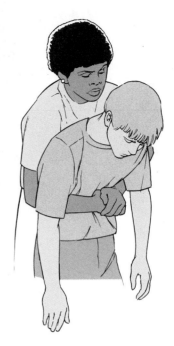

Figure 21.3
The Heimlich maneuver.

After age forty, a yearly preventive exam is recommended for all people. Young adults probably need a regular medical examination less often, but a regular examination is important for all people to help in the early diagnosis of problems. Regular self-examination for breast cancer is recommended, as are periodic mammograms and PAP tests for women (especially after age 40). For men, regular testicular exams and a prostate test are recommended. Other important behaviors that should be considered are listed below:

- Be familiar with the symptoms of the most common medical problems in our culture.
- If symptoms are present, seek medical help. Many deaths could be prevented if the early warning signs of medical problems were heeded.
- If medical advice is given, comply. It is not uncommon for people to stop taking medicine when symptoms stop rather than taking the full amount of medicine prescribed.
- If you doubt the advice given, seek a second opinion.

Being An Informed Consumer

Each year too many people purchase health services and products that are ineffective and often dangerous. Extensive advertising of quack health products, often by celebrities, bombards all of us. It is important to investigate so-called health products and services of all kinds. Information to help you become an effective exercise consumer is presented in Concept 24.

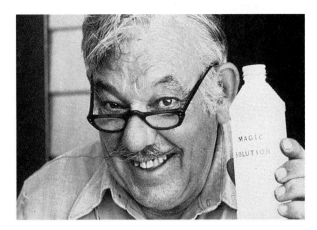
Beware of quacks who promise quick and easy solutions to health problems.

Protecting the Environment

A recent national poll indicated that 70 percent of the adult population felt that the public was not concerned enough about the environment. In fact, more than half felt that there was an immediate need to take drastic action to protect the environment. Concern for the environment has increased in recent years as indicated by the fact that more than eight of ten households now indicate that they voluntarily recycle newspapers, glass, or aluminum. We have not been as actively involved in other life-style changes that would help protect the environment (see table 21.5).

Unlike life-style behaviors such as regular exercise or managing stress, behaviors that help protect the environment may not have immediate wellness benefits. Experts are quick to point out, however, that protecting the environment may be one of the most important things that we can do over time to guarantee quality of living for our children and the generations to come.

Managing Time Effectively

Central to the concept of wellness are working efficiently and making a significant contribution to society. Working effectively requires a commitment of time. A social contribution requires time for special causes, and social wellness requires a commitment of time to family and friends. Similarly, each of the other dimensions of wellness requires a time commitment. A healthy life-style is one that allocates time efficiently to insure that appropriate time is allocated to behaviors that contribute to each wellness dimension, and ultimately to total wellness.

More Facts About Wellness and Healthy Life-Styles

Moderation is a good rule for life-style modification and wellness promotion.

In many ways, the things that enrich your life and lead to quality living can also be the source of problems. Some

Table 21.5

Adult Involvement in Behaviors to Protect the Environment

Life-Style Behavior	Percent of Involvement
• Recycle paper, glass, aluminum, oil, etc.	86%
• Cut energy use.	73%
• Avoid buying or using aerosol sprays.	68%
• Cut water use.	68%
• Replace inefficient automobile.	67%
• Contribute to environmental or conservation group.	51%
• Avoid nonrecyclable goods.	49%
• Car pool or use public transportation.	46%
• Boycott company's unsafe products.	28%
• Use cloth rather than disposable diapers.	25%
• Do environmental or conservation volunteer work.	18%

Source: Data from the Gallup Poll, 1991.

stress (eustress) makes life interesting; too much stress is considered distressful. Regular exercise contributes to good health and wellness. Too little or too much could be detrimental. This is true of almost any life-style. A moderate life-style can make life interesting and enjoyable without creating the risk of health problems.

A balanced life-style is important for promoting wellness.

"All work and no play makes Jack a dull boy" is a saying that illustrates the problem with an unbalanced life-style. If work is the only focus of your life, it detracts from good health and wellness. A balanced life-style includes interesting work and enjoyable leisure as well as balance on the other dimensions of wellness.

Personal control is critical to altering life-styles for wellness promotion.

Many health problems are associated with health behaviors that can be modified through life-style changes. To make positive life-style changes, you must believe that changing your life-style can help you prevent illness and achieve wellness. If you believe that optimal health is outside of your personal control, you will probably not make life-style changes.

Healthy life-styles learned early in life are most likely to be maintained throughout life.

Research suggests that behaviors that are learned at a very young age and that become habit are more likely to be maintained throughout life. For this reason, education concerning healthy life-styles should be started in the formative years. Simple health behaviors such as brushing the teeth, when begun early in life, are often maintained throughout life.

It is never too late to adopt positive life-styles to promote optimal health.

The negative impact of unhealthy living may have effects that are irreversible. Severe malnutrition, for example, could result in stunted growth and other problems that are permanent. Nevertheless, many problems associated with unhealthy life-styles can be improved or eliminated by changing personal living habits. For example, recent research indicates that stopping smoking, even among people who have smoked for years, reduces the risk of heart disease and cancer. Proper exercise and techniques for stress reduction can help reduce back pain and improve the quality of life for people with back problems, even those who have had chronic problems.

Suggested Readings

Bruess, C., and G. Richardson. *Decisions for Health*. 3d ed. Dubuque, IA: Wm. C. Brown Publishers, 1992.
Cancer Facts and Figures—1992. Atlanta: American Cancer Society, 1992.
1992 Heart Facts Reference Sheet. Dallas: American Heart Association, 1992.
Siegel, B. S. *Love, Medicine, and Miracles*. New York: Harper and Row, 1986.
Health Letters Associates. *Wellness Made Easy: 101 Tips for Better Health*. Berkeley: University of California, Berkeley, Wellness Letter, 1990.

LAB RESOURCE MATERIALS

(For use with Lab 21, page L-61)

Chart 21.1   The Healthy Life-Style Questionnaire

Using the Healthy Life-Style Questionnaire

The purpose of this questionnaire is to help you to analyze your life-style and to help you in making decisions concerning good health and wellness for the future. Information on this Healthy LIfe-Style Questionnaire is of a very personal nature. For this reason, this questionnaire is not one that is designed to be handed in to your instructor. **It is for your information only.** Answer each question as honestly as possible and use the scoring information on the next page to help you assess your life-style.

Directions

Select one answer for each question based on your own personal behaviors.

Exercise and Fitness	Never	Sometimes	Often	Regularly
1. I do moderate to vigorous exercise at least three times a week for 15 to 30 minutes.	☐	☐	☐	☐
2. I rate in the good fitness zone on the five components of health-related physical fitness.	No ☐			Yes ☐
Nutrition	Never	Sometimes	Often	Regularly
3. I eat three regular meals daily that contain the recommended servings from the four basic food groups.	☐	☐	☐	☐
4. I limit the amount of saturated fat (solid at room temperature), salt, and simple sugar in my diet.	☐	☐	☐	☐
Stress	Never	Sometimes	Often	Regularly
5. My normal daily activities expose me to stressful situations.	☐	☐	☐	☐
6. I do exercises or other relaxation techniques that help me reduce my stress levels.	☐	☐	☐	☐
Destructive Habits	Never	Sometimes	Often	Regularly
7. I smoke or use other tobacco products.	☐	☐	☐	☐
8. I abuse alcohol or drugs (legal or illegal).	☐	☐	☐	☐
Safe Sex Habits				
9. I abstain from sex or limit sexual activity to a safe partner.	No ☐			Yes ☐
10. I practice other safe procedures for avoiding STDs.	Never ☐	Sometimes ☐	Often ☐	Regularly ☐

continued

Chart 21.1 *continued*

Safety Habits	Never	Sometimes	Often	Regularly
11. I use seat belts and adhere to the speed limit when I drive in an automobile	☐	☐	☐	☐
12. I have a smoke detector in my home and check it regularly to see that it is working effectively.	No ☐			Yes ☐
First Aid	No			Yes
13. I could perform CPR effectively if called on in an emergency.	☐			☐
14. I could perform the Heimlich maneuver effectively if called on in an emergency.	☐			☐
Personal Health Habits	Never	Sometimes	Often	Regularly
15. I brush my teeth at least two times a day and floss at least once a day.	☐	☐	☐	☐
16. I get an adequate amount of sleep each night.	☐	☐	☐	☐
Seeking and Complying with Medical Advice	Never	Sometimes	Often	Regularly
17. I have medical check-ups and seek medical advice when symptoms are present.	☐	☐	☐	☐
18. When I receive advice from a physician including medication, I follow the advice and take the medication as prescribed.	☐	☐	☐	☐
Being an Informed Consumer	Never	Sometimes	Often	Regularly
19. I read product labels and investigate the effectiveness of products before I buy them.	☐	☐	☐	☐
20. I buy and use food supplements and other so-called "health" foods without advice from an M.D. or R.D.	☐	☐	☐	☐
Protecting the Environment	Never	Sometimes	Often	Regularly
21. I recycle paper, glass, or aluminum.	☐	☐	☐	☐
22. I practice other environment protection such as car pooling and conserving energy.	☐	☐	☐	☐
Managing Time Effectively	Never	Sometimes	Often	Regularly
23. I find time for family and friends.	☐	☐	☐	☐
24. I make time for leisure and recreation.	☐	☐	☐	☐

Scoring and Interpreting the Healthy Life-Style Questionnaire

Score the questionnaire using the following method.

1. For questions 1, 3, 4, 6, 10, 11, 15, 16, 17, 18, 19, 21, 22, 23, and 24 assign the following point values to answers: never = 1, sometimes = 2, often = 3, and regularly = 4.

2. For questions 2, 9, 12, 13, and 14 assign the following point values to answers: no = 1 and yes = 4.

3. For questions 5, 7, 8, and 20 assign the following point values to answers: never = 4, sometimes = 3, often = 2, and regularly = 1.

4. Calculate a total Healthy Life-Style Score by adding the number of points for all 24 questions.

5. Subscores for each of the nine different life-style areas can be calculated by summing the scores for the two questions in each area.

Interpret the questionnaire using the following information. In general, a total score of 72 or higher on the Healthy Life-Style Questionnaire would indicate a healthy life-style as it would suggest that you choose the healthy alternative "often." This, however, can be deceiving. You might have a score of 72 or higher and eat high-fat meals regularly or smoke regularly. In other words, scores on individual subscores are also important. For most scales, a score of six or higher merits a "good" rating, though a score of 8 is preferred.

Chart 21.2 Self-Perceptions of Wellness Questionnaire

Using the Self-Perceptions Questionnaire

Directions

There are four possible responses for each question. Place an X in **one** of the four boxes for **each** question.

Sample Question: A person who likes ice cream a lot would mark the box as indicated below.

Some people like ice cream very much.   **but**   Other people do not like ice cream at all.

Especially true for me	True for me		Not true for me	Especially not true for me
☒	☐		☐	☐

1. Some people are happy most of the time   **but**   Other people feel depressed much of the time.

Especially true for me	True for me		Not true for me	Especially not true for me
☐	☐		☐	☐

2. Some people are well informed about health and wellness.   **but**   Other people are ignorant of the facts concerning their health and well-being.

Especially true for me	True for me		Not true for me	Especially not true for me
☐	☐		☐	☐

3. Some people are physically fit.   **but**   Other people are not so fit physically.

Especially true for me	True for me		Not true for me	Especially not true for me
☐	☐		☐	☐

4. Some people have a lot of friends and are very involved socially.   **but**   Other people do not have many friends and are often lonely.

Especially true for me	True for me		Not true for me	Especially not true for me
☐	☐		☐	☐

5. Some people feel fulfilled spiritually.   **but**   Other people are not so fulfilled spiritually.

Especially true for me	True for me		Not true for me	Especially not true for me
☐	☐		☐	☐

6. Some people have a very positive outlook on life—they are optimistic.   **but**   Other people have a more negative outlook on life— they are pessimistic.

Especially true for me	True for me		Not true for me	Especially not true for me
☐	☐		☐	☐

Scoring the Wellness Perceptions Questionnaire

1. Score four points for an X marked in the first box of each row. Score a three for the second box, a two for the third box, and a one for the fourth box in each row.

2. Each question represents one of the wellness dimensions in figure 21.1. The following questions represent these wellness dimensions: 1 = emotional, 2 = intellectual, 3 = physical, 4 = social, 5 = spiritual, and 6 = general.

3. To determine a total wellness score, sum the numbers for the six questions.

4. Use chart 21.1 to determine your wellness ratings.

Chart 21.1 Wellness *Rating Scale*

	Individual Wellness Dimensions	Total Wellness
Excellent	4	21–24
Good	3	18–20
Marginal	2	12–17
Low	1	11 or less

22

Nutrition

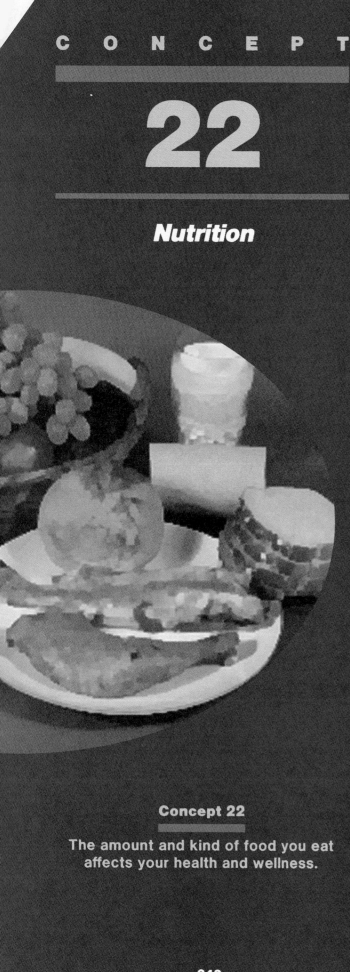

Concept 22

The amount and kind of food you eat affects your health and wellness.

Introduction

In spite of the fact that nutrition is an advanced science, many myths and misconceptions prevail. These are propagated by commercial interests. Product sales are advanced by the public's, and even physicians' and educators', superstitions and ignorance of the facts.

In this Concept some basic nutrition guidelines are presented to inform the reader and dispel various nutrition myths. Since superstition seems to thrive particularly among athletes, coaches, and those interested in high level performance, a special section is presented on nutrition and physical performance.

Because nutrition affects us all, it is important that we are knowledgeable about the subject. It is far too complicated to cover even the fundamentals in these pages; therefore, the reader is encouraged to enroll in a nutrition course taught by a registered dietitian or to study reliable books or journals on the subject, such as those listed in the suggested readings at the end of this Concept.

Health Goals for the Year 2000

- Reduce dietary fat, especially saturated fat intake.
- Increase the complex carbohydrates in the diet.
- Increase the calcium intake in the diet.
- Decrease the salt and sodium in the diet.
- Reduce the incidence of iron deficiency.
- Increase the proportion of people who use food labels.

Terms

- Also see terms in Concept 13.

Amino Acids

Twenty-two basic building blocks of the body that make up proteins.

Basal Metabolic Rate (BMR)

Metabolic rate at rest.

Carbohydrate Loading

Extra consumption of complex carbohydrates in the days prior to a long, sustained performance.

Cellulose

Indigestible fiber (bulk) in foods.

Ergogenic Aid

In this Concept, this term will refer to a nutritional supplement claimed by its promoters to improve performance.

Essential Amino Acids

Eight basic amino acids that the human body cannot produce and that must be obtained from food sources.

Fiber

Indigestible bulk in foods.

Glycogen

A source of energy stored in the muscles and liver that is necessary for sustained physical activity.

Metabolic Rate (MR)

The rate at which the body produces heat that is measured in calories; an indication of the body's activities, including exercise and normal body functions.

Recommended Daily Allowance (RDA)

The minimum amount of a specific nutrient that should be included in the daily diet to meet current health needs.

Saturated Fat

Dietary fat that is usually solid at room temperature and comes primarily from animal sources.

Unsaturated Fat

Monounsaturated or polyunsaturated fat that is usually liquid at room temperature and comes primarily from vegetable sources.

The Facts About Basic Nutrition

The amount and kind of food you eat affects your health and well-being.

There are about forty-five to fifty nutrients in food that are believed to be essential for the body's growth, maintenance, and repair. These are classified into six categories: carbohydrates (and fiber), fats, proteins, vitamins, minerals, and water. The first three provide energy, which is measured in calories.

The Food and Nutrition Board of the National Academy of Sciences—National Research Council has established **recommended daily allowances (RDA)** for each nutrient. To help assure that you select foods containing the essential elements, the board has classified foods into groups, each of which should be included in the daily diet. The quantity of nutrients recommended varies with age and other considerations; for example, a young, growing child needs more calcium than an adult, and a pregnant woman needs more calcium than other women.

Some foods contain some of all six classes of nutrients (e.g, whole-wheat bread) whereas others (e.g., sugar) contain only one. No food is a "complete" food because none contains all the specific essential nutrients.

There are ten "key nutrients" central to human nutrition. They are usually accompanied by other nutrients when obtained through plant and animal sources.

If an adequate supply of the ten "key nutrients" shown in table 22.1 are included in the diet, you will probably receive an ample supply of all the other essential nutrients. Some of the better plant and animal sources of each of the ten is also shown in table 22.1.

Table 22.1

Ten Key Nutrients and Significant Food Sources from Plants and Animals

Nutrient	Plant Source	Animal Source
Fat	Margarine Salad dressings	Fat in meats Butter
Carbohydrate	Breads Cereals Fruits and vegetables	
Protein	Dried beans and peas Nuts	Meat Poultry Fish Cheese Milk
Vitamin A	Dark green, leafy vegetables Yellow vegetables Margarine	Butter Fortified milk Liver
Vitamin C	Citrus fruits Broccoli, potatoes Strawberries, tomatoes Cabbage, dark green, leafy vegetables	Liver
Vitamin B$_1$ (thiamin)	Breads Cereals Nuts	Pork Ham
Vitamin B$_2$ (riboflavin)	Breads Cereals	Milk Cheese Liver
Niacin	Breads Cereals Nuts	Meat Fish Poultry
Iron	Dried peas and beans Spinach, asparagus Prune juice	Meat Liver
Calcium	Turnip greens, okra Broccoli, spinach	Milk Cheese Mackerel Salmon

A nutritionally dense food gives you more nutrients per calorie than a low-density food. It is like "getting more for your money (calorie)." For example, a 200-calorie piece of Boston cream pie has very few vitamins and minerals and is high in fat and refined carbohydrates, whereas 200 calories of tuna has very little fat, 100 percent of the RDA for protein, niacin, vitamin B_{12}, and substantial B_6 and phosphorus.

Eating nutritionally dense food is particularly important for someone on a low-calorie diet. For example, it is difficult to get all the essential nutrients in a 1,000- to 1,200-calorie diet unless foods are chosen carefully.

The Facts About Nutrition and Good Health

The number of calories needed per day depends upon the body's **metabolic rate (MR)**, which, in turn, depends upon such factors as age, sex, size, muscle mass, glandular function, emotional state, climate, and exercise.

Your **basal metabolic rate (BMR)** is the basis for your caloric needs. The higher the BMR, the more calories you burn at rest. Your MR is a combination of your BMR and calories expended in normal daily activities. The MR is usually higher in males, young people, large people, lean and muscular people, and in nervous people; in cold and hot weather; and during exercise.

A moderately active college-age woman needs about 2,000 calories per day, whereas a moderately active man of the same age needs about 2,800 calories. A female athlete in training might burn 2,600 to 4,500 calories; a male athlete in training might expend 3,500 to 6,000. If your weight remains at the optimum, the caloric content of your diet is correct. If weight varies from optimal, the caloric content of the diet may need to be altered.

The three sources of calories in the diet are fat, protein, and carbohydrates. The typical adult consumes too much fat and too little carbohydrate, especially complex carbohydrates. A goal is to reduce the amount of dietary fat and increase the amount of complex carbohydrate in the diet of the average adult (see figure 22.1).

Excess fat in the diet, particularly saturated fat, is associated with the increased risk of disease and is inversely related to optimal health.

Humans need some fat in their diet (see figure 22.2) because fats are carriers of vitamins A, D, E, and K. They are a source of essential linoleic acid, make food taste better, and provide a concentrated form of calories, which

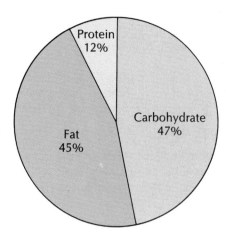

Figure 22.1
Current adult dietary intake.

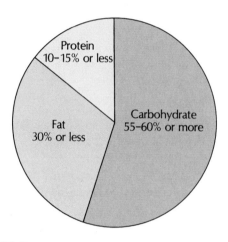

Figure 22.2
Recommended dietary intake.

serve as an important source of energy during moderate to vigorous exercise. Fats have twice the calories per gram as carbohydrates.

There is evidence that excessive total fat in the diet is associated with atherosclerotic cardiovascular disease; breast, prostate, and colon cancer; as well as obesity. **Saturated fats** come primarily from animal sources such as red meat, dairy products, and eggs, but they are also found in some vegetable sources such as coconut and palm oils. They are considered most likely to contribute to the health problems mentioned above. In addition, excess saturated fat in the diet contributes to increased cholesterol, and increased LDL cholesterol in the blood.

Unsaturated fats, also a part of a normal diet, are of two basic types: polyunsaturated and monounsaturated. Polyunsaturated fats are derived principally from vegetable sources such as safflower, cottonseed, soybean, sunflower, and corn oils (Omega-6 fats) and cold water fish sources such as salmon and mackerel (Omega-3 fats). Monounsaturated fats are derived primarily from vegetable sources including olive, peanut, and canola oil.

Unsaturated fats are generally considered to be less likely to contribute to cardiovascular disease, cancer, and obesity than saturated fats. When polyunsaturated fats (Omega-6) are substituted for saturated fats, there is a reduction in cholesterol and LDL cholesterol in the blood, but there may be a decrease in HDL cholesterol as well. However, when monounsaturated fats are substituted for saturated fats, cholesterol and LDL cholesterol are thought to decrease without an accompanying decrease in the desirable HDL. There is very limited evidence that Omega-3 unsaturated fats (fish oils) may inhibit cancers, but Omega-6 fats may not have the same effect. Fish oils have been shown to reduce triglycerides, but there is no conclusive evidence that they are especially successful in reducing blood cholesterol.

Humans produce their own cholesterol even when dietary cholesterol is limited. Still, there is evidence that high dietary cholesterol can increase the risk of atherosclerosis and coronary heart disease. Principal sources of dietary cholesterol are organ meats, some shellfish, and egg yolks.

Dietary Recommendations: Fat

- Total fat in the diet should be limited to 30 percent or less of the total calories consumed.
- Saturated fat in the diet should be limited to 10 percent or less of total calories consumed.
- Polyunsaturated and monounsaturated fats should be substituted for saturated fat in the diet.
- Dietary cholesterol should be limited to 250 to 300 milligrams per day.

Dietary Implementation: Fat

- Substitute lean meat, fish, poultry, nonfat milk, and other low-fat dairy products for high-fat foods.
- Reduce intake of fried foods, especially those cooked in saturated fats (often true of fast-food restaurants), desserts with high levels of fat (many cookies and cakes), and dressings with high-fat levels.
- Limit dietary intake of foods high in cholesterol such as egg yolks, organ meats, and shellfish.
- Use monounsaturated or polyunsaturated fats for cooking.
- Though two or three servings of fish per week may be prudent because of its content of Omega-3 polyunsaturated oils, the experts feel that there is not sufficient evidence to endorse a fish oil dietary supplement.
- Be careful of the total elimination of a single food source from the diet. For example, the elimination of meat and dairy products entirely could result in iron or calcium deficiencies, especially among women and children.

For optimal health, carbohydrates, especially complex carbohydrates, should be the principal source of calories in the diet.

Complex carbohydrates are known as starches and include fruits, vegetables, whole-grain breads, and cereals. These foods are nutritionally dense and also contain **cellulose** (popularly known as **fiber**). Cellulose does not provide nutrition and is not digested, but is considered essential for the bulk it provides for efficient digestion.

Research evidence shows that diets high in complex carbohydrates such as whole-grain cereals, legumes, vegetables, and fruits are associated with a low incidence of lung, colon, esophagus, and stomach cancer as well as coronary heart disease. Some of this benefit may be due to the fact that complex carbohydrate diets are likely to be low in saturated fat. Water-soluble fiber, such as pectin and oat bran, has recently been shown to produce small reductions in total blood cholesterol independent of the effects of reduced dietary fat. Long-term studies indicate that high-fiber diets may also be associated with a lower risk of diabetes mellitus, diverticulosis, hypertension, and gallstone formation. It is not certain whether these health benefits are directly attributable to high dietary fiber or other effects associated with the ingestion of vegetables, fruits, and cereals in the diet.

Complex carbohydrates may also be beneficial to health because they provide rich sources of vitamins and minerals. The possible benefits of consuming a diet high in complex carbohydrates and certain vitamins are discussed in the section on vitamins.

Simple carbohydrates are sugars such as sucrose, lactose, maltose, glucose, and fructose. They are nutritionally low in density and are commonly found in foods considered to possess "empty calories" such as candy and soft drinks.

Simple carbohydrates do not have the same benefits to health as do the complex carbohydrates. Foods high in simple carbohydrates are often high in fat as well. Simple carbohydrates, especially sucrose, a sugar often found in candy and soft drinks, have also been shown to increase the incidence of dental caries. Research has NOT shown that sugar consumption, among those who have an adequate diet, is a risk factor for diseases such as cancer and heart disease.

Dietary Recommendations: Carbohydrates

- Total carbohydrate in the diet should account for 55 percent or more of total calories consumed. (See figure 22.2.)
- Simple carbohydrates should be limited to 15 percent or less of total calories consumed.
- High-fiber foods should be included in the daily diet.

Dietary Implementation: Carbohydrates

- Consume at least five servings of vegetables and/or fruits each day. Servings of green and yellow vegetables as well as citrus fruits are recommended. A serving of vegetables equals approximately one-half cup. A serving of fruit equals one medium-size piece.
- Consume at least six servings of complex carbohydrates such as breads, cereals, and/or legumes. A serving of legumes or cereal equals approximately one-half cup. A serving of bread is one slice, or one roll or muffin.
- Limit intake of desserts, baked goods, and other foods high in simple sugars or empty calories.
- Dietary fiber supplements other than in the form of food (such as oat bran) are not recommended unless prescribed for medical reasons.

Protein is the basic building block for the body, but dietary protein constitutes a relatively small amount of daily calorie intake.

It is said that proteins are the building blocks of your body because all body cells are made of protein. Proteins are formed from twenty-two different **amino acids.** More than 100 proteins are made up of these amino acids. Fourteen of these amino acids are made in your own body, but eight **essential amino acids** are not. You must consume foods that contain these eight essential amino acids if your body is to function properly. Certain foods, called "complete proteins," contain all eight essential amino acids. Examples of complete proteins are meat, dairy products, and fish. Incomplete proteins contain some, but not all, of the essential amino acids. Examples of incomplete proteins are beans, nuts, and rice.

Experts agree that there are no known benefits and some possible risks to consuming diets exceptionally high in animal protein. Certain cancers and coronary heart disease risk have been associated with high dietary intake of animal protein. Researchers are not certain whether the increased risk of contracting these diseases due to a high intake of animal protein is because of the protein itself or the fact that diets high in animal protein are also high in fat. There is evidence that excessive protein intake can lead to urinary calcium loss, which can be dangerous, especially for women.

Some scientists are concerned that restriction of animal protein might result in lower than necessary dietary intake of essential nutrients such as iron, especially for women and children. If the recommendations suggested in this section are followed, this should not be a problem. It is not our intent to suggest that animal protein should not be part of the normal diet, rather that consumption of animal protein be restricted somewhat, especially when the fat content is high.

Dietary Recommendation: Protein

- Protein in the diet should account for 15 percent or less of the total calories consumed.
- Protein in the diet should exceed the RDA of .8 grams per kilogram (2.2 pounds) of a person's desirable weight. This is about 36 grams for a 100-pound person.
- Protein in the diet should NOT exceed twice the RDA (1.6 grams per kilogram of a person's desirable weight).
- Vegetarians or those who severely limit the intake of animal products must be especially careful to eat combinations of foods that assure adequate intake of essential amino acids.

Dietary Implementation: Protein

- Consume at least two servings of lean meat, fish, poultry, and dairy products (especially those low in fat content) or adequate combinations of foods such as beans, nuts, and rice in the diet.
- Dietary supplements of protein such as tablets and powders are NOT recommended.

Adequate vitamin intake is necessary to good health and wellness, but excessive vitamin intake is NOT necessary and can be harmful.

Consuming foods containing the minimum RDA of each of the vitamins is essential to the prevention of disease and maintenance of good health. Consuming foods high in carotinoid and retinoid is recommended because these foods are associated with the reduced risk of some forms of cancer. Carotinoid- and retinoid-rich foods such as green and yellow vegetables, carrots, and sweet potatoes contain high amounts of Vitamin A. Diets high in Vitamin C (citrus fruits and vegetables) and Vitamin E (green leafy vegetables) are also associated with reduced risk of cancer. Some research has suggested that Vitamins C, E, and carotinoid-rich foods act as antioxidants or as substances that can inactivate other substances thought to damage body cells. Most experts point out that selecting more servings from the second level of the food pyramid (see figure 22.3) is wise strategy, but they recommend caution concerning the use of vitamin supplements. Excess doses of vitamins have been shown to cause health problems. For example, excessively high amounts of Vitamin C are dangerous for ten percent of the population who inherit a special gene related to health problems. Excessively high amounts of Vitamin A and D are also associated with various health problems.

Dietary Recommendations: Vitamins

- Vitamins in the amounts equal to the RDAs should be included in the diet each day.

Dietary Implementation: Vitamins

- A diet containing the food servings recommended for carbohydrates, proteins, and fats will more than meet the RDA standards.
- Extra servings of green and yellow vegetables, citrus and other fruits, and other nonanimal food sources high in fiber, vitamins, and minerals is a wise substitute for high-fat foods.
- Those who eat a sound diet as described in this chapter do not need a vitamin supplement. Those who insist on taking a daily vitamin supplement are advised not to take daily amounts larger than the RDA and only after following the guidelines for dietary supplements suggested later in this Concept (see pages 251–52).

Adequate mineral intake is necessary for good health and wellness, but excessive mineral intake is NOT necessary and can be harmful.

Like vitamins, minerals have no calories and provide no energy for the body. They are important in regulating various bodily functions. Two of the ten key nutrients, calcium and iron, are minerals. Calcium is important to bone, muscle, nerve, and blood development and function. Iron is necessary for the blood to carry adequate oxygen. Other important minerals are phosphorus, which builds teeth and bones; sodium, which regulates water in the body; zinc, which aids in the healing process; and potassium, which is necessary for proper muscle function.

RDAs for minerals are established to determine the amounts of each necessary for healthy day-to-day functioning. A sound diet provides all of the RDA for minerals. Evidence indicating that some segments of the population may be mineral deficient have led to the establishment of health goals identifying a need to increase calcium intake, especially among young people and pregnant women, and to reduce the incidence of iron deficiency among very young children and women of childbearing age. Further, the decrease in salt and sodium intake is a health goal established for people of all ages because of the association of dietary salt and sodium with elevated blood pressure. Eating the appropriate number of servings from the food pyramid provides all the minerals necessary for meeting the RDA for minerals. Nutrition goals for the nation emphasize the importance of adequate servings of foods rich in calcium, such as green leafy vegetables and milk products; adequate servings of foods rich in iron, such as beans, peas, spinach, or meat; and reduced salt in the diet.

Dietary Recommendations: Minerals

- Minerals in amounts equal to the RDAs should be taken in the diet each day.
- In general, a dietary supplement of calcium is not recommended; however, it is especially important for women, adolescents, and anyone who restricts calorie intake to make careful food choices to assure adequate calcium in the diet. For post-menopausal women, a calcium supplement is now recommended by some experts. Consult with a registered dietitian or a physician regarding amounts and types of supplements.
- Salt should be limited in the diet to no more than 4 grams per day, and even less would be desirable (3 grams). Three grams equals one teaspoon of table salt.

Dietary Implementation: Minerals

- A diet containing the food servings recommended for carbohydrates, proteins, and fats will more than meet the RDA standards.
- Extra servings of green and yellow vegetables, citrus and other fruits, and other nonanimal sources of foods high in fiber, vitamins, and minerals are recommended as a substitute for high-fat foods.
- In general, people who eat a sound diet as described in this Concept do NOT need a mineral supplement. Those who insist on taking a daily mineral supplement are advised not to take daily amounts larger than the RDA and only after following the guidelines for dietary supplements suggested later in this Concept (see pages 251–52).

Water is a critical component in the healthy diet.

Though water is not on the list of the ten "key nutrients" because it contains no calories, provides no energy, and provides none of the ten key nutrients, it is very important to health and survival. Water is a major component of most of the foods you eat, and more than half of all body tissues are comprised of it. Regular water intake maintains water balance and is critical to many important bodily functions.

Dietary Recommendations and Implementation: Water

- In addition to foods containing water, the average adult needs about two quarts of water every day. Water intake must be increased even more for active people and those in hot environments.

Beverages other than water are a part of many diets. Some beverages can have an adverse effect on good health.

Coffee, tea, soft drinks, and alcoholic beverages are often substituted for water in the diet. Coffee (with caffeine)

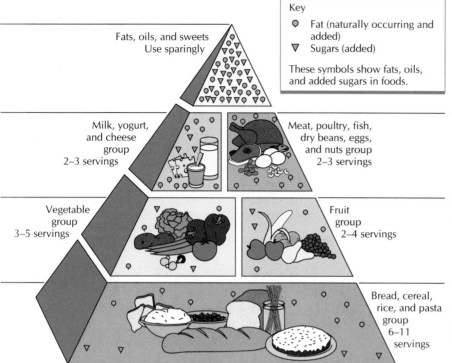

The small tip of the Pyramid shows fats, oils, and sweets. These are foods such as salad dressings and oils, cream, butter, margarine, sugars, soft drinks, candies, and sweet desserts. These foods provide calories and little else nutritionally. Most people should use them sparingly.

On this level of the Food Guide Pyramid are two groups of foods that come mostly from animals: milk, yogurt, and cheese; and meat, poultry, fish, dry beans, eggs, and nuts. These foods are important for protein, calcium, iron, and zinc.

This level includes foods that come from plants – vegetables and fruits. Most people need to eat more of these foods for the vitamins, minerals, and fiber they supply.

At the base of the Food Guide Pyramid are breads, cereals, rice, and pasta – all foods from grains. You need the most servings of these foods each day.

Figure 22.3

The Food Guide Pyramid.

Source: U.S. Department of Agriculture.

consumption has been shown to cause symptoms such as irregular heartbeat in some people. Tea has not been shown to have similar effects, though this may be because tea drinkers typically consume less volume than coffee drinkers and tea has less caffeine per cup than coffee. Both beverages contain caffeine, as do many soft drinks, though drip coffee typically contains two to three times the caffeine of a typical cola drink.

Excessive consumption of alcoholic beverages can have negative health implications because the alcohol often replaces many of the ten "key nutrients." Excessive alcohol consumption is associated with the increased risk of heart disease, high blood pressure, stroke, and osteoporosis. Long-term, excessive alcoholic beverage consumption leads to cirrhosis of the liver, and the increased risk of hepatitis and cancer. Alcohol consumption during pregnancy can result in low birth weight, fetal alcoholism, and other damage to the fetus.

Dietary Recommendations and Implementation: Beverages

- Servings of coffee, tea, and soft drinks should not be substituted for water and/or other beverages or foods such as low-fat milk, fruit juices, or foods rich in calcium, which provide sources of key nutrients.

- Daily servings of beverages containing caffeine should be limited to three or less.
- For good health, alcohol consumption is NOT recommended, but for those who drink it, a maximum of one ounce of alcohol per day is recommended (one ounce equals two beers, small wine drinks, or average-size cocktails).

Facts About Sound Eating Practices

Eating the recommended servings of food from the Food Guide Pyramid will provide the ten key nutrients and enable a person to meet the dietary recommendations outlined in this Concept.

The Food Guide Pyramid (see figure 22.3) was designed to guide people in the selection of nutritious food. A greater number of servings is recommended from the food groups near the base of the pyramid (complex carbohydrates). Active people who expend more than typical amounts of calories in physical activity will need to choose servings near the upper number in the pyramid, whereas sedentary people will need fewer servings. Figure 22.4 provides you with an idea of what constitutes a serving for each food group.

Food Groups

Bread, Cereal, Rice, and Pasta		
1 slice of bread	1 ounce of ready-to-eat cereal	1/2 cup of cooked cereal, rice or pasta

Vegetable		
1 cup of raw leafy vegetables	1/2 cup of other vegetables, cooked or chopped raw	3/4 cup of vegetable juice

Fruit		
1 medium apple, banana, orange	1/2 cup of chopped, cooked, or canned fruit	3/4 cup of fruit juice

Milk, Yogurt, and Cheese		
1 cup of milk or yogurt	1-1/2 ounces of natural cheese	2 ounces of process cheese

Meat, Poultry, Fish, Dry Beans, Eggs, and Nuts	
2–3 ounces of cooked lean meat, poultry, or fish	1/2 cup of cooked dry beans, 1 egg, or 2 tablespoons of peanut butter count as 1 ounce of lean meat

Figure 22.4

What Counts as a Serving?

Source: U.S. Department of Agriculture.

Healthy snacks can be an important part of good nutrition.

Snacking is not necessarily bad. For those interested in losing or maintaining their current weight, small snacks of appropriate foods can help fool the appetite. For those interested in gaining weight, snacks can provide additional calories. The key is selection of the foods for snacking. For those trying to maintain or lose weight, the calories consumed in snacks will probably necessitate limiting the calories consumed at meals.

As with your total diet, the best snacks are those that are nutritionally dense. Too often, snacks are high in calories, fats, simple sugar, and salt. Check the content of snacks. Even foods sold as "healthy snacks," such as granola bars, are often high in fat and simple sugar. Some common snacks such as chips, pretzels, and even popcorn are high in salt and may be cooked in fat.

Some suggestions for healthy snacks include ice milk instead of ice cream, fresh fruits, vegetable sticks, popcorn not cooked in fat and with little or no salt, crackers, and nuts with little or no salt.

Careful selection of food choices is important for those who rely on fast foods as a significant part of their diet.

More and more Americans rely on fast foods as part of their normal diet. Unfortunately, many fast foods are poor nutritional choices. Many hamburgers are high in fat. French fries are high in fat because they are usually cooked in saturated fat. Even choices deemed to be more nutritious, such as chicken or fish sandwiches, are often high in fat and calories because they are cooked in fat and covered with special high-fat/high-calorie sauces.

Dietary Recommendation: Fast Foods

- Become informed about the content of fast foods before you make your selection. For more information see the charts in Appendices C and D, and read the reference at the end of Appendix D. Lab 22B will also help you learn more about the content of fast foods.

Moderation is a good general rule of nutrition.

Too little of important nutrients can lead to health problems. Excluding entire food groups can cause problems and is not advised. People who restrict or eliminate meat from the diet must be sure to carefully select other foods to insure a healthy diet. Just as too little food can cause problems, excessive intake of various nutrients can cause problems. More is not always better. Moderation (neither too much nor too little) in choices of foods is advised.

It is not necessary to permanently eliminate foods that you really enjoy, but some of your favorite food may not be among the best of choices. Enjoying special foods on occasion is part of moderation. The key is to **limit** choices that are not consistent with the recommendations made in this Concept.

Consistency (with variety) is a good general rule of nutrition.

Eating regular meals, including a good breakfast, every day is wise. Many studies have shown breakfast to be an important meal. One-fourth of the day's calories should be consumed at breakfast. Skipping breakfast impairs performance because blood sugar levels drop in the long period between dinner the night before and lunch the following day. Eating every four to six hours is wise.

The Facts About Nutrition and Physical Performance

In general, the nutrition rules described in the previous pages apply to all people, whether active or sedentary. Good nutrition is necessary for all people, but there are some additional nutrition facts that are important for exercisers and athletes. This information is outlined in table 22.2.

Carbohydrate loading and carbohydrate replacement during exercise can enhance sustained aerobic performances exceeding one hour in length.

Athletes and vigorously active people must maintain a high level of readily available fuel especially in the muscles. Adequate complex carbohydrate consumption is the best way to assure this.

Immediately prior to an activity that will require extended duration of physical performance (more than one hour in length, such as a marathon), **carbohydrate loading** can be useful. Carbohydrate loading is accomplished by resting one or two days before the event and eating a higher than normal amount of complex carbohydrates. This procedure helps prevent the depletion of muscle **glycogen,**

Table 22.2
Dietary Recommendations for Athletes and Active People

Fat	Active people, like everyone else, should restrict fat, especially saturated fat.
Protein	The American Dietetics Association (ADA) recommends 1.0 grams per kg of body weight for active people such as athletes. This is higher than the .8 per kg recommended for normal adults. A normal healthy diet easily meets this need so protein above 15 percent of the diet is not recommended, nor are protein supplements (including amino acids).
Carbohydrates	Because active people often expend calories in amounts considerably above normal, extra calories are necessary in the diet. Carbohydrates are the best source. To avoid excess fat and protein intake, carbohydrates (especially complex carbohydrates) may constitute as much as 70 percent of total calorie intake.
Vitamins and Minerals	The best evidence indicates that a sound diet meets the vitamin and mineral needs of active people. Those in activities for which caloric restriction may be encouraged, such as wrestling, must be especially careful in the food choices they make.

which is necessary for sustained performance. However, this procedure could cause problems for those with diabetes, hypertriglycemia, and kidney disorders.

Ingesting carbohydrate solutions during long, sustained exercise can also aid in performance by preventing or forestalling muscle glycogen depletion. Taking in fluids with less than five percent sugar helps prevent dehydration and replenishes energy stores. These solutions should be taken regularly in long, sustained performances. After long, sustained performances, the consumption of carbohydrates within fifteen to thirty minutes can aid in rapid replenishment of muscle glycogen, which may be important to future performances. Carbohydrate drinks are *not* helpful for short (less than an hour) endurance activity.

The timing may be more important than the makeup of the pre-event meal.

It is probably best to eat about three hours before competition or heavy exercise to allow time for digestion. Generally, the athlete can make his or her food selection on the basis of past experience. Tension, anxiety, and excitement are more apt to cause gastric distress than is food selection. It is generally accepted that fat intake should be minimal because it digests more slowly; "gas formers"

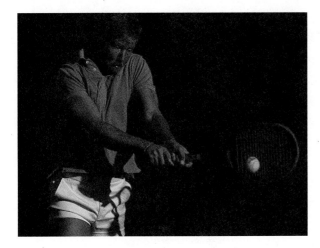
Good nutrition is essential for active people.

should probably be avoided; and proteins and high-cellulose foods should be kept to a moderate amount prior to prolonged events to avoid urinary and bowel excretion. Two or three cups of liquid should be taken to ensure adequate hydration.

Ingestion of simple carbohydrates (sugar, candy) within an hour or two prior to an event is NOT recommended because it may cause an insulin response that results in weakness and fatigue. Sometimes they cause stomach distress, cramps, or nausea.

It should be noted that the excitement associated with competition is probably the main reason for having a special diet before participation. Because many people who exercise regularly usually are not competing, there is little reason to alter normal diet before regular exercise. Likewise, there is no need to delay exercise for long periods after the meal if exercise is moderate and noncompetitive.

The Facts: Nutrition Quackery

The Food and Drug Administration has labeled the "health food" racket as the most widespread quackery in the United States.

Whether athletic or sedentary, the individual on a well-balanced diet does NOT benefit from special organic foods, phosphate, alkaline salts, choline, lecithin, wheat germ, honey, gelatin, aspartates, brewer's yeast, or royal jelly unless prescribed for medical purposes by a physician. Because these products do not produce the special benefits claimed for them, their use and/or sale can be considered nutritional quackery. For more information about quacks and quackery, see pages 271–73 in Concept 24.

Claims for foods in advertisements may NOT provide accurate information about the nutritional value of the foods.

Until recently, food labels have failed to provide useful information concerning the nutritional values of foods. Recently congress enacted laws to make food labels more uniform and to protect consumers. Now products sold in stores must meet specified standards to be able to use words such as "fat free" on the label. For example, a food must have less than one-half of a gram of fat per serving (50 grams) to be considered "fat free," and it must have less than 3 grams per serving to be considered "low fat." To be labeled "low in saturated fat," a food must have less than 15 percent of its calories from saturated fat.

The labels required on foods sold in stores (see figure 22.5 on page 252) provide information based on diets of 2000 calories per day. As noted earlier in this concept, the number of calories you consume depends on your age, body size, gender, metabolic rate, and activity level. The 2000-calorie value is better suited for children and women than for men, who typically consume more calories in a day. Values must be adjusted for those whose daily calorie intake is above 2000 calories.

In spite of recent improvements in food labeling, consumers must continue to be wary of deceptive advertising. While the use of words such as "light" or "low fat" has been regulated to some extent, consumers should be sure that products live up to claims made for them.

Even with recent efforts to regulate dietary supplements, many fall outside the current regulations and use false or deceptive advertising.

It is wise to read food labels, to ask for information about food content in restaurants, and to be wary of claims about supplements advertised for health or fitness improvement.

For most people, dietary supplements, when taken in excess of amounts known to be beneficial to good health, can be considered as nutritional quackery.

As already noted in previous sections of this concept, dietary supplements are not generally necessary for those who eat a sound diet. However, supplements of vitamins and minerals are sometimes recommended by physicians and dietitians. Supplements are most commonly recommended for pregnant women, postmenopausal women, those who restrict dietary intake to less than 1,500 calories daily (such as athletes trying to control weight), those with special medical problems, and those known to have diets deficient in key nutrients.

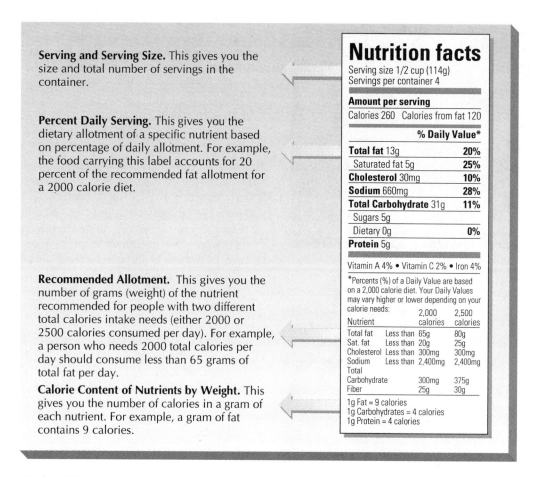

Serving and Serving Size. This gives you the size and total number of servings in the container.

Percent Daily Serving. This gives you the dietary allotment of a specific nutrient based on percentage of daily allotment. For example, the food carrying this label accounts for 20 percent of the recommended fat allotment for a 2000 calorie diet.

Recommended Allotment. This gives you the number of grams (weight) of the nutrient recommended for people with two different total calories intake needs (either 2000 or 2500 calories consumed per day). For example, a person who needs 2000 total calories per day should consume less than 65 grams of total fat per day.

Calorie Content of Nutrients by Weight. This gives you the number of calories in a gram of each nutrient. For example, a gram of fat contains 9 calories.

Nutrition facts

Serving size 1/2 cup (114g)
Servings per container 4

Amount per serving

Calories 260   Calories from fat 120

	% Daily Value*
Total fat 13g	20%
Saturated fat 5g	25%
Cholesterol 30mg	10%
Sodium 660mg	28%
Total Carbohydrate 31g	11%
Sugars 5g	
Dietary 0g	0%
Protein 5g	

Vitamin A 4% • Vitamin C 2% • Iron 4%

*Percents (%) of a Daily Value are based on a 2,000 calorie diet. Your Daily Values may vary higher or lower depending on your calorie needs:

Nutrient		2,000 calories	2,500 calories
Total fat	Less than	65g	80g
Sat. fat	Less than	20g	25g
Cholesterol	Less than	300mg	300mg
Sodium	Less than	2,400mg	2,400mg
Total Carbohydrate		300mg	375g
Fiber		25g	30g

1g Fat = 9 calories
1g Carbohydrates = 4 calories
1g Protein = 4 calories

Figure 22.5

Using food labels.

Source: U.S. Food and Drug Administration.

The most common forms of nutritional quackery involve nutritional supplements containing protein, vitamins, and minerals. Before considering taking any of these supplements, consider the following guidelines:

- *Analyze the content of your diet before making decisions about its quality.* If you assume your current diet is not adequate, on what do you base the assumption? It is recommended that you do a dietary analysis to determine the quality of your diet. This is best done by logging your food intake for several days and determining the content of the foods eaten (see Lab 22A). Expert assistance is useful in conducting a dietary analysis.
- *Have a medical exam to see if you have any symptoms of nutritional deficiencies.*
- *Consult an expert (physician or dietitian) about your nutritional needs.* Most experts will recommend changes in your diet if they decide that you are not getting proper nutrition. Only in special cases will supplements be recommended. Be aware that the term "nutritionist" is one that virtually anyone can use, and the qualifications of such a person should be checked thoroughly before considering him or her an expert. Registered dietitians with a degree (R.D.) in nutrition are considered qualified and recognized as experts.

People who are interested in enhancing physical performance are especially subject to nutrition quackery. A food or nutrition product thought to enhance performance is considered to be an **ergogenic aid.** Many of the products that are alleged to be ergogenic aids can be classified as quack products because they do not enhance performance as promised and are often exceptionally expensive. In some cases so-called "performance-enhancing supplements" are dangerous to health and wellness. Examples of products that are misrepresented in terms of potential performance-enhancing benefits are dietary supplements such as vitamins, minerals, proteins and amino acids, plant steroids, and other dietary supplements. Among the most often misrepresented products are protein and amino acid supplements, sometimes referred to as "steroid alternatives." Table 22.3 lists some of these.

Table 22.3

Some Commonly Misrepresented Dietary Supplements Alleged to Enhance Performance

Product	Claim	The Facts
Plant steroids	• Alleged to promote muscle development similar to animal steroids.	• Plant steroids do not promote muscle mass gains in humans.
Trace elements (ex: chromium picolinate)	• Alleged to promote muscle development.	• No evidence of effectiveness. It could lead to anemia if taken in excess.
Amino acids (ex: arginine, lysine)	• Alleged to promote increases in human growth hormone that lead to increased muscle mass.	• Some evidence that increased HGH results from intake of amino acids, but little evidence of resulting muscle mass increases. There is risk in taking the high doses recommended by sellers. Banned in Canada.
Protein supplements	• Alleged muscle mass gains.	• No evidence of effectiveness, some are not digestible. Not superior to dietary protein as some claim, and far more costly. Overuse can lead to excess loss of body water, diarrhea, abdominal cramps, and altered kidney function.
Caffeine	• Alleged to enhance endurance performance.	• Inconsistent results. Banned by Olympic rules. Some negative health consequences.
Vitamin supplements (ex: B complex, B15)	• Alleged stress reduction and performance enhancement.	• No evidence of benefits to those who are not vitamin deficient. B15 (pangamic acid) is not a vitamin and can be harmful. No evidence of stress-reducing effects.
Minerals (ex: iron)	• Alleged that athletes and active people need more than other people.	• Some evidence that active people have increased need, but the consensus is that a sound diet provides for those needs.

Note: FDA standards have not been set for many advertised products. For this reason the consumer cannot be assured of the exact content of products, and product safety cannot be assured. This is illustrated by the recall of products containing the amino acid L-tryptophan after the deaths of 32 people were linked to its use.

Claims for products alleged to promote weight loss are especially likely to be fraudulent.

Recently the Federal Trade Commission (FTC) studied weight-loss programs, including some of the most famous dietary supplement programs. The FTC forced many of the companies to abandon false claims they used in their advertising. Consumers are urged to ask questions about the health risks of the program, the data supporting program effectiveness, costs of the program, long-term program effectiveness, and expert supervision of the program.

Suggested Readings

National Research Council. *Diet and Health: Implications for Reducing Chronic Disease Risk.* Washington, D.C.: National Academy of Sciences, 1989.

"The Supplement Story: Can Vitamins Help?" *Consumer Reports* 57(1992):12.

Williams, M. H. *Nutrition for Fitness and Sport.* 3d ed. Dubuque, IA: Wm. C. Brown Publishers, 1992.

LAB RESOURCE MATERIALS

(For use with Lab 22A, page L-63)

Chart 22A.1 Dietary Habits Questionnaire

Yes	No	
☐	☐	1. Do you eat regular meals?
☐	☐	2. Do you eat a good breakfast daily?
☐	☐	3. Do you eat lunch regularly?
☐	☐	4. Does your diet contain about 55%–60% carbohydrates with a high concentration of fiber?
☐	☐	5. Are less than one-fourth of the carbohydrates you eat simple carbohydrates?
☐	☐	6. Does your diet contain 10%–15% protein?
☐	☐	7. Does your diet contain less than 30% fat?
☐	☐	8. Do you limit the amount of saturated fat in your diet?
☐	☐	9. Do you limit salt intake to acceptable amounts?
☐	☐	10. Do you get adequate amounts of vitamins in your diet without a supplement?
☐	☐	11. Do you eat regularly from all food groups?
☐	☐	12. Do you drink adequate amounts of water?
☐	☐	13. Do you get adequate minerals in your diet without a supplement?
☐	☐	14. Do you limit your caffeine and alcohol consumption to acceptable levels?
☐	☐	15. Is your average calorie consumption for the three-day period reasonable for your body size and for the amount of calories you normally expend?

_____ Total number of "Yes" answers.

Chart 22A.2 Dietary Habits *Rating Scale*

Score	Rating
14–15	Very Good
12–13	Good
10–11	Marginal
9 or less	Poor

23

Stress Management and Relaxation

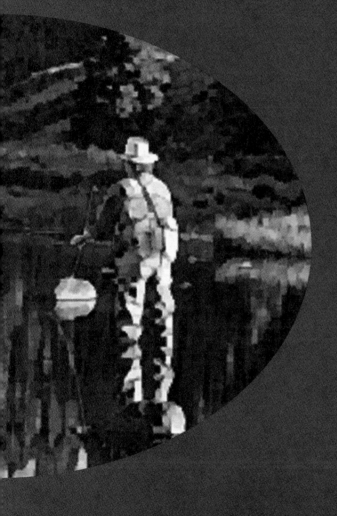

Concept 23

Mental and physical health are affected by an individual's ability to avoid or adapt to stress.

Introduction

Stress can trigger an emotional response that, in turn, evokes the autonomic nervous system to a "fight or flight" response. This adaptive and protective mechanism stimulates the ductless glands to hypo- or hyperactivity in preparation for what is perceived as a threat or assault on the whole organism. In some instances, this **alarm reaction** of the body may be essential to survival, but when evoked inappropriately or excessively, it may be more harmful than the effects of the original stressor. For example, a fight-or-flight response may cause a coronary spasm that could lead to a heart attack.

Health Goals for the Year 2000

- Reduce adverse health effects from stress.
- Help those with stress to reduce or control it.

Terms

Adaptation

The body's efforts to restore normalcy.

Alarm Reaction

The body's warning signal that a stressor is present.

Anxiety

A state of apprehension with a compulsion to do something; excessive anxiety is a tension disorder with physiological characteristics.

Chronic Fatigue

Constant state of entire body fatigue.

Distress

Negative stress, or stress that contributes to health problems.

Eustress

Positive stress, or stress that is mentally or physically stimulating.

Hypostress

Lack of stress.

Neuromuscular Hypertension

Unnecessary or exaggerated muscle contractions; excess tension beyond that needed to perform a given task; also called hypertonus.

Physiological Fatigue

A deterioration in the capacity of the neuromuscular system as the result of physical overwork and strain; also referred to as "true" fatigue.

Psychological Fatigue

A feeling of fatigue usually caused by such things as lack of exercise, boredom, or mental stress that results in a lack of energy and depression; also referred to as "subjective" or "false" fatigue.

Relaxation

The release or reduction of tension in the neuromuscular system.

Stress

The nonspecific response (generalized adaptation) of the body to any demand made upon it in order to maintain physiological equilibrium.

Stressor

Anything that produces stress or increases the rate of wear and tear on the body.

The Facts About Stress and Tension

All living creatures are in a continual state of stress (some more, some less).

There are many kinds of **stressors.** Environmental stressors include heat, noise, overcrowding, climate, and terrain. Physiological stressors may be such things as drugs, caffeine, tobacco, injury, infection or disease, and physical effort.

Emotional stressors are the most frequent and important stressors affecting humans. Some people refer to these as "psychosocial" stressors. These include life-changing events, such as a change in work hours or line of work, family illnesses, problems with superiors, deaths of relatives or friends, and increased responsibilities. In school, pressures such as grades, term papers, and oral presentations may induce stress.

Too little stress (hypostress) is undesirable and distressful.

Stress is not always harmful. In fact, too little stress, sometimes called "rust out," is not best for optimal health. Moderate stress may enhance behavioral adaptation and is necessary for maturation and health. It stimulates psychological growth. It has been said that "freedom from stress is death" and "stress is the spice of life."

Excessive stress reduces the effectiveness of the immune system.

Between 50 and 70 percent of all illnesses are linked to stress response. Too much stress—**distress**—can result in various health disorders. Some mental and physical con-ditions that can be psychosomatic (or stress caused) include high blood pressure and heart disease; psychiatric disorders, such as depression and schizophrenia; indigestion; colitis; ulcers; headaches; insomnia; diarrhea; constipation; increased blood clotting time; increased cholesterol concentration; diuresis; edema; and low back pain. Other serious diseases, such as cancer, can be influenced by a person's state of mind.

In some cases, there is considerable time between a major stressor and the onset of a disease, so we do not always associate the two. With too much stress, rather than "rust out" we "burn out."

Individuals react and adapt differently to different stressors.

What one person finds stressful may not be stressful for another person, and stress affects people differently. It mobilizes some to greater efficiency, while it confuses and disorganizes others. For example, skydiving or riding a roller coaster would be thrilling for some people, but for others it would be a very stressful and unpleasant experience.

An individual's response to stress depends upon the intensity of the threat, the type of situation in which it occurs, and such personal variables as cultural background, tolerance levels, past experience, and personality. You can't make a racehorse out of a turtle and vice versa. Some people react to stress by biting their nails; others eat too much, chain smoke, or drink excessively.

An individual's capacity to adapt is not a static function, but fluctuates with energy, drive, and courage. The better your fitness, the better you can withstand the rigors of tension without becoming susceptible to illness or other disorders.

Individuals tend to adapt best to moderate stress.

You would expect mild stress to produce mild **adaptations,** and strong stress to produce strong adaptive responses, but this is not so. High levels of threat tend to evoke ineffective, disorganized behavior. Figure 23.1 shows this relationship between stress and adaptive responses.

The amount of stress that you can adapt to comfortably is what Hans Selye (1978) calls **eustress** (see figure 23.2) and would, in a sense, be our target zone for stress. Selye is generally regarded as "the father of the modern stress concept."

Stress can be self-induced and pleasurable, or unpleasurable.

Some people may deliberately place themselves in stressful situations; for example, athletes place themselves under maximum strain; lawyers and surgeons are challenged by difficulties; and pregnant women accept the psychological

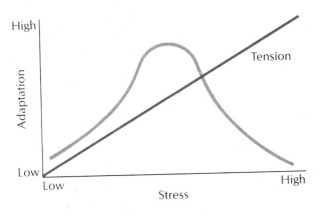

Figure 23.1
Stress and adaptive responses.

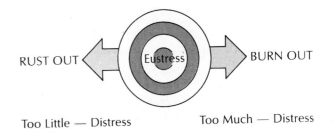

Figure 23.2
Stress target zone.

and physiological stress of bearing children. Self-induced stress may also be an unpleasant but necessary interlude that cannot be avoided. For example, there is a risk of falling that is necessary in learning to ride a bicycle.

Occupations are common sources of stress, and some are more stressful than others.

One study showed that the twelve most stressful jobs were: laborer, secretary, inspector, clinical lab technician, office manager, foreman, manager/administrator, waiter/waitress, machine operator, farm owner, miner, and painter. Air traffic controlling is currently considered a very stressful job. Business and industry often hire psychologists to counsel employees about occupational stress to help reduce absenteeism, boredom, and the number of accidents and resignations.

Fatigue and neuromuscular hypertension are closely related.

High levels of tension are a source of fatigue. Fatigue from lack of rest or sleep, emotional strain, pain, disease, and muscular work may produce too much muscle tension. **Fatigue** may be either **psychological** or **physiological** in origin, but both can result in a state of exhaustion or **chronic fatigue** with neuromuscular hypertension.

Neuromuscular hypertension may be both a cause and an effect of stress.

Anxiety is an emotional response caused by stressors, and it is manifested in muscular tension. Tension is a primary index of stress. One form of this tension is seen in the unnecessary "bracing" or "splinting" action of muscles—the clinched jaw, hunched shoulders, and white knuckles, or muscles contracting where they are not needed. They may stay contracted for long periods, often without your being aware of it. Muscular tension may also be physical in

origin, resulting from overuse of a muscle group. This tension can cause muscle spasms and pain that, in turn, become additional stressors. Trigger points and the myofascial pain syndrome that lead to backache and headache are good examples of excess muscular tension. (See Concept 16 on backache and neckache).

Some tension is normally present in muscles and contributes to the adjustment of the individual to the environment.

Some tension is needed to remain awake, alert, and ready to respond. In fact, a certain degree of tension aids some types of mental activity. It appears that each individual has an optimum level of tension to facilitate the thought process. However, too much tension can inhibit some types of mental activity and physical skills (such as those requiring accuracy and steadiness in postures that must be held for long periods).

The Facts About Stress Management

The first step in managing stress is to recognize the causes and to be aware of the symptoms.

You need to recognize the situations in your life that are the stressors. Try to identify the things that make you feel "stressed-out." Everything from minor irritations, such as traffic jams, to major life changes such as births, deaths, or job loss can be stressors. Or a stress overload of just too many demands on your time can make you feel that you are no longer in control. You may feel so overwhelmed that you become depressed.

Make yourself aware of how your body feels when you are under stress. Are the muscles beginning to tighten? Are you gritting your teeth, gripping the steering wheel tightly, drumming your fingers, patting your foot, or hunching your shoulders? Can you feel your heart beating faster, your breathing rate becoming faster and more shallow? Are you perspiring, shaking, or getting a headache?

The second step is to use some type of **relaxation** technique for relief of symptoms.

When you are aware of what stress does to your body, you can do something to relieve those symptoms immediately as well as on a regular and more long-term basis. You can slow your heart and respiration. You can relax tense muscles. You can clear your mind, and relax mentally and emotionally. Several techniques for relaxing are described later in this Concept.

The third step is to seek solutions for avoiding some of the stressors and for controlling your life-style.

The following are a few suggestions for managing stress:

- Take one thing at a time. You can't do it all at once. Decide which things you can do and which things can be postponed.
- Take action instead of worrying about it. Make a decision about how to solve the problem, then do it.
- If there is no acceptable solution, then accept what cannot be changed. Try to change your feelings about it. Make the best of it and get on with life.
- Think positively. Talk to yourself and visualize yourself succeeding. Think that you WILL pass the exam. You WILL make the free throw. You WILL be cool, calm, and collected as you make your oral presentation. Thinking negative thoughts is distressing in itself and sets you up for failure; it can become a self-fulfilling prophecy.
- Change the way you perceive a stressor. Look at it as a challenge or as a way to learn. Try to see humor in the situation. Look at the bright side.
- Don't try to escape a problem by pretending it doesn't exist. Dulling your senses with alcohol, drugs, or other excesses doesn't make it go away.
- Don't let the little things bother you. Benjamin Franklin reminded us that "Little strokes fell great oaks." Small hassles may not be worth the stress you let them create for you. One cardiologist said: "Rule 1 is don't sweat the small stuff; and rule 2 is, it's all small stuff and if you can't fight it and you can't flee—go with the flow" (American Heart Association 1984).
- Be willing to make adjustments. The old saying, "A branch that is able to bend will not break," is applicable to dealing with stress. Try to be flexible in what you want and when you want it.
- Rank the demands on your time in order of priority, and manage your time effectively so the more important things get done. If you are trying to do too much, you may need to get rid of some responsibilities or delegate them to someone else. You must also learn to say "No" to new responsibilities.

- Balance work with rest and play. "Moderation in all things" is still a good adage. Give some priority to proper rest, recreational activities, and diversion in order to prevent "burn-out." Diversion can be a temporary change from one activity to another (e.g., change from studying to mowing the lawn) or a change of scenery. You may even need a change of job or a vacation.
- Find and use a support system. Everyone needs someone to turn to for support when he/she is feeling overwhelmed. Support can come from friends, family members, clergy, a teacher, a coach, or a professional counselor. One study of athletic injuries has shown that those who were the most stressed were injured more often, and those who had the poorest support system were the most apt to be injured (Andersen and Williams 1988).

A fourth step you can take in managing stress is to be as fit and healthy as possible.

The more fit and healthy you are, the better able you are to cope with stress. Selye (1977) believes physical fitness serves as a sort of "inoculation against stress;" others have called it a "buffer."

Some methods of relieving tension are less desirable or are not recommended.

There is no magic cure for stress or tension, but there are a variety of therapeutic approaches. Some treatments are less desirable than others because they act only as "crutches" or "fire extinguishers" and do not get at the root of the problem. Hypnosis may lead to fantasy and dependency. Alcoholic beverages, tranquilizers, and painkillers may give temporary relief and may be prescribed by a physician as part of the treatment, but they do not resolve the problem and may even mask symptoms or cause further problems like addiction to the medication. Drugs do not provide a long-term solution to chronic tension. Contrary to vitamin and mineral advertisements, there are no proven benefits to supplementing the diet with such products as vitamin C or special "stress" formulations.

Exercise is one of the best ways to relieve stress and aid muscle tension release.

Exercise is especially useful to relieve white-collar job stress. Studies show that regular exercise decreases the likelihood of stress disorders and reduces the intensity of the stress response. It also shortens the time of recovery from an emotional trauma. Its effect tends to be short term, so one must continue to exercise regularly for it to have a continuing effect. Exercise is not like a measles vaccine where one inoculation is good for life.

Aerobic exercise is believed to be especially effective in reducing anxiety and relieving stress (though a wide variety of other activities are also good). It reduces the levels of epinephrine and norepinephrine, the catecholamines that prepare a person for fight or flight, and thus reduces the end result of stress. Exercise can also act as a diversion and as a cathartic, or a release for frustration and anger, and can enhance one's self-esteem. Whatever your choice of exercise, it is likely to be more effective as an antidote to stress if it is something you find enjoyable. (See table 3.3, Concept 3, for some of the other psychological benefits of exercise.)

The Facts About Methods of Relaxation

Stretching exercises and rhythmical exercises especially aid in relaxation.

People who work long hours at a desk can release tension by getting up frequently and stretching, by taking a brisk walk down the hall, or by performing "office exercises." (See Lindsey and Gorrie [1989] and Murphy [1984].)

Exercising to music or to a rhythmic beat has been found to be relaxing and even "hypnotic." Some exercises are designed specifically for relaxation. Examples can be found on pages 260–61.

Massage, heat, and deep breathing aid relaxation of tense muscles.

Gentle effleurage, a type of massage, heat in the form of a hot bath (or shower or sauna), and deep breathing with prolonged exhalation when combined with conscious relaxation techniques described in this Concept, are effective means for relaxing tense muscles for most people.

There are several satisfactory methods of releasing tension through techniques of conscious relaxation.

In some way not fully understood, certain involuntary bodily functions can be controlled by an act of will (voluntarily). Relaxation of the muscles is a skill that can be learned through practice just as other muscle skills are learned, and it works! It is no gimmick.

Conscious relaxation techniques usually employ the "three Rs" of relaxation: (1) reduce mental activity, (2) recognize tension, and (3) reduce respiration.

Five examples of these systems are described here:

- *"The Quick Fix"*—To get relief from a stressful situation during the day, take a "time out" for five or ten minutes; find a quiet place away from the situation with as few distractions as possible. Sit, loosen your clothes, take off your shoes, and close your eyes. Then follow these steps: (1) Inhale deeply for about four seconds; then exhale, letting the air out slowly for about eight seconds (twice as long as the inhalation). Do this several times. (2) Mentally visualize a pleasant image, such as a peaceful lake or stream; continue to relax and breathe deeply. (3) When your time is up, breathe deeply and stretch luxuriously; go back to your work refreshed and with a changed attitude. You may need to do this several times a day.

- *Jacobson's Progressive Relaxation Method*—You must be able to recognize how a tense muscle feels before you can voluntarily release the tension. In this technique, contract the muscles strongly, then relax. Each of the large muscles is relaxed first, and later the small ones. The contractions are gradually reduced in intensity until no movement is visible. Always, the emphasis is placed on detecting the feeling of tension as the first step in "letting go," or "going negative." Jacobson (1961, 1978), a pioneer in muscle relaxation research, emphasized the importance of relaxing eye and speech muscles, because he believed these muscles trigger reactions of the total organism more than other muscles. A sample contract-relax exercise routine for relaxation is presented on page 262.

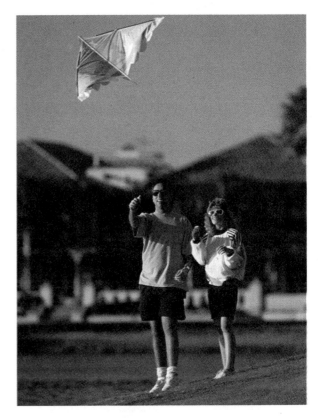

Taking a "time out" to relax is important for good health.

- *Autogenic (Self-generated) Relaxation Training*—
Several times daily, sit or lie in a quiet room with eyes closed. Block out distracting thoughts by passively concentrating on pre-selected words or phrases. This technique has been used to focus on heaviness of limbs, warmth of limbs, heart rate regulation, respiratory rate and depth regulation, and coolness in the forehead. It evokes changes opposite to those produced by stress. Research has shown that people who are skilled in this technique can decrease oxygen consumption, change the electrical activity of the brain, slow the metabolism, decrease blood lactate, lower body temperature, and slow the heart rate.

- *Biofeedback-Autogenic Relaxation Training*—
Biofeedback training utilizes machines that monitor certain physiological processes of the body and provide visual or auditory evidence of what is happening to normally unconscious bodily functions. When combined with autogenic training, subjects have learned to relax and reduce the electrical activity in their muscles, lower blood pressure, decrease heart rate, change their brain waves, and decrease headaches, asthma attacks, and stomach acid secretion. It has also been helpful in treating phobias, stage fright, drug abuse, sexual dysfunction, stuttering, and other psychological problems (Greenberg 1990).

- *Imagery*—Thinking autogenic phrases, you can visualize such feelings as "sinking into a mattress or pillow," or you can think of being a "limp, loose-jointed puppet with no one to hold the strings." You can imagine being a "half-filled sack of flour resting on an uneven surface" or pretend to be "a sack of granulated salt left out in the rain, melting away." Some people seem to respond better to the concept of "floating" than to feeling "heavy." It also includes visualizing pleasant, relaxing scenes as mentioned in the description of "The Quick Fix." You attempt to place yourself in the scene and experience all of the sounds, colors, and scents. Whatever the image you wish to conjure, imagery can help take your mind off anxieties and distractions and, at the same time, release unwanted tension in the muscles using the principle of "mind over matter."

Relaxation Exercises

1. **Neck Stretch**—Roll the head slowly in a half circle from 9:00 to 8:00 to 7, 6, 5, 4, and 3:00, then reverse from 3 to 9:00. Close your eyes and feel the stretch. Do *not* make a full circle by tipping the head back. Repeat several times.

2. **Shoulder Lift**—Hunch the shoulders as high as possible (contract) and then let them drop (relax). Repeat several times. Inhale on the lift; exhale on the drop.

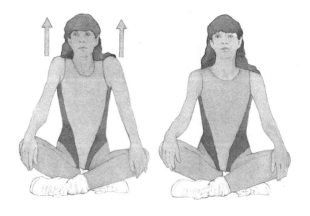

3. **Trunk Stretch and Drop**—Stand and reach as high as possible; tiptoe and stretch every muscle, then collapse completely, letting knees flex and trunk, head, and arms dangle. Repeat two or three times. Inhale on the stretch and exhale on the collapse.

4. **Trunk Swings**—Following the "trunk stretch and drop" (preceding illustration); remain in the "drop" position and with a minimum of muscular effort, set the trunk swinging from side to side by shifting the weight from one foot to the other, letting the heels come off the floor alternately. Keep the entire body (especially the neck) limp.

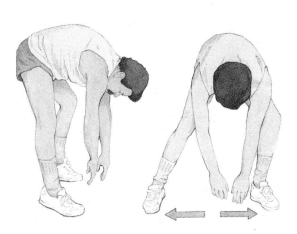

5. **Tension Contrast**—With arms extended overhead, lie on your side. Tense the body as stiff as a board, then let go, and relax, letting the body fall either forward or backward in whatever direction it loses balance. Continue letting go for a few seconds after falling and allow yourself to feel like you are still sinking. Repeat on the other side.

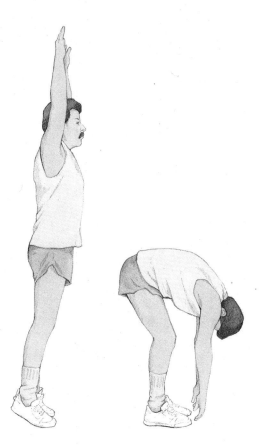

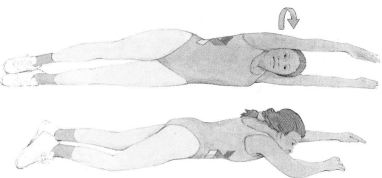

Contract-Relax Exercise Routine for Relaxation*

1. Hand and forearm—Contract your right hand, making a fist; hold 3 counts; relax and keep letting go 6–10 counts. Repeat, then do left fist, then both fists.

2. Biceps—Flex both elbows and contract your biceps; hold 3 counts; relax and continue relaxing 6–10 counts. Repeat.

3. Triceps—Same as biceps except extend both elbows, contract the triceps on the back of the arm. Repeat.

4. Relax both hands, forearms, and upper arms.

5. Forehead—Raise your eyebrows and wrinkle your forehead; hold 3 counts; relax and continue relaxing 6–10 counts.

6. Cheeks and nose—Make a face; wrinkle your nose and squint; hold 3 counts; relax and continue relaxing 6–10 counts.

7. Jaws—Clench your teeth 3 counts; relax for 6–10 counts.

8. Lips and tongue—With teeth apart, press lips together and press tongue to roof of mouth; hold 3 counts; relax 6 to 10 counts.

9. Neck and throat—Push head backward while tucking chin, pushing against floor or pillow if lying; if sitting, push against high chair-back; hold 3 counts; relax for 6–10 counts.

10. Relax forehead, cheeks, nose, jaws, lips, tongue, neck and throat. Relax hands, forearms and upper arms.

11. Shoulder and upper back—Hunch shoulders to ears; hold 3 counts; relax 6–10 counts.

12. Relax lips, tongue, neck, throat, shoulders and upper back.

13. Abdomen—Suck in abdomen; hold for 3 counts; relax for 6–10 counts.

14. Lower back—Contract and arch the back; hold for 3 counts; relax for 6–10 counts.

15. Thighs and buttocks—Squeeze your buttocks together and push your heels into the floor (if lying) or against a chair rung (if sitting); hold 3 counts; relax 6–10 counts.

16. Relax shoulders and upper back, abdomen, lower back, thighs and buttocks.

17. Calves—Pull instep and toes toward shins; hold 3 counts; relax 6–10 counts.

18. Toes—Curl toes; hold 3 counts; relax 6–10 counts.

19. Relax every muscle in your body.

*Note: Eventually, you should progress to a combination of muscle groups and gradually eliminate the "contract" phase of the program. Refer to Jacobson's relaxation method (page 259) for more instructions, or read Jacobson's book or chapter 10 of Greenberg's book (see suggested reading below).

Suggested Reading

Greenberg, J. S. *Comprehensive Stress Management*. 4th ed. Dubuque, Iowa: Wm. C. Brown Communications, Inc., 1993.

LAB RESOURCE MATERIALS

(For use with Labs 23A and 23B, pages L-69 & L-71)

The Life Experience Survey*

Listed below are a number of events that sometimes bring about change in the lives of those who experience them and that necessitate social readjustment. Please check those events that you have experienced in the past year and indicate the time period during which you experienced each event. Be sure that all check marks are directly across from the items to which they correspond.

Also, for each item checked below please indicate the extent to which you viewed the event as having either a positive or negative impact on your life at the time the event occurred. That is, indicate the type and extent of impact that the event had. A rating of −3 would indicate an extremely negative impact. A rating of 0 suggests neither a positive nor a negative impact. A rating of +3 would indicate an extremely positive impact.

Section I of the test is for everyone. It provides three extra blanks (numbers 45, 46, and 47) for you to list any recent experiences that have had an impact on your life but that were not mentioned in the preceding items.

Section II of the test is designed for students only. If there are school-related experiences that have had a noticeable impact on your life but are not listed, you may list them in one or more of the three blanks in Section I.

Note: Some items apply only to males and some apply only to females; these are indicated in the survey.

*From Irwin G. Sarason, James H. Johnson, and Judith M. Siegel. "Assessing the Impact of Life Changes: Development of the Life Experiences Survey" in *Journal of Consulting and Clinical Psychology*, 46(5):932–46. Copyright 1978 by the American Psychological Association. Reprinted by permission.

Section I	0–6 mos.	7–12 mos.	Extremely Negative	Moderately Negative	Somewhat Negative	No Impact	Slightly Positive	Moderately Positive	Extremely Positive
1. Marriage	____	____	−3	−2	−1	0	+1	+2	+3
2. Detention in jail or comparable institution.	____	____	−3	−2	−1	0	+1	+2	+3
3. Death of spouse	____	____	−3	−2	−1	0	+1	+2	+3
4. Major change in sleeping habits (much more or less sleep)	____	____	−3	−2	−1	0	+1	+2	+3
5. Death of close family member:									
a. mother	____	____	−3	−2	−1	0	+1	+2	+3
b. father	____	____	−3	−2	−1	0	+1	+2	+3
c. brother	____	____	−3	−2	−1	0	+1	+2	+3
d. sister	____	____	−3	−2	−1	0	+1	+2	+3
e. child	____	____	−3	−2	−1	0	+1	+2	+3
f. grandmother	____	____	−3	−2	−1	0	+1	+2	+3
g. grandfather	____	____	−3	−2	−1	0	+1	+2	+3
h. other (specify) _____	____	____	−3	−2	−1	0	+1	+2	+3
6. Major change in eating habits (much more or much less food intake)	____	____	−3	−2	−1	0	+1	+2	+3
7. Foreclosure on mortgage or loan	____	____	−3	−2	−1	0	+1	+2	+3
8. Death of a close friend	____	____	−3	−2	−1	0	+1	+2	+3
9. Outstanding personal achievement	____	____	−3	−2	−1	0	+1	+2	+3
10. Minor law violations (traffic ticket, disturbing the peace, etc.)	____	____	−3	−2	−1	0	+1	+2	+3
11. *Male:* Wife's/girlfriend's pregnancy *Female:* Pregnancy	____	____	−3	−2	−1	0	+1	+2	+3
12. Changed work situation (different working conditions, working hours, etc.)	____	____	−3	−2	−1	0	+1	+2	+3
13. New job	____	____	−3	−2	−1	0	+1	+2	+3
14. Serious illness or injury of close family member									
a. father	____	____	−3	−2	−1	0	+1	+2	+3
b. mother	____	____	−3	−2	−1	0	+1	+2	+3
c. sister	____	____	−3	−2	−1	0	+1	+2	+3
d. brother	____	____	−3	−2	−1	0	+1	+2	+3
e. grandfather	____	____	−3	−2	−1	0	+1	+2	+3
f. grandmother	____	____	−3	−2	−1	0	+1	+2	+3

continued

Section I	0–6 mos.	7–12 mos.	Extremely Negative	Moderately Negative	Somewhat Negative	No Impact	Slightly Positive	Moderately Positive	Extremely Positive
g. spouse	____	____	−3	−2	−1	0	+1	+2	+3
h. child	____	____	−3	−2	−1	0	+1	+2	+3
i. other (specify) _____	____	____	−3	−2	−1	0	+1	+2	+3
15. Sexual difficulties	____	____	−3	−2	−1	0	+1	+2	+3
16. Trouble with employer (in danger of losing job, being suspended, demoted, etc.)	____	____	−3	−2	−1	0	+1	+2	+3
17. Trouble with in-laws	____	____	−3	−2	−1	0	+1	+2	+3
18. Major change in financial status (a lot better off or a lot worse off)	____	____	−3	−2	−1	0	+1	+2	+3
19. Major change in closeness of family members (decreased or increased closeness)	____	____	−3	−2	−1	0	+1	+2	+3
20. Gaining a new family member (through birth, adoption, family member moving in, etc.)	____	____	−3	−2	−1	0	+1	+2	+3
21. Change of residence	____	____	−3	−2	−1	0	+1	+2	+3
22. Marital separation from mate (due to conflict)	____	____	−3	−2	−1	0	+1	+2	+3
23. Major change in church activities (increased or decreased attendance)	____	____	−3	−2	−1	0	+1	+2	+3
24. Marital reconciliation with mate	____	____	−3	−2	−1	0	+1	+2	+3
25. Major change in number of arguments with spouse (a lot more or a lot less arguments)	____	____	−3	−2	−1	0	+1	+2	+3
26. *Married Male:* Change in wife's work outside the home (beginning work, ceasing work, changing to a new job) *Married Female:* Change in husband's work (loss of job, beginning new job, retirement, etc.)	____	____	−3	−2	−1	0	+1	+2	+3
27. Major change in usual type and/or amount of recreation	____	____	−3	−2	−1	0	+1	+2	+3
28. Borrowing more than $10,000 (buying home, business, etc.)	____	____	−3	−2	−1	0	+1	+2	+3
29. Borrowing less than $10,000 (buying car, TV, getting school loan, etc.)	____	____	−3	−2	−1	0	+1	+2	+3
30. Being fired from job	____	____	−3	−2	−1	0	+1	+2	+3
31. *Male:* Wife/girlfriend having abortion *Female:* Having abortion	____	____	−3	−2	−1	0	+1	+2	+3
32. Major personal illness or injury	____	____	−3	−2	−1	0	+1	+2	+3
33. Major change in social activities; e.g., parties, movies, visiting (increased, or decreased participation)	____	____	−3	−2	−1	0	+1	+2	+3
34. Major change in living conditions of family (building new home, remodeling, deterioration of home, neighborhood, etc.)	____	____	−3	−2	−1	0	+1	+2	+3

continued

Section I	0–6 mos.	7–12 mos.	Extremely Negative	Moderately Negative	Somewhat Negative	No Impact	Slightly Positive	Moderately Positive	Extremely Positive
35. Divorce	____	____	−3	−2	−1	0	+1	+2	+3
36. Serious injury or illness of close friend	____	____	−3	−2	−1	0	+1	+2	+3
37. Retirement from work	____	____	−3	−2	−1	0	+1	+2	+3
38. Son or daughter leaving home (due to marriage, college, etc.)	____	____	−3	−2	−1	0	+1	+2	+3
39. Ending of formal schooling	____	____	−3	−2	−1	0	+1	+2	+3
40. Separation from spouse (due to work, travel, etc.)	____	____	−3	−2	−1	0	+1	+2	+3
41. Engagement	____	____	−3	−2	−1	0	+1	+2	+3
42. Breaking up with boyfriend/girlfriend	____	____	−3	−2	−1	0	+1	+2	+3
43. Leaving home for the first time	____	____	−3	−2	−1	0	+1	+2	+3
44. Reconciliation with boyfriend/girlfriend	____	____	−3	−2	−1	0	+1	+2	+3
Other recent experiences that have had an impact on your life. List and rate.	____	____	−3	−2	−1	0	+1	+2	+3
45. _____	____	____	−3	−2	−1	0	+1	+2	+3
46. _____	____	____	−3	−2	−1	0	+1	+2	+3
47. _____	____	____	−3	−2	−1	0	+1	+2	+3

Section 2: For Students Only	0–6 mos.	7–12 mos.	Extremely Negative	Moderately Negative	Somewhat Negative	No Impact	Slightly Positive	Moderately Positive	Extremely Positive
48. Beginning new school experience at a higher academic level (college, graduate school, professional school, etc.)	____	____	−3	−2	−1	0	+1	+2	+3
49. Changing to a new school at same academic level (undergraduate, graduate, etc.)	____	____	−3	−2	−1	0	+1	+2	+3
50. Academic probation	____	____	−3	−2	−1	0	+1	+2	+3
51. Being dismissed from dormitory or other residence	____	____	−3	−2	−1	0	+1	+2	+3
52. Failing an important exam	____	____	−3	−2	−1	0	+1	+2	+3
53. Changing a major	____	____	−3	−2	−1	0	+1	+2	+3
54. Failing a course	____	____	−3	−2	−1	0	+1	+2	+3
55. Dropping a course	____	____	−3	−2	−1	0	+1	+2	+3
56. Joining a fraternity/sorority	____	____	−3	−2	−1	0	+1	+2	+3
57. Financial problems concerning school (in danger of not having sufficient money to continue)	____	____	−3	−2	−1	0	+1	+2	+3

Scoring the Life Experience Survey

1. Add all of the negative scores to arrive at your own distress score (negative stress).

2. Add all of the positive scores to arrive at a eustress score (positive stress).

3. It is possible to calculate scores for the last six months, or for the last year. The more recent the incident, the more likely it will be distressful.

Chart 23A.1 *Rating Scale* for Life Experiences and Stress

	Sum of Negative Scores (Distress)	Sum of Positive Scores (Eustress)
May need counseling	14+	
Above average stress	9–13	
Average	6–9	9–10
Below average stress	<6	

Chart 23B.1 Signs of Tension Observed by Tester

	No	Yes
A. Visual Symptoms		
Frowning	☐	☐
Twitching	☐	☐
Eyelids fluttering	☐	☐
Breathing		
shallow	☐	☐
rapid	☐	☐
irregular	☐	☐
Mouth tight	☐	☐
Swallowing	☐	☐
B. Manual Symptoms		
Assistance (subject helps lift arm)	☐	☐
Resistance (subject resists movement)	☐	☐
Posturing (subject holds arm in raised position)	☐	☐
Perseveration (subject continues upward movement)	☐	☐

Total number of "yes" checks _____

Chart 23B.2 Tension-Relaxation *Rating Scale*

Classification	Total Score
Excellent (relaxed)	0
Very good (mild tension)	1–3
Good (moderate tension)	4–6
Fair (tense)	7–9
Poor (marked tension)	10–12

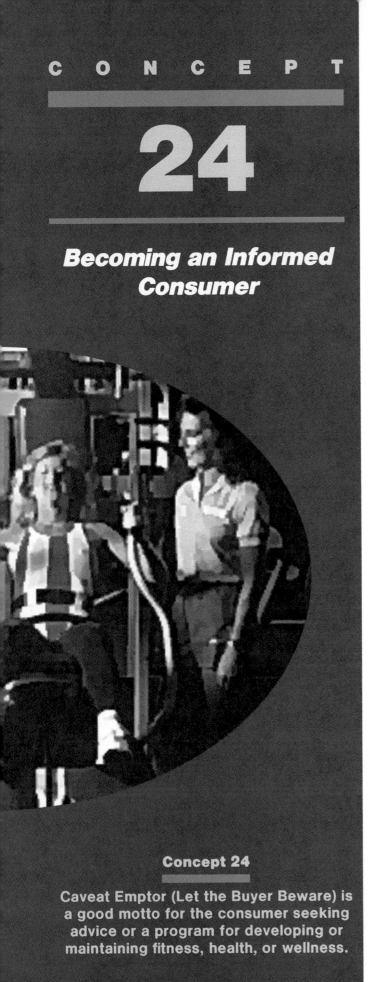

CONCEPT

24

Becoming an Informed Consumer

Concept 24

Caveat Emptor (Let the Buyer Beware) is a good motto for the consumer seeking advice or a program for developing or maintaining fitness, health, or wellness.

Introduction

People have always searched for the fountain of youth and the "easy," "quick," and "miraculous" route to health and happiness. This search has included the area of physical fitness, especially exercise and weight loss. Because of the popularity of these two subjects, the mass media have made it possible to convey as much *misinformation* as information. All people should seek the truth to protect their health as well as their pocketbooks. This Concept discusses some myths and separates fact from fancy. (Also see Concepts 10, 18, and 22 for facts related to misconceptions.)

Health Goal for the Year 2000

- Expand systems for dissemination of health information.

Terms

AMA

Abbreviation for the American Medical Association.

Expert (in exercise and physical fitness)

Person who has a degree(s) in physical education, kinesiology, physical therapy, or kinesiotherapy from an accredited university and has specialized in exercise prescription and physical fitness.

FDA

Abbreviation for the Food and Drug Administration: a federal agency that recommends and enforces government regulations regarding certain foods and drugs.

Panacea

A cure-all; a remedy for all ills.

Passive

A type of exercise in which no voluntary muscle contraction occurs; some outside force moves the body part with no effort by the person.

Tonus

The most frequently misused and abused term in fitness vocabularies. It is "the resistance (tension) developed in a muscle as a result of passive stretch of a muscle. Tonus can not be determined by palpation or inspection of a muscle and has little or nothing to do with the voluntary strength of a muscle" (deLateur 1982).

Facts About Exercise

Exercise has many benefits, but it is not a **panacea**.

There are numerous benefits of exercise, many of which have been described throughout this book. However, some media accounts would have you believe the impossible.

267

People who contemplate beginning a fitness or weight reducing program are reminded of the following:

- The most satisfactory way to lose weight is to combine caloric reduction and exercise.
- Exercise will *not* change the size of bony structures (e.g., ankles).
- Exercise will *not* change the size of glands (e.g., breasts); however, chest/bust girth may be increased by strengthening chest muscles.
- Exercise does *not* break up fatty deposits, though it does burn calories, thus fat will eventually be burned.
- Exercise does *not ensure* good posture or good health, but it does help attain or maintain these attributes.
- There is *no* such thing as "effortless exercise."

Exercise, even of an active nature, is not effective in promoting physical fitness unless it meets the appropriate threshold of training.

Some popular literature suggests that only a few minutes of exercise a day are necessary to develop total physical fitness. Research, however, indicates that total fitness (cardiovascular fitness, strength, muscular endurance, flexibility, and desirable body composition) can be attained only through considerable effort. As mentioned previously, exercise must be of sufficient frequency (daily or every other day), intensity, and time (at least fifteen to thirty minutes *each* day you exercise) for it to be effective. Programs that promise complete fitness but do not meet the necessary levels for frequency, intensity, and time of exercise should be strongly questioned.

Contrary to some claims, Hatha Yoga is not a good program for developing physical fitness.

Some advocates of Hatha Yoga claim that regular practice of the asanas (positions) will bring about improved flexibility, grace, serenity, relaxation, sleep, vitality, endurance, circulation; strength and firmness of muscles; strength of vital organs and glands; taut, smooth skin; ideal body weight; recovery, alertness, and clarity of mind; will cure arthritis, the common cold, diabetes, gallstones, menstrual disorders, piles; and will maintain good vision and hearing.

There is *no* scientific evidence to support most of these claims. Hatha Yoga will not help you lose weight, trim inches, remove flab, improve endurance, maintain proper circulation, strengthen glands and organs, or improve complexion. Neither will it cure diseases.

Hatha Yoga is considered useful for improving flexibility, although some positions are contraindicated (see Concept 19). Hatha Yoga is also useful in reducing stress reactions and in promoting neuromuscular relaxation. In some cases, it may be effective in lowering blood pressure in hypertensives. If a person has very weak muscles to begin with, mild strengthening and muscular endurance may develop from assuming and holding the positions.

Getting rid of cellulite does not require a special exercise, diet, or device, as some books and advertisements insist.

Cellulite is ordinary fat with a fancy name. You do not need a special treatment or device to get rid of it. Fat is fat. To decrease fat, reduce calories and exercise more.

"Spot reducing," or losing fat from a specific location on the body, is not possible. It is a fallacy.

When you exercise, calories are burned and fat is recruited from all over the body in a genetically determined pattern. You can not selectively exercise, bump, vibrate, or squeeze the fat from a particular spot. If you were flabby to begin with, local exercise could strengthen the local muscles, causing a change in the contour and the girth of that body part. But exercise affects the muscles, not the fat on that body part. General aerobic exercises are the most effective for burning fat, but you cannot control where the fat comes off.

Surgically sculpting the body with implants and liposuction to acquire physical beauty will not give you physical fitness and may be harmful.

Rather than doing it the hard way, an increasing number of people are having their "love handles" removed surgically and fake calf and pectoral muscles implanted to improve their physique. Liposuction is not a weight loss technique, but rather is a contouring procedure. Like any surgery, it is not without risks. There have been fatalities and there is a risk of infection, hematoma, skin slough, and other conditions.

The muscle implants give a muscular appearance, but they do not make you stronger or more fit. The implants are not really muscle tissue, but rather silicon gel or a hard substitute. Some complications can occur, such as infection and bleeding, but also, some physicians believe the calf implant may put pressure on the calf muscles and cause them to atrophy. A better way to improve physique and fitness is proper exercise.

The use of hand weights and wrist weights while walking, running, dancing, or bench-stepping can increase the energy cost but requires caution.

The practice of carrying small weights (1–3 pounds) while performing aerobic exercise has been found to increase the metabolic cost of the exercise. When the weight is simply carried, the effect is negligible, but when the arms are pumped (bending the elbow and raising the weight to shoulder height and then extending the elbow as the arm swings down) the energy output can increase enough to make a walk comparable to a slow jog. For the person who does not want to walk or jog faster or farther, it could be an effective way of burning more calories or increasing fitness. It may be better to use wrist weights than to carry a weight, since the act of gripping causes an increase in the diastolic blood pressure. The hand weights or wrist weights are more effective than ankle weights.

It has been suggested that for step-aerobics (bench-stepping), weights should be limited to intermediate and advanced steppers only and that they not exceed one or two pounds. Up to a point, the aerobic intensity can be increased by adding height to the bench (Fox and Broide 1991).

There are hazards to consider in using weights. Coronary patients and hypertensives should be aware that using weights increases both the systolic and diastolic blood pressures. Aerobic dance participants may find it wise to keep the weights below shoulder level if they aggravate the shoulder joint. Anyone with shoulder or elbow joint problems such as arthritis should use weights with caution.

Facts About Passive Exercise and Passive Devices

Passive exercise is not effective in weight reduction, spot reduction, increasing strength, or increasing endurance.

Passive exercise or devices come in a variety of forms.

- *Rolling machines*—These ineffective wooden or metal rollers, operated by an electric motor, roll up and down the body part to which they are applied. They do *not* remove, break up, or redistribute fat.
- *Vibrating belts*—These wide canvas or leather belts may be designed for the chin, hips, thighs, or abdomen. Driven by an electric motor, they jerk back and forth, causing loose tissue of the body part to shake. They do *not* have any beneficial effect on fitness, fat, or figure, and they are potentially harmful if used on the abdomen (especially if used by women during pregnancy, menstruation, or while an IUD is in place). They might also aggravate a back problem.
- *Vibrating tables and pillows*—Some of these quack devices are actually called "toning tables." Contrary to advertisements, these passive devices will *not* improve posture, trim the body, reduce weight, nor will they develop muscle **tonus.** For some people, vibration can help induce relaxation.

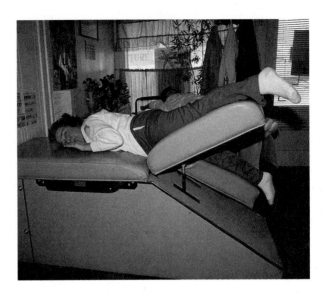
Passive devices are ineffective in improving fitness.

- *Continuous Passive Motion Tables (CPM)*—The CPM table is motor driven, but unlike the vibrating table it moves body parts repeatedly through a range of motion. Tables are designed to do such things as passively extend the leg at the hip joint, raise the upper trunk in a sit-up-like motion, or rotate the legs while the client lies relaxed. Many of the same false claims are made for it as for the vibrating table. It also claims to remove cellulite, increase circulation and oxygen flow, and eliminate excess water retention. None of these claims is true, but the table might be justified in claiming to maintain the range of motion in certain body parts for people who cannot move themselves. A similar concept is incorporated in small, portable machines used in hospitals and rehabilitation centers to maintain range of motion in the leg of knee surgery patients, to maintain integrity of the cartilage, and decrease the incidence of thrombosis. Certainly the normal, healthy person has nothing to gain from using such a device.
- *Motor-driven cycles and rowing machines*—Like all mechanical devices that do the work for the individual, these motor-driven machines are *not* effective in a fitness program. They may help increase circulation, and some may even help maintain flexibility, but they are not as effective as active exercise. *Nonmotorized* cycles and rowing machines are very good equipment for use in a fitness program.
- *Massage*—Whether done by a masseur/masseuse or by a mechanical device, massage is passive, requiring no effort on the part of the individual. It can help increase circulation, induce relaxation, prevent or loosen adhesions, retard muscle

atrophy, and serve other therapeutic uses when administered in the clinical setting for medical reasons, but massage has *no* useful role in a physical fitness program and will *not* alter your shape. There is no scientific evidence that it can hasten nerve growth, remove subcutaneous fat, or increase athletic performance.

- *Electrical muscle stimulators*—Neuromuscular electrical stimulators cause the muscle to contract involuntarily. In the hands of qualified medical personnel, muscle stimulators are valuable therapeutic devices. They can increase muscle strength and endurance selectively and aid in the treatment of edema. They can also help prevent atrophy in a patient who is unable to move, and they may decrease spasticity and contracture, but in a healthy person they do *not* have the same value as exercise. The multiple muscle group stimulation as done in the so-called "toning clinics" or spas has been proven ineffective in muscle strengthening (Lake 1992). These devices can be harmful when used improperly and may induce heart attacks; complicate gastrointestinal, orthopedic, kidney, and other disorders; and aggravate epilepsy, hernias, and varicose veins. They should never be used by the layperson and have *no* place in a reducing or fitness program.

- *Weighted belts*—Claims have been made that these belts reduce waists, thighs, and hips when worn for several hours under the clothing. In reality, they do none of these things and have been reported to cause actual physical harm. When used in a progressive resistance program, wristlet, anklet, or laced-on weights can help produce an overload and, therefore, develop strength or endurance.

- *Inflated, constricting, or nonporous garments*—These garments include rubberized inflated devices ("sauna belts" and "sauna shorts") and paraphernalia that are airtight plastic or rubberized. Evidence indicates that their girth-reducing claims are *unwarranted*. If exercise is performed while wearing such garments, the exercise, *not* the garment, may be beneficial. You can *not* squeeze fat out of the pores *nor* can you melt it!

- *Body wrapping*—Some reducing salons, gyms, or clubs advertise that wrapping the body in bandages soaked in a "magic solution" will cause a permanent reduction in body girth. This so-called "treatment" is pure quackery. Tight, constricting bands can temporarily indent the skin and squeeze body fluids into other parts of the body, but the skin or body will regain its original size within minutes or hours. The solution used is usually something similar to epsom salts, which can cause fluid to be drawn from tissue. The fluid is water, not fat, and is quickly replaced. Body wrapping may be dangerous to your health; at least one fatality has resulted.

- *Elastic tights*—are often worn by athletes such as cyclists for the purpose of decreasing chaffing of the skin. There have been some claims that the tights helped improve venous return and thus recovery from exercise. However, studies have shown that the recovery-response of those who wear tights is no different from that of non-wearers (Berry, et al. 1990).

Having a good tan is often associated with being fit and looking good, but getting tanned can be risky business.

Tanning salons may claim their lamps are safe because they emit only UV-A rays, but these rays can age the skin prematurely and make it look wrinkled and leathery. It may also increase the cancer-producing potential of UV-B rays and cause eye damage. Since there is no warning sign of redness, there is danger of overdosing. Thirty minutes of exposure to UV-A can suppress the immune system. Tanning devices can also aggravate certain skin diseases. The **FDA** advises against the use of any suntan lamp. It is dangerous to use tanning accelerator lotions with the lamps because they can promote burning of the skin. Tanning pills are an even worse choice. They can cause itching, welts, hives, stomach cramps, and diarrhea, and can decrease night vision. Tanning in the sun is also hazardous because it damages the skin, making it age prematurely. It may cause skin cancer. It is best to use products with sun blockers if you must spend long periods in the sun.

Facts About Baths

Saunas, steambaths, whirlpools, and hot tubs are not effective in weight reduction or in the prevention and cure of colds, arthritis, bursitis, backaches, sprains, and bruises.

Baths do *not* melt off fat; fat must be metabolized. The heat and humidity from baths may make you perspire, but it is water, not fat, oozing from the pores.

The effect of such baths is largely psychological, although some temporary relief from aches and pains may result from the heat. The same relief can be had by sitting in a tub of hot water in your bathroom.

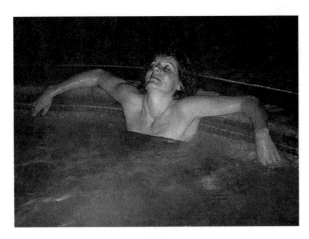

A hot tub may help you relax, but it does not improve fitness.

The so-called baths are potentially dangerous and should be used and maintained properly.

The following guidelines/precautions should be considered before using a sauna, steambath, whirlpool, or hot tub.

- Take a soap shower before and after entering the bath.
- Don't wear makeup or skin lotion/oil.
- Wait at least an hour after eating before bathing.
- Cool down after exercise before entering the bath to avoid overheating.
- Drink plenty of water before or during the bath to avoid dehydration.
- Don't wear jewelry.
- Don't sit on a metal stool; do sit on a towel in the steam or sauna bath.
- Don't bathe alone.
- Don't drink alcohol before bathing.
- Get out immediately if you become dizzy; feel hot, chilled, or nauseous; or get a headache.
- Get permission from your physician if you have heart disease, low or high blood pressure, a fever, kidney disease, or diabetes, are obese or pregnant, or are on medications (especially anticoagulants, stimulants, hypnotics, narcotics, or tranquilizers).
- Prolonged use can be hazardous for the elderly or for children.
- Don't exercise in a sauna or steam bath.
- Skin infections can be spread in a bath; make certain it is cleaned regularly and that the hot tub or whirlpool has proper pH and chlorination.
- Follow these recommendations on temperature and duration of stay:
  Sauna: should not exceed 190 degrees F (88 degrees C) and duration should not exceed ten to fifteen minutes.

Steam Bath: should not exceed 120 degrees F (49 degrees C) and duration should not exceed six to twelve minutes.

Whirlpool/Hot Tub: should not exceed 100 degrees F (37 degrees C) and duration should not exceed five to ten minutes.

Facts About Quacks

You can usually tell the difference between an **expert** and a quack because a quack does not use scientific methods.

Some of the ways to identify quacks, frauds, and ripoffs are to look for these clues:

- They do not use the scientific method of controlled experimentation that can be verified by other scientists.
- To a large extent they use testimonials and anecdotes to support their claims rather than scientific methods. There is no such thing as a convincing testimonial. Anecdotal evidence is no evidence at all.
- They advise you to buy something you would not otherwise have bought.
- They have something to sell.
- They claim *everyone* can benefit from the product or service they are selling. There is no such thing as a simple, quick, easy, painless remedy/tonic or other concoction that is good for many ailments or useful for conditions for which medical science has not yet found a remedy ("Miracle Cures and Other Frauds" 1990).
- They promise "quick," "miraculous" results. There is no such thing as a perfect no-risk treatment.
- The claims for benefits are broad, covering a wide variety of conditions.
- They may offer a money-back guarantee. Note: a guarantee is only as good as the company.
- They may claim the treatment or product is approved by the FDA. Note: federal law does not permit the mention of the FDA in any way that suggests marketing approval.
- They may claim the support of experts. Note: the experts are not identified.
- The ingredients or materials in the product may not be identified.
- They may claim there is a conspiracy against them by "bureaucrats," "organized medicine," the FDA, the **AMA,** and other experts and governmental bodies. Never believe a doctor who claims the medical community is persecuting him/her or that the government is suppressing a wonderful discovery ("Miracle Cures and Other Frauds" 1990).

- Their credentials may be irrelevant to the area in which they claim expertise.
- They use scare tactics, such as "if you don't do this, you will die of a heart attack."
- They may appear to be a sympathetic friend who wants to share with you a "new discovery."
- They may quote from a scientific journal or other legitimate source, but they misquote or quote out of context to mislead you; or they may mix a little bit of truth with a lot of fiction.
- They may cite research or quote from individuals or institutions that have questionable reputations for scientific truth.
- They may claim it is a "new discovery" (usually it is said to have originated in Europe). There is never a great medical breakthrough that debuts in an obscure magazine or tabloid. There are no secret cures or magic formulae which have not been recognized by the scientific community, a picture on the cover of Time magazine, nomination for a Nobel prize, etc., ("Miracle Cures and Other Frauds" 1990).
- The product or organization named is often similar to that of a famous person or creditable institution (e.g., the "Mayo Diet" had no connection with the Mayo Clinic).
- They often sell products through the mail, which does not allow you to examine the product personally. There are no miracle products available only by mail order or from a single source.

There are some common sense precautions one can take to avoid being a victim of a "rip-off."

The following suggestions can help protect you (FDA Consumer, 1986).

- Read the ad carefully, especially the small print.
- Do not send cash; use a check, money order, or credit card so you'll have a receipt.
- Do not order from a company with a P.O. box, unless you know the company.
- Do not let high-pressure sales tactics make you rush into a decision.
- Do not order from a company requiring use of an 800 telephone number and a credit card (they may be trying to avoid federal statutes).
- When in doubt, check out the company through your Better Business Bureau (BBB).
- If you have a complaint, write to the company first, but keep a copy of all receipts, checks, and correspondence.

- If that fails, write to the Direct Marketing Association. You may also report to the BBB, postmaster (if it was a mail order), state attorney general, and/or the Federal Trade Commission (FTC).

Facts About Equipment

The consumer who plans to purchase equipment should keep in mind certain guidelines to get the most for the money.

The following suggestions will help you select equipment:

- Unless you are wealthy or just like to collect gadgets, there is no need to buy a lot of exercise equipment. A complete fitness program can be carried out with *no* equipment. If you learn to depend upon equipment, you may eventually feel that you cannot exercise unless you are at home or at a gym.
- If you do not like jogging or swimming, and you hate calisthenics, then the minimal equipment you may want to consider is a bicycle (regular or stationary), treadmill, or rowing machine for cardiovascular fitness; and a set of weights, pulleys, or isokinetic device for strength and endurance.
- Consult an expert if you want to know the effectiveness of a product. Individuals with college or university degrees in physical education, physical therapy, kinesiotherapy, and kinesiology should be able to give you good advice.
- Buy from a well-established, reputable company that will not disappear overnight and will back up warranties. Avoid mail-order products. If the product is not available in a retail store where it can be examined, you probably should not buy it.

Facts About "Health Clubs"

It is not necessary to join a club, spa, or salon to develop fitness, but if you are considering joining such an establishment, make your choice with care.

The consumer should observe these precautions before becoming a member of a club, spa, or salon.

- Do not expect "miraculous" results as advertised.
- Be prepared to haggle over price and to resist a very hard sell for a long-term contract.

- Choose a no-contract, pay-as-you-go establishment if possible. Otherwise, choose the shortest term contract available.
- If there is a contract, read the fine print carefully and look for:
  1. the interest rate;
  2. "confession of judgment" clauses waiving your right to defend yourself in court;
  3. noncancelable clauses;
  4. "holder-in-due-course" doctrines allowing the establishment to sell your note to a collection agency;
  5. a waiver of the establishment's liability for injury to you on the premises.
- Consult with an independent expert if you have questions about the programs offered by the establishment.
- Do not accept diets, drugs, or food supplements from the club. Your physician will prescribe these if they are needed.
- You do not have to conform to the program the club suggests for you. Do not perform dangerous exercises, passive exercises, or participate in fraudulent "treatments." Choose only those activities that meet the criteria explained in this book.
- Refuse to be pestered by solicitations for new members.
- Make a trial visit to the establishment during the hours when you would normally expect to use the facility to determine if it is open, if it is over-crowded, if the equipment is available, if the attendants are selling rather than assisting, and if you would enjoy the company of the other patrons.
- Determine the qualifications of the personnel, especially of the individual responsible for your program. Is he or she an expert as defined previously?
- Make certain the club is a well-established facility that will not disappear overnight.
- Check its reputation with the Better Business Bureau in your area.
- Investigate the programs offered by the Y, local colleges and universities, and municipal park and recreation departments. These agencies often have excellent fitness classes at lower prices than commercial establishments and usually employ qualified personnel. For weight loss, investigate franchised clubs, such as Weight Watchers or TOPS, or affiliate with a university or a hospital-based program.

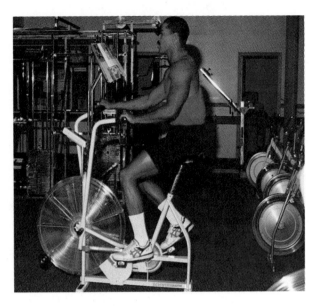

Visit a health club before you join.

Facts About Fitness Books, Magazines, and Articles

All fitness books do not provide scientifically sound, accurate, and reliable information.

Because publishers are motivated by profit and publishing is a highly competitive field, the choice of material to be printed is often selected on the basis of how popular, famous, or attractive the author is, or how sensational or unusual his or her ideas are. Movie stars, models, TV personalities, and even Olympic athletes are rarely experts in biomechanics, anatomy and physiology, exercise, and other foundations of physical fitness. Having a good figure/physique, being fit, or having gone through a training program does not, in itself, qualify a person to advise others.

If you have read the facts presented in the previous concepts, you should be able to distinguish between fact and fiction. To assist you further, however, there are ten guidelines listed in question form that might help you evaluate whether or not a book, magazine, or article on exercise and fitness is valid, reliable, and scientifically sound. (See chart 24.1.) If the answer to each of the questions is not "yes," then you should be suspicious of the material. If in doubt, ask one or more experts, or write to the American Alliance of Health, Physical Education, Recreation and Dance (AAHPERD) or to the American College of Sports Medicine (ACSM) (see addresses in list of references). These organizations will refer your question to an appropriate expert.

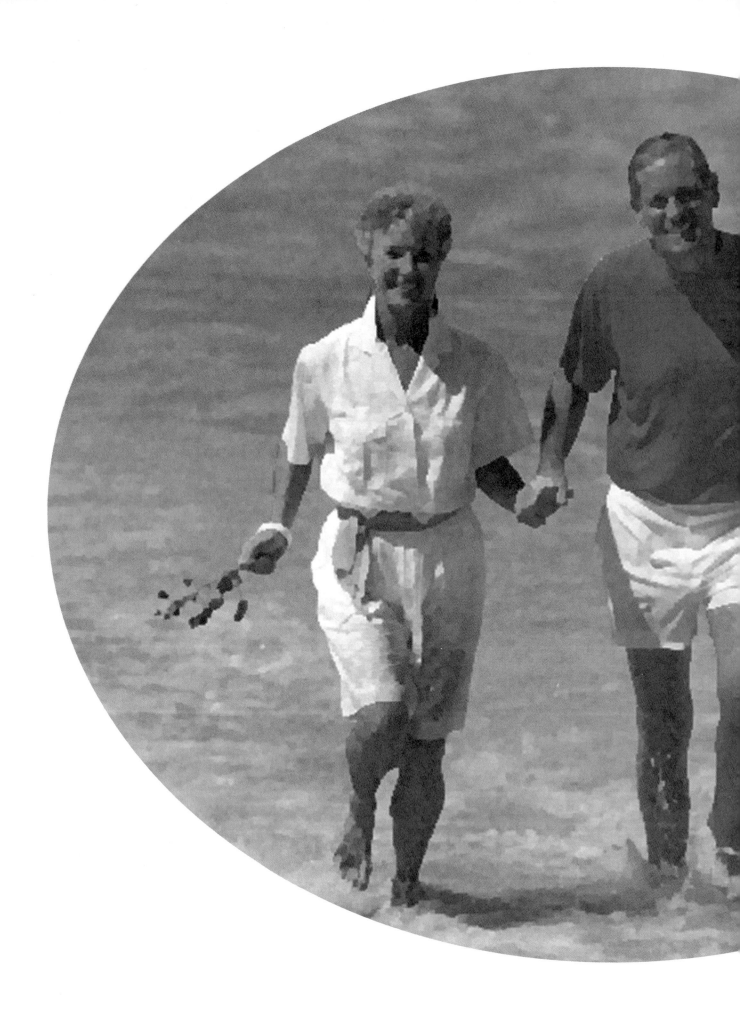

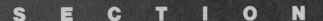

VI

Wellness: Toward a Quality Life-Style

25

Use and Abuse of Tobacco and Alcohol

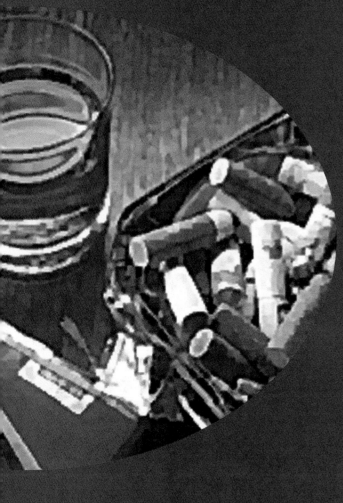

Concept 25

Alcohol and tobacco are the most commonly used drugs in the United States and take the greatest toll in money, health, and lives.

Introduction

Tobacco and alcohol are the two most commonly used and **abused** drugs in the United States. Many people do not associate the word **drug** with tobacco or alcohol because these substances are so commonplace in our society, and both are legal (except for those under the legal age as determined by each state). Yet, these drugs create more medical and socioeconomic problems than any of the so-called "street drugs" that are so much in the news. There are approximately 50 million smokers in the U.S., and it is estimated that at least two-thirds of all adults drink alcoholic beverages. Because use of these two is so widespread in our society, they alone will be discussed in this Concept. Others drugs will be discussed in Concept 26.

Health Goals for the Year 2000

- Reduce drug-related deaths.
- Increase the average age of first use of cigarettes and alcohol.
- Reduce the proportion of young people who have used alcohol.
- Reduce the amount of alcohol consumed per person.
- Reduce the proportion of high school seniors and college students engaging in bouts of heavy drinking of alcoholic beverages.
- Increase the proportion of high school seniors who perceive social disapproval associated with the heavy use of alcohol.
- Increase the proportion of high school seniors who associate physical or psychological harm with the heavy use of alcohol.
- Extend to all states legal blood alcohol concentration tolerance levels of .04 percent for drivers aged 21 and older and to .00 percent for younger drivers.

Terms

Abuse

Using a drug as a habit.

Addiction

The inability to stop using a substance or to stop a behavior.

Alcoholism

The loss of control over drinking behavior and/or the lack of ability to refrain from becoming intoxicated.

Drug

A chemical that changes the way the body works.

Intoxication

Drunkenness, or blood alcohol level above .10 percent (legal intoxication in most states).

Misuse

The use of a drug to help cope with a situation.

The Facts About Tobacco

Tobacco and its smoke contain the addictive drug "nicotine," plus about 400 other chemicals, including 200 known poisons and 50 carcinogens.

Nicotine is a very poisonous chemical (often used in insecticides). It is a potent and powerful psychoactive drug that affects the brain and alters mood and behavior. It is thousands of times more powerful than barbiturates, and five to ten times more potent than cocaine.

Tobacco smoke also contains tar, as well as poisons such as carbon monoxide, formaldehyde, and benzene. Cigarettes have nearly 2,000 times more benzene contamination than the Perrier water that was recalled because it had benzene levels that were above health standards.

When smoke is inhaled, the nicotine reaches the brain in seven seconds, where it acts on highly sensitive receptors and provides a "hit" that then brings about a wide variety of responses throughout the body.

At first there is an increase in heart and breathing rates. Blood vessels constrict, peripheral circulation is slowed, and blood pressure increases. (New users may experience dizziness, nausea, and headache.) Then, feelings of tension and tiredness are relieved.

After a few minutes the feeling wears off and a rebound or withdrawal effect occurs. The smoker may feel depressed and irritable and have the urge to smoke again. **Addiction** occurs with continued use. *Nicotine is one of the most addictive drugs known—even more than heroin or alcohol.*

Nicotine can act as a stimulant or a sedative, depending upon the smoker's circumstances.

As a stimulant, nicotine may cause the smoker to experience an energetic feeling. On the other hand, it may increase the alpha waves in the brain and trigger the release of endorphins, producing feelings of relaxation. Whether it acts as a stimulant or sedative depends on the dose, the smoker's metabolism, the amount of stress the smoker is experiencing, and the time of day. It tends to stimulate in the morning and sedate in the afternoon.

Table 25.1

Health Effects of Smoking

- It is the number one avoidable cause of mortality in the U.S.
- It is the number one cause of lung cancer deaths in the U.S.
- It is the number one cause of cancer in women.
- It is the number one cause of cancer of the esophagus (especially when combined with alcohol).
- It is the number one cause of cancer of the kidney.
- It is the number one cause of pancreatic cancer.
- It increases risk of cancer of the oral cavity.
- It increases risk of cancer of the larynx.
- It increases risk of leukemia.
- It increases the risk of cancer of the urinary bladder.
- It increases risk of heart attack and heart disease.
- It increases risk of atherosclerosis.
- It increases risk of stomach ulcers.
- It increases risk of chronic bronchitis and emphysema.
- It increases risk in pregnant women of miscarriage, infant death, and other complications.
- It causes 88 million more days of sickness per year than for nonsmokers.
- It decreases the HDL in the blood.

It is the long-term effects of smoking that make it a major health problem and the most preventable cause of death in our society.

Smoking is the leading known cause of lung cancer and is related to six other cancers and a number of other medical problems. It causes 370,000 deaths per year; that is, about 1,000 people die per day of the health problems related to smoking. This is more Americans than were killed in World War II. It is not just an American problem. Worldwide, two and a half to three million people die annually from smoking. The effects of smoking on health are listed in table 25.1.

The risk of having health problems increases with the amount of exposure (dosage) to the smoke. This is especially true of lung cancer and heart disease.

Several factors determine the dosage: (1) the number of cigarettes smoked; (2) the length of time one has been smoking; (3) the strength (amount of tar, nicotine, etc.) of the cigarette; (4) the depth of the inhalation; and (5) the amount of exposure to other lung-damaging substances (e.g., asbestos). The greater the dosage of smoke, the greater the risk.

Cigar and pipe smokers have lower death rates than cigarette smokers but still are at great risk.

Cigar and pipe smokers usually inhale less and therefore have less risk of heart and lung disease, but cigarette smokers who switch to cigars and pipes tend to continue inhaling the same way and may not decrease their risk appreciably. Cigar and pipe smoke contains most of the same harmful ingredients of cigarette smoke, sometimes in higher amounts, so that those who do inhale have an even greater risk of dying from lung or heart disease. The little cigars that resemble cigarettes tend to be inhaled like cigarettes, so are especially dangerous because of a very high nicotine and tar content.

Cigar and pipe smokers have higher risks of cancer of the mouth, throat, and larynx than the cigarette smoker. Pipe smokers are especially at risk for lip cancer. Both cigar and pipe smoking are less acceptable socially because of the strong odor and more irritating smoke. One study has shown that in thirty minutes, one cigar can pollute the air more than forty-two cigarettes.

All smokers pollute the air that everyone must breathe. This has become a serious environmental problem.

When the smoker lights up, he/she pollutes the air with "mainstream" smoke that is exhaled (after being filtered by the smoker's lungs). The smoker also pollutes the air with "sidestream" smoke, which comes directly off the burning end of the cigarette/cigar/pipe. The combination of mainstream and sidestream smoke is referred to as "secondhand" smoke.

Sidestream smoke is more dangerous than mainstream smoke because it contains higher concentrations of harmful substances, including nicotine, tar, carbon monoxide, and cadmium. Its carbon monoxide is reported to be from two to fifteen times greater than in the mainstream smoke. Carbon monoxide robs the blood of oxygen. Emphysema, hypertension, and chronic bronchitis have been related to large doses of cadmium. The odor of tobacco smoke clings to hair, skin, and clothes. Smokers tend to be unaware of the odor because of their impaired sense of smell, but to the nonsmoker it is irritating and offensive.

Nonsmokers who must breathe secondhand smoke are in fact "involuntary" or "passive" smokers and can suffer serious health problems.

The Environmental Protection Agency in 1992 estimated as many as 3,800 lung cancer deaths per year that could be attributed to secondhand smoke. It also suggested there was a direct link between secondhand smoke and asthma. It is believed that smoke accounts for serious respiratory ailments in as many as 200,000 children. The National

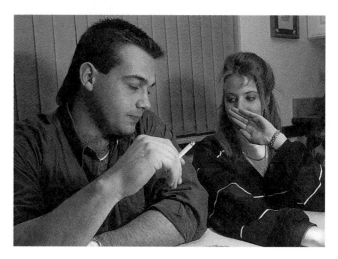
Second-hand smoke makes us all involuntary smokers.

Center for Health Statistics found that children in non-smoking households were likely to be healthier than children who live with smokers.

Some smokers switch to smokeless tobacco because of the misconception that it is a safe substitute for cigarette, cigar, and pipe smoking.

There has been a recent increase in dipping snuff and chewing tobacco. The National Institute of Drug Abuse estimates 22 million Americans (mostly males) have used it. Fifty percent of the users report that they started before the age of 13. Snuff comes in either dry or moist forms. Dry snuff is powdered tobacco mixed with flavorings, designed to be "sniffed," "pinched," or "dipped." Moist snuff is used the same way, but it is moist, finely cut tobacco in a loose form or in a tea-bag-like packet.

Chewing tobacco comes in loose leaf, twist, or plug form. The plug is tightly compacted and the user bites off a "chaw" ("wad" or "quid"). Like snuff, it is held in the mouth for several hours, where it mixes with saliva and is absorbed into the bloodstream. Smokeless tobacco contains about seven times more nicotine than cigarettes, and more of it is absorbed because of the length of time the tobacco is in the mouth. It also contains a higher level of carcinogens than cigarettes.

Like all tobacco, smokeless tobacco is a deadly killer, producing many harmful effects on the health of the user, as well as social restrictions.

Dipping and chewing are as addictive (and maybe more so) as smoking and produce the same kind of withdrawal symptoms upon quitting. It does not pollute the air like smoking, but most nonusers dislike the spitting and the bad breath of users. The health risks of smokeless tobacco are listed in table 25.2.

Table 25.2

Health Risks of Smokeless Tobacco

Smokeless tobacco increases risk of:

- Oral cavity cancer (cheek, gum, lip, palate). It is 4–50 times greater risk, depending on length of time used).
- Cancer of the throat, larynx, and esophagus.
- Precancerous skin changes.
- High blood pressure.
- Rotting teeth, exposed roots, premature tooth loss, worn-down teeth.
- Ulcerated, inflamed, infected gums.
- Slow healing of mouth wounds.
- Decreased resistance to infections.
- Arteriosclerosis, myocardial infarction, and coronary occlusion.
- Widespread hormonal effects, including increased lipids, higher blood sugar, and increased blood clots.
- Increased heart rate.

Table 25.3

Why Teenagers Start Using Tobacco

- Peer pressure.
- Social acceptance.
- Desire to be "mature."
- Desire to be "independent."
- Desire to be like their role models.
- It looks appealing in advertisements.

Most tobacco users began "using" before the age of 14. The reasons for starting are varied, but strikingly similar to reasons given for using alcohol and other drugs (see table 25.3).

Studies show that 60 percent of junior high students and 40 percent of high school seniors do not believe there is a risk in smoking or using smokeless tobacco. The tobacco industry spends $2.6 million per year to make smoking, dipping, and chewing attractive to youth. They portray it as fun, macho, and the "cool" thing to do.

There is a tendency for those who smoke cigarettes to also use alcohol, marijuana, and hard drugs.

More smokers use other drugs than do nonsmokers. This is particularly true of the college age (18–25). The reasons for the relationship are not clear, but it may be that those who do not smoke have a better understanding of the health risks, good self-esteem, a good support system

Table 25.4

Tobacco Withdrawal Symptoms

• Craving for tobacco	• Difficulty sleeping
• Anxiety	• Difficulty concentrating
• Headaches	• Tremors
• Gastrointestinal discomfort	• Changes in appetite
• Mood changes	• Craving for sweets
• Irritability	

of family and friends, and have learned how to say "no" without giving in to the pressures and lures that make the smokers use tobacco in the first place (table 25.3). On the other hand, those who use tobacco have a tendency to use other drugs for the same reasons.

For most users, it is not easy to quit tobacco because nicotine is highly addictive, but there are some techniques and strategies that make it easier.

When a person first stops using tobacco, some of the withdrawal symptoms listed in table 25.4 occur. Because people react differently, a person may experience only a few or all of the symptoms. The length of time it takes to recover from the symptoms varies from days to weeks or months. Most people do not succeed the first time they try to quit. The important thing is to keep trying, because most people who try will eventually succeed. More than 40 million Americans have quit smoking.

The following tips from the American Lung Association and the American Cancer Society should be useful to those who wish to quit using tobacco.

- You must want to quit. This is the most important thing. The reasons could be for health, family, money, etc.
- Remind yourself of the reasons. Each day repeat to yourself the reasons for not using tobacco.
- Decide how to stop. Some ways to stop include counseling, formal programs, "cold turkey," gradually, or with a spouse or friend.
- Remove reminders and temptations. Get rid of ashtrays, tobacco, etc.
- Use substitutes and distractions. Substitute low-calorie snacks or chewing gum, change your routine, try new activities, sit in nonsmoking areas.
- Don't worry about gaining weight. Studies show there is no overall correlation between smoking and body fatness. In one study, one of four ex-smokers lost weight.
- Try a formal "quit smoking program." Examples of these programs are "Freedom from Smoking" (American Lung Association) and "Fresh Start"

(American Cancer Society). Many state, county, and local health departments also sponsor programs. Most colleges and universities have programs associated with the student health center.

- Consider a "crutch." If you choose to taper off, you may want to consider a product that requires a prescription, such as a nicotine transdermal patch or nicotine chewing gum. Because both require a prescription, they should be used with the assistance of a physician and are most effective when used in conjunction with one of the planned programs previously mentioned.

- Alternative tobacco products *may* help. Low-tar or ultra-low-tar cigarettes have helped some people stop smoking. They can, however, be just as harmful as regular cigarettes if use continues. Some people have used clove cigarettes, but some experts feel these may be more harmful than regular cigarettes because of immediate harmful effects to the lungs.

The good news is that when you quit, you may feel better right away and your body will eventually heal most of the damage.

You will begin to feel more energetic, the coughing will stop, you will suddenly begin to taste food again, and your sense of smell will return. Your lungs will eventually heal and look like the lungs of a nonsmoker. Your risk of lung cancer will return to that of the nonsmoker in about fifteen years. There is life after smoking!

Facts About Alcoholic Beverages

Alcoholic beverages contain ethanol (ethyl alcohol)—a drug that is **intoxicating** and addictive and is the drug most often **misused** in the U.S.

Ethanol is a toxic chemical, but unlike methanol (wood alcohol) and isopropyl (rubbing alcohol), it can be used in beverages. As a drug it is classified as a depressant. *It is the most widely used and destructive drug in the United States.* If all of the deaths caused by this drug are counted, it is the third major health problem in the U.S. It is second only to tobacco as a cause of premature death in this country.

The amount of alcohol in distilled spirits (liquor) and wine is listed on the label as its "proof." (Labels on beer and wine coolers are not presently required to list this.) The proof represents approximately double the percentage of alcohol in the beverage; for example, 90 proof

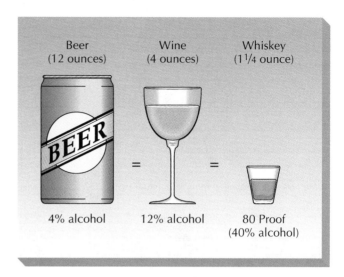

Figure 25.1

Alcohol content of drinks.

Source: Data from the U.S. Surgeon General and the Government Printing Office.

gin is about 45 percent alcohol. Different beverages have different alcohol content, and they also may vary by brand. Beer is usually the lowest percentage at 3–6 percent, depending on state regulations. Wine has approximately 12–22 percent, whereas vodka, gin, scotch, brandy, cognac, and whiskey are the highest, with 40–52 percent.

Beverages are usually served in proportions such that a "drink" of any one of the three categories (beer, wine, or liquor) contains the same amount of alcohol.

Beer is usually served in a twelve-ounce can, bottle, or mug. A typical glass of wine holds four ounces, and a jigger of liquor is one ounce. Even though the percentage of alcohol in the beverages differ, the drinks would be equivalent in alcohol because each would contain about 15 ml of alcohol (see figure 25.1).

The Surgeon General has expressed serious concern about the amount of alcohol drunk in the United States and the consequences of alcohol consumption.

It is estimated that each year Americans drink 378 million gallons of distilled spirits (liquor), 540 million gallons of wine and wine coolers, and six billion gallons of beer. Two-thirds of the adult population drink alcoholic beverages, and one in ten has a chance of becoming an alcoholic. According to a report from Tufts University, 90 percent of all drinkers consume 50 percent of the alcohol served—which means the other 10 percent are very heavy drinkers, consuming the remaining 50 percent.

Table 25.5

Health Effects of Alcohol Consumption

Increased risk of:	• Death
• High blood pressure	• Impaired immune system
• Stroke	• Problems in the reproductive system:
• Cardiac arrhythmias	infertility
• Heart disease	hormonal imbalance
• Blood clotting diseases	menstrual disturbance
• Cirrhosis of the liver	• Fetal Alcohol Syndrome (in pregnant women):
• Cancer:	low birth weight
stomach tongue	physical defects
liver pharynx	brain damage/mental retardation
pancreas larynx	heart defects
colon esophagus	stunted growth
breast	• Malnutrition
	• Decreased health-related physical fitness

College students drink more than the rest of society and are more at risk for alcohol problems than other segments of the population.

Approximately 75 percent of college students drink some alcohol, with 41 percent of the students engaged in heavy drinking (five or more consecutive drinks). Alcoholic beverage consumption on campuses exceeds that of soft drinks, coffee, tea, milk, and juices put together (Eigen 1991).

The average annual consumption of alcoholic beverages for college students is more than 34 gallons per person, and in 1991 they spent more than 4.2 billion dollars on alcohol (more than was spent on operating campus libraries and college scholarships and fellowships by all colleges in the U.S. combined).

Alcohol is absorbed directly into the bloodstream through the walls of the stomach and the small intestines. It then concentrates in various organs in proportion to the amount of water each contains and is eventually oxidized in the liver.

The brain has a high water content, so much of the alcohol goes there, where it will depress the central nervous system. At first it makes the person feel relaxed, maybe happy, and less inhibited. The effects depend upon (1) the drinker's level of fatigue; (2) his/her mood; (3) what and how much food is in the stomach; (4) other drugs/medications consumed; (5) body size/weight; (6) rate of consumption; (7) type of beverage; and (8) individual body chemistry/ genetic predisposition. The more one drinks, the greater the effect.

The effects of alcohol on the health of its consumers is devastating and life threatening.

The greater the alcohol intake and the longer it is used, the higher the risk for health impairment. For example, as few as three drinks per day for men or one and a half drinks per day for women increases the risk of cirrhosis of the liver. There are an estimated 100,000 deaths from alcohol use each year. Some of these are sudden deaths in healthy people! These and other health problems related to alcohol consumption are summarized in table 25.5.

The amount of alcohol in the blood is measured as a percentage and is referred to as "blood alcohol content" (BAC). It is this figure that is used by law enforcement officials to determine if a driver is legally intoxicated.

According to the National Transportation Safety Board, "There is an increased risk in driving when the BAC is between .01 and .04 percent." A BAC of .04 percent is approximately half a drink if you weigh 120 pounds and one drink if you weigh 160. A BAC of .10 percent is the level at which driving becomes illegal in most states. A BAC of .4–.5 percent (approximately 20–25 drinks) would usually be fatal (see table 25.6).

The greatest danger of alcohol-induced impaired motor performance occurs when the drinker gets behind the wheel of a motor vehicle.

Alcohol-related traffic crashes are the leading cause of death and spinal-cord injury for young Americans. The

Table 25.6

Effects of Blood Alcohol Level (BAC) on Driving

BAC .02%	BAC .08%
• Vision impaired: less ability to see objects in motion; less ability to monitor multiple objects	• Slower reflexes and reaction time
• Lowered attention span	• Poor coordination
• Reaction time slows	• Seriously impaired vision, especially at night
• Less critical of own actions	• Overconfidence in driving ability
BAC .05–.06%	• Emotions are exaggerated
• Reaction time noticeably reduced	• Thinking and reasoning powers impaired
• Reduced inhibitions (taking unnecessary chances)	• Less ability to concentrate
• Visual abilities decrease; side vision impaired approximately 30%	• Judgment dulled: careless
• Superficial feelings of relaxation	• Hinders muscle control and coordination
• Judgment is the first function to be impaired	• Distances are misjudged
• Braking distance is extended	• Braking distance exceeded further
• Diminished ability to maneuver through narrow spaces	• Reduced inhibitions (taking unnecessary chances)
• Lowered attention span	• Impaired driving performances at low speeds
• Coordination impaired	• Possible steering inaccuracy
• Information processing impaired	• Increased use of accelerator and brake
• Impaired driving performance at moderate speed	• Less able to see dimly lit objects

Developed by Alaska Chapter of MADD and reprinted in *Orange County (CA) Chapter Newsletter*, Winter 1989–1990, p. 5. Used with permission.

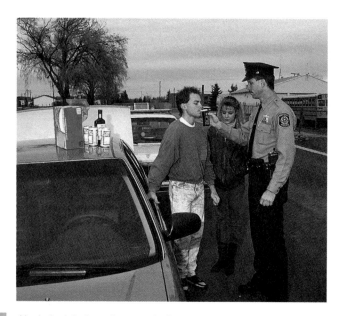

Alcohol-related crashes are the leading cause of death for young people.

driver's likelihood of causing a highway accident increases significantly at a BAC of .04 percent (approximately the level reached by a 180-pound man on two beers). When the BAC reaches .10 percent, the chances have increased by 600 percent. In a 1986 government survey, 70 percent of college students reported driving while under the influence at least once in the past year, and 22 percent said they had done it five times or more.

Two out of five Americans will be involved in an alcohol-related auto crash at some time in their lives.

Alcohol-related problems cost American society an estimated $116–136 billion in 1992.

Alcohol is believed to account for 100,000 deaths per year. Approximately 360,000 students who are now in college will eventually lose their lives due to drinking. National studies conclusively link heavy drinking among youths to physical fights, destroyed property, job troubles, and troubles with the law. Drinking is usually a factor in date rapes and gang rapes. College administrators unanimously agree that it is the cause of most campus crime. A list of some of the alcohol-related problems that contribute to the costs to society are listed in table 25.7 with their percentage of incidence.

The reasons given for starting to drink alcohol are the same or similar to those given for starting to use other drugs; however, the reasons for *starting* are not necessarily the reasons for *continuing* to use alcohol.

Peer pressure and the desire to be accepted are probably the two main reasons people take their first few drinks (usually as a young teenager). Other important influences include the portrayal of drinking as being macho, fun, cool, sexy, mature, elegant and "the thing to do" by role models in the media (slick magazines, movies, television) and in

Table 25.7

Social Problems Associated with Alcohol Abuse

Problems	Percentage of Cases That are Alcohol Related
• Suicides	33
• All deaths from accidents, suicides, murders	50
• All deaths from boating accidents, drownings, and homicides	33
• Deaths from drownings	69
• Deaths from falls	17–53
• Sexual assaults	72
• Child abuse	60
• Family violence	80
• College academic problems	34
• Deaths from college sorority/fraternity hazings	90
• College undergraduates reporting unplanned sexual activity (at least one instance)	29

Table 25.8

Why People Start Drinking

- Peer pressure
- Need to belong and to be accepted
- Media depiction of drinking
- Advertising depiction of drinking
- Lack of knowledge about its effects
- Easy access (especially at home)
- Absence of strong religious attachment
- Male bonding (especially in college)
- Cultural traditions at college
- Social "lubrication"
- It makes them "feel good."

advertising in newspapers and magazines, on billboards, at sports events, and so on. The alcohol industry focuses much of its advertising at young audiences and admits it contributes to underage drinking (Ryan and Mosher 1991). They market heavily on college campuses. In one study, college newspaper space devoted to alcohol advertisements was approximately twenty times greater than the space devoted to books and forty times greater than that devoted to soft drinks. It is estimated that 10 percent of the revenue of the alcohol industry comes from college students.

Another factor contributing to the decision of youth to drink is failure to understand the health effects of alcohol and lack of knowledge about the alcoholic content of beverages. A national survey found that junior high and high school students could not identify the beverage containing the most alcohol when shown beer (4 percent alcohol), malt beverage coolers (4–8 percent), wine coolers (1.5–6.5 percent), mixed drink coolers (4 percent), fruit-flavored wine, such as "Cisco" (20 percent), and nonalcoholic, fruit-flavored mineral water (0 percent). More than one third did not know that "Cisco" contained alcohol (Eigen 1991). Table 25.8 lists the most common reasons people give for starting to drink.

There is no sure way to predict who will become addicted to alcohol because each person is born with a certain level of risk.

Alcoholism is a disease, and it may take a little or a lot to trigger it. Some people seem to have a genetic predispo-

sition for it. There is a one out of ten chance that a person who drinks will become an alcoholic.

Teenagers can quickly become addicted to it because a young person's liver metabolizes the alcohol faster than an adult's. They can reach an advanced stage of alcoholism in just one year, whereas it might take three to fifteen years of heavy drinking for an adult to reach that stage.

Women are more at risk than men because of their lighter weight, and they suffer greater physiological damage from the disease. The death rate among women alcoholics is 50–100 percent higher than for men alcoholics.

It all begins with the first drink. Then there is the "social" drinking, and later it is used as an escape from stress. The more one drinks, the greater the tolerance for alcohol and the more required to feel the effect—and the cycle continues.

There are certain warning signs of alcohol abuse that the drinker should be aware of (but may deny).

Friends and family can help the person recognize these symptoms because the more of them present, the greater the likelihood of alcoholism. Table 25.9 lists the warning signs of alcohol abuse.

Some people should not drink at all, and most people who do drink should drink less.

Some recent studies have suggested that "moderate" drinking (two drinks per day) could reduce your cholesterol and reduce heart attacks. The validity of these studies has been hotly debated, and even if they were valid, it would not change the other uncontested harmful effects of "moderate" drinking such as cardiac arrhythmias, hypertension, and stroke. Dr. Ernest Noble (former director

Table 25.9
Warning Signs of Alcohol Abuse

- Needing a drink to start the day
- Making excuses for drinking
- Sneaking drinks
- Frequent absences from work or school
- Drinking alone
- Gulping drinks
- Financial difficulties
- Guilt feelings after drinking episodes
- Loss of ambition
- Lack of concern for family's welfare
- Memory loss
- Shabby appearance
- Mood changes
- Chronic hangovers

Table 25.10
People Who Should Never Drink

- Those under age 21 (legal age)
- Athletes striving for peak performance
- Women trying to get pregnant or who are pregnant or nursing
- Alcoholics or recovering alcoholics
- Those with a family history of alcoholism
- Those with a medical or surgical problem and/or on medications
- Psychiatric patients or persons experiencing severe psychosis
- Those driving vehicles or operating dangerous machinery or involved in public safety
- People conducting serious business transactions or study

of the National Institute of Alcohol Abuse and Alcoholism and presently director of the U.C.L.A. Alcohol Research Center) believes that some people should abstain completely (see table 25.10).

For those who choose to drink, the National Research Council (1989) recommends a limit of one ounce of alcohol per day (one ounce equals two beers, a small wine drink or an average-sized cocktail). Dr. Noble recommends a more conservative limit of three drinks per week for men and two drinks per week for women, or less—not all on the same day (Noble 1991).

If you drink, be a "responsible drinker" and avoid intoxication.

If you drink (at a party, for example), follow these guidelines from Tufts University:

- Limit alcoholic beverages to no more than one every hour and a half, or two or three drinks over a course of a four or five hour party (to stay within the legal BAC). Note: Between alcoholic beverages, you may wish to carry a nonalcoholic beverage to sip and to prevent friends from pressing a new drink on you.
- Sip the drink slowly.
- Eat foods rich in protein and starch to slow the absorption into the blood.
- Choose noncarbonated drinks (rather than carbonated) for slower absorption.
- Measure your alcohol in a jigger (guessers use too much).
- Never drink and drive. Choose a "designated driver" (who will not drink) before you go to the party.

Contrary to popular opinion, you cannot prevent intoxication by eating a meal or having a glass of milk before drinking alcohol. Neither can you sober up faster by drinking coffee, taking a cold shower, or walking.

If you are giving a party at which alcohol will be served, follow these guidelines.

- Have plenty of nonalcoholic beverages and high protein and starchy foods available for the guests.
- Tactfully remove alcoholic beverages from the hands of overindulgers. (You might give them a job to do and/or substitute a nonalcoholic drink.)
- Close the "bar" an hour or two before the party ends.
- Secure safe transportation for those who are intoxicated. Do not let them drive.

The best advice is to never start drinking, but if you do, there are some positive steps you can take.

Alcoholics need professional help and strong support from friends and family, but they have to want to stop drinking for themselves and must take the proper steps themselves. Others do not help them by denying the problem, nagging them about it, or covering it up for them.

To stop drinking, you may need to find some nondrinking friends and, if necessary, get a job or go to a college where you can get away from the people who influence you to drink. And you may have to practice ways to say "no" so others get the message that you mean it. You may need to get some professional help with assertiveness skills and how to improve your self-esteem. It is important that you develop leisure skills to avoid boredom. Exercise and sports can make you feel good, help you to become more fit and healthy, fill your leisure time, and expose you to new friends. Some professional sources of help include the National Council on Alcoholism (1–800–NCA–Call), Alcoholics Anonymous (AA), and the National Clearinghouse for Alcohol and Drug Abuse Information (Box 2345, Rockville, Md, 20852). Your local health department can also refer you to local support and/or rehabilitation groups. The yellow pages of your telephone book list a number of professional help groups (try looking under alcohol, drugs, and addiction).

Suggested Readings

Drug Use Among American High School Students, College Students and Other Young Adults. National Institute on Drug Abuse, U.S. DHHS, 1987.

Straus, R. H. "Spittin' Image: Breaking the Sports-Tobacco Connection." *Physician and Sportsmedicine* 19(1991):46–48.

U.S. Department of Health and Human Services. *Alcohol and Health.* Seventh Special Report to the U.S. Congress from the Secretary of Health and Human Services. NIAAA, Rockville, MD: 1990.

Wichmann, S. A., and D. R. Martin. "Sports and Tobacco: The Smoke Has Yet to Clear." *Physician and Sportsmedicine* 19(1991):125–31.

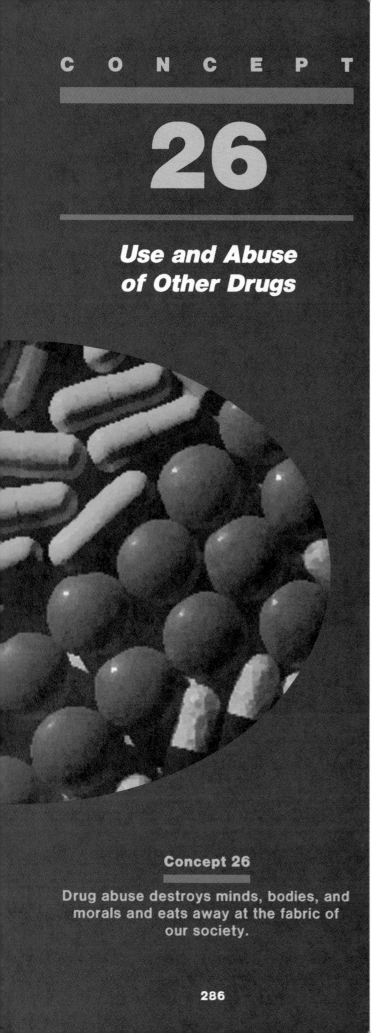

26

Use and Abuse of Other Drugs

Concept 26

Drug abuse destroys minds, bodies, and morals and eats away at the fabric of our society.

Introduction

The estimated cost of drug abuse to the U.S. is about $100 billion, with 72 percent of that cost being for criminal justice (law enforcement, private legal cases, property destruction, and related costs). Lost productivity accounts for $7.2 billion, treatment cost equals $2.7 billion, and early death accounts for $3 billion (see fig. 26.1). America has declared war on drugs because they are eating away at the fabric of our society. Dr. Robert Heath sums up our dilemma in these words:

> When the pleasure a person gains from taking a drug replaces reward for a job well done, we have shoddy workmanship. When puffs from a joint replace the pleasure of a swim on a warm sunny afternoon or a good tennis game, we have apathy and physical deterioration. When the anxiety before an examination is eliminated by the instant pleasure of a drug, the student does not prepare and fails the examination. When ingestion of a chemical substance replaces the satisfaction of solving a problem, being creative, or helping another person, what are the implications for the future of our society—or even our survival as a nation? (Heath n. d., p. 7)

Tobacco and alcohol—the two most commonly used drugs in the U.S.—were discussed in Concept 25. This Concept discusses the misuse and abuse of other drugs, with emphasis on the illegal, so-called "street" drugs.

Health Goals for the Year 2000

- Reduce drug-related deaths.
- Reduce drug-abuse-related visits to hospital emergency departments.
- Increase the average age of first use of marijuana.
- Reduce the proportion of young people who have used marijuana and cocaine in the past month.
- Increase the proportion of high school seniors who perceive social disapproval associated with the occasional use of marijuana and experimentation with cocaine.
- Increase the proportion of high school seniors who associate risk of physical or psychological harm with the regular use of marijuana and experimentation with cocaine.

Terms

Also see Concept 25 terms.

Hallucinations

Seeing, feeling, and or hearing imaginary things.

Physical Dependence

A physiological need to keep using a drug to avoid withdrawal symptoms.

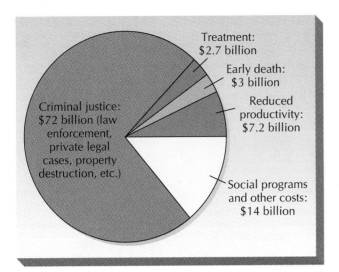

Figure 26.1

Estimated cost of drug abuse in the U.S. is $100 billion dollars.

Source: Data from the National Institutes on Drug Abuse, Department of Health and Human Services.

Psychological Dependence

A psychological need to keep using drugs to obtain pleasurable feelings or to avoid withdrawal symptoms.

Tolerance

Progressively larger doses are required to obtain the same effect as once felt with a smaller dose.

The Facts About Drugs

The abuse of drugs is a particularly serious problem with youth but also invades the workplace.

One in four adolescents is at a very high risk of drug abuse, and one out of three people aged 18–25 use illegal drugs at least once a month. Ten to 25 percent of U.S. workers are estimated to be abusing alcohol or other drugs, and each of these workers costs the employer an average of 25 percent in lost productivity through frequent absences, erratic performance, violence, stealing, bad judgment, and accidents that often endanger others.

It is generally believed that drug use begins (in early teens or younger) with smoking cigarettes. Then users progress to drinking alcohol, and then to smoking marijuana, before graduating to other drugs. This is called the "gateway concept," and tobacco, alcohol, and marijuana are referred to as the "gateway drugs."

In 1988 (the year on which the baseline for the nation's health goals for the year 2000 were established), the average age for starting cigarettes was 11.6. The ages for starting alcohol and marijuana were 13.1 and 13.4, respectively. One in four Americans has tried marijuana, 22 million have tried cocaine (5,000 additional people try it for the first time every day), and 6 million are current cocaine users. The connection between the "gateway drugs" and the "harder" drugs is strong, and it emphasizes the importance of discouraging young people from using them.

Addiction is a disease, not a moral failure. It is being studied by neuroscientists and geneticists, but there is strong evidence that susceptibility to addiction is genetic.

Ten to fifteen percent of Americans are susceptible to the disease of addiction. They will lose control over when they use drugs and how much they use, and they will die from it without outside help. Addiction is called a primary psychosocial and biogenetic disease (Gallagher 1986).

Drugs may be classified in several ways, but the mood-altering or psychoactive drugs are the ones we hear about most.

Mood altering and psychoactive drugs may be placed in five major groups, all of them highly addictive: (1) depressants, (2) narcotics, (3) stimulants, (4) hallucinogens, and (5) designer drugs. Drugs in the same group have similar effects. (A sixth category of misused and abused drugs is prescription drugs.) Each of the five categories of drugs is discussed in this concept, and the effects are described in tables 26.1, 26.2, 26.3, 26.4, and 26.5. The effects are classified as either physiological or psychological (meaning primarily affecting the body versus primarily affecting behavior, respectively). Because the effects of drugs can vary with each individual, and with different doses, it is only possible to generalize about the effects in the tables that follow.

Some examples of depressants (also known as sedatives or "downers") are alcoholic drinks and prescription drugs such as Valium, Xanax, meprobamate (brand names include Miltown or Equanil), sleeping pills, and methaqualone.

These drugs come in the forms of pills, liquids, or injectables. In small doses, they slow the heart rate and respiration. In larger doses (for example alcohol), they act as a poison and damage every organ system in the body. In terms of their effect on behavior, the user might at first feel stimulated because the drugs lower inhibitions, may talk more excitedly, and may experience a sense of well being. Depression, loss of coordination, drop in energy level, mood swings, and confusion occurs after prolonged use.

Table 26.1

Depressants ("Downers," Sedatives)

Examples	Physiological Effects	Psychological Effects
• Alcohol • Sedatives: e.g., Valium, Xanax, meprobamate, sleeping pills, methaqualone	• In small doses slows the heart and respiration. • In large doses acts as a poison and damages every organ system.	• Initially: stimulation, lowered inhibitions, excited talking, sense of well being. • After prolonged use: depression, loss of coordination, drop in energy level, mood swings, confusion, euphoria.

Table 26.2

Narcotics

Examples	Physiological Effects	Psychological Effects
• Heroin • Codeine • Morphine • Methadone	• Narcotics: block pain, chronic constipation, depressed respiration, redness and irritation of nostrils, nausea, lowered sexual drive, impaired immune system. • Heroin causes blood clots, bacterial endocarditis, serum hepatitis, brain abscess, HIV infection (from shared needles). In pregnant users, high risk of miscarriage, stillbirths, birth defects, toxemia, addicted baby.	• Narcotics: euphoria and feeling of pleasure. Nontherapeutic doses may result in mental distress, such as fear and nervousness. In heavy users, drowsiness and apathy may occur.

Narcotics include heroin, codeine, morphine, opium, and methadone.

These drugs are either smoked, injected, sniffed, or swallowed. Heroin has no legal use in medicine and has a very high rate of addiction. It is three times stronger than morphine and the other medicinal narcotics.

Every narcotic, legal or illegal, is a potential poison. A single dose can be fatal. Approximately 60 percent of all deaths related to narcotic abuse are caused by overdose (street narcotics are often impure, increasing the risk of overdose); another 15 percent are the result of infected needles and other contaminated drug paraphernalia. One quarter of the deaths are caused by violence associated with drug trafficking.

Examples of stimulants, also called "uppers," include nicotine, cocaine, amphetamines (diet and pep pills), and "ice."

Cocaine comes in powder form ("coke") and a rocklike form ("crack"). It is inhaled, injected, or smoked. If crack is inhaled, one can use it several months or even years before becoming addicted. In contrast, when it is smoked it produces a very intense and instant "high" that lasts only eight to twenty minutes. The user can become addicted instantly or after as few as four times. "Crack" has been made affordable to virtually everyone and is readily available.

"Ice" comes in rock form or powder. As a powder, it is usually smoked in a glass pipe or cigarette. It is a very

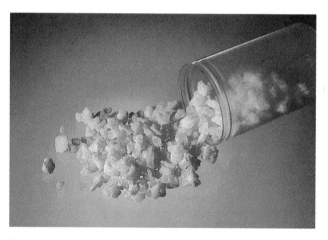

Drug abuse costs the U.S. $100 billion per year.

powerful stimulant with a "high" that lasts from eight to thirty hours. **No other drug damages the body as much as ice!** It may be sold as pure methamphetamine or as a mixture of heroin, crack, and methadrine.

Drugs that cause the user to have **hallucinations** are called hallucinogens or "psychedelics."

Psychedelics include LSD and PCP. The latter is extremely potent. One millionth of a gram can give an eight to twelve hour "trip." It is not addictive, but users develop a **tolerance** to it and thus use increasingly larger doses. A less infamous drug in this category is peyote cactus buttons, which are chewed. It is used legally by some American Indians in religious rites.

Table 26.3
Stimulants

Examples	Physiological Effects	Psychological Effects
• Nicotine • Cocaine (also called coke or crack) • Amphetamines (also called speed or crank); diet and pep pills • Ice (also called glass, L.A. glass, hot ice, or super ice)	• Stimulants: excite central nervous system; increase blood pressure, respiration, and heart rate (sometimes resulting in convulsions and stroke); reduce appetite; highly addictive; overdose is fatal; with increased use: dizziness, headaches, sleeplessness; with long term use: progressive brain damage, malnutrition, HIV infection (from shared needles). • Crack: sore throat, hoarseness, shortness of breath (leads to bronchitis and emphysema), eyes dilate, seeing "lights" around objects. • Ice: extreme energy, thrashing about and running aimlessly, sleeplessness, seizures, flushed skin, constricted pupils of eyes.	• Stimulants: initially feeling of being invincible, alertness, outgoing, excited; with increased use: feeling of anxiety; with long term use: hallucinations, psychosis. • Crack: intense euphoria, then crushing depression, intense feeling of self-hate; as it wears off: depression and sadness, intense anxiety about where to get more drugs, vicious, aggressive, paranoid. • Ice: major effect is toxic psychosis; euphoria, delusions of grandeur, think they are invisible, violent when provoked. • Cocaine: initial rush of energy, feeling confident; as it wears off: depression, moodiness, irritability, severe mental disorders.

Table 26.4
Hallucinogens (Psychodelics)

Examples	Physiological Effects	Psychological Effects
	• Hallucinogens usually: elevate blood pressure, dilate pupils, cause dizziness.	• Hallucinogens: all signs and symptoms very similar to state of temporary insanity and can lead to recurrent and even permanent insanity. Hallucinations, distorted sense of space/time, "bad trips" (panic attacks, delusions, paranoia) that can return as flashbacks months later.
• LSD (also called acid, pearly gates, wedding bells, micro-dot, heavenly blue, royal blue, or window pane)	• LSD: changes chromosomes and may result in birth defects of babies of users; bad trip.	• LSD: vivid hallucinations, feelings of overlapping/merging of the senses, expanded consciousness and mystical experiences, stimulated awareness and desire.
• PCP (also called crystal tea, angel dust, or hog)	• PCP: accumulates in fat cells and may remain in body longer than most drugs; impairs immune system, poor coordination, weight loss, speech problems, heart & lung failure, irreversible brain damage, convulsions, coma & death.	• PCP: Insensitivity to pain can lead to death; euphoria, depersonalization, hallucinations, delirium, amnesia, tunnel vision.
• Marijuana (also called pot, grass, weed, ganja, bhang, Mary Jane, hash, or joint)	• Marijuana long term use: bronchitis, emphysema and lung cancer, permanent memory impairment.	• Marijuana: may *not* hallucinate; pleasant relaxed feeling; giddiness; self-preoccupation; less precise thinking; task performance impaired; inertia develops; with prolonged use: may be withdrawn and apathetic, have anxiety reactions, paranoia. Eventually, decreased motivation and enthusiasm, reduced ability to absorb and integrate effectively, scholastic performance profoundly impaired (Heath n. d.).
• Inhalants (solvents, aerosols, and nitrites)	• Inhalants: slow reaction time; maybe headache, nausea and vomiting; can cause seizure, brain damage, suffocation, heart attack and death; double vision; sensitive to light; dizziness; loss of coordination; weakness; numbness; irregular heart beat; maybe liver and kidney failure; maybe bone marrow damage.	• Inhalants: giddiness, overexcitement, less inhibition, feelings of being all-powerful; powerfulness soon fades and leaves irritability.

Table 26.5
Designer Drugs

Examples	Physiological Effects	Psychological Effects
	• Designer drugs: depress blood pressure, depress respiration, relax muscles, relieve pain.	
• China white	• Nausea, slurred speech, loss of appetite, depressed blood pressure, relaxed muscles, relieves pain (Dye 1988).	
• MDMA (also called ecstasy, XTC, or Adam)	• MDMA: irregular heartbeat, intensifies heart problems, causes exhaustion, liver damage, sometimes brain damage, dilates pupils, dry mouth/throat, nervousness, muscle tension, may deplete neurotransmitters, causes brain damage in rats and monkeys (Dye 1988).	• MDMA: feelings of calm and relaxation, feeling of great insight, may lead to psychosis and psychological ''burnout'' even at moderate doses (Dye 1988).
• DOM (also called STP, Serenity, or Peace)		• DOM: low-dose, high-velocity trips that last a full day or more, high potential for panic reactions.
• DOB	• DOB: can trigger spasms in blood vessels, shutting down blood flow to arms and legs.	
• TMA		• At low dose: produces mescalinelike effects; at high dose: increased aggression, anger, paranoia (Dye 1988).
• PMA		• PMA: triggers panic attacks, fatal dose is equivalent to mild dose of mescaline (Dye 1988).

Marijuana became famous in the 1960s, and there is still political pressure to make it legal; however, the current street marijuana can be three to seven times more potent than the marijuana of the '60s. And extensive research is showing that it can have far-reaching effects.

Inhalants are sometimes listed separately because their effects are so serious. They reach the brain in seconds, and the effect lasts only a few minutes. They come in three types: (1) solvents—such as glue, gasoline, paints, paint thinner, typewriter correction fluid, lighter fluid, shoe polish, and liquid wax; (2) aerosols, such as hair spray, air fresheners, insect spray, and spray paint; and (3) nitrites, including amyl nitrite, nitrous oxide ("laughing gas"), and butyl nitrite (a room odorizer or liquid incense).

Designer drugs are made in laboratories and have many of the same properties as the drugs they simulate, such as pain relievers, anesthetics, or amphetamines.

There are 2,000 to 3,000 potential variations of amphetamines alone, and new drugs are continuously being concocted in illegal labs. These drugs are often extremely potent and can be contaminated or "botched" in the laboratory so that one dose can seriously damage the user. **The risk of overdose is high.**

Designer drugs include China white, which is a synthetic drug but is marketed by some dealers as pure heroin. MDMA was formerly a legal drug but was found to cause brain damage. It then became the "in" drug on the street in the 1980s. MDMA is known as a hallucinogenic amphetamine and is inhaled, injected, or swallowed. DOM was notorious in the 1960s for its low-dose, high-velocity effects. PMA is a toxic amphetamine derivative. TMA produces mescalinelike effects at low doses, whereas high doses are much like high doses of amphetamine (Dye 1988).

Many people unknowingly become drug abusers by failing to carefully follow the prescription on their medications.

Two of the most prevalent occurrences of abuse are: (1) taking prescription drugs (medications) with alcohol or with other medications and (2) taking one medication in quantities out of proportion to the needs for which it was originally prescribed. An example of this is the use of tranquilizers. It has been estimated that 2.4 million people abuse Valium, and even more abuse other prescription drugs (Spence n. d.). Twenty five percent of prescription drugs are capable of interacting with alcohol. Both alcohol and barbiturates slow the central nervous system,

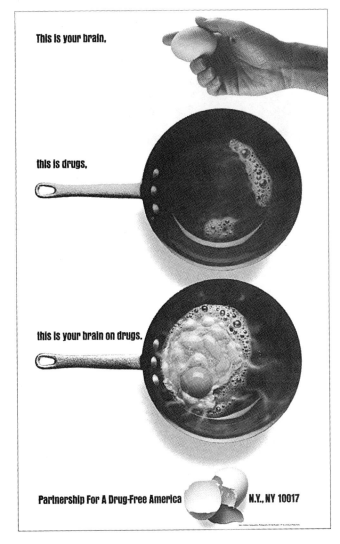

This is your brain.

this is drugs,

this is your brain on drugs.

Partnership For A Drug-Free America   N.Y., NY 10017

Figure 26.2
Any questions?

respiration, and the heart. *Combined, they can multiply the effect to cause death.* Tranquilizers mixed with alcohol can be just as dangerous.

Another unwitting abuse, particularly among the elderly, is overdosing because they forget that they have already taken their medications or they can't read the label and guess at the proper dosage. Some people take several prescriptions at the same time for different ailments, and sometimes these come from different doctors who are unaware that the patient is being treated by another physician. These drugs may interact dangerously or have an additive effect.

Accidental misuse can occur if drugs are taken from the medicine cabinet at night in the dark of if medications are stored in unlabeled bottles so that the wrong drug is taken. Using outdated drugs can also lead to problems. After a medication is no longer needed, any remaining part of it should be destroyed. Because people react differently to drugs, it is possible to become addicted to a prescription drug even when you follow the directions.

Anabolic steroids are prescription drugs that are being sold now on the black market and are being widely misused and abused.

Government studies estimate that there are one million users in the U.S. and that approximately one half of those are adolescents. Anabolic steroid users are likely to misuse or abuse other drugs and frequently share needles, increasing risk of disease transmission. Recent studies are showing **psychological dependence** on this drug. (See Concept 10 for more discussion on steroids and steroid substitutes.)

Women who are pregnant or trying to get pregnant, or who are nursing infants, can cause serious harm to the fetus or baby by using drugs, even prescription drugs.

Each year 375,000 infants are affected by their mothers' drug use. Government surveys estimate that 11 percent of pregnant women use "street drugs." The National Institute on Drug Abuse indicates these effects on the mother and the infant:

- Premature separation of the placenta from the womb and hemorrhage, threatening the lives of both the baby and the mother. (Cocaine use makes mothers twice as likely to have this problem as women on other drugs, and four times as likely as women not on drugs.)
- Miscarriage resulting from increased blood pressure and increasing uterine contractions. Birth defects also occur.
- Decreased oxygen to the baby and possibly a fetal stroke.
- Low birth weight and shorter babies.
- Babies are often born addicted and undergo withdrawal symptoms.
- Increased risk of "sudden infant death syndrome."
- Increased risk of learning disabilities, as well as delayed motor, speech, and language development (National Institute on Drug Abuse 1989).

Drugs can reduce inhibitions and interfere with clear thinking about sexual activity.

Drugs put the user at greater risk for unwanted sex and its consequences—unwanted pregnancies and sexually transmitted disease. There is a misconception that being on drugs makes you sexier. On the contrary, drugs are more likely to have the opposite effect. If you are under the influence of a substance, you may *think* you are cute and sexy when in fact you may just be loud and obnoxious to others. The drug also may make you feel bolder or more aggressive or may make you give in to pressure and do things you normally would not do.

The effects of specific drugs are described elsewhere in Concepts 25 and 26, but remember that they can affect sexual development for the rest of your life. Men can have lowered sperm count or develop feminine characteristics, and women may have menstrual problems. It is also worth reiterating that HIV can be contracted from contaminated needles as well as from sexual activity.

There are some risk factors that make one more likely to misuse or abuse drugs.

The potential for addiction depends on attitude, ease of access, method of use, mental state, and physiological sensitivity. For example, the risk is greater if one has used drugs (including alcohol) recreationally and thinks there is no problem with that. If drugs are readily available—perhaps in the home, dormitory, or sorority/frat house, on campus, or at work, one is more apt to become a user. If when you use a drug you choose the fastest method of getting a "hit," you are in great danger of becoming addicted. Having a history of child abuse or other childhood traumas increases your risk, as do feelings of stress, loneliness, anxiety, and other mental pain. Finally, there seems to be a genetic tendency such that if other members of your family have been alcoholics or abused other drugs, your chances of becoming addicted are significantly greater (Spence n. d., p. 5).

Note: It is possible to get an accidental "trip" by tasting a substance to see what it is, or by putting your hands in your mouth after handling drugs or drug paraphernalia. Remember, for some people, the first trip is the one that starts the addiction. With some drugs, the first trip is the last.

The reasons given for using alcohol and tobacco are very similar to the reasons given for using other drugs.

Typically, the reasons people give when asked why they use drugs or how they got started include the following:

- Everyone is doing it (peer pressure).
- It makes me feel grown up.
- I just want to see what it is like (to experiment).
- To have fun.
- It makes me feel good.
- As a rebellion against parents or authority.
- To cope with pressure/stress.

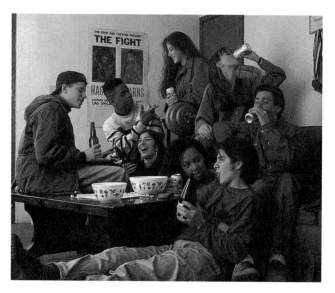

Peer pressure contributes to drug use and abuse.

The Facts: Where to Get Help

At some stage in the recovery process it may be helpful for the user to develop some skills and personal characteristics to avoid resuming old behavior patterns.

One of the characteristics needed is healthy self-esteem. You need to believe that you are important. It is also essential to learn skills to cope with problems and stress. Using a responsible process to make decisions is another skill that needs to be acquired. Knowing the effects and risks of drugs should help you to make more responsible decisions. To combat peer pressure, the ability to clearly and effectively say "no" is necessary. And finally, you need to choose friends whose values support, rather than undermine, your own (Morton 1991).

Denial is a difficult obstacle to overcome and a frequent problem of the abuser. Until it is confronted and controlled, recovery cannot begin. But once the first step is taken, help is available.

To get out of the trap you must seek help. You can talk to someone you trust, such as parent, teacher, or friend. Or you can seek help from a referral source such as an employee assistance program, family or university physician or hospital, or your city or county health department. These sources can help you get into a rehab program or support group. Some of the better-known, nationwide programs include: Alcoholics (or Narcotics or Cocaine) Anonymous and Al-Anon Family Groups. Another option is to look in the yellow pages of the telephone book for rehab programs operated by public and private agencies.

Still another possibility is to call a "hotline," and someone will direct you to help in your area. Three of these include:

National Institute on Drug Abuse (NIDA) Hotline	(1–800–662–HELP)
Cocaine Helpline	(1–800–COCAINE)
Just Say No International	(1–800–258–2766)

Suggested Readings

Avis, H. *Drugs and Life,* 2/e. Dubuque, IA: Wm. C. Brown Communications, Inc., 1993.

Carroll, C. R. *Drugs in Modern Society,* 3/e. Dubuque, IA: Wm. C. Brown Communications, Inc., 1993.

Fields, R. *Drugs and Alcohol in Perspective.* Dubuque, IA: Wm. C. Brown Communications, Inc., 1993.

Gallagher, W. "The Looming Menace of Designer Drugs." *Discover* August 1986: 24–34.

27

Preventing Sexually Transmitted Diseases

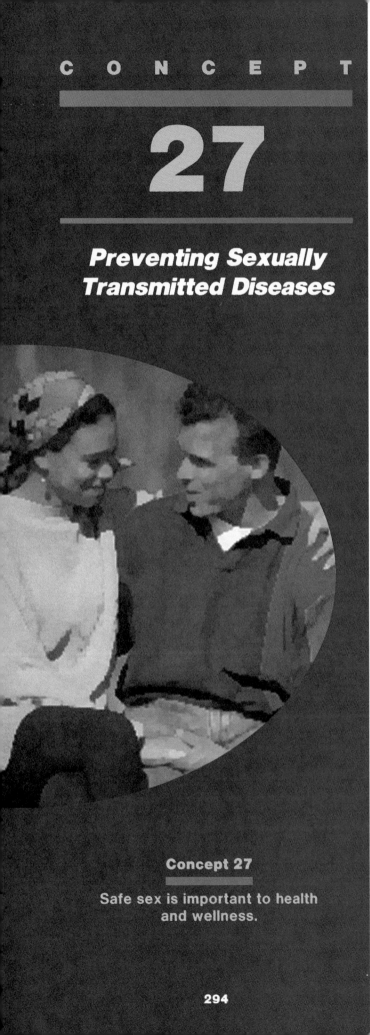

Concept 27

Safe sex is important to health and wellness.

Introduction

The sexual experience is an interpersonal one that influences the actions and behaviors of many people. It is basic to family life and fundamental to the reproduction of the human species. Approached responsibly, the human sexual experience contributes to wellness and quality of life in many ways. When approached irresponsibly, it can result in disease and personal and interpersonal suffering.

Health Goals for the Year 2000

- Prevent and control HIV infection.
- Reduce the incidence of sexually transmitted diseases.

Terms

AIDS (Acquired Immune Deficiency Syndrome)

An individual is said to have AIDS when he/she has developed several conditions (for example, pneumonia, tuberculosis, yeast infections, or other infections) when also infected with the HIV virus.

ARC (Aids Related Complex)

The development of HIV-related immunodeficiency conditions but not those considered to be AIDS.

Antibodies

Bodies in the bloodstream that react to overcome agents that attack the body (e.g., bacteria).

AZT (Antiviral Drug Zidovudine)

The first well-used treatment for those infected with HIV.

Chancre

A sore or lesion commonly associated with syphilis.

Chlamydia

A bacterial infection similar to gonorrhea that attacks the urinary tract and reproductive organs.

Genital Herpes

A viral infection that can attack any area of the body but often causes blisters on sexual organs.

Genital Warts

Warts, caused by a virus, that grow in the genital/anal area (also called condyloma).

Hepatitis B

A virus found in body secretions that causes many symptoms including fever, nausea, jaundice (yellow skin and eyes), and liver enlargement.

Gonorrhea

A bacterial infection of the mucous membranes including the eyes, throat, sexual organs, and other bodily organs.

HIV (Human Immunodeficiency Virus)

A virus that causes a breakdown of the immune system among humans, resulting in the inability of the body to fight infections. It is a precursor to AIDS.

Kaposi's Sarcoma

A type of cancer evidenced by purple sores (tumors) on the skin.

STD (Sexually Transmitted Diseases)

Diseases for which a primary method of transmission is sexual activity.

Pelvic Inflammatory Disease (PID)

An infection of the urethra (urine passage) that can lead to infertility among women.

Pubic Lice

Lice that attach themselves to the base of pubic hairs. Also called crabs.

Syphilis

An infection caused by a corkscrew-shaped bacteria that travels in the bloodstream and embeds itself in the mucous membranes of the body, including those of the sexual organs.

T-Cells

A disease-fighting blood cell that is damaged by the HIV virus.

White Blood Cells (Leucocytes)

A colorless blood cell that destroys disease-causing agents that attempt to invade the body.

General Facts

The healthy sexual experience can contribute to wellness in many ways.

Because it is interpersonal, the human sexual experience is a social one. It affects many more people than a sexual partner. Personal beliefs have much to do with the feelings that participants have toward the sexual experience; thus, spiritual wellness is influenced. Because the sexual experience is often emotionally charged, emotional wellness is also affected. Clearly, intellectual decisions are made concerning the experience, so intellectual well-being is a factor to consider as well. The sexual act is a physical experience that can be pleasurable but that has many long-lasting physical consequences. All five wellness dimensions are involved in decisions concerning participation in, the meaningfulness of, and the long-term consequences of the sexual experience. The healthy sexual experience requires sensitive and thoughtful consideration of the consequences.

Decisions concerning sexual behavior have lifelong consequences.

Positive consequences of a sexual experience include childbearing and an enriched, happy family life. Negative lifelong consequences can include unwanted pregnancy, emotional and physical stress, and strained social relationships, among others. Unsafe sex also takes a toll in disease and death for large numbers of people worldwide.

Unsafe sexual activity can result in disease, poor health, and much pain and suffering.

Until the 1940s, sexually transmitted diseases (STDs) were a major cause of death. The discovery of penicillin and other antibiotics, and improved public health practices, lowered the death rate from STDs, but they remained a significant health problem. In 1992, STDs became one of the ten leading causes of death in the United States, principally because of the high death rate from acquired immune deficiency syndrome (AIDS) caused by the human immunodeficiency virus (HIV). They will continue to be a leading cause of death in the future if a cure is not found soon.

Each year twelve million Americans, mostly teenagers and young adults, are affected by STDs. One quarter of teenagers who are sexually active have need of treatment for STDs annually. Of the more than fifty different STDs, gonorrhea is the most prevalent, but most cases can be treated with antibiotics if detected early. Other common STDs are syphilis, chlamydia, genital herpes, genital warts, pubic lice, and hepatitis B. HIV/AIDS is the most serious STD because there is no known cure.

In addition to the general national health goals designed to prevent, control, and reduce STDs, specific goals include increasing STD education in schools and colleges, extending regulations to protect workers, and improving services through community agencies designed to help the general public.

The Facts About HIV/AIDS

Of all STDs, HIV/AIDS poses the most significant health threat to the nation and the world.

Health experts indicate that we are in the midst of a worldwide HIV/AIDS epidemic. The first known cases of

AIDS were identified in 1981, and in 1984, HIV was identified as the cause. It became one of the ten leading causes of death in 1992, and it is a leading cause of potential years of lost life in the United States.

HIV is the virus that causes AIDS.

When a person "tests positive" for HIV, it means that a blood test has indicated the presence in the body of the human immunodeficiency virus (HIV). HIV invades the body's immune system cells, even killing them. This results in damage to the immune system and the body's ability to fight infections. Typically the **T-cells,** or helper white blood cells, are most affected by HIV. For this reason, a low T-cell count is one method used to determine the progress of the disease.

Antibodies in the blood that normally fight infections are ineffective in stopping the HIV from invading the body. Many researchers believe that HIV has an "assistant," or co-factor, that triggers the HIV to do its damage. At present scientists have yet to identify the co-factor and are unclear of the reasons why HIV affects the immune system as it does.

First HIV infects the body. Over time, **white blood cells** are damaged and antibodies become ineffective. Depending on time elapsed and individual variance in the progression of the disease, AIDS may develop or no symptoms may appear (see figure 27.1).

After HIV enters the body, it takes several months before enough antibodies are developed to be able to detect its presence. For this reason, existing tests may not yet be able to detect HIV. Even in this early period, HIV *can* be transmitted. Of those infected with HIV, five of ten will develop AIDS within ten years. Four of ten will develop **aids related complex** (ARC—other illness associated with HIV), and one in ten will have no apparent ill effects. An individual has AIDS when he or she is infected with HIV and develops various diseases because of impairment of the immune system. Among the conditions that indicate the presence of AIDS are pneumonia, tuberculosis, **Kaposi's sarcoma,** and yeast infections. Other symptoms include fatigue, swollen glands, rashes, weight loss, and loss of appetite. Life expectancy for those with all of the symptoms of AIDS is two to five years on the average, though many have survived as long as ten years.

There is no known cure for AIDS.

For those infected with HIV/AIDS, there is no known cure. The Surgeon General of the United States has indicated that the fatality rate of those diagnosed with AIDS approaches 100 percent. Some treatments, such as **AZT,** though very expensive, may extend survival of those with AIDS, but it is not a cure. Among the drugs showing promise of effectiveness are DDI and DDC. Many others are now being studied. Some work best in combination with

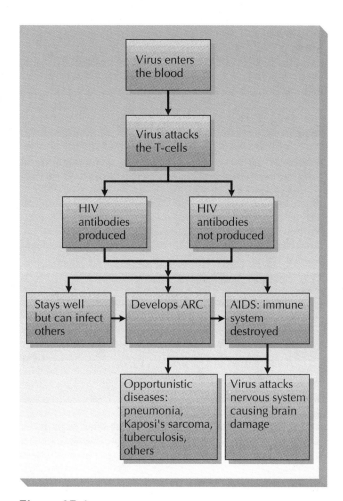

Figure 27.1

Stages of the HIV infection.

From Clint Bruess and Glenn Richardson, *Decisions for Health*, 3d ed. Copyright © 1992 Wm. C. Brown Communications, Inc., Dubuque, Iowa. All Rights Reserved. Reprinted by permission.

others. Because HIV appears to adapt quickly to various medications, periodic changes in medicines are often necessary. A high-priority health goal for the nation is the development of an HIV vaccine.

Many people with HIV do not know they are infected.

Recent public health statistics indicate that many people are HIV positive (have the HIV virus) and do not know it. This complicates efforts to achieve national health goals associated with the condition because HIV can be transmitted by unknowing individuals. Lack of awareness also prevents early treatment.

Only a blood test eight to ten weeks or more after exposure can detect the presence of HIV. More than one test may be necessary to accurately detect HIV in the blood because of the lengthy incubation period. It is especially important that those who are currently at risk or those who may have been at risk in recent years be tested to determine if they have the HIV virus.

Table 27.1
Factors Associated with Reducing Risk of HIV/AIDS.

- Abstain from sexual activity.
- Limit sexual activity to a noninfected partner. A lifetime partner who never has sex with other people or never uses injected drugs (other than medically administered) is the only "safe" partner.
- Avoid sexual activity or other activity that puts you in contact with another person's semen, vaginal fluids, or blood.
- Use a new condom (latex) every time you have sex, especially with a partner who is not known to be "safe."
- Use a water-based lubricant with condoms, because petroleum-based lubricants increase risk of condom failure.
- Abstain from risky sexual activity such as oral and anal sex, and sex with high-risk people (prostitutes, those with HIV or other STD).
- Do not inject drugs.
- Never share a needle or drug paraphernalia.
- Avoid other STDs. Those who have had an STD have increased risk of HIV/AIDS.

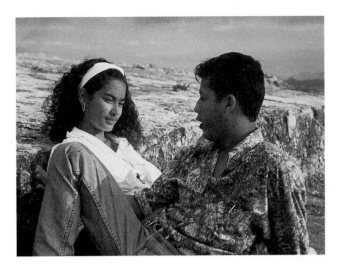

Open communication concerning sexual histories is important in preventing STDs.

Three mechanisms account for virtually all HIV transmission.

The three primary mechanisms responsible for the transmission of HIV are sexual activity, contact with infected blood (sharing needles or transfusion), and transmission from mother to child (before birth, during birth, or through breastfeeding).

Reduced risk of HIV/AIDS will result if exposure to HIV and to the methods of transmission are avoided.

You can lower your risk of HIV infection by adopting lifestyles that are presented in table 27.1

The HIV/AIDS epidemic is a problem that affects all members of society.

HIV is NOT spread through the air or in saliva, sweat, or urine. It does NOT spread by hugging, sharing foods or beverages, or casual kissing. Contact with phones, silverware, or toilet seats does NOT cause the spread of HIV.

HIV must invade the blood system in order for a person to become infected. People who had blood transfusions prior to 1985 had an increased risk of HIV transmission, but since that time the safety of the blood supply has increased dramatically. There is no danger in donating blood, only in receiving HIV-infected blood. Babies born to women with HIV have increased risk of being HIV infected.

The Facts About Other Sexually Transmitted Diseases

The most frequently reported STD in the United States is gonorrhea.

Though the number of cases has dramatically decreased since 1981, gonorrhea is still the most frequently reported STD. There has not been a decline in the incidence of gonorrhea in recent years among ethnic and racial minorities or among teenagers, indicating a need to educate these populations concerning the disease.

Gonorrhea is a bacterial infection that can be treated with modern antibiotics (usually penicillin) if detected early. However, recent strains of the gonorrhea organism have become resistant to antibiotics, causing concern among public health officials.

Sexual activity is the principal method of disease transmission, and penile and vaginal gonorrhea are the most common types. Symptoms usually occur within three to seven days after the bacteria enters the system. Among men the most common symptoms are painful urination and penile drip or discharge. Symptoms are less apparent among women, though painful urination and vaginal discharge are not uncommon. Other types of gonorrhea often have fewer symptoms in both sexes. Chills, fever, painful bowel movements, and sore throat are among the most common.

Early detection by a culture or "smear" test can result in a quick, complete cure. Early cure is especially important for females because gonorrhea can lead to **pelvic inflammatory disease,** which can result in infertility.

Syphilis was a serious national health problem in the 1940s, when it was ten times more prevalent than it is now. In recent years, however, there has been a dramatic increase in this STD. Syphilis was the first STD for which national control measures were initiated.

Like gonorrhea, syphilis is a bacterial infection that can be effectively treated with antibiotics such as penicillin. The corkscrew-shaped bacteria cannot live long outside the human organism. However, it can be easily transmitted from person to person through sexual contact. The bacteria then embeds itself in the walls of the mucous membranes, where it can be transmitted throughout the body. Syphilis can also be transmitted by an infected mother to her unborn child (congenital syphilis).

Once the bacteria invades the body, it typically takes one to three weeks before it can be detected. The symptoms of syphilis include **chancres** that change from a red swelling to a hardened ulcer on the skin. Even if not treated, the sores disappear after a period of one to five weeks. It is important to get treatment even after this primary phase of the disease because it is still contagious and the disease is still present.

After several weeks or longer, secondary symptoms occur, such as rash, loss of hair, joint pain, sore throat, and swollen glands. Even after these symptoms go away, untreated syphilis lingers in a latent phase. Serious health problems may result, including blindness, deafness, tumors, and stillbirth.

Early detection is important and can be diagnosed from chancre discharge or a blood test several weeks after the appearance of chancres. There is an association between syphilis and the spread of HIV. Apparently the presence of chancres greatly increases the risk of transmitting HIV during sexual activity.

Of all STDs, genital herpes is among the most commonly spread because of a lack of awareness of infection.

Genital herpes, one of the most commonly reported STDs, is caused by the herpes simplex virus (HSV). HSV is a family of many viruses that can produce various disorders in humans, such as shingles and chicken pox. HSV Type 1 is often called lip or oral herpes because it causes cold sores and fever blisters on the lips and in the mouth. HSV Type 2 is often referred to as the STD type because it is known to cause genital lesions. These lesions or blisters on the penis, vagina, or cervix usually occur two to twelve days after infection and typically last a week to a month. Swollen glands and headache may also occur.

Though type 2 HSV is generally referred to as the STD type, it is now known that both Types 1 and 2 HSV can cause genital sores, just as either type can cause lip and oral sores. At present there is no cure for genital sores

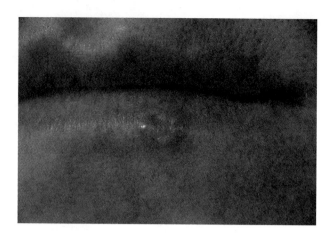

Lip or oral herpes.

caused by HSV, though some prescription drugs can help treat the disease symptoms. HSV can remain dormant in the body for long periods of time, and as a result, symptoms can reoccur at any time.

Genital herpes is especially contagious when the blisters are present. Condom use or abstinence from sexual activity when symptoms are present can reduce the risk of transmission of the disease. Herpes is more dangerous for women than men because of the association between genital herpes and cervical cancer and the risk of transmitting the disease to the unborn.

Some lesser known STDs are significant health problems.

Genital warts, chlamydia, pubic lice, and hepatitis B are examples of lesser known, but very prevalent, STDs. Some general information about these diseases is presented in table 27.2.

Other Important Facts Concerning STDs

Public health statistics indicate that young people are especially at risk for STDs.

Teens and young adults are especially at risk of getting STDs. Almost nine of ten cases of STDs occur among people between the ages of 15–29. One of five people in the U.S. will be treated for an STD by the age of 21. There is evidence that HIV/AIDS incidence on college campuses is significant. One study showed that 40 percent of college women seeking pregnancy tests were infected.

Probable reasons for the high risk among teens and young adults are:

• Perceived immortality. Many teens feel that disease is something that happens to other people, not to them. For example, one study indicates that a large proportion of teens do not feel that they are the "kind of person who would get AIDS."

- Risky sexual activity. Evidence suggests that teens and young adults often do not follow the STD guidelines presented earlier in this concept. For example, data suggest that 70 percent are sexually active by age 20, yet few have used condoms.
- Experimenting with life-styles. Young people are more likely to experiment with drugs and sex than are older people, thus increasing risk of STDs in this population.

Public health statistics indicate that minority groups are especially at risk for STDs.

The incidence of gonorrhea is more than six times higher among blacks than whites, and there is an even higher rate of syphilis among blacks. Blacks and Hispanics are disproportionately represented among those with HIV/AIDS. Many of the minorities with high incidence of STDs are also among those with fewer economic resources and may be unable to obtain adequate medical care. The incidence of STDs, especially HIV/AIDS, is high among homosexuals. Health goals for the nation emphasize the need for education, personal counseling, and medical assistance for these populations. Ignorance about STDs, failure to receive proper treatment, and failure to receive counseling on how to prevent spread of disease among infected people are major reasons why STDs are prevalent today.

STDs can be considered as life-style related conditions.

Most of the risk of STD infection can be eliminated by adopting healthy life-styles as noted in table 27.1. We can control behaviors associated with high risk. Only children born to those with STDs and young children who are not in control of their own behavior lack the ability to alter life-styles to reduce risk of STDs.

A cure for STDs such as HIV/AIDS is a top-priority national health goal. But until cures are found, prevention through healthy life-styles is a key. Sound health practices among those who are infected are also critical to meeting national goals.

Fear of discrimination may limit our effectiveness in dealing with the HIV/AIDS epidemic and the high incidence of other STDs.

Public health sources indicate that some people are reluctant to seek medical assistance, even when symptoms of STDs are present, for fear that detection will result in discrimination. Among the common fears are loss of employment or housing, discrimination in hiring or housing, rejection for medical treatment, and loss of educational opportunities. Overcoming fear of STDs and reducing discrimination among those who may be infected are important steps to reducing the incidence of STDs.

Table 27.2
Facts About Lesser Known STDs.

Genital Warts (Condylomas)
- Are approximately 5% of all reported STDs
- Are most prevalent in ages 15–24
- Are caused by the human papilloma virus (HPV)
- Are linked to cervical and genital cancers
- Are hard and yellow or gray on dry skin
- Are soft and pink, red or dark on moist skin
- There is no known culture test.
- Early diagnosis is important (because of association with forms of cancer).
- The prescription drug Podophyllin is the best treatment.

Chlamydia
- There are 4,000,000 cases annually
- Mostly affects women and children
- May cause pelvic inflammatory disease
- May cause heart, joint, and organ damage
- Hard to detect because of few symptoms
- Can be treated with antibiotics

Pubic Lice (Crabs)
- Are pinhead-sized insects (parasites) that feed on the blood of the host
- Are transmitted by sexual contact and/or contact with contaminated clothes, bedding, and other washable items
- Symptoms include itching; some people have no symptoms.
- Can be controlled by using medicated lotion and shampoos, and by washing contaminated bedding, etc.
- Do NOT transmit other STDs

Hepatitis B (Hepatitis A and C are not STDs)
- Can be spread by sharing needles, sharing eating utensils, or by other personal contact
- Only STD for which there is an effective vaccine
- Can be diagnosed from a blood sample
- Symptoms include fever, vomiting, liver inflammation, jaundice
- Isolation is necessary to avoid transmission to others

Hotlines are available to help those who want information concerning STDs such as HIV/AIDS.

The following National AIDS hotlines are toll free and allow the caller to retain anonymity:

(English) 1–800–342–AIDS (342–2437)
(Spanish) 1–800–344–SIDA (or, 344–7432)

Suggested Readings

Bruess, C., and G. Richardson. *Decisions for Health.* 4th ed. Dubuque, IA: Wm. C. Brown Publishers, 1992.
Food and Drug Administration. *Condoms and Sexually Transmitted Diseases.* Rockville, MD: U.S. Department of Health and Human Services, 1990.
Gorman, C. "Invincible AIDS." *Time* 140(1992):30.
"Teenagers and AIDS." *Newsweek* August 3(1992):44.

28

Preventing Other Health Threats Through Life-Style Change

Concept 28

Many diseases and conditions that cause pain, suffering, and premature death in modern society are associated with unhealthy life-styles.

Introduction

Each year, many deaths and much pain and suffering could be prevented by altering life-styles associated with various diseases and health threats. Among these conditions are cancer, injuries, emotional disorders (including suicide), and diabetes. Cancer is second only to heart disease among the leading causes of death. Deaths from heart disease have decreased in recent years, but deaths from cancer have increased. If this trend continues, cancer will soon become the leading cause of death in North America. Injuries are ranked fourth, diabetes sixth, and suicide eighth as the leading causes of death in our society.

Health Goals for the Year 2000

- Reverse the rise in cancer deaths.
- Reduce the incidence of diabetes.
- Reduce the complications of diabetes.
- Reduce deaths related to diabetes.
- Reduce deaths caused by injuries.
- Reduce hospitalizations resulting from nonfatal injuries.
- Reduce suicides and suicide attempts.
- Reduce the prevalence of mental disorders.

Terms

Benign Tumor

A slow-growing tumor that does not spread to other parts of the body.

Cancer

A disease characterized by abnormal, uncontrolled cell growth that will ultimately spread throughout the body if not treated.

Carcinogen

A substance that tends to produce a tumor or cancer. Examples include asbestos fibers and various substances in tobacco.

Carcinoma

A malignant or invasive form of tumor.

Diabetes (Type I, Insulin-dependent)

A chronic metabolic disease characterized by high blood-sugar (glucose) levels that requires insulin therapy.

Diabetes (Type II, Adult onset)

A chronic metabolic disease characterized by high blood sugar, usually not requiring insulin therapy. Also called adult onset or maturity onset diabetes.

Glucose Tolerance Test

A test used to diagnose diabetes. It consists of a blood-sugar measurement following the ingestion of a standard amount of sugar (glucose) after a period of fasting.

Insulin

A hormone that regulates blood-sugar levels.

Malignant Tumor

Malignant means "growing worse." A malignant tumor is one that is considered to be cancerous and will spread throughout the body if not treated.

Mental Disorders

A problem that results in inability to cope effectively with daily living and is often characterized by the need for special medical or psychological assistance. Also referred to as emotional disorders.

Metastases

The spread of cancer cells to other parts of the body.

The Facts About Cancer

Cancer is a group of more than 100 different diseases (Public Health Service 1991, p. 416).

Throughout the human body, new cells are constantly being created to replace older ones. For reasons unknown, abnormal cells sometime develop that are capable of uncontrolled growth. **Benign tumors** are generally not considered to be cancerous because their growth is restricted to a specific area of the body by a protective membrane. Treatment is important because any tumor can interfere with normal bodily functioning. Once removed, a benign tumor typically will not return.

Malignant tumors are called **carcinomas** because they are capable of uncontrolled growth that can cause death to tissue. Malignant cells invade healthy tissues and deplete them of nutrition and interfere with a multitude of tissue functions. In the early stages of cancer, malignant tumors are located in a small area and can be more easily treated or removed. In advanced cancer (**metastases**), the cells invade the blood or lymph systems and travel throughout the body. When this occurs, cancer becomes much more difficult to treat. Early detection is very important in the treatment and cure of cancer.

Cancer is on the increase in our society.

One of every five deaths in the United States is caused by some form of cancer. One of three people now living will have cancer at some time in his/her life. It is the cause of much suffering and accounts for a large portion of the money spent on health care. Other diseases, such as heart disease and stroke, have decreased in recent years, but the rate of cancer continues to increase. Lung cancer accounts for much of the recent increase in cancer cases in North America.

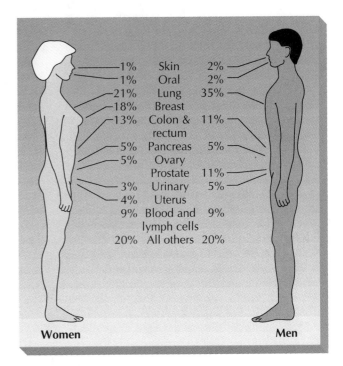

Figure 28.1

Cancer incidence by site and sex.

Source: Data from the American Cancer Society.

Of the more than 100 forms of cancer, four account for more than half of all illness and death.

The four types of cancer that account for the majority of deaths are lung cancer, colorectal cancer, breast cancer, and prostate cancer (see fig. 28.1). For women aged 50–60, breast cancer is the most prevalent form of cancer. Prostate cancer risk for men is especially high after age 55. Cancer risk among blacks is higher than among whites. Nonmalignant skin cancer is the most common form of cancer in the United States, but because it can be relatively easily detected and treated if discovered early, it is not among the leading cancer killers.

Many factors are associated with increased risk of cancer; among them is unhealthy life-styles.

Genetics, environment, and life-style are general categories of risk factors associated with cancer. Those who have a family history of cancer have a greater risk than those who have no family history. Whereas genetic factors are not within your personal control, many environmental and life-style factors are. Figure 28.2 illustrates the contribution of various life-style and environmental factors to cancer mortality. Controlling these risk factors can considerably reduce cancer risk.

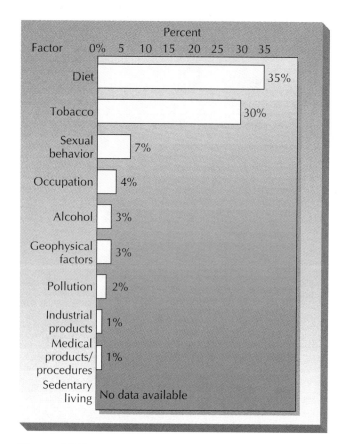

Percent

Factor	0% 5 10 15 20 25 30 35
Diet	35%
Tobacco	30%
Sexual behavior	7%
Occupation	4%
Alcohol	3%
Geophysical factors	3%
Pollution	2%
Industrial products	1%
Medical products/ procedures	1%
Sedentary living	No data available

Figure 28.2

Lifestyle and environmental cancer risk factors.

Source: Data from the American Cancer Society.

Decreasing fat in the diet, increasing complex carbohydrate consumption, and eliminating tobacco use would dramatically reduce cancer risk. Examples of some of the less well-known risk categories include geophysical (radiation), pollution (PCB, a byproduct of the plastic industry), industrial products (asbestos, DDT, and 2-4-5-T [also known as agent orange]), and medical products (X ray). Substances contained in many of these products are considered to be **carcinogens** because exposure to them causes cancer. Avoiding exposure to or consumption of carcinogens reduces the risk of cancer.

It is now known that sedentary living is a risk factor for cancer. Those who are active have less risk of colorectal, breast, and reproductive system cancer. One recent study showed that individuals with low levels of fitness had a greater risk of death from cancer. To date, however, the percentage of risk attributed to sedentary living has not been determined as it has been for other risk factors.

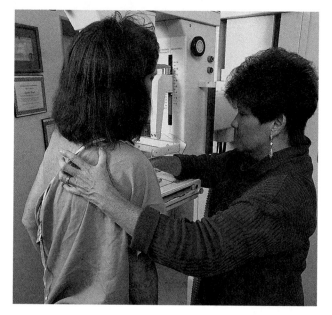

Cancer risk can be reduced by periodic medical tests and self screening.

Recognizing early warning signals can help reduce the risk of cancer.

The acronym CAUTION will help you remember these early warning signs. Look for the following:

C Changes in bowel or bladder habits

A A sore that does not heal

U Unusual bleeding or discharge

T Thickening or lump in the breast or elsewhere

I Indigestion or difficulty swallowing

O Obvious change in a wart or mole

N Nagging cough or hoarseness

Regular self-examinations and periodic medical tests can help reduce risk of cancer.

Self-examination is one screening method that can detect cancer early. In addition, regular medical tests should be sought. Table 28.1 lists some of the tests that should be performed and provides guidelines as to frequency and the type of individual who could most benefit from the test.

Table 28.1
Cancer Screening Guidelines

Test or Procedure	Sex	Age	Frequency
Cancer checkup (exam for cancers of the thyroid, testicles, prostate, ovaries, lymph nodes, mouth, and skin)	Men/women	20 to 40 Over 40	Every 3 years Every year
Testicle self-evaluation	Men	Over 20	Every month
Rectal exam for prostate cancer	Men	Over 40	Every year
Colorectal cancer hemocult test (sample of stool examined for the presence of blood)	Men/women	Over 50	Every year
Sigmoidoscopy (examination of a portion of the large intestine)	Men/women	50 and over	Every 3 to 5 years
Pap test	Women	Sexually active women over 18 should have an annual Pap test and pelvic exam.	
Pelvic exam	Women		
Breast self-exam	Women	20 and over	Every month
Breast exam by physician	Women	Over 20	Every year
Mammogram	Women	35 to 39 40 to 49 50 and over	Baseline Every 1 to 2 years Every year
Endometrial tissue sample (sample of tissue from the lining of the uterus)	Women	At menopause for women at high risk (history of infertility, obesity, failure to ovulate, abnormal uterine bleeding, or estrogen therapy)	At menopause for women at high risk
Skin cancer check	Men/women	At any age if at high risk because of lengthy exposure to sun	As recommended by your physician. See your doctor if changes occur in warts or moles.

Source: *Healthplex Magazine,* 8, 1992, with data from the American Cancer Society.

Table 28.2
Strategies for Preventing Cancer

- Eat a healthy diet: reduce fat to less than 30%, increase complex carbohydrates, decrease simple carbohydrates, avoid junk food, and eat green and yellow vegetables
- Eliminate tobacco use: cigarettes, other smoking, and smokeless tobacco
- Perform regular activity: be physically fit, do daily exercise, and avoid obesity
- Reduce sun and ultraviolet light exposure: use sunscreen, wear protective clothing, and avoid exposure to sun and tanning lights
- Do regular self-screening and medical testing (see table 28.1)
- Avoid carcinogens in food (such as sodium nitrate in bacon) and in other sources (such as insecticides)
- Use moderation if you drink alcohol
- Avoid breathing polluted air
- Avoid excessive X rays

There are several strategies that can be followed to help prevent cancer.

The national health goals focus on altering life-styles to improve health and well-being. Some of the strategies that can help prevent cancer are shown in table 28.2

The Facts About Diabetes

There are two general classifications of diabetes that cause health risk to many individuals.

Glucose is a sugar in the blood that is a source of energy. Normally, glucose levels range from 50 to 100 mg per each 100 ml of blood. Diabetes is a disease that occurs when the blood glucose is chronically high. There are as many as thirty different reasons for high blood sugar. Therefore, diabetes is really many different diseases, not just one. There is no cure for diabetes, but in most cases it can be controlled with proper medication and a healthy life-style.

Insulin, a hormone produced by the pancreas, regulates the glucose in the blood. When a person's body fails to produce adequate insulin and the individual needs to take insulin (oral or injection) to regulate blood-glucose levels, he or she is said to have **Type I (insulin-dependent) diabetes.** About ten percent of all diabetics have Type I diabetes.

Type II (adult-onset) diabetes is typically noninsulin dependent and can often be controlled with significant life-style changes and drugs other than insulin. There is a familial predisposition to both Type I and Type II, though the predisposition is greater for Type I diabetes. Some people with Type II diabetes do not produce enough insulin to regulate their blood-sugar levels, but more commonly they are "insensitive" to insulin, so the body cannot effectively use available blood sugar.

Diabetes and related conditions are a leading cause of death in our society.

Twelve million people have diabetes in the United States. Of those, seven million are aware of their condition and the other five million are not. People with diabetes have a shortened life as well as many short-term and long-term complications associated with the disease. It is especially important for them to recognize their illness because proper medication and changes in life-style can greatly reduce the complications of the disease and the death rate associated with it.

Blacks and American Indians are especially at risk of diabetes. Not only is the death rate higher among these groups, but so are the health problems associated with the disease.

Diabetes is associated with other health problems.

Those with diabetes have an increased risk of additional health problems. For example, diabetes is considered to be a risk factor for heart disease and high blood pressure. Diabetics have a higher rate of kidney failure (including the need for kidney transplants and kidney dialysis), a high incidence of blindness, and a high incidence of lower limb amputation. Women with diabetes also have a high rate of pregnancy complications.

Life-style changes can help reduce the symptoms and complications typically associated with diabetes.

Three of the health goals for the nation for the year 2000 reflect life-style changes that can help reduce health problems associated with diabetes. These goals are:

- Reduce overweight (fatness) in the general population. Reducing body fat is probably the most significant way to reduce the incidence of diabetes in our society.
- Increase daily exercise. Regular exercise results in calories expended and is one way to help reduce overfatness. It also helps regulate blood-sugar levels and helps body cells become more sensitive to insulin.
- Reduce dietary fat intake, increase intake of complex carbohydrates, and decrease total calorie intake. Particularly important is the value of a sound diet in reducing body fatness.

Once diabetes is recognized, adherence to a treatment program is essential to prevent related conditions.

Controlling weight, eating properly, and performing regular exercise can help prevent the symptoms of Type II diabetes in particular. In addition to these strategies, adherence to a regular medication schedule and stress management are important. However, if symptoms such as nausea, fatigue, weakness, excessive thirst, and loss of weight occur, as they often do in Type I diabetics, or if blurred vision, numbness of the limbs, and skin or gum infections occur, medical help should be sought. A **glucose tolerance test** can be performed to help detect the existence of diabetes. Early diagnosis resulting from attention to the symptoms described above can expedite successful treatment.

The Facts About Other Health Threats

Injuries are a major cause of death and suffering.

Not only are injuries the fourth leading cause of death among people of all ages; they claim more lives than chronic and infectious diseases among people aged 40 and younger. The major causes of injuries are shown in table 28.3.

Injuries also account for much pain and suffering. Of all hospital stays, one in six results from a nonfatal injury. Injury rates are higher among males than females, and they are quite high among ethnic and racial minority groups.

Table 28.3
Major Causes of Injuries

- Motor vehicle crashes
- Falls
- Poisoning
- Drowning
- Residential fires

Source: Public Health Service, 1991.

Table 28.4

Steps to Reduce Injuries

Reduce Motor Vehicle Accidents
- Reduce driving under the influence of alcohol.
- Increase use of shoulder seat belts and air bags.
- Reduce driving speed.
- Use motorcycle helmets.
- Improve safety of off-road vehicles.
- Increase safety programs for pedestrians and cyclists.
- Establish more effective licensing for very young and older drivers.

Improve Home and Neighborhood Environments
- Enact laws requiring new handguns be designed to minimize discharge by children.
- Extend laws requiring sprinkler systems in homes with high risk of fire.
- Increase presence of functional smoke detectors in homes.
- Increase injury education in schools.
- Require effective face, head, eye, and mouth protection in sports.
- Improve pool and boat safety education.
- Learn cardiopulmonary resuscitation.
- Properly mark poisons and prescription drugs.
- Properly package and store poisons and prescription drugs (childproof).
- Shift to nontoxic fuels for cooking.
- Provide poison education for children and older populations.

Changes in life-styles can reduce injury rates.

A major conclusion of the Public Health Service is that the prevention of injuries requires the combined efforts of many fields, including health, education, transportation, law, engineering, architecture, and safety science.

The second major conclusion of the Public Health Service is that alcohol is "intimately associated" with the causes and severity of injuries (see Concept 25). Other life-style behaviors are also associated with reducing injury incidence, and some of the steps that can be taken to reduce these injuries are listed in table 28.4.

Improved occupational safety could help reduce injury rates.

Many of the nation's health goals focus on improving occupational safety, especially among construction, health care (nurses, etc.), farm, transportation, and mine workers. (For more details, see the suggested readings at the end of this Concept.)

Many **mental disorders** pose threats to health and wellness.

The health goals for the nation identify suicide, schizophrenia, and depression as the most serious mental disorders needing attention. (Though the Public Health Service uses the term mental disorders, they are sometimes called emotional disorders.) Other common mental disorders are sleep disturbances, panic disorders, antisocial personality disorders, fears, and phobias.

Mental disorders result in loss of life, injury, and inability to function, and they cost the public millions of dollars annually.

Nearly one in ten among the adult population suffers from a mental disorder that limits ability to function effectively and requires special assistance. Depression and other mood disorders affect one in twenty people. These disorders cost $73 billion dollars annually, primarily from loss of productivity. The most serious outcome of mental disorders is suicide (30,000 annually).

Reducing the incidence of suicide and serious injury from suicide attempts is an important national health goal.

Suicide attempts are common among all age groups. Men are more likely to commit suicide than women. Among male teenagers, it is the second leading cause of death, and male teenagers with antisocial personality disorders are especially susceptible.

Depression is closely associated with suicide, as are alcohol and drug abuse. Inability to cope with stressful life events may contribute to suicide. Examples of precipitating events are divorce, separation, loss of a loved one, unemployment, and financial setbacks.

The best chance for reducing suicides appears to be early detection and treatment of mental disorders such as depression. Professional help should be sought, and as many concerned people as possible should be recruited to help the suicidal individual seek professional assistance. Experts suggest that threats of suicide must not be taken lightly.

Depression is a common mental disorder that most often can be treated effectively.

At some time in life, most people occasionally feel depressed or "blue." This type of depression is usually not a mental disorder. People with clinical depression (classified as a mental disorder) have chronic feelings of guilt, hopelessness, low self esteem, and dejection. They frequently have trouble sleeping, loss of appetite, lack of interest in social activities, lack of interest in sex, and inability to concentrate.

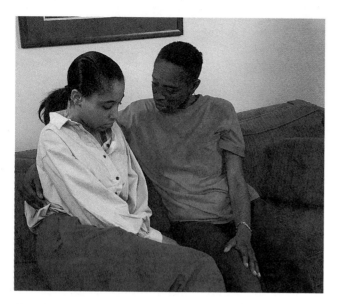

The help of a professional is often necessary to treat depression.

Among the life-style changes that can help relieve symptoms are regular exercise, increased social contact, realistic goal setting, and removing oneself from situations that contribute to depression. These changes, however, must often be accompanied by professional therapy and/or medication. Helping an individual to change lifestyles and to seek professional help are important because depression is often associated with suicide.

Sleep disorders can often be helped by life-style changes.

Sleep disorders, especially insomnia (long-term problems with sleep) can result in depression and other dysfunctions. Physiological problems in the brain can cause sleep disorders, but most often they are a result of depression, stress, chronic pain, or abuse of alcohol/drugs. Severe sleep disorders will require professional help. However, there are some guidelines to aid one in sleeping. Examples are: avoid excessive caffeine or alcohol, exercise regularly, and use stress-management techniques. Establishing a regular routine for sleeping can also be helpful and should include regular sleeping hours, a stress-reduction time before bedtime, and a healthy sleeping environment.

Suggested Readings

American Cancer Society. *Cancer Facts and Figures—1991*. New York: The American Cancer Society, 1992.

Bruess, C., and G. Richardson. *Decisions for Health*. Dubuque, IA: Wm. C. Brown Publishers, 1992.

Levy, M., et al. *Life and Health: Targeting Wellness*. New York: McGraw Hill, 1992.

Public Health Service. *Healthy People 2000: National Health Promotion and Disease Prevention Objectives*. Washington, D.C.: U.S. Government Printing Office, 1991.

29

Leisure, Recreation, and Effective Time Management

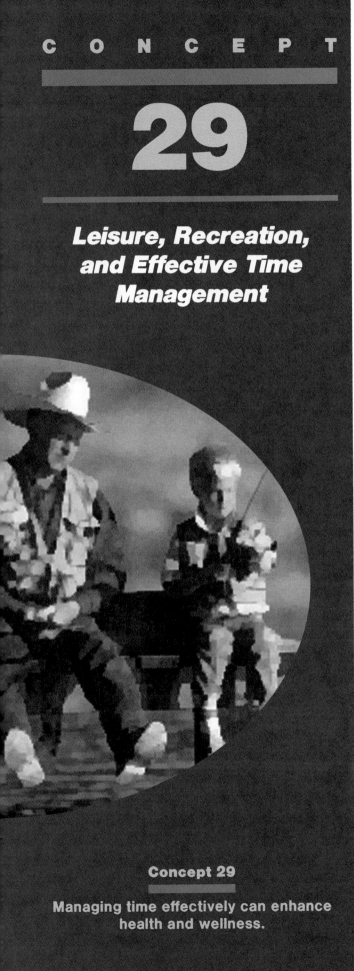

Concept 29

Managing time effectively can enhance health and wellness.

Introduction

Throughout this book, life-style modification has been endorsed as a means of achieving optimal health as evidenced by absence of disease, quality living, and a general sense of well-being. Many people in our culture see the need for life-style changes but fail to carry out their plans for many reasons. Most often mentioned is the lack of time. "I would like to exercise, but I don't have the time." "My two jobs don't allow me as much time as I would like to spend with my family." "I know I need to relax and enjoy myself, but I just can't find the time." These are a few of the common reasons given for failing to make life-style changes. You may never find time to do all of the things you want to do, but you can learn to manage time more effectively.

Health Goals for the Year 2000

- Increase the span of healthy life.
- Decrease the proportion of people reporting high levels of stress.
- Increase community availability of pools, parks, trails, and recreational open space.
- Reduce the proportion of people who do not engage in free-time activity.

Terms

Committed Time

Time that is committed to specific activity or purpose.

Free Time

Time not committed to work or other duties of the day.

Leisure

Time that is free from the demands of work is often called leisure time. Leisure is more than free time; it is also an attitude. Leisure activities need not be means to ends (purposeful) but are ends in themselves.

Play

Play is something one does of his/her own free will. The play experience is fun, intrinsically rewarding, and a self-absorbing means of self-expression. It is characterized by a sense of freedom or escape from normal life's rules.

Recreation

Recreation literally means creating something anew. In this book it refers to something that you do for your amusement or for fun to help you divert your attention and to refresh your self (recreate yourself).

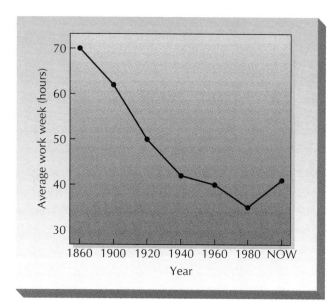

Figure 29.1

Decreases in working time since 1860.

Source: Data from G. Bammel and L. Burris-Bammel, *Leisure and Human Behavior*, 2d ed., 1992, and L. Hugick and J. Leonard, "Job Dissatisfaction Grows: Moonlighting on the Rise" in *The Gallup Poll Monthly*, 312:2–15, 1991.

The Facts About Work and Free Time

In the last 100 years, the average work week has been greatly reduced, netting the average person many hours of nonwork time annually.

Laws restricting work week length and mechanization of industry and farming are two of the many reasons why the amount of time spent on work is less now than at the turn of the century. Figure 29.1 illustrates the dramatic drop in time spent working since 1860. Child labor laws have also changed, reducing the working hours of children. Added hours of nonwork time have allowed most adults to have a better quality of life than their parents and grandparents.

The amount of time the average person spends at work has increased rather than decreased in the last decade.

The most recent statistics indicate that a reversal has occurred in recent years in the trend toward reduced work time. A major reason for the recent increase in work time is that many more people now hold second jobs than in the past. Also, some jobs of modern society have increasing rather than decreasing time demands. For example, medical doctors and other professionals often work many more hours than the 35–44 hours that the majority of people work.

Unenjoyable work detracts from a person's sense of well being and quality of life.

Many people enjoy the hours they spend at work more than the hours off the job. It is interesting to note, however, that satisfaction at work has dramatically decreased in the last forty years. The number of people who enjoy work more than nonwork time was twice as high in 1950 as it is in the 1990s. Nevertheless, work is still important to well-being as indicated by the fact that more than 73 percent of all adults would continue to work even if they had enough money to live without working.

Job satisfaction is important to quality living, but an overcommitment to work can result in decreased well-being. When work conflicts with family or personal relationships, five out of six times the family or personal relationships will suffer rather than work. At least a third of all people report that work conflicts significantly with their family and personal relationships. Most likely to be affected negatively are personal health, marriage or romantic relationships, and relationships with children.

All nonwork time is NOT free time.

Among some workers the demands of "other duties" have increased, allowing fewer hours of truly free time each year. **Committed time** has increased for many people; for example, travel to and from work, extra time at work-related activities that are unpaid, home management and care in addition to work outside the home, and transporting children.

Free time is very important to the average person.

Most people say that free time is important, but surveys indicate that more than half of all adults feel that they get too little of it. Many adults report that they get too little time for **recreation** or to simply relax and "do nothing" (leisure).

Recreation and leisure are important contributors to wellness (quality of life).

Leisure is time spent "doing things I just want to do" or "doing nothing." Recreation, on the other hand, is often purposeful. Both leisure and recreation can contribute to wellness (see table 29.1), though leisure activities are not done specifically to achieve these benefits.

The value of recreation and leisure in the busy lives of those in Western culture is evidenced by the emphasis public health officials place on availability and accessibility of recreational facilities in the future.

Table 29.1

Contributions of Recreation to Wellness

Contributions of Recreation	Wellness Dimensions
Refreshes person and provides balance to meaningful work.	Work
Provides fun and meaningful use of free time.	Free time
Appropriate activities will enhance all aspects of physical fitness.	Physical fitness
Can reduce life stress and provides a source of refreshment that helps avoid depression. A source of fun and happiness.	Mental/Emotional
Provides opportunities for social interactions, including family relationships.	Social
Spiritual activities are often free time activities that could be considered to be leisure and, in some cases, recreation.	Spiritual
The impact on each wellness dimension can provide a cumulative improvement in one's total outlook on life.	Total life outlook

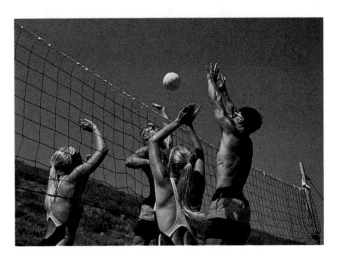

True play is done just for the fun of it.

To achieve wellness benefits, recreation should provide a sense of play.

Play is done of one's own free will. It is done for fun for intrinsic rather than extrinsic reasons, although it can be done for extrinsic reasons as well. Activities performed for material things such as trophies and medals can be considered as recreational as long as the principal reason for doing the activity is a sense of fun and playfulness. If the activity is done primarily for extrinsic reasons, it may not provide wellness benefits and is probably not true recreation. For example, to play golf to impress the boss is an extrinsic reason that may increase life stress rather than decrease it.

There are many meaningful types of recreation.

Many recreational activities involve moderate to vigorous physical activity. If fitness is the goal, these activities should be chosen. Involvement in nonphysical activities also constitutes recreation. For example, reading is a participation activity that can contribute significantly to other wellness dimensions, such as emotional/mental and spiritual. Passive involvement (spectating) is a third type of participation. Passive participation has been criticized by some people who feel that active participation is an important ingredient of meaningful recreation. Experts are quick to point out that spectating can be very refreshing and meaningful. For example, watching a good play at the theater qualifies as meaningful recreation and could be true leisure. Likewise, active participation in community theater can be meaningful recreation. To achieve the wellness benefits of recreation, liberal participation and meaningful passive involvement (spectating) are encouraged. Involvement as a spectator does not preclude active participation. However, since free time available for recreation is often limited, excessive spectating can result in decreased active participation. Examples of some of the most popular recreational activities are listed in table 29.2.

Television viewing has its limitations but is not without its advantages as a recreational activity.

Television is a free-time activity that deserves special mention. Evidence presented elsewhere in this book shows that those who spend a great deal of time watching television tend to be fatter and less physically active than those who spend less time watching television. On the other hand, 58 percent of adults feel that watching television is a "good" use of free time. Nevertheless, as many as four in ten people feel that they watch too much television. Television is still the "favorite way to spend an evening" (Gallup 1990, p. 11) for most Americans and, more people feel that television is good for society than bad. Like other activities, it can qualify as leisure and recreation.

Table 29.2
Popular Recreational Activities: Types of Involvement Available

Category	Personal Physical Activity	Personal Participation	Participation by Others (Spectator)
Water Activity			
• Swimming	Yes	Yes	Maybe
• Boating	Maybe	Yes	Maybe
• Water skiing	Yes	Yes	Maybe
Outdoor Activity			
• Fishing	Maybe	Yes	Rarely
• Gardening	Maybe	Yes	No
• Hunting	Yes	Yes	No
• Hiking	Yes	Yes	No
• Camping	Maybe	Yes	No
Sports/Games			
• Bowling	Maybe	Yes	Yes
• Baseball	Yes	Yes	Yes
• Football	Yes	Yes	Yes
• Softball	Yes	Yes	Maybe
• Golf	Yes	Yes	Yes
Winter Sports			
• Skiing	Yes	Yes	Maybe
• Skating	Yes	Yes	Yes
Fitness Activities			
• Aerobic dance	Yes	Yes	Rarely
• Weight training	Yes	Yes	No
• Running/jogging	Yes	Yes	Rarely
• Home calisthenics	Yes	Yes	No
• Bicycling	Yes	Yes	Rarely
Arts and Crafts			
• Crafts	No	Yes	Yes
• Dance	Yes	Yes	Yes
• Drama	Maybe	Maybe	Yes
• Drawing/painting	No	Yes	Yes
• Movies	No	No	Yes
• Music	Maybe	Yes	Yes
• Television	No	No	Yes
Others			
• Auto racing	Maybe	Maybe	Yes
• Board games	No	Yes	Maybe
• Cards (nongambling)	No	Yes	Maybe
• Games of chance	No	Yes	Yes
• Horse/dog racing	No	No	Yes
• Pool/billiards	Yes	Yes	Maybe
• Reading	No	Yes	No
• Travel/tourism	Maybe	Yes	No

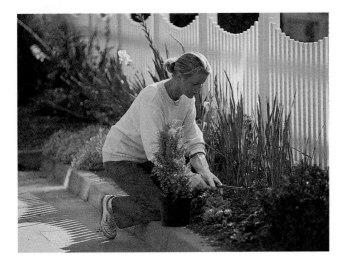

Your choice of recreation should reflect your personal interests.

Choice of recreational activities depends on many factors.

The reasons why people choose different recreational activities are many. Some of the more important reasons that influence choices are outlined in table 29.3.

Facts About Time Management

There are some steps that can be followed to help you manage your time effectively.

Step 1—Establish Priorities

Analyze what you value in life. Most Americans indicate that they want to reduce time spent in work-related activities and spend more time in recreation, at leisure, and with family or friends. Make a list of your priorities. Are these priorities currently being met? Are there activities for which you would like to have more time? Are there people with whom you would like to spend more time?

Step 2—Monitor Your Current Time Use

What we say we value does not always provide the basis for the way we spend our time. Keep a daily log of actual time expenditures to help you see how you could save time to devote to activities you value.

Table 29.3

Reasons for Choices of Recreational Activities

Reason	Rationale
Socioeconomic status	• Some activities are high in cost (example: golf, theater)
Vocation/profession	• Some have more free time than others • Peer pressures vary with jobs
Sex	• Women have fewer free hours than men • Women and men's interests vary
Age	• Retirees have more free hours • More activity limitations occur with age
Ethnic	• Peer pressures vary by group • Cultural interests may vary
Residence	• Location may limit availability • Weather affects activity choices
Disabilities	• Some disabilities limit availability or success

Step 3—Analyze Your Current Time Use

Each day has only 24 hours, and time available for daily activities is fixed. To have more time for priorities, schedules must be modified. Analysis of daily logs can help you determine how you spend your time. Ask yourself these questions.

- In what activities can I spend less time?
  Be honest. It's easy to say you'll spend less time on work, but can you really do it? Sometimes committed time other than work can be the problem. For example, some joggers spend so much time running that they have less time to spend with family.
- What can I do to reduce time spent in these activities?
  Maybe you can "kill two birds with one stone." For example, recreational time could be used to build fitness. Recreational time could also be family time (e.g., jog with the family). The key is finding activities that truly fulfill priorities for everyone involved. Finding work or recreational activities closer to home may save time.

Step 4—Make a Schedule

Writing a daily schedule can help you use time more effectively. This will allow you to enjoy life as a result of meeting priorities and spending time doing the things that enrich life for you and others important to you. A schedule should not be a rigid plan; it should be flexible enough to allow spontaneous activities.

If you cannot adhere to your time schedule, it should be modified. Your plan may not be realistic, and trying to adhere to it could cause you stress. In that case, the schedule is a problem rather than a solution to a problem.

Committed time can also be free time. It is possible to make a commitment to reserve time for activities that are important to you. Taking the time to re-create yourself or to enjoy family and friends is important. Sometimes the only way to "find the time" is to plan for it. Charts for helping you manage time effectively are provided in Lab 29.

Suggested Readings

Bammel, G., and L. Burrus-Bammel. *Leisure and Human Behavior* 2d ed. Dubuque, IA: Wm. C. Brown Publishers, 1992.

Csikszentmihalyi, M., and R. Graef. "Feeling Free." *Psychology Today* 12(1979):90.

LAB RESOURCE MATERIALS

(For use with Lab 29, p. L-85)

Chart 29.1 Time Management

Step 1: Establishing Priorities

1. Check your priorities from the list below. Add priorities as necessary.

2. Rank each of the priorities you checked. Use a 1 for the highest priority, a 2 for the second highest priority, and so on.

	Rank		Rank		Rank
☐ more time with family	_____	☐ more time with boy/girlfriend	_____	☐ more time with spouse	_____
☐ more time for leisure	_____	☐ more time to relax	_____	☐ more time to study	_____
☐ more time for work success	_____	☐ more time for physical activity	_____	☐ more time to improve myself	_____
☐ more time for other recreation	_____	☐ other _____	_____	☐ other _____	_____

Step 2: Monitor Current Time Use

1. On the daily calendar, keep track of daily time expenditure.

2. Write in exactly what you did for each time block.

7–9 AM	9–11 AM	11 AM–1 PM	1–3 PM
3–5 PM	**5–7 PM**	**7–9 PM**	**9–11 PM**

Step 3: Analyze Your Current Time Use

Where can I spend less time? (write below)	What can I do to reduce time spent in these activities? (write below)

Step 4: Make a Schedule. Write in Your Planned Activities for the Day

7–9 AM	9–11 AM	11 AM–1 PM	1–3 PM
3–5 PM	**5–7 PM**	**7–9 PM**	**9–11 PM**

CONCEPT

30

Planning Life-Styles for Optimal Health and Wellness

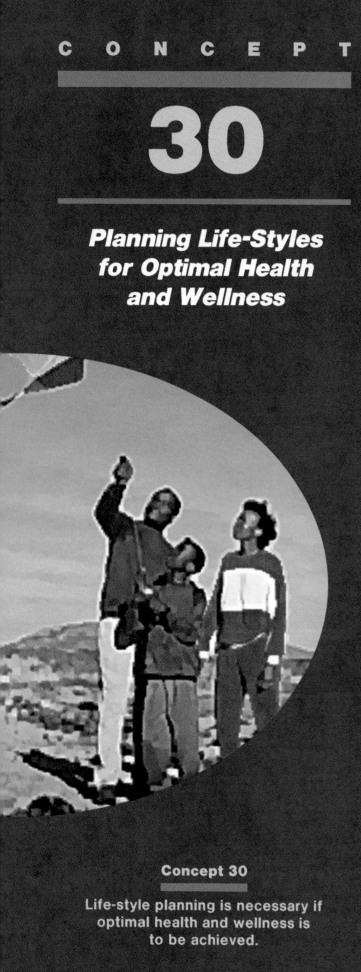

Concept 30

Life-style planning is necessary if optimal health and wellness is to be achieved.

Introduction

The nation's foremost health goal for the year 2000 is to increase the *optimally healthy* span of life for all of us. Living a long time, by itself, is not as important as living a healthy life that is full and rewarding. When they established the health goals for the year 2000, the nation's health leaders pointed out that health is more than preventing death and disease, it is also ". . . improved quality of life. . . . Health is thus best measured by citizens' sense of well-being" (Public Health Service 1991, p. 6).

If the goals of increased length of life and increased quality of life are to be achieved, it is important that we practice healthy life-styles. Unhealthful life-styles account for more than one half of the early death in our society. Unhealthy environment is another significant source of early death and less than quality living. It is for this reason that practicing healthy life-styles is so important. Suggestions for effective life-style planning are outlined in this concept.

Health Goals for the Year 2000

▬ Increase the span of optimally healthy life.

Terms

Behavioral Goal

A statement of intent to perform a specific behavior. A behavioral goal is associated with changing a life-style. An example is: "I will reduce the fat consumed in my diet to 30 percent or less."

Outcome Goal

A statement of intent to achieve a specific performance or standard associated with good health or wellness. An example is: "I will achieve a systolic blood pressure of 140 or less."

The Facts

There are certain areas of living that have great potential for improving wellness.

Some of the life-styles identified in this book that have potential for improving health and wellness are outlined in table 30.1. Taking action to modify life-styles in any of these areas that need attention can be useful for enhancing health and wellness.

Table 30.1

Healthy Life-Styles

- Exercising regularly
- Eating properly
- Controlling stress
- Avoiding destructive habits
- Practicing safe sex
- Adopting safety habits
- Learning first aid
- Adopting personal health behaviors
- Seeking and complying with medical advice
- Becoming an informed consumer
- Protecting the environment
- Managing time effectively

There are several steps that you can take to help change your life-style for better health and wellness.

Step 1—Identify areas of possible change.

Consider possible life-style changes in the areas outlined in Table 30.1. Are changes in any of these areas appropriate for you? (A checklist is provided in Lab 30.)

Step 2—Establish goals.

Establishing goals can help you effectively change your life-style for health and wellness. There are several guidelines that can help you establish meaningful goals.

- Set goals that are attainable. It is easier to attain small goals. Each small success encourages you to persist in your long term efforts to change your life-style.
- Set only a few goals at one time. Too many goals can lead to failure.
- For most people, **behavioral goals** are better than **outcome goals,** especially for the short term. A goal such as reducing your caloric intake by 200 calories every day is a behavior goal. Trying to lose 20 pounds is an outcome goal. If you do the process (changing your life-style) on a consistent basis you *will* meet your outcome goals.
- Make your goals specific. Specific goals help you evaluate to keep records and to determine if you have been successful in meeting your goals.
- Put your goals in writing. Making a written statement of goals allows you to keep records and can provide motivation for making life-style changes.

Step 3—Develop a plan for meeting your goals.

Based on the areas of change identified in Step 1 and the goals established in Step 2, write out a plan for meeting your goals. Typically a plan includes a schedule (days and times) for performing the behavior outlined in your goals. For example, if you establish the goal of doing relaxation exercises for 15 minutes, five days a week, you should write out a calendar indicating the days you plan to do the exercises and the time of the day you plan to perform them. If your goal is to learn CPR, you should write down a date for calling to schedule a CPR class and a tentative date for going to the class.

Reminders can be useful in keeping with your plan. For example, if your plan calls for you to floss your teeth each night before you go to bed, you might tape a message to your mirror to remind you to do the flossing *behavior.*

Step 4—Keep records.

Use your written plan to keep records. If you perform the life-style behavior as planned, make a check on the calendar. If you did not do the behavior as scheduled, reschedule it on your calendar. At the end of a specified period (a week or two), check to see if your plan is working. If, in the scheduled time, you have check marks for most of the days in your life-style plan, you will be well on the way to life-style change. You will be ready to develop a new plan (see Step 5). If you have only a few checks by the life-style behaviors in your plan, you will need to identify why you are not meeting your goals. The most common reasons for failure are:

- You established goals that were too hard or unrealistic.
- You established too many goals to accomplish during one short period of time.
- Your schedule may not have been well suited to your daily routine and may need modification.
- You lack commitment to the goals. If this is the case, you may need the assistance of a professional in meeting your goals.

Step 5—Evaluate and modify.

If you were successful in performing most of the life-style behaviors that you wrote in your plan, go back to Step 2 and re-establish new short-term goals. Repeat Steps 3 and 4. After you have met your short-term goals several times, you may want to check to see if you are coming close to setting your long-term goals. By this time you will be well on your way to significant life-style change. Once you have made the new behaviors into "good habits," you may not need to continue to include them in your life-style plan. You may, at this time, want to start to work on meeting some new life-style goals.

If you have failed to live up to your plan, you may want to modify it to make it more realistic and to increase your chances of success. Go back to Step 1 and begin again. Try to determine why your previous plan was not successful (see Lab 30).

Sometimes life-style changes cannot be made without the assistance of others.

The support of friends and family can be very important in helping you to accomplish life-style changes. Friends and family play a significant role in exercise adherence. The same is true for other behaviors. For example, family members can help you reduce the fat calories in your diet by cooking special foods and not preparing high-fat meals. Friends can encourage friends to fasten their seat belts.

There are some life-style changes that may require the assistance of a professional. If your attempts to change your life-style meet with failure, don't set yourself up for repeated failure. Get help!

Most colleges have programs through their health center that provide free, confidential assistance or referral. Many businesses now have Employee Assistance Programs (EAP). The programs have counselors who will help you or your family members find help with a particular problem. EAP staff are dedicated to help you *without revealing personal information to your employer*. These programs have a strong record for helping people with problems ranging from small to very serious, such as drug addiction or smoking cessation. Many other programs and support groups are now available to help you change your life-style. For example, most hospitals and many health organizations now have hotlines that provide you with referral services for establishing healthy life-styles.

One positive life-style change often leads to another.

People who make one significant life-style change to enhance wellness are likely to make other changes. For example, people who begin a regular exercise program and adhere to it over a period of time are also likely to make modifications in diet and adopt effective stress-reduction procedures. Those who smoke are more likely to stop if they have been successful in becoming a regular exerciser or a healthy eater.

The wellness life-style seems to be contagious. The key is to start slowly to increase the chance of success. Remember, the ultimate goal for the year 2000 of increasing the span of optimally healthy life, is best accomplished by altering life-styles in a consistent and regular manner. The nation's health leaders have indicated that a commitment by each individual combined with scientific knowledge, professional skills, community support, and political effort will ". . . enable the people to achieve their potential to live full, active lives" (Public Health Service 1991, p. 6).

Suggested Readings

Bruess, C., and G. Richardson. *Decisions for Health.* 3d ed. Dubuque, IA: Wm. C. Brown Communications, Inc., 1992.
Public Health Service. *Healthy People 2000: National Health Promotion and Disease Prevention Objectives.* Washington, DC: U. S. Government Printing Office, 1991.

LAB 2A

A Physical Activity Questionnaire

Name   Section   Date

PURPOSE

The purposes of this laboratory are:
1. To evaluate your feelings concerning physical activity.
2. To determine the specific reasons why you do or do not participate in regular physical activity.

PROCEDURE

1. Read each of the fourteen items in the physical activity questionnaire, chart 2.1 shown here or in the Lab Resource Materials for Concept 2 on page 16.
2. After each statement, check one box indicating whether you strongly agree, agree, disagree, or strongly disagree with it. If you are unsure of your answer, check "undecided."
3. When all fourteen items have been answered, use the scoring procedure on page 17 to score the physical activity questionnaire.

RESULTS

1. After you have determined seven different physical activity questionnaire scores and a total score, use chart 2.2, also in the Lab Resource Materials for Concept 2, to determine your rating for each score.
2. Check your rating for each of the seven reasons for exercising and your total score here.

	Excellent	Good	Fair	Poor	Very Poor
Health and fitness	☐	☐	☐	☐	☐
Fun and enjoyment	☐	☐	☐	☐	☐
Relaxation and tension release	☐	☐	☐	☐	☐
Challenge and achievement	☐	☐	☐	☐	☐
Social	☐	☐	☐	☐	☐
Appearance	☐	☐	☐	☐	☐
Competition	☐	☐	☐	☐	☐
Total Score	☐	☐	☐	☐	☐

CONCLUSIONS AND IMPLICATIONS

■ Read Concept 2 before completing this section. The seven scores on the physical activity questionnaire should reflect your reasons for participating in physical activity.

1. Do you think that the scores on which you were rated "excellent" or "good" accurately reflect the reasons why you might do regular exercise? Explain.

2. Do you think that the scores on which you were rated "poor" or "very poor" might be reasons why you would avoid physical activity? Explain.

3. Those who are physically active should score high on the total score. Is your total score a good reflection of your overall attitude about physical activity? Explain.

Chart 2.1 The Physical Activity Questionnaire						
The term "physical activity" in the following statements refers to all kinds of activities, including sports, formal exercises, and informal activities, such as jogging and cycling. Check your answers first, then read the directions for scoring, found in the Lab Resource Materials for Concept 2 on page 17.						
	Strongly Agree	**Agree**	**Undecided**	**Disagree**	**Strongly Disagree**	**Score**
1. Doing regular physical activity can be as harmful to health as it is helpful.	☐	☐	☐	☐	☐	_____
2. One of the main reasons I do regular physical activity is because it is fun.	☐	☐	☐	☐	☐	_____
3. Participating in physical activities makes me tense and nervous.	☐	☐	☐	☐	☐	_____
4. The challenge of physical training is one reason why I participate in physical activity.	☐	☐	☐	☐	☐	_____
5. One of the things I like about physical activity is the participation with other people.	☐	☐	☐	☐	☐	_____
6. Doing regular physical activity does little to make me more physically attractive.	☐	☐	☐	☐	☐	_____
7. Competition is a good way to keep a game from being fun.	☐	☐	☐	☐	☐	_____
8. I should exercise regularly for my own good health and physical fitness.	☐	☐	☐	☐	☐	_____
9. Doing exercise and playing sports is boring.	☐	☐	☐	☐	☐	_____
10. I enjoy taking part in physical activity because it helps me to relax and get away from the pressures of daily living.	☐	☐	☐	☐	☐	_____
11. Most sports and physical activities are too difficult for me to enjoy.	☐	☐	☐	☐	☐	_____
12. I do not enjoy physical activities that require the participation of other people.	☐	☐	☐	☐	☐	_____
13. Regular exercise helps me look my best.	☐	☐	☐	☐	☐	_____
14. Competing against others in physical activities makes them enjoyable.	☐	☐	☐	☐	☐	_____

Physical Fitness

Name   Section   Date

■ Read Concept 2 before completing this lab.

PURPOSE

The purposes of this laboratory session are:
1. To help you identify different components of physical fitness. It is hoped that, through participation, you can begin to see the differences between the various aspects of physical fitness, especially the differences between health-related and skill-related physical fitness.
2. To help you to gain insight into the importance of various components of physical fitness and to help you evaluate them.

PROCEDURE

Perform all the physical fitness stunts described in chart 2.3 in the Lab Resource Materials for Concept 2 on pages 17–19. Record your results in the appropriate blank opposite each item.

RESULTS

The stunts you tried are *not* good tests of fitness, but attempting the stunts may help you see that fitness is not just one thing; it is many different things. Circle the numbers of the skill-related and health-related items you passed.

Skill related   1   2   3   4   5   6

Health related   7   8   9   10   11

CONCLUSIONS AND IMPLICATIONS

To really test your fitness, you will need to do many of the tests presented later in this text. Therefore, you may be especially interested in testing yourself in those areas in which you did not do well on various stunts. For your own well-being, you should want to do well in health-related fitness.

How did you do on the health-related fitness stunts?

Were you surprised or disappointed in your performance?
Yes ☐ No ☐ Explain.

How did you do on the skill-related fitness stunts?

Were you surprised or disappointed in your performance? Yes ☐ No ☐ Explain.

Assessing Heart Disease Risk Factors

Name	Section	Date

■ Read Concept 3 before completing this lab.

PURPOSE

The purpose of this lab is to assess your risk of developing coronary heart disease.

PROCEDURE

1. Complete the ten questions on the Heart Disease Risk Factor Questionnaire (shown here or on page 33 in the Lab Resource Materials for Concept 3) by circling the answer that is most appropriate for *you*.
2. Look at the top of the column for each of your answers. In the space provided at the right of each question, write down the number of risk points for that answer.
3. Determine your unalterable risk score by adding the risk points for questions 1, 2, and 3.
4. Determine your alterable risk score by adding the risk points for questions 4 through 10.
5. Determine your total heart disease risk score by adding the scores obtained in steps 3 and 4.
6. Look up your risk ratings on chart 3.1.

RESULTS

Write your risk scores and risk ratings in the appropriate blanks below.

	Score	Rating
Unalterable risk		
Alterable risk		
Total heart disease risk		

Chart 3.1 Heart Disease Risk *Rating Scale*			
Rating	**Unalterable Score**	**Alterable Score**	**Total Score**
Very high	9 or More	21 or More	31 or More
High	7–8	15–20	26–30
Average	5–6	11–14	16–25
Low	4 or Less	10 or Less	15 or Less

The higher your score on the Heart Disease Risk Factor Questionnaire, the greater your heart disease risk. Which of the risk factors do you need to try to control to reduce your risk of heart disease? Why?

LAB 3

Heart Disease Risk Factor Questionnaire

Circle the appropriate answer to each question.

	Risk Points				
	1	**2**	**3**	**4**	**Score**
Unalterable Factors					
1. How old are you?	30 or less	31–40	41–54	55+	_____
2. Do you have a history of heart disease in your family?	none	grandparent with heart disease	parent with heart disease	more than one with heart disease	_____
3. What is your sex?	female		male		_____
				Total Unalterable Risk Score	_____
Alterable Factors					
4. What is your percent of body fat?	F = 20%↓ M = 15%↓	25%↓ 20%↓	30%↓ 25%↓	35%↑ 30%↑	_____
5. Do you have a high-fat diet?	no	slightly high in fat	above normal in fat	eat a lot of meat, fried and fatty foods	_____
6. What is your blood pressure? (systolic, or upper, score)	120↓	121–140	141–160	160↑	_____
7. Do you have other diseases?	no	ulcer	diabetes	both	_____
8. Do you exercise regularly?	4–5 days a week	3 days a week	less than 3 days a week	no	_____
9. Do you smoke?	no	cigar or pipe	less than ½ pack a day	more than ½ pack a day	_____
10. Are you under much stress?	less than normal	normal	slightly above normal	quite high	_____
				Total Alterable Risk Score	_____
				Grand Total Risk Score	_____

LAB 4A

Physical Activity Readiness

Name _____   Section _____   Date _____

■ Read Concept 4 before completing this lab.

PURPOSE

The purpose of this lab is to help you determine your physical readiness for participation in a program of regular exercise.

PROCEDURE

1. Read the directions on "The PAR-Q and You" form shown here and in the Lab Resource Materials for Concept 4, page 42.
2. Answer each of the seven questions on the form.
3. If you answered "yes" to one or more of the questions, follow the directions in the lower left-hand corner of the PAI regarding medical consultation.
4. If you answered "no" to all seven questions, follow the directions at the lower right-hand corner of the PAR-Q.
5. If you plan to participate in competitive sports or vigorous training, answer the five questions in chart 4.2 (see Lab Resource Materials, p. 43).

RESULTS

Physical Activity Readiness Questionnaire (PAR-Q)*

Circle the number of "yes" answers that you had for the physical activity readiness questionnaire.

    0   1   2   3   4   5   6   7

Physical Readiness for Sports or Vigorous Training

Circle the number of "yes" answers that you had for the Physical Readiness for Sports or Vigorous Training Questionnaire from chart 4.2.

    0   1   2   3   4   5

CONCLUSIONS AND IMPLICATIONS

Based on the answers to the PAR-Q, should you seek medical consultation before beginning or modifying your exercise program? Why or why not?

Based on answers to the Physical Readiness for Sports or Vigorous Training Questionnaire, do you feel that you are physically ready for sports and vigorous training? Why or why not?

Chart 4.1 Physical Activity Readiness Questionnaire (PAR-Q) *
A Self-Administered Questionnaire for Adults

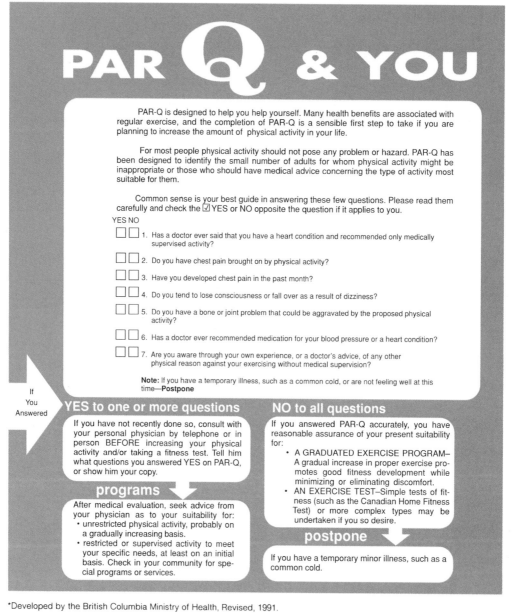

PAR Q & YOU

PAR-Q is designed to help you help yourself. Many health benefits are associated with regular exercise, and the completion of PAR-Q is a sensible first step to take if you are planning to increase the amount of physical activity in your life.

For most people physical activity should not pose any problem or hazard. PAR-Q has been designed to identify the small number of adults for whom physical activity might be inappropriate or those who should have medical advice concerning the type of activity most suitable for them.

Common sense is your best guide in answering these few questions. Please read them carefully and check the ☑ YES or NO opposite the question if it applies to you.

YES NO

☐ ☐ 1. Has a doctor ever said that you have a heart condition and recommended only medically supervised activity?

☐ ☐ 2. Do you have chest pain brought on by physical activity?

☐ ☐ 3. Have you developed chest pain in the past month?

☐ ☐ 4. Do you tend to lose consciousness or fall over as a result of dizziness?

☐ ☐ 5. Do you have a bone or joint problem that could be aggravated by the proposed physical activity?

☐ ☐ 6. Has a doctor ever recommended medication for your blood pressure or a heart condition?

☐ ☐ 7. Are you aware through your own experience, or a doctor's advice, of any other physical reason against your exercising without medical supervision?

Note: If you have a temporary illness, such as a common cold, or are not feeling well at this time—Postpone

If You Answered

YES to one or more questions

If you have not recently done so, consult with your personal physician by telephone or in person BEFORE increasing your physical activity and/or taking a fitness test. Tell him what questions you answered YES on PAR-Q, or show him your copy.

programs

After medical evaluation, seek advice from your physician as to your suitability for:
• unrestricted physical activity, probably on a gradually increasing basis.
• restricted or supervised activity to meet your specific needs, at least on an initial basis. Check in your community for special programs or services.

NO to all questions

If you answered PAR-Q accurately, you have reasonable assurance of your present suitability for:
• A GRADUATED EXERCISE PROGRAM— A gradual increase in proper exercise promotes good fitness development while minimizing or eliminating discomfort.
• AN EXERCISE TEST—Simple tests of fitness (such as the Canadian Home Fitness Test) or more complex types may be undertaken if you so desire.

postpone

If you have a temporary minor illness, such as a common cold.

*Developed by the British Columbia Ministry of Health, Revised, 1991.

Reference: PAR-Q Validation Report, British Columbia Ministry of Health, May, 1978.

Produced by the British Columbia Ministry of Health and the Department of National Health & Welfare.

Note: It is important that you answer all questions honestly. The PAR-Q is a scientifically and medically researched preexercise selection device. It complements exercise programs, exercise testing procedures, and the liability considerations attendant with such programs and testing procedures. PAR-Q, like any other preexercise screening device, will misclassify a small percentage of prospective participants, but no preexercise screening method can entirely avoid this problem.

The Warm-up and Cool-down

LAB
4B

Name   Section   Date

■ Read Concept 4 before completing this lab.

PURPOSE

The purpose of this lab is to familiarize you with a sample group of exercises that can be used as a warm-up or cool-down for aerobic types of workout.

PROCEDURE

Perform the exercises described in Concept 4 on pages 37–38.

RESULTS

1. In which of the stretches did you feel the most tightness?

	None	Moderate	Severe
Calf stretcher	☐	☐	☐
Back saver toe touch	☐	☐	☐
Leg hug	☐	☐	☐
Side stretch	☐	☐	☐
Zipper	☐	☐	☐

2. Did you notice an increase in heart rate during the cardiovascular warm-up? Yes ☐ No ☐

CONCLUSIONS AND IMPLICATIONS

Do you think that the sample warm-up and cool-down program is adequate for the activities you plan to do as part of your exercise program? Yes ☐ No ☐ Explain.

Does the sport or activity you plan to do involve vigorous use of muscles not stretched by this program? Yes ☐ No ☐ If so, what muscles or body parts will need special attention?

Read Concept 9 and consider those stretching exercises for your warm-up and cool-down.

Counting the Target Heart Rate

Name _____ Section _____ Date _____

■ Read Concept 6 before completing this lab.

PURPOSE

The purposes of this laboratory session are:
1. To learn to count carotid pulse.
2. To learn to count radial pulse.
3. To understand the threshold of training and target zone concepts.
4. To establish a personal minimal cardiovascular threshold of training.
5. To establish a personal target zone for cardiovascular fitness.
6. To determine the specific jogging speed necessary to elevate your heart rate to threshold of training and target zones.

PROCEDURE

1. Practice counting the number of pulses felt for a given period of time at both the carotid and radial locations (see pages 59–60 for directions on counting the pulse). Use a clock or watch to count for fifteen, thirty, and sixty seconds. To establish your heart rate in beats per minute, multiply your fifteen-second count by four, and your thirty-second count by two.
2. Practice locating your carotid and radial pulses quickly. This is important when trying to count your pulse after exercise.
3. Practice counting the pulse of another person using both the wrist and carotid locations (do not use your thumb).
4. One partner should run a quarter-mile, then the other partner should count her or his heart rate at the end of the run (use carotid pulse). Try to run at a rate that you think will keep the rate of the heart above the threshold of training and in the target zone. Use fifteen-second pulse counts and multiply by four to get heart rate in beats per minute (bpm). Record the bpm in the results section.
5. Repeat, alternating roles, the second person running and the first person counting heart rate. Record the results.
6. Repeat the test so each person runs a second time. Record the results.

RESULTS

Record the various **resting** pulse counts for carotid and radial pulses in the spaces provided here.

Carotid Pulse Count (Self)	Heart Rate per Minute	Carotid Pulse Count (Partner)	Heart Rate per Minute
_____ 15 seconds × 4	_____	_____ 15 seconds × 4	_____
_____ 30 seconds × 2	_____	_____ 30 seconds × 2	_____
_____ 60 seconds × 1	_____	_____ 60 seconds × 1	_____

Radial Pulse Count (Self)	Heart Rate per Minute	Radial Pulse Count (Partner)	Heart Rate per Minute
_____ 15 seconds × 4	_____	_____ 15 seconds × 4	_____
_____ 30 seconds × 2	_____	_____ 30 seconds × 2	_____
_____ 60 seconds × 1	_____	_____ 60 seconds × 1	_____

What is your threshold of training (from chart 6A, page 64)? _____ bpm

What is your target zone (from chart 6A, p. 64)? _____ bpm

What was your heart rate for the first run? (fifteen seconds) _____ × 4 = _____ bpm

What was your heart rate for the second run? (fifteen seconds) _____ × 4 = _____ bpm

How fast do you have to run to get your heart rate above threshold and into the target zone? Check the following.

First run speed just right ☐   Faster than the first run ☐   Slower than the first run ☐

Second run speed just right ☐   Faster than the second run ☐   Slower than the second run ☐

LAB 6A

CONCLUSIONS AND IMPLICATIONS

1. Which resting pulse did you find easiest to locate on yourself?   (circle one)   Carotid   Radial
2. Which resting pulse did you find easiest to locate on your partner? (circle one)   Carotid   Radial
3. Which of the two methods of counting the pulse do you think you would prefer to use when counting exercise heart rate? (circle one)   Carotid   Radial   Why?

4. Do you achieve the cardiovascular threshold in the course of a normal day? Yes ☐ No ☐
5. What would you suggest for yourself as a regular (three to five times per week) cardiovascular exercise program?

LAB 6A SUPPLEMENT*

You may want to keep track of your exercise heart rate over a week's time or longer to see if you are reaching the target zone in your workouts. Shade your target zone with a highlight pen and plot your exercise heart rate for each day of the week (see sample).

Exercise Heart Rate								Sample	
200									
190									
180									
170									
160									
150									
140									
130									
120									
110									
100									
90									
80									
	Monday	Tuesday	Wednesday	Thursday	Friday	Saturday	Sunday	Day 1	Day 2
	_____	_____	_____	_____	_____	_____	_____	155	162

Write in your daily exercise heart rate on the lines above.

*Thanks to Ginnie Atkins for suggesting this lab supplement.

LAB 6B

Evaluating Cardiovascular Fitness

Name _____   Section _____   Date _____

■ Read Concept 6 before completing this lab.

PURPOSE

The purposes of this laboratory are:
1. To acquaint you with several methods for evaluating cardiovascular fitness.
2. To help you evaluate and rate your own cardiovascular fitness.

PROCEDURE

Perform one or more of the three cardiovascular fitness tests described in the Lab Resource Materials for Concept 6 on pages 64–67. Determine your ratings on the test(s) using the rating charts provided.

RESULTS

Record the information obtained from taking the cardiovascular fitness test(s) (one or more) in the space provided.

Twelve-Minute Run

(Distance) _____ miles

Rating _____

Rockport Walking Test

(Time) _____ minutes

Heart rate _____ bpm

Rating _____

The Step Test

Heart rate _____ bpm

Rating _____

The Bicycle Test

Workload _____ kpm

Heart rate _____ bpm

Weight _____ lbs

Weight in kg* _____

ml/O$_2$/kg _____

Rating _____

*Weight in lbs ÷ 2.2

CONCLUSIONS AND IMPLICATIONS

If you took more than one test, were the ratings for each similar? Yes ☐ No ☐ If so, were the ratings what you expected them to be? Yes ☐ No ☐ Explain.

If not, which rating do you think is really the best indicator of your cardiovascular fitness? Explain.

If you took only one test, explain why.

If you took only one test, estimate how you would have performed on one additional test.
Check one: ☐ 12-minute run ☐ Step test ☐ Bicycle test ☐ Walking test

Is your cardiovascular fitness what you think it ought to be? Yes ☐ No ☐ Explain.

LAB 6C

Ratings of Perceived Exertion

Name _____ Section _____ Date _____

■ Read Concept 6 before completing this lab.

PURPOSE

The purpose of this laboratory session is to learn to accurately perceive the intensity of exercise so that you can reduce the number of times that you must stop and count your heart rate during exercise workouts.

PROCEDURE

1. Find your threshold of training and target heart rates using chart 6A on page 64 and record it in the Results section below.
2. Perform the following exercise bouts:
   a. Walk for 3 minutes at a brisk pace.
   b. Jog for 3 minutes at a slow pace.
   c. Jog for 3 minutes at a pace that you feel will elevate your heart rate to your threshold level.
3. After each exercise bout, count your heart rate (see Lab 6A). Record the heart rates in the Results section.
4. After each exercise bout, rate the intensity of the exercise using the Rating of Perceived Exertion Scale on the back of this sheet. Rate the intensity of the exercise by number but use the reference words to help you. Record your ratings for each exercise bout in the Results section.
5. Repeat the threshold jog again followed by a more intense run. After each run, count your heart rate and make a rating of perceived exertion. Make sure that each of these two runs elevates your heart rate above threshold and into the target zone

RESULTS

Threshold heart rate _____ (bpm)   Target heart rate _____ (bpm)

Activity	Heart Rate (bpm)	Rating of Perceived Exertion (Numerical Rating)
Walk	_____	_____
Slow jog	_____	_____
Threshold jog	_____	_____
Threshold jog 2	_____	_____
Above threshold jog	_____	_____

Ratings of perceived exertion were originally planned to correspond to heart rates. Adding a zero to a numerical rating would produce the expected heart rate for that rating. However, people perceive exertion differently depending on age, level of training, and experience in exercise, so ratings do not always correspond to heart rate values. The important thing to learn is the RPE number that corresponds to your threshold of training heart rate and the RPE that represents the upper limit heart rate of your target zone. Typically, numerical RPE ratings for exercise in the target zone will range from 12 to 16. With practice (such as you have done here), you can learn to make accurate ratings. More practice than is provided in this lab is necessary. Answering the questions below may help you in learning to make accurate ratings of perceived exertion.

LAB 6C

	Yes	No
1. Did the walk or slow jog elevate your heart rate to threshold level?	☐	☐
2. Was your RPE number less than 12 for the walk and slow jog?	☐	☐
3. Did the two threshold runs get your heart rate near your threshold heart rate?	☐	☐
4. Was your RPE number for threshold heart rate in the range of 12–14?	☐	☐
5. Did your final run get your heart rate well into your target heart rate zone?	☐	☐
6. Was your RPE number in the final run in the range of 12–16?	☐	☐

Chart 6.C Ratings of Perceived Exertion (RPE)

Scale	Verbal Rating
6	
7	Very, very light
8	
9	Very light
10	
11	Fairly light
12	
13	Somewhat hard
14	
15	Hard
16	
17	Very hard
18	
19	Very, very hard
20	

From G. Borg, "Psychological Bases of Perceived Exertion" in *Medicine and Science in Sports and Exercise,* 14:377, 1982, © by The American College of Sports Medicine.

With practice, do you think you could learn to use RPE to determine if you are exercising with enough intensity to build cardiovascular fitness? Yes ☐ No ☐ Explain.

Note: If the last three runs did not elevate the heart rate into the target zone, it will be difficult to learn to make accurate ratings of perceived exertion.

Jogging/Running

Name _____ Section _____ Date _____

■ Read Concept 7 before completing this lab.

PURPOSE

The purposes of this laboratory session are:
1. To give you an opportunity to experience one type of jogging program that can be used to develop and maintain cardiovascular fitness.
2. To acquaint you with basic jogging techniques.

PROCEDURE

1. Work with a partner and evaluate each other on jogging techniques.
   a. Stand twenty yards in front of your partner while he/she jogs toward you; watch his/her arm and leg swing and foot placement.
   b. Jog along ten yards behind your partner while he/she is jogging and watch for arm and leg swing and foot placement.
   c. Stand ten yards to one side as your partner jogs past you; watch for body position and foot placement.
2. Check the appropriate Correct or Incorrect boxes in chart 7A.1.
3. Using proper jogging technique, jog for fifteen minutes at your own individual cardiovascular threshold of training. (Determine your threshold of training using chart 6A, page 64.)

RESULTS

Have your partner evaluate your jogging technique using chart 7A.1. Give an overall evaluation of your jogging technique. Is it good or bad?

What is your cardiovascular target zone heart rate? _____ bpm

What was your heart rate after your fifteen-minute jog? _____ bpm

During your fifteen-minute jog, did you reach your threshold of training? Yes ☐ No ☐

With the help of a partner, note on chart 7A.1 any problems in technique. (Read the information on jogging in Concept 7, page 73, before evaluating your partner's jogging technique.)

Chart 7A.1   Jogging Technique

Body Segment	Technique (Check Appropriate Boxes Below)		
	Correct	Incorrect	
Foot placement	☐	☐	Heel hits ground first
	☐	☐	Rock forward, push off ball of foot
	☐	☐	Toes point straight ahead
	☐	☐	Feet under knees, do not swing side to side
Length of stride	☐	☐	Stride is several inches longer than regular step
Arm movement	☐	☐	Arms bent at 90°
	☐	☐	Arms swing front to back, not side to side
	☐	☐	Arms alternate opposite striding leg
	☐	☐	Hands and arms are relaxed
Body position	☐	☐	Upper body nearly erect
	☐	☐	Head and chest are up

CONCLUSIONS AND IMPLICATIONS

Do you have any jogging problems? Yes ☐ No ☐

Do you feel that you can solve any jogging problems you have? Yes ☐ No ☐ Explain.

Do you think that jogging is a good type of exercise for you? Yes ☐ No ☐ Explain.

Do you think that you will include jogging in your exercise program for use in later life? Yes ☐ No ☐ Explain (if different from answer above).

Aerobic and Anaerobic Exercises

Name _____ Section _____ Date _____

■ Read Concept 7 before completing this lab.

PURPOSE

The purposes of this laboratory session are:
1. To give you an opportunity to experience an aerobic or anaerobic exercise program that is particularly good for developing cardiovascular fitness and aiding in fat reduction.
2. To familiarize you with an exercise program that can be continued as part of your life's normal routine.

PROCEDURE

1. Select a sample program for some form of aerobic or anaerobic exercise and try it out. It can be earning points according to Cooper's Aerobics Chart (table 7.4), Dance Aerobics, (appendix E, p. A.11), or performing a sample of any of the other forms of aerobic or anaerobic exercise discussed in Concept 7. For example, you may want to try a walking program, an interval training program, a rope jumping routine, or a circuit weight program.
2. If you would like to repeat this lab more than once doing a different activity each time, space is provided in the results section for four descriptions.

RESULTS

Name the activity in which you participated, and briefly describe and evaluate your experience.

Activity name _____

Time spent _____ minutes
Description and evaluation

Activity name _____

Time spent _____ minutes
Description and evaluation

Activity name _____

Time spent _____ minutes
Description and evaluation

Activity name _____

Time spent _____ minutes
Description and evaluation

CONCLUSIONS AND IMPLICATIONS

Did you like the activity or activities you performed? Yes ☐ No ☐
Do you think you would choose to make one or more of these activities part of your regular exercise program? Yes ☐ No ☐
Explain.

If you did more than one activity, which one did you most enjoy? _____
Why?

Of all the activities discussed in Concept 7, which ones do you think you would be most likely to include in your regular exercise program?

LAB 8

Evaluating Flexibility

Name _____ Section _____ Date _____

■ Read Concept 8 before completing this lab.

PURPOSE

The purpose of this laboratory experience is to evaluate your flexibility in several joints.

PROCEDURE

1. Take the flexibility test as outlined on pages 84–85 of the Lab Resource Materials for Concept 8.
2. Record your scores in the Results section.
3. Use chart 8.1 in the Lab Resource Materials for Concept 8 to determine your rating on the test, then record your rating in the Results section.

RESULTS

	Test 1		Test 2		Test 3	
	Left	Right	Right up	Left up	Left	Right

What were your flexibility scores? _____ _____   _____ _____   _____ _____

Check your rating below.

Flexibility *Ratings* on Selected Joints				
	High Performance	**Good Fitness**	**Marginal**	**Poor**
Test 1 Left	☐	☐	☐	☐
Right	☐	☐	☐	☐
Test 2 Right Up	☐	☐	☐	☐
Left Up	☐	☐	☐	☐
Test 3 Left	☐	☐	☐	☐
Right	☐	☐	☐	☐

Do any of these muscle groups need stretching?

	Yes	No
Back of the thighs and knees (hamstrings)	☐	☐
Calf muscles	☐	☐
Lower back (lumbar region)	☐	☐
Front of right shoulder	☐	☐
Back of right shoulder	☐	☐
Front of left shoulder	☐	☐
Back of left shoulder	☐	☐
Most of the body	☐	☐

Note: Read Concept 9 and Lab 9 for exercises to improve your flexibility.

CONCLUSIONS AND IMPLICATIONS

Discuss your current flexibility and your flexibility needs for the future.

LAB
8

Stretching Exercises

Name _____ Section _____ Date _____

■ Read Concept 9 before performing this lab. Also review Concept 8.

PURPOSE

The purposes of this laboratory experience are:
1. To give you an opportunity to experience different flexibility exercises.
2. To acquaint you with a flexibility program that can be continued throughout your life.
3. To help you distinguish between the types of flexibility exercises.

PROCEDURE

1. Review the stretching exercises in Concept 9 on pages 87–93.
2. Perform each of the exercises to your threshold (or slightly below if you have not been exercising regularly). See Concept 8 for your threshold level.
3. Answer the questions in the results section.

RESULTS

See reverse side.

CONCLUSIONS AND IMPLICATIONS

In what areas of the body do you most need to do muscle stretching based on your results (see next page)? Discuss.

Place a check beside several exercises (at least five) you think you would include in your exercise program. Place a check in the appropriate box if you did or did not experience muscle tightness when doing the exercises. List reasons for your exercise choices on the chart on the following page.

Name of Exercise	Tightness		Ex. Choice	Reason for Choosing the Exercise
	Yes	No		
1. Lower leg stretcher	☐	☐	_____	_____
2. Sitting stretcher	☐	☐	_____	_____
3. One-leg stretcher	☐	☐	_____	_____
4. Leg hug	☐	☐	_____	_____
5. Pectoral stretch	☐	☐	_____	_____
6. Billig's exercise	☐	☐	_____	_____
7. Lateral trunk stretcher	☐	☐	_____	_____
8. Hip and thigh stretcher	☐	☐	_____	_____
9. Arm stretcher	☐	☐	_____	_____
10. Shin stretcher	☐	☐	_____	_____
11. Hamstring stretcher	☐	☐	_____	_____
12. Trunk twister	☐	☐	_____	_____
13. Rectus femoris stretch	☐	☐	_____	_____
14. Lateral thigh and hip stretch	☐	☐	_____	_____
15. Arm pretzel	☐	☐	_____	_____
16. Spine twist	☐	☐	_____	_____
17. Neck rotation	☐	☐	_____	_____
18. Wand exercise	☐	☐	_____	_____
19. Calf stretcher	☐	☐	_____	_____
20. Back-saver toe touch	☐	☐	_____	_____
Stunts				
1. Two hand ankle wrap	☐	☐	_____	_____
2. Wand step-through	☐	☐	_____	_____
3. Wring the dishrag	☐	☐	_____	_____
Sport-specific ballistic exercises				
1. Trunk motions	☐	☐	_____	_____
2. Arm and trunk motions	☐	☐	_____	_____

Evaluating Muscular Strength and Power

Name _____ Section _____ Date _____

■ Read Concept 10 before completing this lab.

PURPOSE

The purposes of this lab are:
1. To evaluate your isotonic and isometric strength in selected muscle groups.
2. To evaluate leg muscle power.
3. To have fun.

PROCEDURE

I. Isotonic Strength
   1. Use an appropriate warm-up before attempting these stunts.
   2. Choose a partner to assist you in performing and scoring.
   3. Attempt the stunt groups found in the Lab Resource Materials for Concept 10, pages 110–113; within each grouping, *start with the stunt that you believe is the most difficult one that you can pass.* If you pass that one, try the next most difficult one in the same grouping. If you cannot pass it, try the next lower stunt, and so on.
   4. You receive the score of the most difficult stunt you can perform in each grouping.
   5. Record your scores, totals, and ratings in the Results section of this report.
II. Isometric
   1. Follow the directions on page 113 in Concept 10.
   2. If time and equipment permit, take three measures of each hand and record the best score on each, along with your total score and rating.
III. Power
   1. Follow the directions on page 113 in Concept 10.
   2. If time and equipment permit, take two trials and record your best score and your rating.

RESULTS

Isotonic Strength		Isometric Strength		Power	
Test I	_____	Right Grip	_____		
Test II	_____	Left Grip	_____	Best Score	_____
Test III	_____				
Test IV	_____				
Total Score	_____	Total Score	_____		
Rating	_____	Rating	_____	Rating	_____

List the muscle groups involved in each of the tests.

Test I _____

Test II _____

Test III _____

Test IV _____

Isometric Grip _____

Power Jump _____

CONCLUSIONS AND IMPLICATIONS

On which measure of strength did you score the poorest? Isometric strength ☐ Isotonic strength ☐ Power ☐ Explain your results.

On which measure of strength did you score the best? Isometric strength ☐ Isotonic strength ☐ Power ☐ Explain your results.

Evaluating Muscular Endurance

Name _____ Section _____ Date _____

■ Read Concept 11 before proceeding with this lab.

PURPOSE

The purposes of this laboratory session are:
1. To evaluate the dynamic muscular endurance of two muscle groups and the static endurance of the arms and trunk muscles.
2. To get acquainted with some exercises to improve endurance.
3. To have fun.

PROCEDURE

1. Perform the sitting tucks, push-ups, and flexed arm support tests described in the Lab Resource Materials for Concept 11 on page 121.
2. When not being tested, you may wish to perform the muscular endurance exercises in Lab 12B using a light weight and up to 25 repetitions.
3. Record your tests scores in the Results section. Determine and record your rating from charts 11.1, 11.2, and 11.3 in the Lab Resource Materials for Concept 11.

RESULTS

Record your scores below.

Sitting tucks _____ Push-ups _____ Flexed Arm Support _____ (seconds)
Check your ratings below.

	High Performance	Good Fitness	Marginal	Poor
Sitting tucks	☐	☐	☐	☐
Push-ups	☐	☐	☐	☐
Flexed-arm support	☐	☐	☐	☐

On which of the tests of muscular endurance did you score the poorest? Sitting tucks ☐ Push-ups ☐ Flexed-arm support ☐
Explain your results.

On which of the tests of muscular endurance did you score the best? Sitting tucks ☐ Push-ups ☐ Flexed-arm support ☐
Explain your results.

Determining One Repetition Maximum (1RM) and Resistance Training for Strength

Name   Section   Date

■ Read Concepts 10, 11, and 12 before proceeding with this lab.

PURPOSE

The purposes of this lab are:
1. To determine your one repetition maximum for various strength exercises.
2. To determine the best amount of weight to use for various strength exercises.

PROCEDURE

1. One repetition maximum (1RM) refers to the maximum amount of weight you can lift one time for a specific exercise. Testing yourself to determine how much you can lift only one time using traditional methods can be fatiguing and even dangerous. This procedure allows you to estimate 1RM based on the number of times you can lift a weight that is less than 1RM. For example, begin with the curl exercise. Estimate how much weight you can lift two or three times. Be conservative; it is best to start with too little weight than too much. This procedure will work if you select a weight heavier than you can lift ten times. If you lift more than ten times, the procedure should be done again on another day when you are rested.
2. Using correct form, curl the weight as many times as you can.
3. Use Chart 12A.2 (see Lab Resource Materials, p. 146) to determine your 1RM for the curl exercise. Find the weight used in the left hand column and then find the number of repetitions you performed across the top of the chart.
4. Your 1RM score is the value where the weight row and the repetitions column intersect.
5. Repeat this procedure for each of the exercises in the sample strength program listed in Chart 12A.1. (Choose either the free-weight or machine exercises. The names and numbers of the exercises shown in Chart 12A.1 correspond with the exercises shown in Concept 12 on pages 129–136.) Record these 1RM scores in the results section.
6. Calculate a percentage of 1RM for each exercise. If you are a beginner, use 50 percent to 65 percent. If you have been doing some strength training, select 65 percent to 80 percent, and if you are experienced select 80 percent to 90 percent.
7. On another day, perform three sets of six repetitions of each of the exercises in Chart 12A.1, using the percentage of 1RM you have selected. *Note:* This is meant to be a sample exercise program. When you actually plan your own program, you will probably decide to use different percentages of 1RM (see Concept 10).

Chart 12A.1   Sample Weight/Resistance Training Program

Free Weight Exercise				Machine Exercise			
Name	**Number**	**1RM**	**% 1RM Selected**	**Name**	**Number**	**1RM**	**% 1RM Selected**
Shoulder shrug	17	_____	_____	Hamstring curl	32	_____	_____
Military press	18	_____	_____	Bench press	29	_____	_____
Half squat	19	_____	_____	Leg press	26	_____	_____
Biceps curl	20	_____	_____	Biceps curl	24	_____	_____
Triceps curl	21	_____	_____	Triceps curl	28	_____	_____
Toe raise	22	_____	_____	Ankle press	30	_____	_____
Upright row	23	_____	_____	Seated rowing	25	_____	_____

Which exercises did you select? free weights ☐ machine weights ☐ Why?

What percentage of 1RM did you select? _____ Discuss your reasons.

LAB 12A

Were the weights/resistance suggested too heavy for you? Yes ☐ No ☐
Were the weights/resistance suggested too light for you? Yes ☐ No ☐
Briefly give your reaction to weight/resistance training as a potential program for you to use to develop your own fitness (strength).

Circuit Resistance Training for Endurance

Name   Section   Date

■ Read Concepts 10, 11, and 12 before proceeding with this lab.

PURPOSE

The purposes of this lab are:

1. To become familiar with a program of Circuit Resistance Training for muscular endurance.
2. To have fun.

PROCEDURE

1. Perform an appropriate warm-up and stretch.
2. Perform the following exercises in Concept 12. (*Note:* You or your instructor may prefer to substitute other resistance machine stations or use calisthenics.) If desired, you may also include a cardiovascular station such as jog-in-place or rope-jump. If there is a shortage of equipment, the instructor may wish to assign each person a partner and have the partner jump rope while the other person works on the machine, and then trade places before moving on to each new station.

Arm	Leg	Trunk
1. lat pull-down	2. knee extensions	3. abdominal board curls
4. seated rowing	5. toe raises	6. back extensions
7. shoulder press	8. leg press (high)	9. hand gripper or tennis ball squeeze

3. Rotate in the order listed above or as designated by your instructor, alternating arm, leg, and trunk exercises.
4. On the first set (circuit), perform twenty reps at 30 to 40 percent 1 RM, or 20 RM for forty-five seconds (this allows approximately two seconds for each rep.). Use the procedure described in Lab 12A to determine percentage of 1RM.
5. On the signal at the end of the forty-five seconds, move to the next station, adjust the resistance and get ready in fifteen seconds.
6. Continue around the circuit, performing forty-five seconds work and fifteen seconds rest periods. Perform a second circuit and increase your reps at each station to twenty-five. If time permits, perform a third circuit of twenty-five reps.
7. Perform an appropriate cool-down and stretch.

RESULTS

	Yes	No
1. Were you able to complete twenty to twenty-five reps in forty-five seconds?	☐	☐
2. Were you able to change stations in fifteen seconds?	☐	☐
3. Was this your first experience with circuit resistance training?	☐	☐
4. Did you like the workout?	☐	☐

In the space below, describe your reactions to circuit resistance training for muscular endurance as a potential program for use to develop your own fitness.

Describe any changes you might make in the program to make it better fit your needs.

LAB
12B

Evaluating Body Fatness and Waist-to-Hip Ratios

Name _____ Section _____ Date _____

■ Read Concept 13 before completing this lab.

PURPOSE

The purposes of this laboratory session are:
1. To learn to use skinfold calipers to make skinfold measurements.
2. To determine your percent body fat using skinfold measurements.
3. To assess your waist-to-hip ratio using circumference measurements.

PROCEDURE

1. Read the directions for making skinfold and/or body circumference measurements described on pages 156–157.
2. If possible, observe a demonstration of the proper procedures for measuring skinfolds and body circumferences at each of the different body locations. In the future, you may wish to help a person of the same or opposite sex take measurements, so you may wish to learn how to make all the measurements.
3. Work with a partner if possible. Take several measurements on your partner at each of the different skinfold and body circumference locations. Allow your partner to make the appropriate measurements on you.
4. If possible, have an expert make measurements on you and your partner so that you can compare your measurements.
5. Record each of the measurements in the Results section.
6. Calculate your body fatness from skinfolds by summing the appropriate skinfold values (chest, abdominal, and thigh for men; triceps, iliac crest, and thigh for women). Using your age and the sum of the appropriate skinfolds, determine your body fatness using charts 13A.1 (men), page 158, and 13A.2 (women), page 159.
7. Rate your fatness using chart 13A.3 on page 160.
8. If different types of calipers are available to you, practice making measurements with each type so that comparisons of results can be made.
9. Calculate your waist-to-hip ratio from body circumferences. Rate yourself using chart 13A.4, page 160.
10. Remember that body composition measurements are confidential information. Care should be taken not to discuss another person's results. Results are intended to be useful information to the people being tested. Take the skinfold testing seriously.

RESULTS

Write your skinfold measurements in the blanks provided on the following page. In some cases, all measurements may not be possible. Provide results for the tests you were able to complete. List the name of the caliper used.

Males (Skinfolds)

Measurement by Partner (or self)

Chest _____ mm

Abdominal _____ mm

Thigh _____ mm

Sum _____

Percent Body Fat _____

Rating _____

Caliper Used _____

Measurement by Instructor (if possible)

Chest _____ mm

Abdominal _____ mm

Thigh _____ mm

Sum _____

Percent Body Fat _____

Rating _____

Caliper Used _____

Males (Circumferences)

Measurement by Partner (or self)

Waist Circumference _____ in./mm

Hip Circumference _____ in./mm

Waist-to-Hip Ratio _____

Rating _____

Measurement by Instructor (if possible)

Waist Circumference _____ in./mm

Hip Circumference _____ in./mm

Waist-to-Hip Ratio _____

Rating _____

Females (Skinfolds)

Measurement by Partner (or self)

Tricep _____ mm

Iliac Crest _____ mm

Thigh _____ mm

Sum _____

Percent Body Fat _____

Rating _____

Caliper Used _____

Measurement by Instructor (if possible)

Tricep _____ mm

Iliac Crest _____ mm

Thigh _____ mm

Sum _____

Percent Body Fat _____

Rating _____

Caliper Used _____

Females (Circumferences)

Measurement by Partner (or self)

Waist Circumference _____ in./mm

Hip Circumference _____ in./mm

Waist-to-Hip Ratio _____

Rating _____

Measurement by Instructor (if possible)

Waist Circumference _____ in./mm

Hip Circumference _____ in./mm

Waist-to-Hip Ratio _____

Rating _____

LAB
13A

CONCLUSIONS AND IMPLICATIONS

Is your fatness (percent body fat) what you like it to be? Yes ☐ No ☐ Explain.

Is your waist-to-hip ratio what you would like it to be? Yes ☐ No ☐ Explain.

What do you think you will need to do in the future to obtain or maintain a desirable level of body fatness and a desirable waist-to-hip ratio?

Determining "Desirable" Body Weight and Body Mass Index

Name _____ Section _____ Date _____

■ Read Concept 13 and complete Lab 13A before doing this lab.

PURPOSE

The purposes of this laboratory session are:
1. To determine desirable weight.
2. To compare two different methods for determining desirable body weight.
3. To determine body mass index (BMI).

PROCEDURE

1. Determine percent body fat (see Lab 13A). Measure height and weight (see Lab Resource Materials, pages 160–161).
2. Determine your frame size (small, medium, large) using the procedures in the Lab Resource Materials (page 161).
3. Determine your desirable weight using height-weight charts in the Lab Resource Materials (page 161).
4. If your percentage of body fat is more than 20 percent for females or 16 percent for males, use charts 13B.4 and 13B.5 to determine your desirable weight based on your current weight and your current percentage of body fat. Locate your current body weight in the left column and your percent of fat across the top of the chart. Your desirable weight is located at the point where the row and column intersect. If your body fat is less than 16 percent for males, and less than 20 percent for females, you do not need to use tables 13B.4 or 13B.5, but it is important for you to read the notes at the bottom of these tables.
5. Calculate your BMI and determine your rating using Chart 13B.6.

RESULTS

Record your scores below:

Percent body fat _____ (from charts 13A.1 and 13A.2)

Weight _____ lbs Weight _____ kg (weight in lbs/2.2)

Height _____ in Height _____ meters (height in inches × .0254)

Frame size small _____ medium _____ large _____ (chart 13B.1)

Desirable weight (chart 13B.2 or 13B.3) _____ lbs/kg

Desirable weight (skinfolds)

Above 16% men and 20% women _____ lbs (charts 13B.4 and 13B.5)

BMI weight (kg) _____ ÷ height (meters) $\left(\dfrac{\text{weight}}{\text{height}^2}\right)$

BMI = _____

BMI Rating _____ (chart 13B.6)

Is your desirable weight as determined from the height-weight chart what it should be? Yes ☐ No ☐ Explain.

Is your desirable weight as determined from percent body fat (skinfolds) what it should be? Yes ☐ No ☐ Explain.

Is your Body Mass Index what it should be? Yes ☐ No ☐ Explain.

LAB 13B

Is there a discrepancy between your answers? Yes ☐ No ☐ If so, explain it. If not, describe the measurement in which you have the most confidence. Explain the reasons for your answer.

Note: If you can't explain it, you may need to consult with your instructor and/or retake your measurements.

Keeping Records for Fat Control

Name _____   Section _____   Date _____

■ Read Concept 14 before completing this lab.

PURPOSE

1. To learn to keep records of calories consumed.
2. To learn to keep records of calories expended.
3. To learn to keep records of fat and weight changes.
4. To learn to chart behavior (diet and exercise) and fat and weight changes over time.

PROCEDURE

1. Write your daily calorie intake goal (the number of calories you would like to consume each day) and your daily calorie expenditure goal (the number of calories you would like to expend each day) in chart 14.1.
2. Keep a dietary log for one day to learn how it is done (use chart 14.1). If you have already completed a three-day diet recall in Lab 22B, you may use the same information here. Record the food eaten, the time eaten, and the calories in the food. Use the calorie chart in Appendix C.
3. Keep an exercise log for one day to learn how it is done (see chart 14.2). Record the activity, the length of time each activity was done, and the calories expended in each activity. Use table 13.3 on page 155.
4. Record your current weight in the results section. Also record your goal weight for fourteen days from now.
5. Record your current percent fat in the results section (see Lab 13A). Also record your goal percent fat for fourteen days from now.
6. This one-day record-keeping effort will get you started. If you really want to lose fat, you should make extra copies of logs and keep records for fourteen days. If you do this for fourteen days, determine your weight and percent fat to see if you met your goals.

RESULTS

Starting weight _____   Goal weight _____

Starting fat % _____   Goal fat % _____

OPTIONAL RESULTS

Weight after fourteen days _____ Percent fat after fourteen days _____

Number of days your exercise goals were met _____ Number of days your dietary goals were met _____

Chart 14.1 Diet Log		
Food Eaten and Amount	**Calories**	**Time of Day**
_____	_____	_____
_____	_____	_____
_____	_____	_____
_____	_____	_____
_____	_____	_____
_____	_____	_____
_____	_____	_____
_____	_____	_____
_____	_____	_____
_____	_____	_____
_____	_____	_____
_____	_____	_____
_____	_____	_____
_____	_____	_____
_____	_____	_____
_____	_____	_____
_____	_____	_____
_____	_____	_____
_____	_____	_____
_____	_____	_____
_____	_____	_____
_____	_____	_____
Total Calories	_____	
Daily Calorie Goal	_____	

Chart 14.2 Exercise Log		
Activity	**Time (min.)**	**Calories**
_____	_____	_____
_____	_____	_____
_____	_____	_____
_____	_____	_____
_____	_____	_____
_____	_____	_____
_____	_____	_____
_____	_____	_____
_____	_____	_____
_____	_____	_____
_____	_____	_____
_____	_____	_____
_____	_____	_____
_____	_____	_____
_____	_____	_____
_____	_____	_____
_____	_____	_____
_____	_____	_____
_____	_____	_____
_____	_____	_____
_____	_____	_____
Total Calories	_____	
Daily Calorie Goal	_____	

CONCLUSIONS AND IMPLICATIONS

Do you think that record keeping would be useful to you? Yes ☐ No ☐ Explain why or why not.

Evaluating Skill-Related Physical Fitness

Name _____ Section _____ Date _____

■ Read Concept 15 before completing this lab.

PURPOSE

The purpose of this lab is to help you evaluate your own skill-related fitness, including agility, balance, coordination, power, speed, and reaction time. This information may be of value in planning your personal fitness program and in deciding which sports may be best, based on your own skill-related fitness.

PROCEDURE

1. Read the directions for each of the skill-related fitness tests presented on pages 180–182 of the Lab Resource Materials for Concept 15.
2. Take as many of the tests as possible, given the time and equipment available.
3. Be sure to warm up before and to cool down after the tests.
4. It is all right to practice the tests before trying them. However, you should decide ahead of time which trial you will use to test your skill-related fitness.
5. After completing the tests, write your scores in the appropriate places in the Results section.
6. Determine your rating for each of the tests from the rating charts on pages 180–182 of the Lab Resource Materials for Concept 15.

LAB
15A

RESULTS

Place a check in the box for each of the tests you completed.

Agility (Illinois run)   ☐

Balance (Bass test)   ☐

Coordination (stick test)   ☐

Power (vertical jump)   ☐

Reaction time (stick drop test) ☐

Speed (three-second run)   ☐

Record your score and rating (from charts 15.1–15.6 in the Lab Resource Materials for Concept 15) in the following spaces.

	Score	Rating	
Agility	_____	_____	(chart 15.1, page 180)
Balance	_____	_____	(chart 15.2, page 180)
Coordination	_____	_____	(chart 15.3, page 181)
Power	_____	_____	(chart 15.4, page 181)
Reaction time	_____	_____	(chart 15.5, page 182)
Speed	_____	_____	(chart 15.6, page 182)

Discuss your strengths and weaknesses in these skill-related fitness tests.

How do you account for your strengths and what can you do to eliminate your weaknesses?

Sports require different components of skill-related fitness. Which sports seem best suited for you, given your skill-related fitness scores? Why?

Sports and Preplanned Programs for Physical Fitness

Name _____ Section _____ Date _____

■ Read Concept 15 before completing this lab.

PURPOSE

The purpose of this lab is to explore the use of different sports or preplanned programs as a part of your personal physical fitness program.

PROCEDURE

1. On chart 15B.1, check any of the ten most popular sports in America in which you especially like to participate.
2. Also on chart 15B.1, check the sports in which you feel you are skilled (ones in which you have enough skill to enjoy playing a game without more lessons).
3. Perform, in or out of class, two or three different sports, or a preplanned program (see Appendixes E and F), each for thirty to sixty minutes.
4. On chart 15B.2 in the Results section list the activity you performed.
5. Check the fitness parts in which you think you might improve by doing the sport or preplanned program. Refer to table 15.2, page 174.

RESULTS

Chart 15B.1 Sports Interests and Proficiencies		
Sport or Program	**Check if Interested**	**Check if Proficient**
Bowling	☐	☐
Tennis	☐	☐
Basketball	☐	☐
Softball	☐	☐
Baseball	☐	☐
Golf	☐	☐
Volleyball	☐	☐
Football	☐	☐
Frisbee	☐	☐
Table tennis	☐	☐
Preplanned program	☐	☐
Others (write in)	☐	☐
_____	☐	☐
_____	☐	☐

Chart 15B.2 Fitness Benefits			
Benefit	**Sport** _____	**Sport** _____	**Preplanned Program** _____
Cardiovascular fitness	☐	☐	☐
Flexibility	☐	☐	☐
Body leanness	☐	☐	☐
Strength	☐	☐	☐
Muscular endurance	☐	☐	☐

CONCLUSIONS AND IMPLICATIONS

Which sports or preplanned program do you feel you might actually include in your exercise program for a lifetime?

Why did you choose them?

LAB
15B

Evaluating Posture

Name   Section   Date

■ Read Concept 16 before completing this lab.

PURPOSE

The purposes of this laboratory session are as follows:
1. To learn to recognize postural deviations and thus become more posture conscious.
2. To determine your posture limitations in order to institute a preventive and corrective program.

PROCEDURE

1. Wear as little clothing as possible (bathing suits are recommended) and remove shoes and socks.
2. Work in groups of two or three, with one person acting as the "subject" while partners serve as "examiners;" alternate roles. *Note:* The instructor may prefer to conduct all examinations by individual screening exams or posture photographs.
   a. Stand by a vertically hung plumb line.
   b. Use chart 16.1. Check any deviations and indicate their severity as follows: 0—none; 1—slight; 2—moderate; 3—severe.
   c. Total the score and determine your posture rating from chart 16.2.
3. If time permits, perform the back and posture exercises from Concept 17, pages 197–206.

RESULTS

Record your posture score. _____
Record your posture rating from chart 16.2.

CONCLUSIONS AND IMPLICATIONS

Were you aware of the deviations that were found? Yes ☐ No ☐
List the deviations that were moderate or severe.

What program will you follow to build or maintain good posture? List specific exercises from Concept 17 that you need to practice to correct each deviation you have identified.

If you were checked as having some of the symptoms of scoliosis, see your instructor for a more thorough examination and possible referral to a physician.

Healthy Back Test

Name   Section   Date

■ Read Concept 16 before completing this lab.

PURPOSE

The purpose of this laboratory session is to determine if you have some muscle imbalance and potential for back problems.

PROCEDURE

1. Secure a partner and administer the Healthy Back Tests to each other. (Details appear in chart 16.3, pages 193–194 of the Lab Resource Materials for Concept 16.) Record results of tests in the results section of this laboratory. If you failed a test, write in the muscles involved.
2. Determine your rating by circling your score on chart 16.4. Record your rating below.

RESULTS

Test	Pass	Fail	If you failed, what were the tight muscles involved?
1. Back to wall	☐	☐	_____
2. Straight-leg lift	☐	☐	_____
3. Thomas test	☐	☐	_____
4. Ely's test	☐	☐	_____
5. Ober's test	☐	☐	_____
6. Press-up	☐	☐	_____
7. Knee roll	☐	☐	_____
Total	____	____	_____

Chart 16.4 Healthy Back Test Ratings	
	Number of Tests Passed
Excellent	7
Very good	6
Good	5
Fair	4
Poor	1–3

CONCLUSIONS AND IMPLICATIONS

Discuss your need to do exercises for care of the back.

LAB
16B

Backache Risk Assessment

Name _____   Section _____   Date _____

■ Read Concept 16 before completing this lab.

PURPOSE

The purpose of this lab is to evaluate your risk of having back and neck problems now or in the future, based upon your work and play habits.

PROCEDURE

1. Answer the questions in the Backache Risk Assessment below (chart 16.5).
2. Total your score according to directions.
3. Circle your rating on chart 16.6.

Chart 16.5 Backache Risk Assessment		
Check "yes" if the statement applies to you; check "no" if it does not apply. Total the number of "yes" answers.		
	Yes	**No**
1. I often have a backache at the end of the day.	☐	☐
2. I usually don't think of my back when I lift and carry things.	☐	☐
3. I often move heavy loads without getting help.	☐	☐
4. I'm not sure I use good body mechanics when I work.	☐	☐
5. I frequently push and pull things.	☐	☐
6. I do a lot of bending over.	☐	☐
7. I do a lot of reaching in work or exercise and sports.	☐	☐
8. I do a lot of twisting in work or exercise and sports.	☐	☐
9. I do a lot of lifting and carrying.	☐	☐
10. I don't do strength exercises for my back and abdomen regularly.	☐	☐
11. I don't do stretching exercises for my trunk, hips, and legs regularly.	☐	☐
12. I sit for long periods without a break.	☐	☐
13. I spend a lot of time leaning over my work.	☐	☐
14. I do exercises that are considered "questionable."	☐	☐
Total	_____	_____

RESULTS

What were the number of "yes" answers? _____
Circle your rating in chart 16.6.

Chart 16.6 Back Risk Rating	
	Number of Yes Answers
Extremely high risk	10–14
High risk	7–9
Moderate risk	4–6
Some risk	1–3
Low risk	0

CONCLUSIONS AND IMPLICATIONS

Based on the Healthy Back Test results and on your Backache Risk Assessment results, suggest some changes you believe are indicated for you.

LAB
16C

Preventive and Therapeutic Exercises for Posture, Neck, and Back

Name _____ Section _____ Date _____

■ Read Concept 17 before completing this lab.

PURPOSE

1. Under the direction and supervision of the instructor, perform the exercises described in Concept 17.
2. In the following list, place a check beside the exercise that you think that you would most likely include in your program.
3. In the Conclusion and Implications section, explain why you chose the exercise.

RESULTS

Exercises from Concept 17

1. Wand Exercise	☐	15. Reverse Curl	☐
2. Pectoral Stretch	☐	16. Crunch a and b	☐
3. Side Bender	☐	17. Crunch Twist/Bench	☐
4. Isometric Neck Ex.	☐	18. Sitting Tucks	☐
5. Neck Rotation Ex.	☐	19. Standing Crunch	☐
6. Back-Saver H.S. Str.	☐	20. Arm Lift	☐
7. Hip and Thigh Stretch	☐	21. Seated Rowing	☐
8. Low Back Stretcher	☐	22. Upper Trunk Lift	☐
9. Single Knee-to-Chest	☐	23. Lower Trunk Lift	☐
10. Dbl. Knee-to-Chest	☐	24. Press-Up	☐
11. Calf Stretcher	☐	25. Bridging	☐
12. Lower Leg Stretch	☐	26. Wall Slide	☐
13. Half Squat (Wts.)	☐	27. Supine Trunk Twist	☐
14. Pelvic Tilt	☐		

(a) Name the postural, neck, and/or back problem(s) you want to prevent or alleviate; (b) tell which exercises you would choose for each (designate these by number); and (c) briefly explain why you selected each.

LAB
17

Questionable Exercises

Name   Section   Date

■ Read Concept 18 before performing this lab.

PURPOSE

To experience some "good" exercises that can accomplish the purpose of some "questionable" exercises.

PROCEDURE

1. Look at the illustrations of questionable exercises in Concept 18, then review the exercises suggested as good alternatives.
2. For each questionable exercise listed, there is one (or more) good alternative to accomplish the same purpose without harm to the individual. Perform the good exercises listed.

RESULTS

Record your results on the following page.
1. How many "questionable" exercises could you find mentioned in Concept 18? List them in the first column.
2. How many good "alternative" exercises could you find mentioned in Concept 18? List them in the second column opposite the exercise for which they are an alternative.

"Questionable" Exercises

1. _____
2. _____
3. _____
4. _____
5. _____
6. _____
7. _____
8. _____
9. _____
10. _____
11. _____
12. _____
13. _____
14. _____
15. _____
16. _____
17. _____

Good "Alternative" Exercises

1. _____
2. _____
3. _____
4. _____
5. _____
6. _____
7. _____
8. _____
9. _____
10. _____
11. _____
12. _____
13. _____
14. _____
15. _____
16. _____
17. _____

"Questionable" Exercises	Good "Alternative" Exercises
18. _____	18. _____
19. _____	19. _____
20. _____	20. _____
21. _____	21. _____
22. _____	22. _____
23. _____	23. _____
24. _____	24. _____
25. _____	25. _____
26. _____	26. _____
27. _____	27. _____
28. _____	28. _____
29. _____	29. _____
30. _____	30. _____
31. _____	31. _____
32. _____	32. _____
33. _____	33. _____
34. _____	34. _____
35. _____	35. _____
36. _____	36. _____
37. _____	37. _____
38. _____	38. _____
39. _____	39. _____
40. _____	40. _____

CONCLUSIONS AND IMPLICATIONS

Could you find forty "questionable" exercises? _____
If not, compare notes with someone or reread the Concept.
Circle the number of those "questionable" exercises you have performed in the past.
What conclusions do you draw from this experience?

What will you do in the future?

The Exercise Adherence Questionnaire

Name _____   Section _____   Date _____

■ Read Concept 19 before completing this lab.

PURPOSE

The purposes of this laboratory are:
1. To help you understand the factors that lead to exercise adherence.
2. To help you see which of these factors may keep you from adhering to exercise.
3. To help you see which factors you might change to improve your chances of adhering to exercise.

PROCEDURE

1. Read each of the fourteen items in the Exercise Adherence Questionnaire, chart 19.1 in the Lab Resource Materials for Concept 19 on page 225.
2. After each statement, check the box indicating whether you think the item is Very True, Somewhat True, or Not True of you.
3. When you have answered all fourteen items, use the scoring procedures on page 226 to score the questionnaire.

RESULTS

After you have scored the questionnaire, record your scores for each of the three scales and your total score in the spaces provided below. Use chart 19.2 on page 226 to determine your rating for each score. Write the ratings in the appropriate blanks.

	Score	**Rating**
Predisposing factors	_____	_____
Enabling factors	_____	_____
Reinforcing factors	_____	_____
Total	_____	_____

CONCLUSIONS AND IMPLICATIONS

You may want to look over Concept 19 before completing this section. The scores on the Exercise Adherence Questionnaire should give you an idea of your tendency to do regular exercise.

1. Which Predisposing Factors are most likely to help you get started in regular exercise or keep you from starting an exercise program? Explain.

2. Which Enabling Factors are most likely to help you stick with exercise or keep you from sticking with it once you start? Explain.

3. Which Reinforcing Factors are most likely to help you stick with exercise or keep you from sticking with it once you start? Explain.

4. A high score should reflect a general tendency to be active on a regular basis. Is your total score a good reflection of your overall exercise adherence? Yes ☐ No ☐ Explain.

LAB
19

Planning Your Personal Exercise Program

Name   Section   Date
_____

■ Read Concept 20 before completing this lab.

PURPOSE

The purpose of this lab is to plan a personal fitness program using the seven steps outlined in Concept 20.

PROCEDURE AND RESULTS

Answer the questions and fill in the charts following the seven steps outlined below.

1. Establish the Reasons for Your Program
In the space provided, write your principal reasons for wanting to start an exercise program. Consider using the results of the Physical Activity Questionnaire (Lab 2A) to help you.

2. Identify Your Personal Fitness Needs
In chart 20.1, darken the boxes of your self-test rating for each of the tests you have taken. (Refer to the appropriate rating charts to determine your ratings.) If you did not take a test, darken the "no result" box.

In chart 20.2, darken one box for each component of fitness. Record only *one* rating for each by averaging ratings from chart 20.1. If you took more than one test for a particular fitness component, use your own judgment in determining your average rating. Use ratings 1–4 for cardiovascular fitness, 5 for flexibility, 6–7 for strength, 8 for muscular endurance, and 9 for fatness. Record one average rating for skill-related fitness using ratings 10–15 from chart 20.1. Record one average rating for fitness of the back and posture using ratings 16–17 from chart 20.1. Connect the darkened boxes to create your own personal fitness profile. The completed profile will give you important information for planning your program.

Chart 20.1 *Ratings* for Fitness Self-Tests

Fitness Tests	Rating				
	High Performance Zone	Good Fitness Zone	Marginal Zone	Low Zone	No Results
1. Twelve-Minute Run Chart 6B.1, page 65	☐	☐	☐	☐	☐
2. Step Test Chart 6B.2, page 65	☐	☐	☐	☐	☐
3. Bicycle Test Chart 6B.4, page 66	☐	☐	☐	☐	☐
4. Rockport Walking Test Charts 6B.5 and 6B.6, page 67	☐	☐	☐	☐	☐
5. Flexibility Test 1	☐	☐	☐	☐	☐
Chart 8.1 Test 2	☐	☐	☐	☐	☐
page 85 Test 3	☐	☐	☐	☐	☐
6. Isotonic Strength Chart 10.1 or 10.2, page 114	☐	☐	☐	☐	☐
7. Isometric Strength (average) Chart 10.3, page 114, or 10.4, page 115	☐	☐	☐	☐	☐
8. Muscular Endurance Chart 11.1 or 11.2, page 122	☐	☐	☐	☐	☐
9. Fatness Rating (skinfold) Chart 13A.3, page 160	☐	☐	☐	☐	☐
10. Agility Chart 15.1, page 180	☐	☐	☐	☐	☐
11. Balance Chart 15.2, page 180	☐	☐	☐	☐	☐
12. Coordination Chart 15.3, page 181	☐	☐	☐	☐	☐
13. Power Chart 15.4, page 181	☐	☐	☐	☐	☐
14. Reaction Time Chart 15.5, page 182	☐	☐	☐	☐	☐
15. Speed Chart 15.6, page 182	☐	☐	☐	☐	☐
16. Fitness of the Back Chart 16.4, page 194	☐	☐	☐	☐	☐
17. Posture Chart 16.2, page 192	☐	☐	☐	☐	☐

LAB
20

Chart 20.2	A Profile of Personal Fitness Needs				
	Rating				
Fitness Component	**High Performance Zone**	**Good Fitness Zone**	**Marginal Zone**	**Low Zone**	**No Rating**
Cardiovascular	☐	☐	☐	☐	☐
Endurance	☐	☐	☐	☐	☐
Strength	☐	☐	☐	☐	☐
Flexibility	☐	☐	☐	☐	☐
Fat control	☐	☐	☐	☐	☐
Skill-related fitness	☐	☐	☐	☐	☐
Posture and fitness of the back	☐	☐	☐	☐	☐

3. **Establish Your Exercise and Fitness Goals**
   A. *Short-Term Goals*

   Exercise Goals: Give the length of time for your typical workout (in minutes) and the number of workouts per day and per week.

   Length of workout _____ minutes

   Workouts per day _____

   Workout days per week _____

   Weeks of program _____ no more than four

   Fitness Goals: Beginners should omit this section. If you have been exercising regularly, write down the specific goals you expect to accomplish in the number of weeks specified in your exercise goals. Example: perform ten pull-ups or perform twenty-five crunches. Consider goals for each component of fitness.

   B. *Long-Term Goals*

   Exercise Goals: Designate the number of months for which you are making a commitment to exercise.

   Months _____ (no more than twelve)

   Fitness Goals: Write your specific performance goals for the number of months specified above. Indicate expected scores on fitness tests. For example: Run one and one-half miles in twelve minutes or attain 21 percent body fatness.

4. **Select Your Activities**

Complete chart 20.3. In the top part of the chart, list the activities you currently do on a regular basis that you would like to continue. In the middle section, indicate some new activities that would be especially good for developing your fitness goals or meeting a weakness or special need (see chart 20.2). Finally, in the bottom section of the chart, list some new activities you would especially like to try because you enjoy them (even if they do not meet your special fitness needs). After each, note the component of fitness developed by the activity. You should have at least one activity for each of the health-related fitness components. You should be especially careful to include exercise for the components of fitness for which you have low ratings.

Chart 20.3 Personal Physical Activities

Current Activities
(List activities in which you currently participate.)

Activity	Fitness Components Developed by Activity
1. _____	_____
2. _____	_____
3. _____	_____
4. _____	_____
5. _____	_____

Proposed New Activities for Fitness
(List new activities for meeting fitness needs.)

Activity	Fitness Components Developed by Activity
1. _____	_____
2. _____	_____
3. _____	_____
4. _____	_____
5. _____	_____

New Activities Just for Fun
(List new activities that you think you might especially enjoy, but that may not be good for developing fitness.)

Activity
1. _____
2. _____
3. _____

5. Prepare A Personal Weekly Exercise Schedule

Complete chart 20.4. For each day of the week, write in the activities you plan to do on that particular day. Select the activities from chart 20.3. A special place is provided for your warm-up and cool-down activities. In this section, write in the activities you will do to warm up and cool down each day. (You do not need to list these each day on the daily schedules. Another section is provided for "special exercises" that you may do on a regular basis.) These may include exercises for the back, or just a set of calisthenics or exercises you plan to do. Once you list these activities in the "special exercise section," you need only refer to them in your daily schedule as "special exercises," rather than write them on each day's schedule. Table 20.1 on page 229 is a sample program that you might want to consult before preparing your personal schedule.

6. Keep Exercise and Fitness Records

Record keeping can help you stick with your exercise program and can help you attain your fitness goals. Use a one-month calendar or chart 20.5 to keep track of your regular exercise and fitness changes. Follow these steps in using the calendar.

- Write the month at the top and the dates on the calendar beginning on the day you expect to begin your program (yellow).
- Place an X in the appropriate box of the dates you expect to do your program (green).
- Write fitness goals on the calendar on the day you expect to accomplish them.
- Place an X in the appropriate box each time you do your exercise as planned (blue).
- Test your fitness on dates with goals. Set new goals for the future.
- Prepare a new record-keeping calendar when the current one expires.

7. Evaluate and Modify Your Program

After you have tried your program, either in class or on your own, evaluate it. Note your comments in the appropriate section of chart 20.4. *Remember, even the best program needs periodic reevaluation and modification.*

Chart 20.4 Weekly Exercise Program

Daily Schedules
(List the activities and times of day for each activity.)

Monday	Tuesday	Wednesday

Thursday	Friday	Saturday

Sunday	Warm-Up and Cool-Down Activities	Program Evaluation (Fill in after trying out your program.)

Special Exercises

Chart 20.5 Record-Keeping Calendar

	Sunday		Monday		Tuesday		Wednesday		Thursday		Friday		Saturday
Date	Goals:	Date	Goals:	Date	Goals:	Date	Goals:	Date	Goals:	Date	Goals:	Date	Goals:
Date	Goals:	Date	Goals:	Date	Goals:	Date	Goals:	Date	Goals:	Date	Goals:	Date	Goals:
Date	Goals:	Date	Goals:	Date	Goals:	Date	Goals:	Date	Goals:	Date	Goals:	Date	Goals:
Date	Goals:	Date	Goals:	Date	Goals:	Date	Goals:	Date	Goals:	Date	Goals:	Date	Goals:

Assessing Personal Wellness

Name _____ Section _____ Date _____

■ Read Concept 21 before completing this lab.

PURPOSE

The purpose of this laboratory experience is to make you aware of your own perceptions of personal wellness.

PROCEDURE

1. Answer the questions in the Self-Perceptions of Wellness Questionnaire on the following page.
2. Score the questionnaire using the procedures outlined in the Lab Resource Materials on page 241.
3. Record your scores in the spaces provided in the results section.
4. Determine your ratings for each wellness score using Chart 21.3 in the Lab Resource Materials on page 241.

RESULTS

Write your scores and ratings in the appropriate blanks below.

Wellness Dimension (Perceptions)	Score	Rating	
Emotional wellness	_____	_____	(question 1)
Intellectual wellness	_____	_____	(question 2)
Physical wellness	_____	_____	(question 3)
Social wellness	_____	_____	(question 4)
Spiritual wellness	_____	_____	(question 5)
General wellness	_____	_____	(question 6)
Total wellness	_____	_____	(all questions)

LAB
21

CONCLUSIONS AND IMPLICATIONS

Do you think the first five ratings (one for each dimension of wellness) reflect your true state of wellness? ☐ Yes ☐ No
Explain.

Do you think your general wellness score (question 6) and/or your total wellness rating (sum of 6 questions) reflect your overall state of wellness? Check one: ☐ Both ☐ General ☐ Total ☐ Neither Explain.

Do you think that your current life-style will help you improve your wellness ratings in the years ahead? ☐Yes ☐No Explain.

Chart 21.2 Self-Perceptions of Wellness Questionnaire

Using the Self-Perceptions Questionnaire

Directions

There are four possible responses for each question. Place an X in **one** of the four boxes for **each** question.

Sample Question: A person who likes ice cream a lot would mark the box as indicated below.

Some people like ice cream very much.   **but**   Other people do not like ice cream at all.

Especially true for me   True for me   Not true for me   Especially not true for me
        ☒   ☐   ☐   ☐

1. Some people are happy most of the time.   **but**   Other people feel depressed much of the time.

Especially true for me   True for me   Not true for me   Especially not true for me
        ☐   ☐   ☐   ☐

2. Some people are well informed about health and   **but**   Other people are ignorant of the facts concerning
wellness.   their health and well-being.

Especially true for me   True for me   Not true for me   Especially not true for me
        ☐   ☐   ☐   ☐

3. Some people are physically fit.   **but**   Other people are not so fit physically.

Especially true for me   True for me   Not true for me   Especially not true for me
        ☐   ☐   ☐   ☐

4. Some people have a lot of friends and are very involved   **but**   Other people do not have many friends and are often lonely.
socially.

Especially true for me   True for me   Not true for me   Especially not true for me
        ☐   ☐   ☐   ☐

5. Some people feel fulfilled spiritually.   **but**   Other people are not so fulfilled spiritually.

Especially true for me   True for me   Not true for me   Especially not true for me
        ☐   ☐   ☐   ☐

6. Some people have a very positive outlook on life—they   **but**   Other people have a more negative outlook on life—
are optimistic.   they are pessimistic.

Especially true for me   True for me   Not true for me   Especially not true for me
        ☐   ☐   ☐   ☐

Nutrition Analysis

Name _____ Section _____ Date _____

■ Read Concept 22 before proceeding with this lab.

PURPOSE

The purposes of this laboratory are:
1. To determine the nutritional quality of your diet.
2. To determine your average daily caloric intake.
3. To determine necessary changes in eating habits.

PROCEDURE

1. a. Record your dietary intake for two days using the dietary record sheet (chart 22A.3). Record intake for one weekday (p. L-65) and one weekend day (p. L-66).
   b. Include the actual foods eaten, the amount (size of portion in teaspoons, tablespoons, cups, oz., or other standard units of measurement). Be sure to include all drinks (coffee, tea, soft drinks, etc.).
   c. Include *all* foods eaten including sauces, gravies, dressings, toppings, spreads, etc.
   d. Determine your calorie consumption for each of the two days. Use Appendix C to assist you.
   e. Check the number of servings from each food group.
   f. Estimate the proportion of complex carbohydrate, simple carbohydrate, protein, and fat in each meal and in snacks.
2. a. Answer the questions in chart 22A.1 using information from each of the three dietary record sheets.
   b. Score one point for each "yes" answer on chart 22A.1.
   c. Use chart 22A.2 to rate your dietary habits. Circle the appropriate rating.

RESULTS

Record the number of calories consumed for each of the two days.

Day 1 _____ Day 2 _____

Chart 22A.1 Dietary Habits Questionnaire

Yes	No	
☐	☐	1. Do you eat regular meals?
☐	☐	2. Do you eat a good breakfast daily?
☐	☐	3. Do you eat lunch regularly?
☐	☐	4. Does your diet contain about 55%–60% carbohydrates with a high concentration of fiber?
☐	☐	5. Are less than one-fourth of the carbohydrates you eat simple carbohydrates?
☐	☐	6. Does your diet contain 10%–15% protein?
☐	☐	7. Does your diet contain less than 30% fat?
☐	☐	8. Do you limit the amount of saturated fat in your diet?
☐	☐	9. Do you limit salt intake to acceptable amounts?
☐	☐	10. Do you get adequate amounts of vitamins in your diet without a supplement?
☐	☐	11. Do you eat regularly from all food groups?
☐	☐	12. Do you drink adequate amounts of water?
☐	☐	13. Do you get adequate minerals in your diet without a supplement?
☐	☐	14. Do you limit your caffeine consumption to acceptable levels?
☐	☐	15. Is your average calorie consumption for the three-day period reasonable for your body size and for the amount of calories you normally expend?

_____ Total number of "Yes" answers.

Chart 22A.2 Dietary Habits *Rating Scale*

Score	Rating
14–15	Very Good
12–13	Good
10–11	Marginal
9 or less	Poor

CONCLUSIONS AND IMPLICATIONS

Are changes in your eating habits necessary? Yes ☐ No ☐ If so, what changes? If not, explain.

Chart 22A.3 Diet Record

Day 1

Breakfast Food	Amount	Calories	Basic Food Servings	Food Content
			Dairy Group ☐ ☐ Meat/Fish/Eggs ☐ ☐ Vegetables/Fruits ☐ ☐ ☐ ☐ Breads/Cereals ☐ ☐ ☐ ☐	% Protein _____ % Fat _____ % Complex Carbohydrate _____ % Simple Carbohydrate _____

Lunch Food	Amount	Calories	Basic Food Servings	Food Content
			Dairy Group ☐ ☐ Meat/Fish/Eggs ☐ ☐ Vegetables/Fruits ☐ ☐ ☐ ☐ Breads/Cereals ☐ ☐ ☐ ☐	% Protein _____ % Fat _____ % Complex Carbohydrate _____ % Simple Carbohydrate _____

Dinner Food	Amount	Calories	Basic Food Servings	Food Content
			Dairy Group ☐ ☐ Meat/Fish/Eggs ☐ ☐ Vegetables/Fruits ☐ ☐ ☐ ☐ Breads/Cereals ☐ ☐ ☐ ☐	% Protein _____ % Fat _____ % Complex Carbohydrate _____ % Simple Carbohydrate _____

Snack Food	Amount	Calories	Basic Food Servings	Food Content
			Dairy Group ☐ ☐ Meat/Fish/Eggs ☐ ☐ Vegetables/Fruits ☐ ☐ ☐ ☐ Breads/Cereals ☐ ☐ ☐ ☐	% Protein _____ % Fat _____ % Complex Carbohydrate _____ % Simple Carbohydrate _____
		Total Calories for Day		

Chart 22A.3 Diet Record

Day 2

Breakfast Food	Amount	Calories	Basic Food Servings	Food Content
			Dairy Group ☐ ☐ Meat/Fish/Eggs ☐ ☐ Vegetables/Fruits ☐ ☐ ☐ ☐ Breads/Cereals ☐ ☐ ☐ ☐	% Protein _____ % Fat _____ % Complex Carbohydrate _____ % Simple Carbohydrate _____

Lunch Food	Amount	Calories	Basic Food Servings	Food Content
			Dairy Group ☐ ☐ Meat/Fish/Eggs ☐ ☐ Vegetables/Fruits ☐ ☐ ☐ ☐ Breads/Cereals ☐ ☐ ☐ ☐	% Protein _____ % Fat _____ % Complex Carbohydrate _____ % Simple Carbohydrate _____

Dinner Food	Amount	Calories	Basic Food Servings	Food Content
			Dairy Group ☐ ☐ Meat/Fish/Eggs ☐ ☐ Vegetables/Fruits ☐ ☐ ☐ ☐ Breads/Cereals ☐ ☐ ☐ ☐	% Protein _____ % Fat _____ % Complex Carbohydrate _____ % Simple Carbohydrate _____

Snack Food	Amount	Calories	Basic Food Servings	Food Content
			Dairy Group ☐ ☐ Meat/Fish/Eggs ☐ ☐ Vegetables/Fruits ☐ ☐ ☐ ☐ Breads/Cereals ☐ ☐ ☐ ☐	% Protein _____ % Fat _____ % Complex Carbohydrate _____ % Simple Carbohydrate _____
		Total Calories for Day		

Selecting Nutritious Foods

Name _____ Section _____ Date _____

■ Read Concept 22 and have your book handy before proceeding with this lab.

PURPOSE

The purposes of this lab are:

1. To learn to select a nutritious diet.
2. To determine the nutritive value of favorite foods.
3. To compare a nutritious food's values to a favorite food's values.

PROCEDURE

1. Use Appendix D to determine values of foods. You may select a food more than once.
2. Select a breakfast, lunch, and dinner from the favorite foods list (see Appendix D). Include between-meal snacks with nearest meal. If you cannot find foods you would normally choose, select those most similar to choices you might make.
3. Select a breakfast, lunch, and dinner from foods you feel would make the most nutritious meals. Include between-meal snacks with nearest meal.
4. Record the foods you list in the "favorite foods" and "nutritious foods" in chart 22B on the back of this sheet. Record the calories for proteins, carbohydrates, and fats for each of the foods you choose.
5. Total each column for the "favorite" and the "nutritious" meal.
6. Determine the percentages of your total calories that are protein, carbohydrate, and fat by dividing each column total by the total number of calories consumed.
7. Answer the questions in the conclusions section below.

RESULTS

Record results in the charts on the following page and summarize below.

Favorite Foods

Protein Calories	_____	÷	Total Calories	_____ = % Protein	_____
Carboh. Calories	_____	÷	Total Calories	_____ = % Carboh.	_____
Fat Calories	_____	÷	Total Calories	_____ = % Fat	_____

Nutritious Foods

Protein Calories	_____	÷	Total Calories	_____ = % Protein	_____
Carboh. Calories	_____	÷	Total Calories	_____ = % Carboh.	_____
Fat Calories	_____	÷	Total Calories	_____ = % Fat	_____

CONCLUSIONS AND IMPLICATIONS

Was your "favorite" one-day diet nutritious? Yes ☐ No ☐ Were you able to select a "nutritious" diet that meets the standards outlined in Concept 22? Yes ☐ No ☐ Discuss your results.

Chart 22B "Favorite" versus "Nutritious" Food Choices for Three Daily Meals

Breakfast

Food No.	Favorite				Food No.	Nutritious			
	Cal.	Pro. Cal.	Car. Cal.	Fat Cal.		Cal.	Pro. Cal.	Car. Cal.	Fat Cal.
Totals					Totals				

Lunch

Food No.	Favorite				Food No.	Nutritious			
	Cal.	Pro. Cal.	Car. Cal.	Fat Cal.		Cal.	Pro. Cal.	Car. Cal.	Fat Cal.
Totals					Totals				

Dinner

Food No.	Favorite				Food No.	Nutritious			
	Cal.	Pro. Cal.	Car. Cal.	Fat Cal.		Cal.	Pro. Cal.	Car. Cal.	Fat Cal.
Totals					Totals				
Daily Totals	□	□	□	□	Daily Totals	□	□	□	□
Daily %		□	□	□	Daily %		□	□	□

LAB 22B

Evaluating Your Stress Level

Name _____ Section _____ Date _____

■ Read Concept 23 before proceeding with this lab.

PURPOSE

The purpose of this lab is to evaluate your stress during the past year and determine its implications. Research shows that when people become too stressed, they are more susceptible to certain diseases such as heart disease, ulcers, allergies, hypertension, and insomnia. There are also some psychological implications, as this lab will show. People with high stress need to recognize its causes and effects, and find ways of coping with or reducing stress.

PROCEDURE

1. Look at the Life Experience Survey in the Lab Resource Materials on pages 262–265. Indicate with a check whether the experience (if it occurred in the past year) occurred during the first six months or the last six months. Circle the score representing the impact the experience had on you.
2. Add all of the negative numbers and record your score (distress) in the Results section below. Add the positive numbers and record your score (eustress) in the Results section below. Use all of the events in the last year.
3. Find your scores on the rating scale (chart 23A.1 below) and record your ratings.
4. Interpret the results by answering the questions, and discussing the conclusions and implications in the space provided.
5. You may also want to calculate your distress and eustress scores over the last six months rather than the last year. The more recent the event, the greater the likelihood that it will be stressful.

Chart 23A.1 *Rating Scale* for Life Experiences and Stress	Sum of Negative Scores (Distress)	Sum of Positive Scores (Eustress)
May need counseling	14+	
Above average stress	9–13	>10
Average	6–9	9–10
Below average stress	<6	<8

RESULTS

Sum of negative scores   _____ (distress)

Sum of positive scores   _____ (eustress)

Rating on negative scores _____

Rating on positive scores _____

CONCLUSIONS AND IMPLICATIONS

The higher the negative score, the greater the distress and the more likely you are to:

1. have high anxiety;
2. have some personal maladjustments, psychological problems, and/or neuroticism;
3. be depressed;
4. feel less capable of exerting control over your environment;
5. have academic problems; lower GPA.

A high positive score (eustress) suggests that your life's experiences are enriching your quality of life.

What do your stress ratings imply?

Do you need to seek professional help? Yes ☐ No ☐

What strategies will you try to reduce your negative stress?

What strategies will you use to enrich your life's experience?

Evaluating Neuromuscular Tension

Name _____   Section _____   Date _____

■ Read Concept 23 before proceeding with this lab.

PURPOSE

The purpose of this laboratory session is to learn to recognize signs of excess tension in yourself and in others by symptomatic mannerisms and by manually testing your ability to relax. If time permits, perform the relaxation exercises in Concept 23 before executing the lab. A trained person can diagnose neuromuscular hypertension by observation and by manual testing. While there is insufficient time in this course to master either the technique of relaxing or the techniques of evaluation, it is possible to learn the procedures for both.

PROCEDURE

1. Choose a partner. Designate one partner as the subject and the other as the tester. Alternate roles.
2. The subject should lie supine in a comfortable position and consciously try to relax as described in Concept 23. This may be done alone, or the instructor may wish to direct the entire group in this procedure.
3. The tester should kneel beside the subject's right hand and remain very still and quiet while the subject is concentrating.
4. After five minutes have elapsed, the tester should observe the subject for signs of tension in Part A of chart 23B.1 and check "yes" or "no" for symptoms of visual tension.
5. Quietly and gently, the tester should grasp the subject's right wrist with his or her fingers, and slowly raise it about three inches from the floor, letting it hinge at the elbow, then let the hand drop. Observe the signs of tension outlined in section B of chart 23B.1. *Caution:* Make no movement or sound to disturb your partner's concentration and relaxation. Check the chart to indicate manual symptoms of tension.
6. You may wish to repeat this after another minute or two.
7. Arouse the subject at the end of the testing and total the number of "yes" checks.
8. Find the rating in chart 23B.2 and record it below.
9. Change places and repeat the evaluation with a new subject and tester.
10. Draw conclusions and discuss the implications by answering the questions that follow.

RESULTS

What is your tension score? _____

What is your tension-relaxation rating? ____

Chart 23B.1 Signs of Tension Observed by Tester	No	Yes
A. Visual Symptoms		
Frowning	☐	☐
Twitching	☐	☐
Eyelids fluttering	☐	☐
Breathing:		
shallow	☐	☐
rapid	☐	☐
irregular	☐	☐
Mouth tight	☐	☐
Swallowing	☐	☐
B. Manual Symptoms		
Assistance (subject helps lift arm)	☐	☐
Resistance (subject resists movement)	☐	☐
Posturing (subject holds arm in raised position)	☐	☐
Perseveration (subject continues upward movement)	☐	☐
Total number of "yes" checks _____		

Chart 23B.2 Tension-Relaxation *Rating Scale*	
Classification	**Total Score**
Excellent (relaxed)	0
Very good (mild tension)	1–3
Good (moderate tension)	4–6
Fair (tense)	7–9
Poor (marked tension)	10–12

CONCLUSIONS AND IMPLICATIONS

Were you aware of your own tension?	Yes _____	No _____
Was it more difficult to relax than you expected?	Yes _____	No _____
Did your awareness of your partner make it more difficult to concentrate?	Yes _____	No _____
Can you concentrate on your breathing without altering its rhythm?	Yes _____	No _____
Could you learn to release muscular tension and help manage your stress with additional practice?	Yes _____	No _____
Could you learn to release tension while sitting or standing with your eyes open?	Yes _____	No _____
Do you think your score today is typical of your normal tension level?	Yes _____	No _____

What implications does this concept have for you in terms of your daily life (e.g., sleeping, studying, taking exams, performing on stage, etc.)?

LAB
23B

LAB 23C

Relaxing Tense Muscles

Name _____

■ Read Concept 23 before completing this lab.

PURPOSE

The purpose of this lab is to learn how to relax tense muscles.

PROCEDURE

Part 1
Perform each of the exercises on the following page.

Part II
1. Sit in a chair or lie on your back in a quiet, nondistracting atmosphere while you are learning this relaxation technique. (Later you will want to be able to use the technique in public, everyday situations, while you are at work, or any time you are under stress.) Get as comfortable as possible.
2. Do the contract-relax routine for relaxation on the following page. Contract the muscles to a moderate level of tension (do not use maximum contractions) as you inhale for five to seven seconds. Study where you are feeling the tension. Try to keep the tension isolated to the designated muscle group without allowing it to spill over to other muscles. Use the dominant side of body first; repeat on the nondominant side.
3. Next, release the tension completely, instantly relaxing the muscles, and exhale. Extend the feeling of relaxation throughout your muscles for twenty to thirty seconds before contracting again. Think of relaxing expressions like "warm," "calm," "peaceful," and "serene."
4. If time permits, you should practice each muscle group two to five times (until tension is gone) before going on to the next group. In a class, you may have time for only one trial. For home practice, do the routine twice a day for fifteen minutes.

RESULTS, CONCLUSIONS, AND IMPLICATIONS

Did you find the relaxation exercises effective? Yes ☐ No ☐
Do you think you would find them useful as part of your normal daily routine or as a "quick fix" for stress? Yes ☐ No ☐
Explain.

Did you find the contract-relax exercise routine relaxing? Yes ☐ No ☐
Do you think you would find them useful as part of your normal daily routine or as a "quick fix" for stress?
Yes ☐ No ☐ Explain.

LAB
23C

Relaxation Exercises*

1. **Neck Stretch**—Roll the head slowly in a half circle from 9:00 to 8:00 to 7, 6, 5, 4, and 3:00, then reverse from 3 to 9:00. Close your eyes and feel the stretch. Do *not* make a full circle by tipping the head back. Repeat several times.

2. **Shoulder Lift**—Hunch the shoulders as high as possible (contract) and then let them drop (relax). Repeat several times. Inhale on the lift; exhale on the drop.

3. **Trunk Stretch and Drop**—Stand and reach as high as possible; tiptoe and stretch every muscle, then collapse completely, letting knees flex and trunk, head, and arms dangle. Repeat two or three times. Inhale on the stretch and exhale on the collapse.

4. **Trunk Swings**—Following the "trunk stretch and drop," remain in the drop position and with a minimum of muscular effort, set the trunk swinging from side to side by shifting the weight from one foot to the other, letting the heels come off the floor alternately. Keep the entire body (especially the neck) limp.

5. **Tension Contrast**—With arms extended overhead, lie on your side. Tense the body as stiff as a board, then let go, and relax, letting the body fall either forward or backward in whatever direction it loses balance. Continue letting go for a few seconds after falling and allow yourself to feel like you are still sinking. Repeat on the other side.

*For illustrations, see pages 260–261.

Contract-Relax Exercise Routine for Relaxation*

1. Hand and forearm—Contract your right hand, making a fist; hold 3 counts; relax and keep letting go 6–10 counts. Repeat, then do left fist, then both fists.

2. Biceps—Flex both elbows and contract your biceps; hold 3 counts; relax and continue relaxing 6–10 counts. Repeat.

3. Triceps—Same as biceps except extend both elbows, contract the triceps on the back of the arm. Repeat.

4. Relax both hands, forearms, and upper arms.

5. Forehead—Raise your eyebrows and wrinkle your forehead; hold 3 counts; relax and continue relaxing 6–10 counts.

6. Cheeks and nose—Make a face; wrinkle your nose and squint; hold 3 counts; relax and continue relaxing 6–10 counts.

7. Jaws—Clench your teeth 3 counts; relax for 6–10 counts.

8. Lips and tongue—With teeth apart, press lips together and press tongue to roof of mouth; hold 3 counts; relax 6 to 10 counts.

9. Neck and throat—Push head backward while tucking chin, pushing against floor or pillow if lying; if sitting, push against high chair-back; hold 3 counts; relax for 6–10 counts.

10. Relax forehead, cheeks, nose, jaws, lips, tongue, neck and throat. Relax hands, forearms and upper arms.

11. Shoulder and upper back—Hunch shoulders to ears; hold 3 counts; relax 6–10 counts.

12. Relax lips, tongue, neck, throat, shoulders and upper back.

13. Abdomen—Suck in abdomen; hold for 3 counts; relax for 6–10 counts.

14. Lower back—Contract and arch the back; hold for 3 counts; relax for 6–10 counts.

15. Thighs and buttocks—Squeeze your buttocks together and push your heels into the floor (if lying) or against a chair rung (if sitting); hold 3 counts; relax 6–10 counts.

16. Relax shoulders and upper back, abdomen, lower back, thighs and buttocks.

17. Calves—Pull instep and toes toward shins; hold 3 counts; relax 6–10 counts.

18. Toes—Curl toes; hold 3 counts; relax 6–10 counts.

19. Relax every muscle in your body.

*Note: Eventually, you should progress to a combination of muscle groups and gradually eliminate the "contract" phase of the program. Refer to Jacobson's relaxation method (page 259) for more instructions, or read Jacobson's book or chapter 10 of Greenberg's book (see p. 262).

LAB
23C

Evaluating Fitness Literature and Devices

Name _____ Section _____ Date _____

■ Read Concept 24 before completing this lab.

PURPOSE

The purpose of this lab is to practice evaluating exercises found in popular literature.

PROCEDURE

1. Read a popular book or magazine and find what you believe to be a poor exercise or device that claims to improve your health, fitness, figure, or posture. If possible, attach a copy of the description of the exercise/device to this lab sheet.
2. Use chart 24A.1 to evaluate the exercise/device. Check "yes" or "no" for each item. Then record your scores in the Results section.
3. Describe the exercise/device you evaluated in the space provided in chart 24A.2.

Chart 24A.1 Exercise/Device Evaluation*

	Yes	No		Yes	No
1. Is the article or book written by an expert as defined in Concept 24?	☐	☐	7. Does it employ "active" exercise in which your own muscles contract?	☐	☐
2. Does the exercise/device employ the overload principle?	☐	☐	8. Are the benefits claimed for it reasonable?	☐	☐
3. Does it employ the progression principle?	☐	☐	9. Are the authors trying to help you (rather than selling a product)?	☐	☐
4. Does it employ the F.I.T. formula?	☐	☐	10. Do they refrain from using terms such as "quick," "miraculous," "tone," "remove fat," "new discovery," or other gimmick words?	☐	☐
5. Does it employ the principle of specificity?	☐	☐			
6. Is it a safe exercise? (See Concept 18.)	☐	☐			

*If in doubt, you may seek an expert's opinion on some of these questions.

Chart 24A.2 Exercise/Device Description

1. Give the exercise/device you are evaluating one point for each "yes" answer on questions 1, 8, 9, and 10. _____ (Score 1)

2. Give it one point for each "yes" answer on questions 2, 3, 4, 5, 6, and 7. _____ (Score 2)

3. Total of score 1 and score 2. _____ (Total score)

CONCLUSIONS AND IMPLICATIONS

1. A high score 1 total (3 or 4) in the Results section indicates that the authors of the exercise or device know what they are talking about.
2. A high score 2 total (5 or 6) indicates that it is consistent with good exercise theory.
3. A high total score (8 to 10) suggests that it is sound for at least some aspects of fitness.

Using this information, write an assessment here of the exercise or device.

LAB
24

Being an Informed Consumer

Name _____ Section _____ Date _____

■ Read Concept 24 before completing this lab.

PURPOSE

The purpose of this lab is to practice evaluating a "health club."

PROCEDURE

1. Visit a health club and pretend to be interested in becoming a member. (*Note:* Only one or two class members should go to each club to avoid suspicion.)
2. Listen carefully to all that is said and ask lots of questions (without exposing your real motives).
3. Look carefully all around you as you are given the tour of the facilities; ask what the exercises or the equipment does for you or ask leading questions such as "Will this take inches off my hips?", etc.
4. As soon as you leave the club, jot some notes before you forget what you heard and saw or complete this report immediately. Do not take notes while you are in the club. Space is provided in chart 24B.1 for notes.

RESULTS

1. Check the evaluation list on chart 24B.1 by checking on the "yes" or "no" answers, and add any special notes opposite each item.
2. Score the chart as follows:
   a. Give one point for each "no" answer for items 1, 2, 3, 4, 5, 7, 8, 10, 13, and 14, and place the score in the blank.   Total A _____
   b. Give one point for each "yes" answer for items 6, 9, 11, 12, and 17, and place the score in the blank.   Total B _____
   c. Total a and b above and place the score in the blank.   Total A and B _____
   d. Give one point for each "yes" answer on 14, 15, and 16, and place the score in the blank.   Total D _____

Chart 24B.1 Health Club Evaluation

	Yes	No	Notes
1. Were claims for improvement in weight, figure/physique, or fitness realistic?	☐	☐	_____
2. Was a long-term contract (1–3 years) encouraged?	☐	☐	_____
3. Was the sales pitch high-pressure to make an immediate decision?	☐	☐	_____
4. Were you given a copy of the contract to read at home?	☐	☐	_____
5. Did the fine print include objectionable clauses?	☐	☐	_____
6. Did they recommend a physician's approval prior to joining?	☐	☐	_____
7. Did they sell diet supplements as a side line?	☐	☐	_____
8. Did they have passive equipment?	☐	☐	_____
9. Did they have cardiovascular training equipment or facilities (cycles, track, pool, aerobic dance)?	☐	☐	_____
10. Did they make unscientific claims for the equipment, exercise, baths, or diet supplements?	☐	☐	_____
11. Were the facilities clean?	☐	☐	_____
12. Were the facilities crowded?	☐	☐	_____
13. Were there days and hours when facilities were open but would not be available to you?	☐	☐	_____
14. Were there limits on the number of minutes you could use a piece of equipment?	☐	☐	_____
15. Did the floor personnel closely supervise and assist clients?	☐	☐	_____
16. Were the floor personnel qualified "experts"?	☐	☐	_____
17. Were the managers/owners qualified "experts"?	☐	☐	_____
18. Has the club been in business at this location for a year or more?	☐	☐	_____

CONCLUSIONS AND IMPLICATIONS

1. A total score of 12–15 points on items *A* and *B* suggests the club rates at least "fair" compared to other clubs.
2. A score of 3 on item *D* indicates that the personnel are qualified and suggests that you could expect to get accurate technical advice from the staff.
3. Regardless of the total scores, you would have to decide the importance of each item in the evaluation chart to you personally, as well as evaluate other considerations such as cost, location, personalities of the clients and the personnel, and so on, to decide if this would be a good place for you or your friends to join.

In the space below, discuss your conclusion about the quality of this club and whether you think it would fit your needs if you wanted to belong to a club.

Blood Alcohol Level

Name _____ Section _____ Date _____

■ Read Concept 25 before completing this lab.

To learn to calculate your (or a friend's) blood alcohol level (BAC).

PROCEDURE

1. Assume a "drink" is a twelve-ounce can or bottle of 4% beer or a four-ounce glass (a small glass) of 12% alcohol wine, or a mixed drink with a one-ounce shot glass (jigger) of 100 proof liquor (or one and one-fourth of a jigger of 80 proof).
   Case A. Assume you consumed two drinks within one hour.
   Case B. Assume you consumed two drinks over a period of one hour and twenty minutes.
   Case C. Assume you had two six-packs of beer (twelve cans) over five hours.
   Case D. Same as C, but if you weigh less than 150 pounds, assume you weigh 50 more pounds than you now weigh, and if you weigh more than 150 pounds, assume you weigh 50 pounds less.
2. Divide 3.8 by your weight in pounds to obtain your "BAC maximum per drink," or refer to chart 25.1, column one (one drink consumed in one hour). You should obtain a number between .015 and .04.

$$\text{Approximate BAC over time} = \frac{(3.8 \times \# \text{ of drinks})}{(\text{body weight})} - \frac{(.01 \times \# \text{ min.} - 40)}{40}$$

3. *After* forty minutes have passed, your body will begin eliminating alcohol from the bloodstream at the rate of about .01% for each *additional* forty minutes. Multiply the number of drinks you've had by your "BAC maximum per drink" and subtract .01% from the number for each forty minutes that have passed since you began drinking—but don't count the first forty minutes. Compute your BAC for cases A, B, C, and D.

   Example: Case A. Mary weighs 100 pounds. $\dfrac{3.8 \times 2}{100} = \dfrac{7.6}{100} = .076\% \text{ BAC}$

   Case B. Mary takes 80 minutes. $.076\% - \dfrac{(.01 \times 80 - 40)}{40} = .066\% \text{ BAC}$

4. Record your results below by writing the formula and computing the BAC for each case.

RESULTS

Case A $\dfrac{(3.8 \times \underline{\quad} \# \text{ drinks})}{\underline{\quad} \text{ lbs.}} - \dfrac{(0.1 \times \underline{\quad} \# \text{ min.} - 40)}{40}$

$\underline{\hspace{3cm}} \quad \underline{\hspace{2cm}} = \underline{\hspace{2cm}} \text{ (BAC)}$

Case B $\dfrac{(3.8 \times \underline{\quad} \# \text{ drinks})}{\underline{\quad} \text{ lbs.}} - \dfrac{(0.1 \times \underline{\quad} \# \text{ min.} - 40)}{40}$

$\underline{\hspace{3cm}} \quad \underline{\hspace{2cm}} = \underline{\hspace{2cm}} \text{ (BAC)}$

Case C $\dfrac{(3.8 \times \underline{\hspace{1cm}} \text{ # drinks})}{\underline{\hspace{1cm}} \text{ lbs.}} - \dfrac{(0.1 \times \underline{\hspace{1cm}} \text{ # min.} - 40}{40}$

$$\underline{\hspace{4cm}} \quad \underline{\hspace{2cm}} = \underline{\hspace{2cm}} \text{ (BAC)}$$

Case D $\dfrac{(3.8 \times \underline{\hspace{1cm}} \text{ # drinks})}{\underline{\hspace{1cm}} \text{ lbs.}} - \dfrac{(0.1 \times \underline{\hspace{1cm}} \text{ # min.} - 40}{40}$

$$\underline{\hspace{4cm}} \quad \underline{\hspace{2cm}} = \underline{\hspace{2cm}} \text{ (BAC)}$$

CONCLUSIONS AND IMPLICATIONS

1. Would you be able to drive legally according to your state laws? Circle yes or no.
   Case A. Yes   No
   Case B. Yes   No
   Case C. Yes   No
   Case D. Yes   No

2. Would you be able to drive legally if the Health Goals for the Year 2000 were put into effect? Circle yes or no.
   Case A. Yes   No
   Case B. Yes   No
   Case C. Yes   No
   Case D. Yes   No

3. What have you learned by doing this exercise?

Chart 25.1 Maximum Blood Alcohol Level (%)*					
Your Weight in Pounds	Drinks Consumed in One Hour				
	1	2	3	4	5
100	0.038%	0.076	0.114	0.152	0.190
120	0.032	0.064	0.096	0.128	0.160
140	0.027	0.054	0.081	0.108	0.135
160	0.024	0.048	0.072	0.096	0.120
180	0.021	0.042	0.063	0.084	0.105
200	0.019	0.038	0.057	0.076	0.095
220	0.017	0.034	0.051	0.068	0.085
240	0.016	0.032	0.048	0.064	0.080

Reprinted with permission from *Fight Your Ticket* by Attorney David Brown (Nolo Press, Berkeley, CA).

Note: Percentages obtained by dividing the number 3.8 by the body weight in pounds. This factor takes into account various English-to-metric and other conversion factors, the body's typical weight-percentage of blood (per pound of body weight) in which the alcohol will be mixed, and the proportion of alcohol that will wind up in the blood.

Use and Abuse of Other Drugs

Name _____ Section _____ Date _____

■ Read Concept 26 before completing this lab.

PURPOSE

The purposes of this laboratory are to help you to evaluate your own (or a friend or family member's) behavior and potential for becoming an abuser of drugs. This is for your own information and need not be submitted to the instructor or shared with other persons.

PROCEDURE

Answer these questions to determine if you are (or the person you are evaluating could be) an abuser of medications. Circle the answer that applies to you.

A. Prescription Drug Abuse

Yes No 1. Do you/they take more medicine than prescribed per dosage?
Yes No 2. Do you/they feel more nervous than ever when your medicine wears off?
Yes No 3. Do you/they hoard medicine?
Yes No 4. Do you/they gulp pills?
Yes No 5. Do you/they hide the amount of medicine taken from friends, family or your/their doctors?
Yes No 6. Does your/their doctor know you/they have other doctors, and do they have a list of all the medications you/they are taking from all sources (dentist, family physician, specialists)?

The more questions to which you answered "yes," the more apt you/they are to be a drug abuser.

B. Risk Factors for Becoming Addicted

Yes No 1. Have any members of your/their family ever abused drugs?
Yes No 2. Were you/they abused as a child, or did you/they go through other trauma during childhood?
Yes No 3. Are you/they now undergoing unusual stress or mental pain?
Yes No 4. Do you/they have easy access to drugs?
Yes No 5. Have or do you/they used drugs recreationally?
Yes No 6. If you/they have or do now use drugs recreationally, did or do you/they choose the fastest method of getting a "hit"?

The more "yes" answers you have, the greater your/their risk of addiction. (Remember that alcohol is a drug, too.)

C. Signs and Symptoms That a Problem with Drugs Exists

Yes No 1. Do you/they use drugs as an "escape" or to help cope with a stressful situation?
Yes No 2. Do you/they become depressed easily?
Yes No 3. Do you/they use drugs the first thing in the morning?
Yes No 4. Have you/they ever tried to quit and resumed using again?
Yes No 5. Do you/they do things under the influence of a drug that you/they would not normally do?
Yes No 6. Have you/they had any drug-related "close calls" with the police, or any arrests?
Yes No 7. Do you/they think a party or social gathering isn't fun unless drugs are served?
Yes No 8. Do you/they feel proud of an increased tolerance to drugs?
Yes No 9. Do you/they use drugs when alone?
Yes No 10. Have or do you/they use a wide variety of drugs?
Yes No 11. Are you/they constantly thinking about being "high"?
Yes No 12. Do you/they avoid people or places that oppose or "frown on" usage?
Yes No 13. Have your/their friends, family, teachers, or employer expressed concern about your/their use?

Yes No 14. Is your/their usage causing you/them to neglect responsibilities?
Yes No 15. Have you/they ever had blackouts from times of using?
Yes No 16. Have you/they stolen to get money for drugs?
Yes No 17. Have you/they seriously considered that you might have a drug problem?

The more questions to which you answer "yes," the more apt you/they are to have a serious problem with drugs.

RESULTS

A. Do you/they abuse prescription drugs (medications)?   Yes No
B. Are you/they at considerable risk for addiction?   Yes No
C. Do you/they have a serious problem with drugs?   Yes No

CONCLUSIONS AND IMPLICATIONS

If you/they do abuse medications or are at risk for addiction or have a serious problem with drugs, indicate in this space what you intend to do about it.

If you feel that you/they are not at risk for addiction, discuss the reasons that your/their risk is low.

**LAB
26**

Determining Your Cancer Risk

Name _____ Section _____ Date _____

■ Read Concept 28 before completing this lab.

PURPOSE

The purpose of this laboratory experience is to make you aware of your cancer risk for various types of cancer.

PROCEDURE

1. Answer the questions in the Cancer Risk Factors Questionnaire on the back of this sheet.
2. Total the number of risk factors for each cancer type. If you possess one or more risk factors, you increase your risk of developing that type of cancer.

RESULTS

Record the information as requested on the back of this sheet.

CONCLUSIONS AND IMPLICATIONS

For which type of cancer do you feel you are at greatest risk? Explain.

What life-styles could you modify to reduce your risk? Explain the reasons for your choice.

Directions for Scoring

The Cancer Risk Factor Questionnaire helps you identify three of the key risk factors for several of the most prevalent types of cancer. All risk factors are not of equal importance in determining risk of developing cancer. Nevertheless, you can get an idea of the factors that are likely to put you at risk by counting your risk factors. To score the questionnaire:

- Count your risk for each of the forms of cancer. Only females count risk for breast and uterine/cervical cancer. Only males count risk for prostate cancer. Note: males can develop breast cancer, though the risk is considerably less than for females.
- If you have one or more of the risk factors, you have an increased risk of developing that form of cancer. You should do additional reading to determine which of the factors for that type of cancer puts you at greatest risk.

CANCER RISK FACTOR QUESTIONNAIRE

Opposite each risk factor draw an X in the boxes under each type of cancer for which it is a risk factor. If the box is darkened, do not place an X in the box. Count the Xs in each column and write the total in the total column below each type.

Risk factor

Type of Cancer

Risk factor	Skin	Oral	Lung	Breast (Female)	Colo-rectal	Prostate (Male)	Uterine/ Cervical (Female)
1. Smoking							
2. Smokeless tobacco use							
3. Secondary smoking (smoking environment)							
4. Industrial exposure (coal miner, etc.)							
5. Radiation exposure							
6. Family history of specific type cancer							
7. High-fat diet							
8. Low-fiber diet							
9. Obesity							
10. Failure to ovulate (females)							
11. Estrogen irregularity (females)							
12. No children or late first pregnancy (females)							
13. Excessive alcohol use							
14. Age over 50							
15. Excessive sun exposure							
16. Fair complexion							
Total risk factors:							

L-84   Lab 28

Concepts of Recreation, Leisure, and Time Management

Name _____   Section _____   Date _____

■ Read Concept 29 before completing this lab.

PURPOSE

The purpose of this laboratory is to help you learn to manage time to meet personal priorities.

PROCEDURE

1. Follow the four steps outlined on the back of this sheet.
2. Answer the questions in the conclusions and implications section below.

RESULTS

Record the information as requested on the back of this sheet.

CONCLUSIONS AND IMPLICATIONS

Were you able to modify your schedule to find more time for important priorities? ☐ Yes ☐ No Explain.

Sometimes people feel that NOW IS NOT THE TIME for taking time out for priorities. The feeling is that at some future time ("when I graduate" or "when I have more experience on my job") they will have more time. Do you feel this way? ☐ Yes ☐ No Explain your answer.

Often delaying things until a future time is just a way to avoid making tough decisions. Is this true for you? ☐ Yes ☐ No Explain your answer.

Chart 29.1 Time Management

Step 1: Establishing Priorities

1. Check your priorities from the list below. Add priorities as necessary.

2. Rank each of the priorities you checked. Use a 1 for the highest priority, a 2 for the second highest priority, and so on.

	Rank		Rank		Rank
☐ more time with family	_____	☐ more time with boy/girlfriend	_____	☐ more time with spouse	_____
☐ more time for leisure	_____	☐ more time to relax	_____	☐ more time to study	_____
☐ more time for work success	_____	☐ more time for physical activity	_____	☐ more time to improve myself	_____
☐ more time for other recreation	_____	☐ other _____	_____	☐ other _____	_____

Step 2: Monitor Current Time Use

1. On the daily calendar, keep track of daily time expenditure.

2. Write in exactly what you did for each time block.

7–9 AM	9–11 AM	11 AM–1 PM	1–3 PM
3–5 PM	5–7 PM	7–9 PM	9–11 PM

Step 3: Analyze Your Current Time Use

Where can I spend less time? (write below)	What can I do to reduce time spent in these activities? (write below)

Step 4: Make a Schedule. Write in Your Planned Activities for the Day

7–9 AM	9–11 AM	11 AM–1 PM	1–3 PM
3–5 PM	5–7 PM	7–9 PM	9–11 PM

Planning for Life-Style Change

Name _____   Section _____   Date _____

■ Read Concept 30 before completing this lab.

PURPOSE

The purpose of this lab is to make plans for life-style change using the five steps outlined in Concept 30.

PROCEDURE

Answer the questions and fill in the spaces following the five steps outlined below.

1. Identify Areas of Possible Change
Place an X in the box beside the areas in chart 30.1 in which you would like to make changes.

Chart 30.1   Areas of Possible Life-Style Change

☐ Managing time effectively   ☐ Learning first aid

☐ Eating properly   ☐ Adopting personal health behaviors

☐ Controlling stress   ☐ Seeking and complying with medical advice

☐ Avoiding destructive habits   ☐ Becoming an informed consumer

☐ Practicing safe sex   ☐ Protecting the environment

☐ Adopting safety habits   ☐ Other (designate) _____

2. Establish Your Goals
In chart 30.2, write your goals for the next month. Write the date by which the goal is to be accomplished. Do not include physical activity or fitness goals. They were included in Lab 20.

Chart 30.2 Life-Style Goals			
Goal	Date to Be Met	Goal	Date to Be Met

LAB
30

3. Write Your Plan

If appropriate, write a specific plan for meeting your goals. For example, if you plan to do daily relaxation exercises write the exercises, the days of the week, and the time of the day that they will be performed.

Chart 30.3 Plans for Life-Style Change

4. Keep Records

Use the monthly calendar below or make one like it on a full sheet of paper to keep track of your goals and life-style changes. Write in the dates on the calendar (yellow) beginning on the day you plan to begin modifying your life-style. Write goals on the calendar. Place an X in the green boxes for dates goals are to be met or programs are planned. Place an X in the blue boxes each time you carry out your program or meet your goals.

Chart 30.4 Life-Style Record-Keeping Calendar

MONTH _____

Sunday	Monday	Tuesday	Wednesday	Thursday	Friday	Saturday	
Date	Date	Date	Date	Date	Date	Date	GOAL 1:
Goals:	Goals:	Goals:	Goals:	Goals:	Goals:	Goals:	
Date	Date	Date	Date	Date	Date	Date	GOAL 2:
Goals:	Goals:	Goals:	Goals:	Goals:	Goals:	Goals:	
Date	Date	Date	Date	Date	Date	Date	GOAL 3:
Goals:	Goals:	Goals:	Goals:	Goals:	Goals:	Goals:	
Date	Date	Date	Date	Date	Date	Date	GOAL 4:
Goals:	Goals:	Goals:	Goals:	Goals:	Goals:	Goals:	

5. Periodically Revise

Check to see how successful you have been in meeting your goals and revise your plan if necessary.

LAB
30

Approximate Conversions from Metric to Traditional Measures

LENGTH
  centimeters to inches: cm $\times$ .39 = in
  meters to feet: m $\times$ 3.3 = ft
  meters to yards: m $\times$ 1.09 = yd
  kilometers to miles: km $\times$ 0.6 = mi

MASS (WEIGHT)
  grams to ounces: g $\times$ 0.0352 = oz
  kilograms to pounds: kg $\times$ 2.2 = lbs

AREA
  square centimeters to square inches: $cm^2 \times 0.16 = in^2$
  square meters to square feet: $m^2 \times 11.11 = ft^2$
  square meters to square yards: $m^2 \times 1.02 = yd^2$

VOLUME
  milliliters to fluid ounces: ml $\times$ 0.03 = fl oz
  liters to quarts: 1 $\times$ 1.06 = qt
  liters to gallons: 1 $\times$ 0.264 = gal
  cubic meters to cubic feet: $m^3 \times 33 = ft^3$
  cubic meters to cubic yards: $m^3 \times 1.3 = yd^3$

Approximate Conversions from Traditional to Metric Measures

LENGTH
  inches to centimeters: in $\times$ 2.54 = cm
  feet to centimeters: ft $\times$ 30.48 = cm
  yards to meters: yd $\times$ 0.92 = m
  miles to kilometers: mi $\times$ 1.6 = km

MASS (WEIGHT)
  ounces to grams: oz $\times$ 28.41 = gm
  pounds to kilograms: lbs $\times$ 0.45 = kg

AREA
  square inches to square centimeters: $in^2 \times 6.5 = cm^2$
  square feet to square meters: $ft^2 \times 0.09 = m^2$
  square yards to square meters: $yd^2 \times 0.76 = m^2$

VOLUME
  quarts to liters: qt $\times$ 0.95 = 1
  gallons to liters: gal $\times$ 3.8 = 1
  cubic feet to cubic meters: $ft^3 \times 0.03 = m^3$
  cubic yards to cubic meters: $yd^3 \times 0.76 = m^3$

Metric Conversions of Selected Charts and Tables

Chart 6B.1 Twelve-Minute Run Test (Scores in Meters)				
Men (age)				
Classification	**17–26**	**27–39**	**40–49**	**50+**
High performance zone	2880+	2560+	2400+	2240+
Good fitness zone	2480–2779	2320–2559	2240–2399	2000–2239
Marginal zone	2160–2479	2080–2319	2000–2239	1760–1999
Low zone	< 2160	< 2080	< 2000	< 1760
Women (age)				
Classification	**17–26**	**27–39**	**40–49**	**50+**
High performance zone	2320+	2160+	2000+	1840+
Good fitness zone	2000–2319	1920–2159	1840–1999	1680–1839
Marginal zone	1840–1999	1680–1919	1600–1839	1520–1679
Low zone	< 1840	< 1680	< 1600	< 1520

Table 7.4
Aerobic Points Chart

Points	Walking-Running Time for 1 Mile (1.6 kg)	Cycling Time for 2 Miles (3.2 km)	Swimming Time for 300 yds (275 m)	Handball, Basketball	Stationary Running for 5 Minutes	Stationary Running for 10 Minutes	Points
0	> 20 min.	> 12 min.	> 10 min.	< 10 min.	< 60 steps/min.	< 50 steps/min.	0
1	20:00–14:30 min.	8–12 min.	8–10 min.	> 10 min.	60–70 steps/min.	50–65 steps/min.	1
2	14:29–12:00 min.	6–8 min.	7:30–8 min.	> 20 min.	80–90 steps/min.	65–70 steps/min.	2
3	11:59–10:00 min.	< 6 min.	6–7:30 min.	> 30 min.		70–80 steps/min.	3
4	9:59–8:00 min.		< 6 min.	> 40 min.		80–90 steps/min.	4
5	7:59–6:30 min.			> 50 min.			5
6	< 6:30 min.			> 60 min.			6

Charts 10.2 and 10.3 Isometric Strength *Rating Scales*

	Strength *Rating Scale* for Men (kg)		
Classification	Left Grip	Right Grip	Total Score
High performance zone	57+	61+	118+
Good fitness zone	45–56	50–60	95–117
Marginal zone	41–44	43–49	84–94
Low zone	< 41	< 43	< 84

	Strength *Rating Scale* for Women (kg)		
Classification	Left Grip	Right Grip	Total Score
High performance zone	34+	39+	73+
Good fitness zone	27–33	32–38	59–72
Marginal zone	20–26	23–31	43–58
Low zone	< 20	< 23	< 43

These rating charts are suitable for use by young adults between eighteen and thirty years of age. After thirty, an adjustment of 0.5 of 1 percent per year is appropriate because some loss of muscle tissue typically occurs as you grow older.

Chart 15.5 Reaction Time *Rating Scale*

Classification	Score in Inches	Score in Centimeters
Excellent	21 +	53 +
Very good	19–21	48–52
Good	16–18¾	41–47
Fair	13–15¾	33–40
Poor	< 13	< 33

Chart 15.6 Speed *Rating Scale*

Classification	Men		Women	
	Yards	Meters	Yards	Meters
Excellent	24+	22+	22+	20+
Very good	22–23	20–21.9	20–21	18–19.9
Good	18–21	16.5–19.9	16–19	14.5–17.9
Fair	16–17	14.5–16.4	14–15	13–14.4
Poor	< 16	< 14.5	< 14	< 13

Chart 15.4 Power *Rating Scale*

Classification	Men	Women
Excellent	68 cm +	60 cm +
Very good	53–67 cm	48–59 cm
Good	42–52 cm	37–47 cm
Fair	32–41 cm	27–36 cm
Poor	< 32 cm	< 27 cm

APPENDIX C

*Calorie Guide to Common Foods**

Beverages

Coffee (black)	0
Coke (12 oz.)	137
Hot chocolate, milk (1 cup)	247
Lemonade (1 cup)	100
Limeade, diluted to serve (1 cup)	110
Soda, fruit flavored (12 oz.)	161
Tea (clear)	0

Breads and Cereals

Bagel (1 half)	76
Biscuit (2″ × 2″)	135
Bread, pita (1 oz.)	80
Bread, raisin (½″ thick)	65
Bread, rye	55
Bread, white enriched (½″ thick)	64
Bread, whole wheat (½″ thick)	55
Bun (hamburger)	120
Cereals, cooked (½ cup)	80
Corn flakes (1 cup)	96
Corn grits (1 cup)	125
Corn muffin (2½″ diam.)	103
Crackers, graham (1 med.)	28
Crackers, soda (1 plain)	24
English muffin (1 half)	74
Macaroni, with cheese (1 cup)	464
Muffin, plain	135
Noodles (1 cup)	200
Oatmeal (1 cup)	150
Pancakes (1–4″ diam.)	59
Pizza (1 section)	180
Popped corn (1 cup)	54
Potato chips (10 med.)	108
Pretzels (5 small sticks)	18
Rice (1 cup)	225
Roll, plain (1 med.)	118
Roll, sweet (1 med.)	178
Shredded wheat (1 med. biscuit)	79
Spaghetti, plain cooked (1 cup)	218
Tortilla (1 corn)	70
Waffle (4½″ × 5″)	216

Dairy Products

Butter, 1 pat (1½ tsp.)	50
Cheese, cheddar (1 oz.)	113
Cheese, cottage (1 cup)	270
Cheese, cream (1 oz.)	106
Cheese, Parmesan (1 tbsp.)	29
Cheese, Swiss natural (1 oz.)	105
Cream, sour (1 tbsp.)	31
Dairy Queen Cone (med.)	335
Frozen custard (1 cup)	375
Frozen yogurt, vanilla (1 cup)	180
Ice cream, plain (prem.) (1 cup)	350
Ice cream soda, choc. (large glass)	455
Ice milk (1 cup)	184
Ices (1 cup)	177
Milk, chocolate (1 cup)	185
Milk, half-and-half (1 tbsp.)	20
Milk, malted (1 cup)	281
Milk, skim (1 cup)	88
Milk, skim dry (1 tbsp.)	28
Milk, whole (1 cup)	166
Sherbet (1 cup)	270
Whipped topping (1 tbsp.)	14
Yogurt (1 cup)	150

Desserts and Sweets

Cake, angel (2″ wedge)	108
Cake, chocolate (2″ × 3″ × 1″)	150
Cake, plain (3″ × 2½″)	180
Chocolate, bar	200–300
Chocolate, bitter (1 oz.)	142
Chocolate, sweet (1 oz.)	133
Chocolate, syrup (1 tbsp.)	42
Cocoa (1 tbsp.)	21
Cookies, plain (1 med.)	75
Custard, baked (1 cup)	283
Doughnut (1 large)	250
Gelatin, dessert (1 cup)	155
Gelatin, with fruit (1 cup)	170
Gingerbread (2″ × 2″ × 2″)	180
Jams, jellies (1 tbsp.)	55
Pie, apple (1/7 of 9″ pie)	345
Pie, cherry (1/7 of 9″ pie)	355
Pie, chocolate (1/7 of 9″ pie)	360
Pie, coconut (1/7 of 9″ pie)	266
Pie, lemon meringue (1/7 of 9″ pie)	302
Sugar, granulated (1 tsp.)	27
Syrup, table (1 tbsp.)	57

*Note: For a complete listing of foods, the reader is referred to: *Nutritive Value of Foods,* U. S. Department of Agriculture, Washington, D. C., Home and Gardens Bulletin, No. 72. (Available in most libraries, university bookstores, and Home Economics departments.)

Fruit

Apple, fresh (med.)	76
Applesauce, unsweetened (1 cup)	184
Avocado, raw (½ peeled)	279
Banana, fresh (med.)	88
Cantaloupe, raw (½, 5″ diam.)	60
Cherries (10 sweet)	50
Cranberry sauce, unsweetened (1 tbsp.)	25
Fruit cocktail, canned (1 cup)	170
Grapefruit, fresh (½)	60
Grapefruit juice, raw (1 cup)	95
Grape juice, bottled (½ cup)	80
Grapes (20–25)	75
Nectarine (1 med.)	88
Olives, green	72
Olives, ripe (10)	105
Orange, fresh (med.)	60
Orange juice, frozen diluted (1 cup)	110
Peach, fresh (med.)	46
Peach, canned in syrup (2 halves)	79
Pear, fresh (med.)	95
Pears, canned in syrup (2 halves)	79
Pineapple, crushed in syrup (1 cup)	204
Pineapple (½ cup fresh)	50
Prune juice (1 cup)	170
Raisins, dry (1 tbsp.)	26
Strawberries, fresh (1 cup)	54
Strawberries, frozen (3 oz.)	90
Tangerine (2½″ diam.)	40
Watermelon, wedge (4″ × 8″)	120

Meat, Fish, Eggs

Bacon, drained (2 slices)	97
Bacon, Canadian (1 oz.)	62
Beef, hamburger chuck (3 oz.)	316
Beef, pot pie	560
Beef steak, sirloin or T-bone (3 oz.)	257
Beef and vegetable stew (1 cup)	185
Chicken, fried breast (8 oz.)	210
Chicken, fried (1 leg and thigh)	305
Chicken, roasted breast (2 slices)	100
Chili, without beans (1 cup)	510
Chili, with beans (1 cup)	335
Egg, boiled	77
Egg, fried	125
Egg, scrambled	100
Fish and chips (2 pcs. fish; 4 oz. chips)	275
Fish, broiled (3″ × 3″ × ½″)	112
Fish stick	40
Frankfurter, boiled	124
Ham (4″ × 4″)	338
Lamb (3 oz. roast, lean)	158
Liver (3″ × 3″)	150
Luncheon meat (2 oz.)	135
Pork chop, loin (3″ × 5″)	284
Salmon, canned (1 cup)	145
Sausage, pork (4 oz.)	510

Shrimp, canned (3 oz.)	108
Tuna, canned (½ cup)	185
Veal, cutlet (3″ × 4″)	175

Nuts and Seeds

Cashews (1 cup)	770
Coconut (1 cup)	450
Peanut butter (1 tbsp.)	92
Peanuts, roasted, no skin (1 cup)	805
Pecans (1 cup)	752
Sunflower seeds (1 tbsp.)	50

Sandwiches
(2 slices of bread—plain)

Bologna	214
Cheeseburger (small McDonald's)	300
Chicken salad	185
Egg salad	240
Fish filet (McDonald's)	400
Ham	360
Ham and cheese	360
Hamburger (small McDonald's)	260
Hamburger, Burger King Whopper	600
Hamburger, Big Mac	550
Hamburger (McDonald's Quarter Pounder)	420
Peanut butter	250
Roast beef (Arby's Regular)	425

Sauces, Fats, Oils

Catsup, tomato (1 tbsp.)	17
Chili sauce (1 tbsp.)	17
French dressing (1 tbsp.)	59
Margarine (1 pat)	50
Mayonnaise (1 tbsp.)	92
Mayonnaise-type (1 tbsp.)	65
Vegetable, sunflower, safflower oils (1 tbsp.)	120

Soup, Ready to Serve (1 cup)

Bean	190
Beef noodle	100
Cream	200
Tomato	90
Vegetable	80

Vegetables

Alfalfa sprouts (½ cup)	19
Asparagus (6 spears)	22
Bean sprouts (1 cup)	37
Beans, green (1 cup)	27
Beans, lima (1 cup)	152
Beans, navy (1 cup)	642
Beans, pork and molasses (1 cup)	325
Broccoli, fresh cooked (1 cup)	60
Cabbage, cooked (1 cup)	40
Cauliflower (1 cup)	25
Carrot, raw (med.)	21
Carrots, canned (1 cup)	44

Celery, diced raw (1 cup)	20	Pickles, sweet (med.)	22
Coleslaw (1 cup)	102	Potato, baked (med.)	97
Corn, sweet, canned (1 cup)	140	Potato, french fried (8 stick)	155
Corn, sweet (med. ear)	84	Potato, mashed (1 cup)	185
Cucumber, raw (6 slices)	6	Radish, raw (small)	1
Lettuce (2 large leaves)	7	Sauerkraut, drained (1 cup)	32
Mushrooms, canned (1 cup)	28	Spinach, fresh, cooked (1 cup)	46
Onions, french fried (10 rings)	75	Squash, summer (1 cup)	30
Onions, raw (med.)	25	Sweet pepper (med.)	15
Peas, field (½ cup)	90	Sweet potato, candied (small)	314
Peas, green (1 cup)	145	Tomato, cooked (1 cup)	50
Pickles, dill (med.)	15	Tomato, raw (med.)	30

Calories of Protein, Carbohydrates, and Fats in Foods*

Food No./Food Choice	Total Calories	Protein Calories	Carbohydrate Calories	Fat Calories
Breakfast				
1. Scrambled Egg (1 1g)	111	29	7	75
2. Fried Egg (1 1g)	99	26	1	72
3. Pancake (1–6")	146	19	67	58
4. Syrup (1 T)	60	0	60	0
5. French Toast (1 slice)	180	23	49	108
6. Waffle (7-inch)	245	28	100	117
7. Biscuit (medium)	104	8	52	44
8. Bran Muffin (medium)	104	11	63	31
9. White Toast (slice)	68	9	52	7
10. Wheat Toast (slice)	67	14	52	6
11. Peanut Butter (1 T)	94	15	11	68
12. Yogurt (8 oz. plain)	227	39	161	27
13. Orange Juice (8 oz.)	114	8	100	6
14. Apple Juice (8 oz.)	117	1	116	0
15. Soft Drink (12 oz.)	144	0	144	0
16. Bacon (2 slices)	86	15	2	70
17. Sausage (1-link)	141	11	0	130
18. Sausage (1 patty)	284	23	0	261
19. Grits (8 oz.)	125	11	110	4
20. Hash Browns (8 oz.)	355	18	178	159
21. French Fries (reg.)	239	12	115	112
22. Donut Cake	125	4	61	60
23. Donut Glazed	164	8	87	69
24. Sweet Roll	317	22	136	159
25. Cake (medium slice)	274	14	175	85
26. Ice Cream (8 oz.)	257	15	108	134
27. Cream Cheese (T)	52	4	1	47
28. Jelly (T)	49	0	49	0
29. Jam (T)	54	0	54	0
30. Coffee (cup)	0	0	0	0
31. Tea (cup)	0	0	0	0
32. Cream (T)	32	2	2	28
33. Sugar (t)	15	0	15	0
34. Corn Flakes (8 oz.)	97	8	87	2
35. Wheat Flakes (8 oz.)	106	12	90	4
36. Oatmeal (8 oz.)	132	19	92	21
37. Strawberries (8 oz.)	55	4	46	5
38. Orange (medium)	64	6	57	1
39. Apple (medium)	96	1	86	9
40. Banana (medium)	101	4	95	2
41. Cantaloupe (half)	82	7	73	2
42. Grapefruit (half)	40	2	37	1

*Notes:
1. FF by a food indicates that it is typical of a food served in a fast food restaurant.
2. Your portions of foods may be larger or smaller than those listed here. For this reason you may wish to select a food more than once (i.e., two hamburgers) or select only a portion of a serving (i.e., divide the calories in half for a half portion).
3. An oz. equals an ounce or 28.4 grams.
4. T = Tablespoon and t = teaspoon.
The principal reference for the calculation of values used in this appendix were the *Nutritive Value of Foods,* published by the United States Department of Agriculture, Washington, D. C., Home and Gardens Bulletin, No. 72, although other published sources were consulted, including Jacobson, M., and S. Fritschner, *The Fast-Food Guide* (an excellent source of information about fast foods), New York, Workman Publishing Company, 1986.

Food No./Food Choice	Total Calories	Protein Calories	Carbohydrate Calories	Fat Calories
43. Custard Pie (slice)	285	20	188	77
44. Fruit Pie (slice)	350	14	259	77
45. Fritter (medium)	132	11	54	67
46. Skim Milk (8 oz.)	88	36	52	0
47. Whole Milk (8 oz.)	159	33	48	78
48. Butter (pat)	36	0	0	36
49. Margarine (pat)	36	0	0	36
Lunch				
1. Hamburger (reg. FF)	255	48	120	89
2. Cheeseburger (reg. FF)	307	61	120	126
3. Doubleburger (FF)	563	101	163	299
4. ¼ lb. Burger (FF)	427	73	137	217
5. Doublecheese Burger (FF)	670	174	134	362
6. Doublecheese Baconburger (FF)	724	138	174	340
7. Hot Dog (FF)	214	36	54	124
8. Chili Dog (FF)	320	51	90	179
9. Pizza, Cheese (slice FF)	290	116	116	58
10. Pizza, Meat (slice FF)	360	126	126	108
11. Pizza, Everything (slice FF)	510	179	173	158
12. Sandwich, Roast Beef (FF)	350	88	126	137
13. Sandwich, Bologna	313	44	106	163
14. Sandwich, Bologna-Cheese	428	69	158	201
15. Sandwich, Ham-Cheese (FF)	380	91	133	156
16. Sandwich, Peanut Butter	281	39	118	124
17. Sandwich, PB and Jelly	330	40	168	122
18. Sandwich, Egg Salad	330	40	109	181
19. Sandwich, Tuna Salad	390	101	109	180
20. Sandwich, Fish (FF)	432	56	147	229
21. French Fries (reg. FF)	239	12	115	112
22. French Fries (lg. FF)	406	20	195	191
23. Onion Rings (reg. FF)	274	14	112	148
24. Chili (8 oz.)	260	49	62	148
25. Bean Soup (8 oz.)	355	67	181	107
26. Beef Noodle Soup (8 oz.)	140	32	59	49
27. Tomato Soup (8 oz.)	180	14	121	45
28. Vegetable Soup (8 oz.)	160	21	107	32
29. Small Salad, Plain	37	6	27	4
30. Small Salad, French Dressing	152	8	50	94
31. Small Salad, Italian Dressing	162	8	28	126
32. Small Salad, Bleu Cheese	184	13	28	143
33. Potato Salad (8 oz.)	248	27	159	62
34. Cole Slaw (8 oz.)	180	0	25	155
35. Macaroni and Cheese (8 oz.)	230	37	103	90
36. Taco Beef (FF)	186	59	56	71
37. Bean Burrito (FF)	343	45	192	106
38. Meat Burrito (FF)	466	158	196	112
39. Mexican Rice (FF)	213	17	160	36
40. Mexican Beans (FF)	168	42	82	44
41. Fried Chicken Breast (FF)	436	262	13	161
42. Broiled Chicken Breast	284	224	0	60
43. Broiled Fish	228	82	32	114
44. Fish Stick (1 stick FF)	50	18	8	24
45. Fried Egg	99	26	1	72
46. Donut	125	4	61	60
47. Potato Chips (small bag)	115	3	39	73
48. Soft Drink (12 oz.)	144	0	144	0
49. Apple Juice (8 oz.)	117	1	116	0
50. Skim Milk (8 oz.)	88	36	52	0
51. Whole Milk (8 oz.)	159	33	48	78
52. Diet Drink (12 oz.)	0	0	0	0
53. Mustard (t)	4	0	4	0
54. Catsup (t)	6	0	6	0
55. Mayonnaise (T)	100	0	0	100
56. Fruit Pie	350	14	260	77

Food No./Food Choice	Total Calories	Protein Calories	Carbohydrate Calories	Fat Calories
57. Cheese Cake	400	56	132	212
58. Ice Cream (8 oz.)	257	15	108	134
59. Coffee (8 oz.)	0	0	0	0
60. Tea (8 oz.)	0	0	0	0

Dinner

Food No./Food Choice	Total Calories	Protein Calories	Carbohydrate Calories	Fat Calories
1. Hamburger (reg. FF)	255	48	120	89
2. Cheeseburger (reg. FF)	307	61	120	126
3. Doubleburger (FF)	563	101	163	299
4. ¼ lb. Burger (FF)	427	73	137	217
5. Doublecheese Burger (FF)	670	174	134	362
6. Doublecheese Baconburger (FF)	724	138	174	412
7. Hot Dog (FF)	214	36	54	124
8. Chili Dog (FF)	320	51	90	179
9. Pizza, Cheese (slice FF)	290	116	116	58
10. Pizza, Meat (slice FF)	360	126	126	108
11. Pizza, Everything (slice FF)	510	179	173	158
12. Steak (8 oz.)	880	290	0	590
13. French Fried Shrimp (6 oz.)	360	133	68	158
14. Roast Beef (8 oz.)	440	268	0	172
15. Liver (8 oz.)	520	250	52	218
16. Corned Beef (8 oz.)	493	242	0	251
17. Meat Loaf (8 oz.)	711	228	35	448
18. Ham (8 oz.)	540	178	0	362
19. Spaghetti, No Meat (13 oz.)	400	56	220	124
20. Spaghetti, Meat (13 oz.)	500	115	230	155
21. Baked Potato (medium)	90	12	78	0
22. Cooked Carrots (8 oz.)	71	12	59	0
23. Cooked Spinach (8 oz.)	50	18	18	14
24. Corn (one ear)	70	10	52	8
25. Cooked Green Beans (8 oz.)	54	11	43	0
26. Cooked Broccoli (8 oz.)	60	19	26	15
27. Cooked Cabbage	47	12	35	0
28. French Fries (reg. FF)	239	12	115	112
29. French Fries (lg. FF)	406	20	195	191
30. Onion Rings (reg. FF)	274	14	112	148
31. Chili (8 oz.)	260	49	62	148
32. Small Salad, Plain	37	6	27	4
33. Small Salad, French Dressing	152	8	50	94
34. Small Salad, Italian Dressing	162	8	28	126
35. Small Salad, Bleu Cheese	184	13	28	143
36. Potato Salad (8 oz.)	248	27	159	62
37. Cole Slaw (8 oz.)	180	0	25	155
38. Macaroni and Cheese (8 oz.)	230	37	103	90
39. Taco Beef (FF)	186	59	56	71
40. Bean Burrito (FF)	343	45	192	106
41. Meat Burrito (FF)	466	158	196	112
42. Mexican Rice (FF)	213	8	160	36
43. Mexican Beans (FF)	168	42	82	44
44. Fried Chicken Breast (FF)	436	262	13	161
45. Broiled Chicken Breast	284	224	0	60
46. Broiled Fish	228	82	32	116
47. Fish Stick (1 stick FF)	50	18	8	24
48. Soft Drink (12 oz.)	144	0	144	0
49. Apple Juice (8 oz.)	117	1	116	0
50. Skim Milk (8 oz.)	88	36	52	0
51. Whole Milk (8 oz.)	159	33	48	48
52. Diet Drink (12 oz.)	0	0	0	0
53. Mustard (t)	4	0	4	0
54. Catsup (t)	6	0	6	0
55. Mayonnaise (T)	100	0	0	100
56. Fruit Pie (slice)	350	14	259	77
57. Cheese Cake (slice)	400	56	132	212

Food No./Food Choice	Total Calories	Protein Calories	Carbohydrate Calories	Fat Calories
58. Ice Cream (8 oz.)	257	15	108	134
59. Custard Pie (slice)	285	20	188	77
60. Cake (slice)	274	14	175	85
Snacks				
1. Peanut Butter (1 T)	94	15	11	68
2. Yogurt (8 oz. plain)	227	39	161	27
3. Orange Juice (8 oz.)	114	8	100	6
4. Apple Juice (8 oz.)	117	1	116	0
5. Soft Drink (12 oz.)	144	0	144	0
6. Donut, Cake	125	4	61	60
7. Donut, Glazed	164	8	87	69
8. Sweet Roll	317	22	136	159
9. Cake (medium slice)	274	14	175	85
10. Ice Cream (8 oz.)	257	15	108	134
11. Soft Serve Cone (reg.)	240	10	89	134
12. Ice Cream Sandwich Bar	210	40	82	88
13. Strawberries (8 oz.)	55	4	46	5
14. Orange (medium)	64	6	57	1
15. Apple (medium)	96	1	86	9
16. Banana (medium)	101	4	95	2
17. Cantaloupe (half)	82	7	73	2
18. Grapefruit (half)	40	2	37	1
19. Celery Stick	5	2	3	0
20. Carrot (medium)	20	3	17	0
21. Raisins (4 oz.)	210	6	204	0
22. Watermelon (4″ × 6″ slice)	115	8	99	8
23. Chocolate Chip Cookie	60	3	9	48
24. Brownie	145	6	26	113
25. Oatmeal Cookie	65	3	13	49
26. Sandwich Cookie	200	8	112	80
27. Custard Pie (slice)	285	20	188	77
28. Fruit Pie (slice)	350	14	259	77
29. Gelatin (4 oz.)	70	4	32	34
30. Fritter (medium)	132	11	54	67
31. Skim Milk (8 oz.)	88	36	52	0
32. Diet Drink	0	0	0	0
33. Potato Chips (small bag)	115	3	39	73
34. Roasted Peanuts (1.3 oz.)	210	34	25	151
35. Chocolate Candy Bar (1 oz.)	145	7	61	77
36. Choc. Almond Candy Bar (1 oz.)	265	38	74	164
37. Cracker Saltine	18	1	1	16
38. Popped Corn	40	7	33	0
39. Cheese Nachos	471	63	194	214

Dance Aerobics

Dance Aerobic Routine

16 counts	Jog in place. Clap your hands.	32 counts	16 Backward lunges.
32 counts	8 Schottische steps, alternate right and left.	32 counts	8 Schottische steps, alternate right and left.
32 counts	8 Jesse polka steps, alternate right and left.	32 counts	8 Jesse polka steps, alternate right and left.
32 counts	8 Schottische steps, alternate right and left.	32 counts	16 Twists, alternate right and left.
		32 counts	Jog and double-time clap.
32 counts	8 Jesse polka steps, alternate right and left.	32 counts	8 Schottische steps, alternate right and left.
32 counts	16 Side lunges, alternate left and right.	32 counts	8 Jesse polka steps, alternate right and left.
32 counts	16 Ponies.		

Dance Aerobic Skills*

To do this routine, you will need to perform the following skills. Learn these skills first, then put them together in a routine. A routine is a series of skills done to music or to a count. Perform to Lionel Richie's "Dancing on the Ceiling" or another 4-count song.

Schottische Step

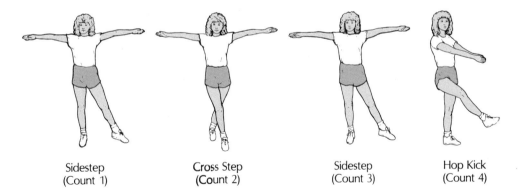

Sidestep
(Count 1)

Cross Step
(Count 2)

Sidestep
(Count 3)

Hop Kick
(Count 4)

The Schottische Step can be done to the right or to the left. On count 1, sidestep; on 2, cross step; on 3, sidestep again; and on 4, hop kick. Practice doing the step in each direction. Hold your arms out to your sides at shoulder level. After you have learned the Schottische Step, you can add a clap of the hands on the hop kick (count of 4).

*Credit is extended to Donna Landers, creator of this routine.

Jesse Polka Kick

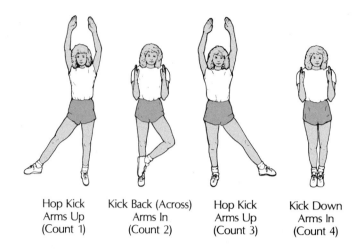

Hop Kick   Kick Back (Across)   Hop Kick   Kick Down
Arms Up   Arms In   Arms Up   Arms In
(Count 1)   (Count 2)   (Count 3)   (Count 4)

The Jesse Polka Kick can be done while standing (hopping) on either foot. On count 1, hop kick; on 2, kick back so that your heel crosses on the opposite side of the hopping leg; on 3, hop kick again; on 4 kick down (return to standing position). When you have learned the step well, add the arm movements. On 1, the arms are over the head; on 2, the arms are at shoulder level; on 3, the arms are over the head; on 4, the arms are back at shoulder level. You may want to say "up, in, up, in" as you practice moving your arms. Practice the step while hopping on the right then on the left foot.

Side Lunge

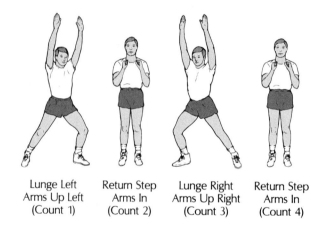

Lunge Left   Return Step   Lunge Right   Return Step
Arms Up Left   Arms In   Arms Up Right   Arms In
(Count 1)   (Count 2)   (Count 3)   (Count 4)

On count 1, face left and push your arms up above your head to the left while your right leg steps behind you; on 2, face forward, bring your arms in to your shoulders and return your right foot to the starting position; on 3, face right and push your arms above your head to the right while your left leg steps behind you; on 4, face forward, bring your arms in to your shoulders and return your left foot to the starting position. As you get better, you can hop rather than step when doing the lunge.

Ponies

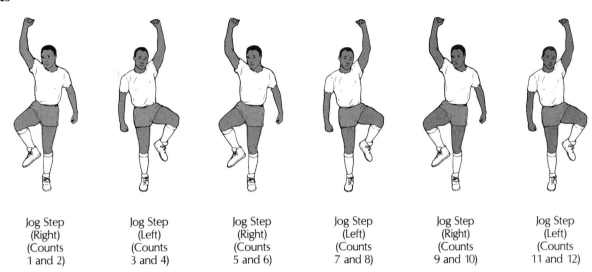

| Jog Step (Right) (Counts 1 and 2) | Jog Step (Left) (Counts 3 and 4) | Jog Step (Right) (Counts 5 and 6) | Jog Step (Left) (Counts 7 and 8) | Jog Step (Right) (Counts 9 and 10) | Jog Step (Left) (Counts 11 and 12) |

On counts 1 and 2, jog step right-left-right (three steps in two counts); on counts 3 and 4, jog step left-right-left (three steps in two counts). Face slightly to the right when doing the three steps starting with the right foot; and face slightly to the left when doing the three steps starting with the left foot. After you learn the step, lift the right arm with the right leg and the left arm with the left leg on each step.

Backward Lunges

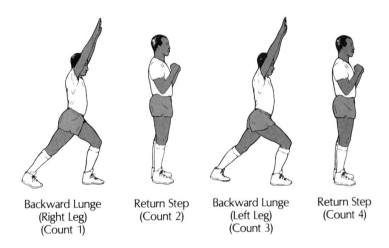

| Backward Lunge (Right Leg) (Count 1) | Return Step (Count 2) | Backward Lunge (Left Leg) (Count 3) | Return Step (Count 4) |

On count 1, step backward with your right leg; on 2, return to starting position; on 3, step backward with your left leg; and on 4, return to the starting position. When you have learned the step, reach upward and forward with the arms on the back lunges and bring the arms to the shoulders when you return to the starting position.

Twists

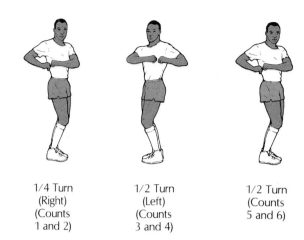

1/4 Turn
(Right)
(Counts
1 and 2)

1/2 Turn
(Left)
(Counts
3 and 4)

1/2 Turn
(Counts
5 and 6)

On counts 1 and 2, hop in the air and make a 1/4 turn to the right; hold your arms at shoulder height with your elbows up and swing them in the opposite directions of the leg twist. On counts 3 and 4, hop in the air and make a 1/2 turn to the left; turn your arms and shoulders in the opposite direction. Repeat, alternating twists to the left and right every two counts. On the last twist, a 1/2 turn is used to get back to the starting position.

APPENDIX F

Royal Canadian XBX and 5BX Programs

The Royal Canadian XBX and 5BX programs are progressive exercise plans designed to build total physical fitness. These plans, originally developed for use by the Royal Canadian Air Force, require eleven to twelve minutes a day. Like the Aerobics Program, they were originally designed to develop and maintain the physical fitness of military personnel. However, the programs have been widely received by the public. This sample from the Royal Canadian Program is one of the many included in the program, and is of moderate intensity. Some exercises have been modified to improve them. This sample is presented so that you can try a preplanned program to see if you might like to include one in your personal program.

Perform each exercise the number of repetitions indicated.

Sample Program	Number of Repetitions
Exercise 1**	10
Exercise 2**	16
Exercise 3	12
Exercise 4**	24
Exercise 5**	26
Exercise 6**	28
Exercise 7	28
Exercise 8	22
Exercise 9	8
Exercise 10	140

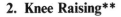

1. Back-Saver Toe Touch**

Purpose

To stretch the muscles on the back of the thigh (hamstrings).

This exercise is part of the sample warm-up in Concept 4, and described and illustrated on p. 37.

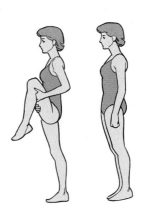

2. Knee Raising**

Start. Stand erect, feet together, arms at sides. Raise left knee as high as possible, grasping behind the upper leg with hands. Pull leg against body. Keep straight throughout. Lower foot to floor. Repeat with right leg. Continue by alternating legs.
Count. Left knee raise plus right knee raise counts as one repetition.

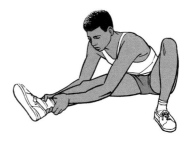

3. Lateral Bending

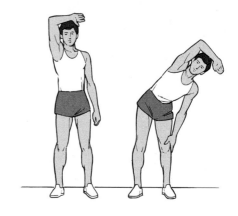

Start. Stand erect, feet twelve inches apart, right arm extended over head, bent at elbow. Bend sideward from waist to left. Slide left hand down leg as far as possible, and at the same time press to left with right arm. Return to starting position and change arm positions. Repeat to right. Continue by alternating to left, then right. (*Caution:* Do not arch the back).

Count. Bend to left plus bend to right counts as one repetition.

4. Arm Circling**

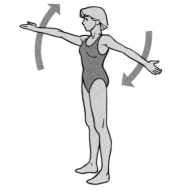

Start. Stand erect, feet twelve inches apart, arms at sides. Make large circles with arms in a windmill action—one arm following the other and both moving at the same time. Make backward circles only. Keep palms up.

Count. Each full circle by both arms counts as one repetition.

5. Crunch (Curl-Up)**

Purpose

Develop the upper abdominal muscles and correct abdominal ptosis.

Position

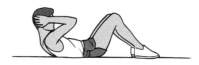

Assume a hook-lying position with arms crossed and hands on shoulders, or palms on ears. If desired, legs may rest on bench to increase difficulty. For less resistance, place hands at side of body (do not put hands behind neck).

Movement

Curl up until shoulder blades leave floor then roll down to the starting position. Repeat. (See station 9.)
Note: Twisting the trunk on the curl-up develops the oblique abdominals.

6. Arm and Leg-Lift**

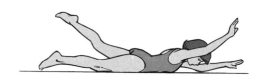

Start. Lie face down, legs straight and together; arms straight, together, and forward. First, lift the left leg and the right arm. Return to starting position. Next, lift the right leg and the left arm. Return to starting position. Keep the chin on the floor. (*Caution:* Do not arch the back).

Count: Each return to the starting position counts as one repetition.

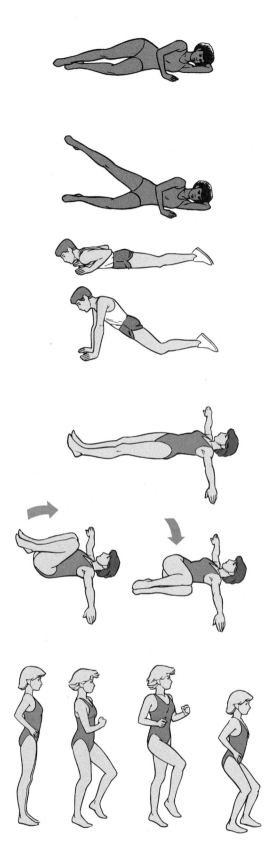

7. Side Leg Raising

Start. Lie on side with the top leg straight and the bottom leg slightly bent. Raise upper leg until it is at a 45-degree angle. Lower to starting position. (*Caution:* Keep knee caps pointed forward.)

Count. Each leg raise counts as one. Do half the number of repetitions raising the left leg. Roll to the other side and do half with the right leg.

8. Modified Push-Up

Start. Lie face down, hands directly under shoulders, knees on the floor. Raise body from floor by straightening it from head to knees. In the "up" position, the body should be in a straight line with palms of hands and knees in contact with floor. Lower to starting position. Keep head up throughout.

Count. Each return to the starting position counts as one repetition.

9. Leg-Overs—Tuck

Start. Lie on back, legs straight and together, arms stretched sidewards at shoulder level, palms down. Raise both legs from floor, bending at hips and knees until in a tuck position. Lower legs to left, keeping knees together and both shoulders on floor. Twist hips and lower legs to floor on right side. Twist hips to tuck position and return to starting position. Keep knees close to abdomen throughout.

Count. Each return to the starting position counts as one repetition.

10. Run and Half Knee Bends

Start. Stand erect, feet together, arms at sides. Starting with left leg, run in place raising feet at least six inches from the floor.

Count. Each time the left foot touches the floor counts as one repetition. After each set of fifty counts do ten half knee bends.

Half Knee Bends. Start with hands on hips, feet together, body erect. Bend at knees and hips, lowering body until thigh and calf form an angle of about 90 degrees. Do not bend knees past a right angle. Keep back straight. Return to starting position.

*Used by permission Royal Canadian Air Force, *Exercise Plans for Physical Fitness*. Queen's Printer, Ottawa, Canada: Revised U. S. Edition, 1962. By special arrangement with *This Week Magazine*.
**Exercises with double asterisks have been modified by the authors to improve them and to make them safer.

REFERENCES

A Guide to Managing Stress. Daly City, Calif.: Krames Communications, n.d.

"A Primer on Food Additives." *FDA Consumer* 22(1988):13.

"A Prudent Toast to Your Health." *Tufts University Diet & Nutrition Letter* (December 1989):3.

AAHPERD. *Technical Manual: Health Related Physical Fitness.* Reston, Va.: AAHPERD, 1984.

Aarons, S. "Smoking: Implications for Weight." San Francisco, CA: NASPE Session, AAHPERD National Convention, 1991.

About Inhalants. South Deerfield, MA: Channing L. Bete Co., Inc., 1992.

Adams, K., et al. "The Effect of Six Weeks of Squat, Plyometric and Squat-Plyometric Training on Power Production." *Journal of Applied Sport Science Research* 6(1992):36–41.

"Adverse Social Consequences of Alcohol Use and Alcoholism." *Alcohol and Health: Fifth Special Report to the U.S. Congress.* Washington, DC: Public Health Service, NIAA, 1984.

"Aerobicizers Getting More Than They Asked For?" *Journal of Physical Education, Recreation and Dance* 62(1991):16.

Aisenbrey, J., and J. L. DePaepe. "A Review of Osteoporosis Research: Implications for Exercise Education and Future Inquiry." *Clinical Kinesiology* 46(1992):2–12.

Aleshire, P. "Fourteen in State Tell of Side Effects from Diet Aid L-Tryptophan." *The Arizona Republic,* November 15, 1989.

"Alcohol and Cognition." *Alcohol Alert.* Washington, DC: National Institute on Alcohol Abuse and Alcoholism, 1989. Produced for the U.S. Department of Health and Human Services; Public Health Service; Alcohol, Drug Abuse, and Mental Health Administration.

Alcohol and Health. Seventh Special Report to the U.S. Congress from the Secretary of Health and Human Services, NIAAA. Rockville, MD: U.S. Department of Health and Human Services, 1990.

"Alcohol and Prescription Drugs." Reprint. *SRX—Medication Education for Seniors of San Francisco Health Department.* San Francisco, CA: Office of Senior Health Services, n.d.

Allman, F. L. "Rehabilitation Following Athletic Injuries." In O'Donoghue, D. H., *Treatment of Injuries to Athletes.* 4th ed. Philadelphia: Saunders, 1984, p. 677.

Allsen, P. E., and P. Witbeck. *Racquetball.* 5th ed. Dubuque, Iowa: Wm. C. Brown Publishers, 1992.

Alon, G., et al. "Comparison of the Effects of Electrical Stimulation and Exercise on Abdominal Musculature." *Journal of Orthopaedic and Sports Physical Therapy* 8(1987):567.

Alpert, J. S., et al. "Athletic Heart Syndrome." *Physician and Sportsmedicine* 17(1989):103.

Alsop, K. "Potential Hazards of Abdominal Exercises." *JOPERD* 42(1971):89.

Alter, M. J. *Sports Stretch.* Champaign, IL.: Human Kinetics Publishers, 1990.

Alter, M. J. *The Science of Stretching.* Champaign, Ill: Human Kinetics Publishers, 1988.

Althoff, S. A., et al. "Back to the Basics—Whatever Happened to Posture." *Journal of Physical Education, Recreation and Dance* 59(1988):20.

Alvarado, D. "Survey of Exercises Determines Skating a High-Risk Activity." *The Arizona Republic* (June 11, 1992):D7.

"Alzado Tribute Called off at Last Minute." *Los Angeles Times,* Jan. 12, 1992.

American Alliance of Health, Physical Education, Recreation and Dance. 1900 Association Drive, Reston, Va. 22091.

American Cancer Society. "Alcohol-Nutrient Interactions in Cancer Etiology." Second National Conference on Diet, Nutrition and Cancer (Sept. 5–7):1985.

American College of Sports Medicine. P. O. Box 1440, Indianapolis, Ind. 46206–1440.

American College of Sports Medicine. "Position Stand on the Use of Anabolic-Androgenic Steroids in Sports." *Sports Medicine Bulletin* (1984):1.

American College of Sports Medicine. "The Recommended Quantity and Quality of Exercise for Developing and Maintaining Cardiorespiratory and Muscular Fitness in Healthy Adults." *Medicine and Science in Sports and Exercise* 22(1990):2.

American College of Sports Medicine. *Guidelines for Exercise Testing and Exercise Prescription.* 4th ed. Philadelphia: Lea & Febiger, 1991.

American College of Sports Medicine. "Weight Loss in Wrestlers: Position Stand of American College of Sports Medicine." In P. E. Allsen, ed. *Conditioning and Physical Fitness.* Dubuque, Iowa: Wm. C. Brown Publishers, 1978.

American College of Sports Medicine. "Proper and Improper Weight Loss Programs." *Medicine and Science in Sports and Exercise* 15(1983):ix.

American Dietetic Association. "Position of the American Dietetic Association: Nutrition for Physical Fitness and Athletic Performance for Adults." *Journal of the American Dietetic Association* 87(1987):933.

American Heart Association (Greater Long Beach Chapter). "Stress—Bona Fide A.H.A. Risk Factor." *Heart Lines* 41:1(1984).

American Heart Association. "Dietary Guidelines." *Modern Maturity* 35(1992):59.

American Heart Association. *1992 Heart Facts Reference Sheet.* Dallas: American Heart Association, 1992.

American Institute of Stress. "Signs and Symptoms of Stress." In *Aviation Medical Bulletin.* Atlanta, GA.: Harvey W. Watt and Co., March, 1991.

American Thoracic Society, Medical Section of American Lung Association. "Health Effects of Smoking on Children: The Official Statement of the American Thoracic Society." *American Review of Respiratory Disease* 5 (1985):1137.

Anderson, K. M., et al. "Cholesterol and Mortality: Thirty Years of Follow-up from the Framingham Study." *Journal of the American Medical Association* 257(1987):2, 176.

Anderson, M. B., and J. M. Williams. "A Model of Stress and Athletic Injury: Prediction and Prevention." *Journal of Sport and Exercise Psychology* 10(1988):294–306.

Anderson, S. D. "Drugs Affecting the Respiratory System with Particular Reference to Asthma." *Medicine and Science in Sports and Exercise* 13(1981):259.

Anderson, T., and J. T. Kearney. "Effects of Three Resistance Training Programs on Muscular Strength and Absolute and Relative Endurance." *Research Quarterly for Exercise and Sport* 53(1982):1.

"Are Sports Drinks Better Than Water?" *Physician and Sportsmedicine* 20(1992):33.

Ashton-Miller, J. A., and A. B. Schultz. "Biomechanics of the Human Spine and Trunk." *Exercise and Sports Sciences Reviews* 16(1988):169–204.

Aspinall, W. "Clinical Testing for Cervical Mechanical Disorders Which Produce Ischemic Vertigo." *Journal of Orthopaedic and Sports Physical Therapy* 11(Nov. 1989):176–82.

Astrand, P. O., and K. Rodahl. *Textbook of Work Physiology.* 3d ed. New York: McGraw-Hill, 1986.

Auble, T. E., et al. "Aerobic Requirement for Moving Handweights through Various Ranges of Motion While Walking." *Physician and Sportsmedicine* 15(1987):133.

Avery, C. "Abdominal Obesity: Scaling Down This Deadly Risk." *Physician and Sportsmedicine* 19(1991):137.

Back Exercises for a Healthy Back. Daly City, Calif.: Krames Communications, 1988, 8 pp.

Back Pain: How to Control a Nagging Backache. Daly City, Calif.: Krames Communications, 1987, 16 pp.

"Back Specialists Hit 'Inversion Fad.'" *Medical World News* 28(1983).

Back Tips for Health Care Providers. Daly City, Calif.: Krames Communications, 1986, 16 pp.

Back Tips for People Who Sit. Daly City, Calif.: Krames Communications, 1985, 9 pp.

Bammel, G., and L. Burrus-Bammel. *Leisure and Human Behavior.* 2d ed. Dubuque, IA: Wm. C. Brown Communications, Inc., 1992.

Barnard, R. J. "The Heart Needs a Warm-Up Time." *Physician and Sportsmedicine* 4(1976):40.

Barnes, W. S. "The Relationship between Maximum Isokinetic Strength and Isokinetic Endurance." *Research Quarterly for Exercise and Sport* 51(1980):714.

Barrack, R. L., et al. "Joint Laxity and Proprioception in the Knee." *Physician and Sportsmedicine* 11(1983):130.

Barrett, S. *The Health Robbers.* Philadelphia: George F. Stickley Co., 1980.

Barrett, S., and Editors of Consumers Reports. *Health Schemes, Scams and Frauds.* Fairfield, OH: Consumer Report Books, 1991.

Bartels, R. L. "Weight Training: How to Lift and Eat for Strength and Power." *Physician and Sportsmedicine* 20(1992):233–34.

Basmajian, J. V. *Therapeutic Exercise.* 5th ed. Baltimore: Williams & Wilkins, 1990.

Basmajian, J. V., ed. *Manipulation, Traction and Massage.* Baltimore: Williams & Wilkins, 1985.

Bazzoli, A. S. "Chronic Back Pain: A Common Sense Approach." *American Journal of Physical Medicine and Rehabilitation* 71(1992):53–54.

Bazzoli, A. S., and F. S. Pollina. "Heel Pain in Recreational Runners." *Physician and Sportsmedicine* 17(1989):55.

"Beating Depression." *U. S. News and World Report* 108(1990):48.

Beaulieu, J. E. "Developing a Stretching Program." *Physician and Sportsmedicine* 9(1981):59.

Beck, J. L. "Overuse Injuries." *Clinics in Sports Medicine: Rehabilitation of the Injured Athlete* 4(1985):533.

Beighton, P. H. "Dominant Inheritance in Familial Generalized Articular Hypermobility." *Journal of Bone and Joint Surgery* 52B(1970):145–47.

Bember, M. G., et al. "The Effect of the Rate of Muscle Contraction on the Force-Time Curve Parameters of Male and Female Subjects." *Research Quarterly for Exercise and Sports* 61(1990):96–99.

Benda, C. "Stepping Into the Right Sock." *Physician and Sportsmedicine* 19(1991):125–28.

Benson, H. *Beyond the Relaxation Response.* New York: Berkley Publishing Group, 1985.

Berger, B. G., and D. R. Owen. "Anxiety Reduction with Swimming: Relationship between Exercises and State, Trait and Somatic Anxiety." *International Journal of Sport Psychology* 18(1988):286.

Berger, B. G., and D. R. Owen. "Stress Reduction and Mood Enhancement in Four Exercise Modes: Swimming, Body Condition, Hatha Yoga and Fencing." *Research Quarterly for Exercise and Sport* 59(1988):148.

Berger, B. G., et al. "Comparison of Jogging, the Relaxation Response, and Group Interaction for Stress Reduction." *Journal of Sport and Exercise Psychology* 10(1988):431.

Berlin, J., et al. "A Meta-analysis of Physical Activity in the Prevention of Heart Disease." *American Journal of Epidemiology* 132(1990):612.

Berry, M. J., et al. "The Effects of Elastic Tights on the Post-Exercise Response." *Canadian Journal of Applied Sports Sciences* 15(1990): 244.

Bertera, R. "The Effects of Workplace Health Promotion on Absenteeism and Employee Costs in a Large Industrial Population." *American Journal of Public Health* 80(1990):1101.

Bishop, K. N., et al. "The Effect of Eccentric Strength Training as Various Speeds on Concentric Strength of the Quadriceps and Hamstring Muscles." *Journal of Orthopaedic and Sports Physical Therapy* 13(1991):226–30.

Black, D. R., and Burckes-Miller, M. E. "Male and Female College Athletes: Use of Anorexia Nervosa and Bulimia Nervosa Weight Loss Methods." *Research Quarterly for Exercise and Sports* 59(1988):252.

Blackburn, S. E., and I. G. Portney. "Electromyographic Activity of Back Musculature during Williams' Flexion Exercises." *Physical Therapy* 61(1981):878.

Blair, S. "Science, Medicine and Health: Risk of Sedentary Living." *ARAPCS Newsletter* 12(1990):1.

Blair, S., et al. "Physical Activity and Health: A Lifestyle Approach." *Medicine, Exercise, Nutrition and Health* 1(1992):54.

Blair, S., et al. "Physical Fitness and All-Cause Mortality." *Journal of the American Medical Association* 262(1989):2395.

Blair, S. N. "Exercise within A Healthy Life-Style." In Dishman, R. K., *Exercise Adherence.* Champaign, Ill.: Human Kinetics Publishers, 1988.

Blair, S. N., and A. Oberman. "Epidemiological Analysis of Coronary Heart Disease." *Cardiology Clinics* 5(1987):271.

Blair, S. N., and R. S. Paffenbarger. "Physical Activity and Risk of Cancer." (ab.) *Medicine and Science in Sports and Exercise* 19(1987):418.

Bland, J. *Disorders of the Cervical Spine: Diagnosis and Medical Management.* Philadelphia: W. B. Saunders Company, 1987.

Blumenthal, D. "A Simple Guide to Complex Carbohydrates." *FDA Consumer* 23(1989):13.

Boone, T., et al. "A Physiological Evaluation of the Sports Massage." *Athletic Training* 26(1991):51–54.

"Booze for Health: Let the Drinker Beware." San Rafael, CA: The Marin Institute for the Prevention of Alcohol and Other Drug Problems (Summer 1991):4.

Borms, J., et. al. "Optional Duration of Static Stretching Exercises for Improvement of Coxo-Femoral Flexibility." *Journal of Sports Science* 16(1988):152–61.

Botvin, G. "Prevention of Adolescent Substance Abuse Through the Development of Personal and Social Competence." *Preventing Adolescent Drug Abuse: Intervention Strategies.* Rockville, MD: National Institute on Drug Abuse (1983):121. Research Monograph 47, DHHS Publication (ADM)83–1280.

Bouchard, C. "Heredity and the Path to Overweight and Obesity." *Medicine and Science in Sports and Exercise* 23(1991):285.

Bouchard, C., et al. "Genetics of Aerobic and Anaerobic Performances." *Exercise and Sport Sciences Reviews* 20(1992):27.

Bouchard, C., et al., eds. *Exercise, Fitness, and Health.* Champaign, Ill.: Human Kinetics Publishers, 1990.

Bourey, R. E., et al. "Interactions of Exercise, Coagulation, Platelets, and Fibrinoysis: A Brief Review." *Medicine and Science in Sports and Exercise* 20(1988):439.

Boyce, R., and S. Jackson. "One-Arm Lifting for a Healthy Back." *Strategies* (Jan. 1991):19–22.

Bracker, M. D., S. R. Garfin, and S. A. Singer. "Low Back Pain in a Tennis Player." *Physician and Sportsmedicine* 16(1988):75.

Braude, M. C., and H. M. Char. *Genetic and Biological Markers in Drug Abuse and Alcoholism.* National Institute on Drug Abuse Research Monograph (1986):66.

Bray, G. A. "Obesity: A Blueprint for Progress." *Contemporary Nutrition* 12(1987):1.

"Break the Habit, Not Bones." *Health Digest* (May/June 1992):7.

Brill, P. A., et al. "Recruitment, Retention, and Success in Worksite Health Promotion: Association with Demographic Characteristics." *American Journal of Health Promotion* 5(1991):215.

Brittenham, G. "Plyometric Exercise: A Word of Caution." *JOPERD* (Jan. 1992): 20–23.

Brodie, D. A., et al. "Joint Laxity in Selected Athletic Populations." *Medicine and Science in Sports and Exercise* 14(1982):190.

Brooks, C. M., "Adult Participation in Physical Activities Requiring Moderate to High Levels of Energy Expenditure." *Physician and Sportsmedicine* 15(1987):119.

Brower, K. J., et al. "Evidence for Physical and Psychological Dependence on Anabolic Androgenic Steroids in Eight Weight Lifters." *American Journal of Psychiatry* 147(1990):510–12.

Brown, B. B. *Between Health and Illness: New Notions on Stress and the Nature of Well-Being.* New York: Bantam Books, 1985.

Brown, B. S., et al. "Anaerobic Power Changes Following Short Term Task Specific, Dynamic and Static Loading." *Journal of Applied Sport Science Research* 2(1988):35–38.

Brown, S., et al. "Injury Prevention and Control: Prospects for the 1990s." *Annual Review of Public Health* 11(1990):251.

Brown, S. P., and D. E. Cundiff. "Exercise, Aging, and Longevity." *Health Education* 19(1988):4.

Brownell, K., et al. "Matching Weight Control Programs to Individuals." *The Weight Control Digest* 1(1991):65.

Brownell, K. D. *The LEARN Program for Weight Control.* Philadelphia: University of Pennsylvania, 1987.

Brownson, R., et al. "Physical Activity on the Job and Cancer in Missouri." *American Journal of Public Health* 81(1991):639.

Bruess, C., and G. Richardson. *Decisions for Health.* 3d ed. Dubuque, IA: Wm. C. Brown Publishers, 1992.

Brunick, T. "Choosing the Right Shoe." *Physician and Sportsmedicine* 18(1990):104.

Bureau of Labor Statistics. *Annual Survey of Occupational Injuries and Illness.* Washington, DC: Department of Labor, 1989.

Burkett, L. N., and P. W. Darst. *Cycling.* Glenview, Ill.: Scott, Foresman and Co., 1987.

Buroker, K. C., and J. A. Schwane. "Does Post-Exercise Static Stretching Alleviate Delayed Muscle Soreness?" *Physician and Sportsmedicine* 17(June 1989):65–83.

Butterfield, G. "Letter to the Editor-in-Chief." *Medicine and Science in Sports and Exercise* 20(1988):415.

Butterfield, G. E. "Whole-body Protein Utilization in Humans." *Medicine and Science in Sports and Exercise* 19(1987):Supplement, 157.

Buyze, M. T., et al. "Comparative Training Responses to Rope Skipping and Jogging." *Physician and Sportsmedicine* 14(1986):65.

Byers, T. "Food, Additives, and Cancer." *Postgraduate Medicine* 84(1988):275.

Cailliet, R. *Knee Pain and Disability.* 2d ed. Philadelphia: F. A. Davis, Co., 1983.

Cailliet, R. *Low Back Pain Syndrome.* 4th ed. Philadelphia: F. A. Davis, Co., 1988.

Cailliet, R. *Neck and Arm Pain.* 3d ed. Philadelphia: F. A. Davis, Co., 1990.

Cailliet, R. *Shoulder Pain.* 2d ed. Philadelphia: F. A. Davis, Co., 1981.

Cailliet, R. *Soft Tissue Pain and Disability.* 2d ed. Philadelphia: F. A. Davis, Co., 1988.

"Can One Train Cardiorespiratory and Muscular Fitness Simultaneously?" (Editorial). *Canadian Journal of Sport Science* 16(1991):167–68.

"Can You Live Longer?" *Consumer Reports* 57(1992):7.

Cancer Facts and Figures—1991. New York: The American Cancer Society, 1992.

"Cancer Screening Guidelines." *Healthplex* 8(1992):17.

Carrol, C. R. *Drugs in Modern Society.* 3d ed. Dubuque, IA: Wm. C. Brown Communications, Inc., 1993.

Carruthers, C. P., and C. D. Hood. "Alcoholics and Children of Alcoholics: The Role of Leisure in Recovery." *Journal of Physical Education, Recreation and Dance* (April 1992):48.

Casperson, C. J. "Physical Activity Epidemiology: Concepts, Methods, and Applications to Exercise Science." *Exercise and Sport Sciences Reviews* 17(1989):423.

Casperson, C. J. "Physical Inactivity and Coronary Heart Disease." *Physician and Sportsmedicine* 15(1987):43.

Casperson, C. J., et al. "Physical Activity, Exercise, and Physical Fitness: Definitions and Distinctions for Health-Related Research." *Public Health Reports* 100(1985):126.

Casperson, C. J., et al. "Physical Activity, Exercise, and Physical Fitness: Concepts, Methods, and Application to Exercise Science." *Exercise and Sports Sciences Review* 17(1989):126.

Cates, W. "The Other STD's: Do They Really Matter?" *Journal of the American Medical Association* 259(1988):3606.

Center for Disease Control. "Vigorous Physical Activity Among High School Students." *Morbidity and Mortality Weekly Report* 41(1992):1.

Centers for Disease Control. "Years of Potential Life Lost Before Age 65— United States 1987." *Morbidity and Mortality Weekly Report* 38(1989):27.

Centers for Disease Control. *HIV/AIDS Surveillance Report.* Atlanta, GA: U.S. Department of Health and Human Services, 1991.

Centers for Disease Control. *Morbidity and Mortality Weekly Report* 39(1990):110.

Chadbourne, R. "A Hard Look at Running Surfaces." *Physician and Sportsmedicine* 18(1990):103.

Chambers, M. "Exercise: A Prescription for a Good Night's Sleep?" *Physician and Sportsmedicine* 19(1991):107.

Chandler, T. J., and M. H. Stone. "The Squat Exercise in Athletic Conditioning: A Review of the Literature." *National Strength and Conditioning Association Journal* 13(1991):52–60.

Chandler, T. J., et al. "The Effect of the Squat Exercise on Knee Stability." *Medicine and Science in Sports and Exercise* 21(June 1989):299–303.

Chandrashekkhar, Y., et al. "Exercise as a Coronary Protective Factor." *American Heart Journal* 122(1991):1723.

Changing Your Mind: Drugs That Alter Your Moods. Center City, MN: Hazelden Educational Materials, 1991.

Chemical Dependency: Is There a Problem? San Bruno, CA: Krames Communications, 1987.

Cho, A. K. "Ice: A New Dosage Form of an Old Drug." *Science.* August 10, 1990, 631.

Chodak, G. W., et al. "Routine Screening for Prostate Cancer Using the Digital Rectal Examination." *Progress and Clinical and Biological Research* 269(1988):87.

Cigarette Smoking: The Facts About Your Lungs. New York, NY: American Lung Association, 1987.

Cinque, C. "Are Americans Fit? Survey Data Conflict." *Physician and Sportsmedicine* 14(1986):24.

Clark, N. "Case Studies in Sports Nutrition." *Physician and Sportsmedicine* 16(1988):131.

Clark, N. "Fueling Up With Carbs: How Much is Enough?" *Physician and Sportsmedicine* 19(1991):68.

Clark, N. "How to Gain Weight Healthfully." *Physician and Sportsmedicine* 19(1991):53.

Clark, N. "Protein Myths: The Meat of the Matter." *Sportcare and Fitness* 2(1989):53.

Clarkson, P. "Minerals, Exercise Performance and Supplementation." *Journal of Sport Sciences* 9(1991):91.

Clouet, D., K. Asghar, and R. Brown. "Mechanisms of Cocaine Abuse and Toxicity." Rockville, MD: National Institute on Drug Abuse (1988):ix. Research Monograph 88, U.S. Department of Health and Human Services, Public Health Service.

Cocaine in the Workplace: What You Can Do. Daly City, CA: Krames Communications, 1986.

Cohen, J. S., et al. "Hypercholesterolemia in Male Power Lifters Using Anabolic-Androgenic Steroids." *Physician and Sportsmedicine* 16(1988):49.

Cohen, S. *The Substance Abuse Problems Vol. Two.* New York: The Haworth Press, 1985.

Coleman, B. C. "Parade to Target 'Joe Camel' Ads." Santa Ana, CA: *Orange County Register,* June 21, 1992.

Collingwood, T. R., et al. "Enlisting Physical Education for the War on Drugs." *Journal of Health, Physical Education, Recreation and Dance* 63(1992).

Colucci, D., et al. "Comparison of Static versus PNF Stretching on Shoulder ROM in Intercollegiate Baseball Players." *Athletic Training* 24(1989):116.

Commandre, F. A., et al. "Lumbar Spine, Sport and Actual Treatment." *Journal of Sports Medicine and Physical Fitness* 31(1992):129–35.

Condon, S. A., and R. S. Hutton. "Soleus Electromyographic Activity and Ankle Dorsiflexion Range of Motion during Four Stretching Procedures." *Physical Therapy* 67(1987):24–30.

"Congressional Panel to FDA: Get Tough with Medical-Device Makers." *Medical World News* (August 16, 1982):15.

Consumer Union. *Health Quackery.* Orangeburg, N.Y.: Consumer Reports Books, 1980.

Cooper, E. "Statement on Physical Activity and Heart Disease." American Heart Association News Release. July 1, 1992, pp. 1–2.

Cooper, K. H. *Running Without Fear.* New York: M. Evans & Co., Inc., 1988.

Cooper, K. H. *The Aerobics Program for Total Well-Being.* New York: M. Evans & Co., Inc., 1982.

Corbin, C. B. "Self-Confidence of Women in Sports." In W. M. Walsh, ed. *Clinics in Sports Medicine: Women in Sports.* Philadelphia: W. B. Saunders Co., 1984.

Corbin, C. B. "Youth Fitness, Exercise, and Health." *Research Quarterly for Exercise and Sport* 58(1987):308.

Corbin, C. B., and Pangrazi, R. "The Health Benefits of Exercise." *Research Digest for Physical Activity and Fitness* 1(1993):1.

Corbin, C. B., and R. Lindsey. *Fitness for Life.* 3d ed. Glenview, Ill.: Scott, Foresman and Co., 1993.

Corbin, C. B., and R. Pangrazi. "Are American Children and Youth Fat?" *Research Quarterly for Exercise and Sport* 63(1993):96.

Corbin, C. B., et al. "Commitment to Physical Activity." *International Journal of Sport Psychology* 18(1987):215.

Corbin, D. E. *Jogging.* Glenview, Ill.: Scott, Foresman and Company, 1987.

Corbin, D. E., and J. Metal-Corbin. *Reach for It: A Handbook of Health, Exercise and Dance Activities, for Older Adults.* 2d ed. Dubuque, Iowa: E. Bowers, 1990.

Cordain, L., et al. "The Effects of an Aerobic Running Program on Bowel Transit Time." *Journal of Sports Medicine* 26(1986):101.

Cornelius, W. L. "Modified PNF Stretching: Improvement in Hip Flexion." *National Strength and Conditioning Association Journal* 12(1990):44–46.

Cornelius, W. L. "PNF Ankle Stretching: Partner/No-Partner Procedures." *National Strength and Conditioning Association Journal* 13(1991):59–63.

Cornelius, W. L., and K. Craft-Hamm. "Proprioceptive Neuromuscular Facilitation Flexibility Techniques: Acute Effects on Arterial Blood Pressure." *Physician and Sportsmedicine* 16(1988):152–61.

Costello, F. *Bounding to the Top: The Complete Book on Plyometric Training.* West Bowie, Md.: Athletic Training Consultants, Inc., 1986.

Couldry, W., et al. "Carotid vs. Radial Pulse Counts." *Physician and Sportsmedicine* 10(1982):67.

Cousins, N. *Head First—The Biology of Hope.* New York: Dutton, 1989.

Couzens, G. S. "Surgically Sculpting Athletic Physiques: Liposuction and Calf and Pectoral Implants." *Physician and Sportsmedicine* 20(1992):153–66.

Cowart, V. "Dietary Supplements." *Physician and Sportsmedicine* 20(1992):189.

Cowart, V. "Human Growth Hormone: The Latest Ergogenic Aid?" *Physician and Sportsmedicine* 16(1988):175.

Cowart, V. "If Youngsters Overdose with Anabolic Steroids, What's the Cost Anatomically and Otherwise?" *Journal of the American Medical Association* 261(1989):1856.

Cowart, V. "Steroids in Sports: After Four Decades Time to Return These Genies To Bottle?" *Journal of the American Medical Association* 257(1987):421.

Cowart, V. S. "Can Exercise Help Women with PMS?" *Physician and Sportsmedicine* 17(1989):169.

Crack Kills, Don't Do It. Skill Builder. St. Rose, LA: SYNDISTAR, Inc., n.d.

Croce, P. *Stretching for Athletics.* 2d ed. Champaign, Ill.: Leisure Press, 1984.

Cross, T. "Speed/Strength Exercise: The Lateral Squat." *National Strength and Conditioning Association Journal* 13(1991):56–58.

Cross, T. "Strength Exercise: The Angle Lunge." *National Strength and Conditioning Association Journal* 13(1991):51–58.

Cryer, P. "Glucose Counterregulation, Hypoglycemia, and Intensive Insulin Therapy in Diabetes Mellitus." *New England Journal of Medicine* 313(1985):232.

Csikszentmihalyi, M., and R. Graef. "Feeling Free." *Psychology Today* 12(1979):84.

Culhane, C. "Ice Spreads to West Coast Area." *U.S. Journal of Drug and Alcohol Dependence 14* 1(1990):16.

Cureton, K. J., et al. "Muscle Hypertrophy in Men and Women." *Medicine and Science in Sports and Exercise* 20(1988):338.

Cureton, T. K. *Physical Fitness and Dynamic Health.* New York: Dial Press, 1965.

Curran, J. W., et al. "Epidemiology of HIV Infection and AIDS in the United States." *Science* 239(1988):610.

Davis, A. A., and Carragee, E. J. "Sciatica: Treating a Painful Symptom." *Physician and Sportsmedicine* 20(Jan. 1992):126–35.

Day, N. *Shoulder Owner's Manual.* Daly City, Calif.: Krames Communications, 1984.

DeBenedette, V. "Getting Fit for Life: Can Exercise Reduce Stress?" *Physician and Sportsmedicine* 16(1988):185.

DeBenedette, V. "Health Club Tanning Booths: Risky Business." *Physician and Sportsmedicine* 15(1987):59.

DeBenedette, V. "Keeping Pace with the Many Forms of Walking." *Physician and Sportsmedicine* 16(1988):145.

DeBusk, R., et al. "Training Effects of Long Versus Short Bouts of Exercise in Healthy Subjects." *American Journal of Cardiology* 65(1990):1010.

Deitz, W. H., et. al. "Do We Fatten Our Children at the Television Set?" *Pediatrics* 75(1985):807.

deLateur, B. J., and J. F. Lehmann. "Therapeutic Exercise To Develop Strength and Endurance." In *Krusen's Handbook of Physical Medicine and Rehabilitation.* 4th ed. Kotke & Lehman, Eds. Philadelphia: W. B. Saunders, 1990, pp. 480–95.

deLateur, B. J., et al. "Footwear and Posture: Compensatory Strategies for Heel Height." *American Journal of Physical Medicine and Rehabilitation* 70(1991):246.–54.

Delitto, R., and S. J. Rose. "An Electromyographic Analysis of Two Techniques for Squat Lifting and Lowering." *Physical Therapy* 72(June 1992):438–48.

DePiccoli, B., et al. "Anabolic Steroid Use in Body Builders: An Echocardiographic Study of Left Ventricle Morphology and Function." *International Journal of Sports Medicine* 4(1991):408–12.

DiCicco, L., et al. "Evaluation of CASPAR Alcohol Education Curriculum." *Journal of Alcohol Studies* 2(1984):160.

Dickinson, A., and K. M. Bennett. "Therapeutic Exercise." In J. S. Harvey, ed. *Clinics in Sports Medicine: Rehabilitation of the Injured Athlete* 4(1985):420.

DiClemente, R. J., et al. "Adolescents and AIDS: A Survey of Knowledge, Attitudes, and Beliefs About AIDS in San Francisco." *American Journal of Public Health* 76(1986):1443.

Dietary Guidelines and Your Diet. Hyattsville, MD: USDA, 1992, No. HG–232, 1–11.

Dintiman, G. B., and J. S. Greenberg. *Health through Discovery.* New York: Random House, 1989.

Direct and Indirect Costs of Diabetes in the United States in 1987. Alexandria, VA: American Diabetes Association, 1988.

Direct Marketing Association. 6 East 43rd St., New York, N.Y. 10017.

Dishman, R., et al. "Health Locus of Control Predicts Free-living, But Not Supervised, Physical Activity." *Research Quarterly for Exercise and Sport* 61(1990):383.

Dishman, R. K. (ed.) *Exercise Adherence.* Champaign, Ill.: Human Kinetics Publishers, 1988.

Dishman, R. K., et al. "The Determinants of Physical Activity and Exercise." *Public Health Reports* 100(1985):158.

Donatelle, R. J., et al. *Access to Health.* Englewood Cliffs, N.J.: Prentice-Hall, 1988.

Donatelli, R., and B. Greenfield. "Case Study: Rehabilitation of a Stiff and Painful Shoulder: A Biomechanical Approach." *Journal of Orthopaedic and Sports Physical Therapy* 9(1987):118.

Dondero, T. J., et al. "Monitoring the Levels and Trends of HIV Infection: The Public Health Service's HIV Surveillance Program." *Public Health Reports* 103(1988):213.

Dowdy, D. B., et al. "Effects of Aerobic Dance on Physical Work Capacity, Cardiovascular Fitness, and Body Composition of Middle-aged Women." *Research Quarterly* 56(1985):227.

"Drug Abuse and Pregnancy." *NIDA Capsules.* Washington, DC: National Institute on Drug Abuse; U.S. Department of Health and Human Services; Public Health Service; Alcohol, Drug Abuse and Mental Health Administration, June 1989.

Drugs of Abuse 6, No. 2. Washington, DC: Drug Enforcement Agency, July 1979.

Drug Use Among American High School Students, College Students and Other Young Adults. Washington, DC: National Institute on Drug Abuse, U.S. Department of Health and Human Services, 1987.

Duda, M. "Elite Lifters at Risk for Spondylolysis." *Physician and Sportsmedicine* 15(1987):57.

Duda, M. "Plyometrics: A Legitimate Form of Power Training." *Physician and Sportsmedicine* 16(1988):213.

Duda, M. "The Medical Risks and Benefits of Sauna, Steam Bath and Whirlpool Use." *Physician and Sportsmedicine* 15(1987):170.

Dudley, G. A. "Metabolic Consequences of Resistance-Type Exercise." *Medicine and Science in Sports and Exercise* 20(1988):Supplement, 158.

Duncan, P. W., et al. "Mode and Speed Specificity of Eccentric and Concentric Exercise Training." *Journal of Orthopaedic and Sports Physical Therapy* 11(1989):70–75.

Dunn, A., et al. "Exercise and the Neurobiology of Depression." *Exercise and Sport Sciences Reviews* 19(1991):41.

Durant, R. H., et al. "Use of Multiple Drugs Among Adolescents Who Use Anabolic Steroids." *New England Journal of Medicine* 328(1993):922.

Dye, C. *"'Adam' & 'Eve' & 'Ecstasy': Facts About MDMA."* Tempe, AZ: D.I.N. Publications, 1988.

Dzewaltowski, D., et al. "Physical Activity Participation: Social Cognitive Theory Versus the Theories of Reasoned Action and Planned Behavior." *Journal of Sport and Exercise Psychology* 12(1990):388.

Early Signs of Addiction: Are the Illusions Taking Over? San Bruno, CA: Krames Communications, 1990.

Eddy, D. M., et al. "The Value of Mammography Screening in Women under 50 Years." *Journal of the American Medical Association* 259(1988):187.

Eichner, E. R. "Does Running Cause Osteoarthritis?" *Physician and Sportsmedicine* 17(1989):147.

Eichner, E. R., et al. "Exercise, Lymphokines, Calories, and Cancer." *Physician and Sportsmedicine* 15(1987):109.

Eigen, L. D. "Alcohol Practices, Policies and Potentials of American Colleges and Universities: An OSAP White Paper." Washington, DC: Office for Substance Abuse and Prevention; Alcohol, Drug Abuse and Mental Health Administration; U.S. Department of Health and Human Services, 1991.

Eitner, D., et al. *Physical Therapy for Sports.* Philadelphia: W. B. Saunders Co., 1982.

Ekoe, J. "Overview of Diabetes Mellitus and Exercise." *Medicine and Science in Sports and Exercise* 21(1989):353.

Elliot, D. L., et al. "Effect of Resistance Training on Excess Post-exercise Oxygen Consumption." *Journal of Applied Sport Science Research* 6(1992):77–81.

Entyre, B. R., and E. J. Lee. "Comments on Proprioceptive Neuromuscular Facilitation Stretching Techniques." *Research Quarterly for Exercise and Sport* 58(1987):184–88.

Entyre, B. R., and L. D. Abraham. "Antagonist Muscle Activity during Stretching: A Paradox Reassessed." *Medicine and Science in Sports and Exercise* 20(1988):285–89.

Epstein, F. H. "Beyond Cholesterol: Modification of Low Density Lipoprotein That Increases Its Athrogenicity." *New England Journal of Medicine* 320(1989):915.

Epstein, L., et al. "Ten-year Follow-up of Behavioral, Family-Based Treatment for Obese Children." *Journal of the American Medical Association* 264(1990):2519.

"Estimated U.S. Costs of Drug Abuse." Chapel Hill, NC: Research Triangle Institute, 1990.

Evans, W. J. "Exercise-Induced Skeletal Muscle Damage." *Physician and Sportsmedicine* 15(1987):89.

Ewing, A., et al. "Effect of Exercise with Light Hand Weights on Strength." *Journal of Orthopaedic and Sports Physical Therapy* 8(1987):533.

Facts About Cigarette Smoking. New York, NY: American Lung Association, n.d.

Facts About Nicotine Addiction and Cigarettes. New York, NY: American Lung Association, 1990.

Facts About Second Hand Smoke. New York, NY: American Lung Association, 1990.

Facts About the Nicotine Transdermal Patch. New York, NY: American Lung Association, 1992.

Fahrni, W. H. "Deep-Bending Exercises May Be the Lower Back's Last Straw." *Medical World News* 8(1967):96.

Ferenchick, G. S., et al. "Steroids and Cardiomyopathy: How Strong a Connection?" *Physician and Sportsmedicine* 19(1991):107–10.

"FDA Examines Danger of Patch Plus Cigarettes." Santa Ana, CA: *Orange County Register,* June 19, 1992.

Field, R. "How Humans Sit." *The American Way* (April 15, 1988): 28–29.

Fisher, A. G., and P. E. Allsen. *Jogging.* 2d ed. Dubuque, Iowa: Wm. C. Brown Publishers, 1987.

Fisk, J. W. *A Practical Guide to Management of the Painful Neck and Back.* Springfield, Ill.: Charles C. Thomas, Publisher, 1977.

Fitnessgram: Test Administration Manual. Dallas: Cooper Institute for Aerobics Research, 1992.

Fitness Canada. *Canada Fitness Survey—Highlights.* Ottawa, Ontario: Government of Canada, 1990.

"Fitness Improves Driving." *Senior World of Orange County* 17(Jan. 1991).

"Fitness: Working Out the Facts." *Consumer Reports Health Letter.* 3(July 1991):49, 52.

Fleck, S. J. "Cardiovascular Adaptations to Resistance Training." *Medicine and Science in Sports and Exercise* 20(1988):Supplement, 146.

Fleck, S. J., and W. J. Kraemer. "Resistance Training: Basic Principles (Part 1 of 4)." *Physician and Sportsmedicine* 16(1988):160.

Fleck, S. J., and W. J. Kraemer. "Resistance Training: Exercise Prescription (Part 4 of 4)." *Physician and Sportsmedicine* 16(1988):68.

Fleck, S. J., and W. J. Kraemer. "Resistance Training: Physiological Responses (Part 3 of 4)." *The Physician and Sportsmedicine* 16(1988):63.

Fleck, S. J., and W. J. Kraemer. "Resistance Training: Physiological Responses and Adaptations (Part 2 of 4)." *The Physician and Sportsmedicine* 16(1988):108.

Fletcher, G. F., et al. "American Heart Association Statement on Exercise: Benefits and Recommendations for Physical Activity Programs for All Americans." *Circulation* 86(1992):2726.

Flint, M. "Selecting Exercises." *JOPERD* 35(1964):19.

Flint, M., and J. Gudgell. "Electromyographic Study of Abdominal Muscular Activity during Exercise." *Research Quarterly* 36(1965):1.

Folkenberg, J. "Reporting Reactions to Additives." *FDA Consumer* 22(1988):16.

"Focus: Stress Management Overview," *Fitness Leader* 1:1(1982):1.

Food and Drug Administration. *Condoms and Sexually Transmitted Diseases.* Rockville, MD: U.S. Department of Health and Human Services, 1990.

"Foods, Drugs or Frauds?" *FDA Consumer,* May, 1985 (reprint).

Foreyt, J. "Factors Common to Successful Therapy for the Obese Patient." *Medicine and Science in Sports and Exercise* 23(1991):292.

Forman, J. W. *The Personal Stress Reduction Program.* Englewood Cliffs, N.J.: Prentice-Hall, Inc., 1987.

Fox, K., et al. "The Physical Self-Perception Profile." *Journal of Sport and Exercise Psychology* 11(1989):408.

Fox, M., and D. Broide. *Molly Fox's Step On It.* New York: Avon Books. (1991):5.

Frankle, M., and D. Leffers. "Athletes on Anabolic-Androgenic Steroids: New Approach Diminishes Health Problems." *Physician and Sportsmedicine* 20(1992):75–87.

Franklin, B. "Exercise Training and Coronary Collateral Circulation." *Medicine and Science in Sport and Exercise* 23(1991):648.

Franklin, B., et al. "Exercise Testing Update." *Physician and Sportsmedicine* 19(1991):111.

Franks, B. D., et al. *Fitness Leader's Handbook.* Champaign, IL: Human Kinetics, 1989.

Freudenberg, H. *Burnout: The High Cost of High Achievement.* New York: Anchor Press: Doubleday, 1980.

Friedl, K., and R. J. Moore. "Steroid Replacers: Let The Athlete Beware." *National Strength and Conditioning Association Journal* 14(1992):14–19.

Friedl, K. E., and C. E. Yesalis. "Self-Treatment of Gynecomastia in Bodybuilders Who Use Anabolic Steroids." *Physician and Sportsmedicine* 17(1989):67.

Friedman, J. M. W., et al. "Prevalence of Specific Suicidal Behaviors in a High School Sample." *American Journal of Psychiatry* 144(1987):1203.

Frisch, R. E. "Lower Prevalence of Breast Cancer and Cancers of the Reproductive System Among Former College Athletes Compared to Non-Athletes." *British Journal of Cancer* 52(1985):885.

Frisch, R. E., et al. "Lower Lifetime Occurrence of Breast Cancer and Cancers of the Reproductive System Among Former College Athletes." *American Journal of Clinical Nutrition* 45(1987):328.

"FYI: Technology." *Orange County Register.* Jan. 1, 1990.

Gajdosik, R. L. "Effects of Static Stretching on the Maximal Length and Resistance to Passive Stretch of Short Hamstring Muscles." *Journal of Orthopaedic and Sports Physical Therapy* 14 (Dec. 1991):250–55.

Gallagher, W. "The Looming Menace of Designer Drugs." *Discover,* August 1986:24.

Gallup, G. "Importance of Social Values." *Gallup Report* (March 1989):282.

Gallup, G. "Leisure: Swimming, Fishing, Bicycling Are Top Sports Activities." *Gallup Report* 281(1989):28.

Gallup, G., and F. Newport. "Gallup Leisure Audit." *The Gallup Poll Monthly* 295(1990):27.

Gallup, G., and F. Newport. "Despite Dissatisfaction with Way Things Are Going, Americans Remain Positive." *The Gallup Poll Monthly.* 298(1990):10.

Gallup, G., and F. Newport. "Americans Have Love-Hate Relationship with Their TV Sets." *The Gallup Poll Monthly* 301(1990):2.

Gallup, G., and F. Newport. "Americans Now Drinking Less Alcohol." *Gallup Poll Monthly,* Dec. 1990:2–6.

Gallup, G., and F. Newport. "Many Americans Favor Restrictions on Smoking in Public Places." *Gallup Poll Monthly* 301(1990):19.

Gallup, G., and F. Newport. "Gallup Leisure Poll." *The Gallup Poll Monthly* 295(1990):27.

Garbutt, G., et al. "Running Speed and Spinal Shrinkage in Runners With and Without Low Back Pain." *Medicine and Science in Sports and Exercise* 22(1990):769–72.

Garcia, A., et al. "Predicting Long-term Adherence to Aerobic Exercise: A Comparison of Two Models." *Journal of Sport and Exercise Psychology* 13(1991):394.

Garhammer, J. *Sports Illustrated Strength Training.* New York: Harper & Row, Publishers, 1986.

Garnica, R. A. "Muscular Power in Young Women After Slow and Fast Isokinetic Training." *Journal of Orthopaedic and Sports Physical Therapy* 8(1986):1.

Garrett, W. E. "Muscle Strain Injuries: Clinical and Basic Aspects." *Medicine and Science in Sports and Exercise* 22(1990):436–43.

Garrick, J. G., et al. "The Epidemiology of Aerobic Dance." *American Journal of Sports Medicine* 14(1986):67.

Gauthier, M. M. "Can Exercise Reduce the Risk of Cancer?" *Physician and Sportsmedicine* 14(1986):171.

Gauthier, M. M. "Continuous Passive Motion: The No-Exercise Exercise." *Physician and Sportsmedicine* 15(1987):142.

Gauthier, M. M. "Soda Pop May Increase Fracture Risk." *Physician and Sportsmedicine* 17(1989):46.

George, F. J. "Exercise Physiology and Medicine" in *Year Book of Sports Medicine.* Chicago: Year Book Medical Publishers, Inc. (1988):42.

Gerhardsson, M., et al. "Sedentary Jobs and Colon Cancer." *American Journal of Epidemiology* 123(1986):775.

Giel, D. "Is There a Crisis in Youth Fitness—or Fatness?" *Physician and Sportsmedicine* 16(1988):145.

Gilbert, D. A. *Compendium of American Public Opinion.* New York: Facts on File Publications, 1988.

Gillespie, J. *Drugs and Fitting In.* Center City, MN: Hazelden Publishing, 1989.

Gillespie, J. *Drugs Mean Alcohol Too!* Center City, MN: Hazelden Publishing, 1989.

Gillespie, J. *Drugs Mean Nicotine Too!* Center City, MN: Hazelden Publishing, 1989.

Gillette, T. M. et al. "Relationship of Body Core Temperature and Warm-Up to Knee Range of Motion." *Journal of Orthopaedic and Sports Physical Therapy* 13(Mar. 1991): 126–31.

Gleim, G. W., et al. "Influence of Flexibility on Economy of Walking and Jogging." *Journal of Orthopaedic Research* 8(1990):814–23.

Godges, J. J., et al. "The Effects of Two Stretching Procedures on Hip Range of Motion and Gait Economy." *Journal of Orthopaedic and Sports Physical Therapy* 11(1989):350–57.

Goldfine, H., et al. "Exercising to Health." *Physician and Sportsmedicine* 19(1991):81.

Goldman, R. M. "Dr. Goldman Replies." *Physician and Sportsmedicine* 13(1985):15.

Goldstein, D. "Clinical Applications for Exercise." *Physician and Sportsmedicine* 17(1989):83.

Goode, E., ed. *Annual Editions: Drugs, Society and Behavior.* Guilford, CT: Dushkin Publishing Company, 1991.

Goodman, C. E. "Low Back Pain in the Cosmetic Athlete." *Physician and Sportsmedicine* 15(1987):97.

Gorman, C. "Invincible AIDS." *Time* 140(1992):30.

Gorman, D., and B. Brown. "Fitness and Aging: An Overview." *JOPERD* 57(1986):50.

Gorman, M., et al. "Position of the American Dietetic Association: Health Implications of Dietary Fiber." *Journal of the American Dietetics Association* 88(1988):216.

Grahame, R., and J. M. Jenkins. "Joint Hypermobility—Asset or Liability." *Annals of Rheumatic Disease* 31(1972):109.

Grandjean, E. *Ergonomics of the Home.* London: Taylor and Francis, Ltd., 1973.

Grandjean, E. *Fitting the Task to the Man.* 4th ed. London: Taylor and Francis, Ltd., 1988.

Graves, J. E., et al. "Physiological Responses to Walking with Hand Weights, Wrist Weights and Ankle Weights." *Medicine and Science in Sports and Exercise* 20(1988):265.

Graves, J. E., et al. "The Effect of Hand-Held Weights on the Physiological Responses to Walking Exercise." *Medicine and Science in Sports and Exercise* 19(1987):260.

Greenberg, J. S. *Comprehensive Stress Management.* 3d ed. Dubuque, IA: Wm. C. Brown Publishers, 1990.

Greenberg, J. S. *Coping With Stress: A Practical Guide.* 2d ed. Dubuque, Iowa: Wm. C. Brown Publishers, 1990.

Griffith, D. "It's Not the Creep in a Trench Coat. . . ." *The Cutting Edge.* Riverside, CA: Teen Challenge 3(1992):1.

Grigg, W. "Quackery: It Costs More Than Money." *FDA Consumer* 22(1988):30.

Grossman, M. R., et al. "Review of Length Associated Changes in Muscle." *Physical Therapy* 62(1982):1799.

Groves, D. "Is Childhood Obesity Related to TV Addiction?" *Physician and Sportsmedicine* 11(1988):117.

Guilland, J., et al. "Vitamin Status of Young Athletes Including the Effects of Supplementation." *Medicine and Science in Sports and Exercise* 21(1989):441.

Gunderson, E., and R. Rahe, eds. *Life Stress and Illness.* Springfield, Ill.: Charles C. Thomas, 1979.

"Gymnastics Might Put a Nasty Twist on Back Problems." *Orange County Register,* Jan. 4, 1990.

Haennel, R., et al. "Effects of Hydraulic Circuit Training on Cardiovascular Function." *Medicine and Science in Sports and Exercise* 21(1989): 605–11.

Haldeman, S. "Spinal Manipulative Therapy in Sports Medicine." *Clinics in Sports Medicine: Injuries to the Spine* 5(1986):277.

"Hanging A Health Hazard?" *Medical World News,* August 22, 1983.

Hannam, S., et al. "The Jump Training Program: In-Season Conditioning for Women's Basketball." *JOPERD* 59(Oct. 1988):76–79.

Hardy, L., and D. Jones. "Dynamic Flexibility and Proprioceptive Neuromuscular Facilitation." *Research Quarterly for Exercise and Sport* 57(1986):150.

Harman, E. A., et al. "Effects of a Belt on Intra-Abdominal Pressure during Weight Lifting." *Medicine and Science in Sports and Exercise* 21(1989):186.

Harmer, P. A. "The Effect of Pre-Performance Massage on Stride Frequency in Sprinters." *Athletic Training* 26(1991):55–59.

Harris, K. A., and R. G. Holly. "Physiological Response to Circuit Weight Training in Borderline Hypertensives Subjects." *Medicine and Science in Sports and Exercise* 19(1987):246.

Harris, L. *Inside America.* New York: Vintage Books, 1987.

Harris, L. "Possible Changes in Life-Style." *The Harris Survey* 27(1987):2.

Harris, L. "Sports." *Harris Poll* (April 1989):1.

Harris, T. G., and J. Gurin. "The New Eighties Life-Style: Look Who's Getting It All Together." *American Health* 4(1985):46.

Hartz, A. J., et al. "The Association of Girth Measurements with Disease in 32,856 Women." *American Journal of Epidemiology* 119(1984):71.

Harvey, J., and S. Tanner. "Low Back Pain in Young Athletes: A Practical Approach." *Sports Medicine* 12(1991):394–406.

Harwood, H. J., et al. *Economic Costs to Society of Alcohol and Drug Abuse and Mental Illness: 1980.* Research Triangle Park, NC: Research Triangle Institute, 1984.

Haskell, W., et al. "Cardiovascular Benefits and Assessment of Physical Activity and Physical Fitness in Adults." *Medicine and Science in Sports and Exercise* 24(1992):S201 (Supplement).

Haupt, H. A., and G. D. Rovere. "Anabolic Steroids: A Review of the Literature." *American Journal of Sports Medicine* 12(1984):469.

Hauri, P., et al. "Slumber Strategies." *Health* 22(1990):57.

Hawkins, D. J., D. M. Lishner, and R. F. Catalano. "Childhood Predictors of Adolescent Substance Abuse." *Etiology of Drug Abuse: Implications for Prevention.* Washington, DC: National Institutes of Drug Abuse, 1985. Research Monograph 56. DHHS Publication (ADM) 85–1335.

Haymes, E. M. "Nutritional Concerns: Need for Iron." *Medicine and Science in Sports and Exercise* 19(1987): Supplement, 197.

Heath, R. G. "Marijuana and the Brain." Reprint. Topsfield, MA: Committees of Correspondence, Inc., n.d.

Hebert, H. J. "Secondhand Smoke Hurts Children, EPA Says." Santa Ana, CA: *Orange County Register,* June 18, 1992.

Heino, J. G., et al. "Relationship Between Hip Extension Range of Motion and Postural Alignment." *Journal of Orthopaedic and Sports Physical Therapy* 12(1990):243–48.

Heinrich, C., et al. "Bone Mineral Content of Cyclically Menstruating Female Resistance and Endurance Trained Athletes." *Medicine and Science in Sports and Exercise* 22(1990):558.

Helmrich, S., et al. "Physical Activity and Reduced Occurrence of Non-Insulin-Dependent Diabetes Mellitus." *New England Journal of Medicine* 325(1991):147.

Hempel, L. S., and C. L. Wells. "Cardiorespiratory Cost of the Nautilus Express Circuit." *Physician and Sportsmedicine* 13(1985):83.

Hiatt, W., et al. "Benefits of Exercise Conditioning for Patients with Peripheral Arterial Disease." *Circulation* 81(1990):602.

Hickson, R. C. "Interference of Strength Development by Simultaneously Training for Strength and Endurance." *European Journal of Applied Physiology* 45(1980):255.

Higgins, M., et al. "Rectus Femoris and Erector Spinae Activity During Simulated Knees-Bent and Knees-Straight Lifting." (Abstract of platform presentation at 1991 Section Meeting of APTA.) *Journal of Orthopaedic and Sports Physical Therapy* 13(May 1991):257.

Hingson, R., et al. "Acquired Immunodeficiency Syndrome Transmission: Changes in Knowledge and Behaviors Among Teenagers." *Pediatrics* 85(1990):24.

Hoeger, W. W. K., and D. R. Hopkins. "A Comparison of the Sit-and-Reach and the Modified Sit-and-Reach in the Measurement of Flexibility in Women." *Research Quarterly for Exercise and Sport* 31(June 1992): 191–95.

Hoffman, J. "Growth Hormone." *National Strength and Conditioning Association Journal* 12(1990):78–81.

Holbrook, T., et al. "The Association of Lifetime Weight and Weight Control Patterns with Diabetes among Men and Women in an Adult Community." *International Journal of Obesity* 13(1989):723.

Hole, J. W. *Essentials of Human Anatomy and Physiology.* 4th ed. Dubuque, Iowa: Wm. C. Brown Publishers, 1992.

Holmstrom, E., et al. "Trunk Muscle Strength and Back Muscle Endurance in Construction Workers With and Without Low Back Disorders." *Scandinavian Journal of Rehabilitation Medicine* 24(1992): 3–10.

Hooper, P. L. "Aerobic Dance Program Improves Cardiovascular Fitness in Men." *Physician and Sportsmedicine* 12(1984):132.

Hopkins, D. R., and W. W. K. Hoeger. "A Comparison of the Sit-and-Reach Test and the Modified Sit-and-Reach Test in the Measurement of Flexibility for Males." *Journal of Applied Sport Science Research* 6(1992):7–10.

Hortobagyi, T., et al. "Effects of Simultaneous Training for Strength and Endurance on Upper and Lower Body Strength and Running Performance." *Journal of Sports Medicine and Physical Fitness* 31(1991):20–30.

Houmard, J. "The Effects of Warm-Up on Responses to Intense Exercise." *International Journal of Sports Medicine* 12(1991):480.

Hubbard, R. W., and L. E. Armstrong. "Hyperthermia: New Thoughts on an Old Problem." *Physician and Sportsmedicine* 17(1989):97.

Hueber, G. "Americans Report High Levels of Environmental Concern." *The Gallup Poll Monthly* 307(1991):6.

Hugick, L., and J. Leonard. "Job Dissatisfaction Grows; 'Moonlighting' on the Rise." *The Gallup Poll Monthly* 312(1991):2.

Hugick, L., et al. "The Perfect Meal: Something Old, Something New." *The Gallup Poll Monthly* 314(1991):35.

"Human Growth Hormone." *Sports Medicine Digest* 6(1984):13.

Humphrey, D. "Strength and Endurance of Lower Arm Muscles." *Physician and Sportsmedicine* 16(1988):157.

Humphrey, D. "Strength and Endurance of the Thigh Muscles." *Physician and Sportsmedicine* 17(1989):185.

Humphrey, D. "Strength and Endurance of Upper Arm Muscles." *Physician and Sportsmedicine* 16(1988):181.

Humphrey, D. "Strengthening the Gluteus Maximus." *Physician and Sportsmedicine* 17(1989):217.

Humphrey. D. "Exercises for the Upper Thigh Muscles." *Physician and Sportsmedicine* 17(1989):213.

Hurley, B. F., et al. "Resistive Training Can Reduce Coronary Risk Factors without Altering V

Ice: The Cold Hard Facts. Skill Builder. St. Rose, LA: SYNDISTAR INC., n.d.

Ike, R. W. "Arthritis and Aerobic Exercise: A Review." *Physician and Sportsmedicine* 17(1989):128.

International Federation of Sports Medicine. "Physical Exercise: An Important Factor for Health." *Physician and Sportsmedicine* 18(1990):155.

International Society of Sport Psychology. "Physical Activity and Psychological Benefits: Position Statement" 20(1992):179.

Is There a Safe Tobacco? Take a Look at the Facts. New York, NY: American Lung Association, 1990.

Ivy, J. L., et al. "Muscle Glycogen Synthesis after Exercise: Effect of Time of Carbohydrate Ingestion." *Journal of Applied Physiology* 64(1988):1480.

Jackson, A. S., et al. "Generalized Equations for Predicting Body Density of Women." *Medicine and Science in Sports and Exercise* 12(1980):175.

Jacobson, B. "Effects of Amino Acids on Growth Hormone Release." *Physician and Sportsmedicine* 18(1990):63.

Jacobson, E. *You Must Relax*. New York: McGraw-Hill, 1978.

Jacobson, M. F. "Alcohol Deaths: Sharing the Blame." *Nutrition Action Healthletter* (April 1989):6.

James, J. "Smokeless Tobacco." *DATAFAX*. Tempe, AZ: Do It Now Foundation, 1990.

James, J. *Peyote & Mescaline: History & Use of the "Sacred Cactus."* Tempe, AZ: D.I.N. Publications, 1990.

Jarvis, W. T. *Quackery and You*. Washington, D.C.: Review and Herald Publishing Association, 1983.

Jeffrey, R., et al. "Weight Cycling and Cardiovascular Risk Factors in Obese Men and Women." *American Journal of Clinical Nutrition* 55(1992):641.

Jenkins, W. L., et al. "Speed Specific Isokinetic Training." *Journal of Orthopaedic and Sports Physical Therapy* 6(1984):181–84.

Johnson, E. (Magic). *What You Can Do To Avoid AIDS*. New York: Times Books, 1992.

Johnson, J. D. *Tennis*. 5th ed. Dubuque, Iowa: Wm. C. Brown Publishers, 1988.

Jone, D. A., et al. "Physiological Changes in Skeletal Muscles as a Result of Strength Training." *Quarterly Journal of Experimental Physiology* 74(1989):233–56.

Jones, L. "The Pulling Movement." *National Strength and Conditioning Association Journal* 13(1991):14–17.

Jones, R., et al. "A Study of Worksite Health Promotion Programs and Absenteeism." *Journal of Occupational Medicine* 32(1990):95.

Kalfas, I. H., et al. "Spondylotic C–3 Radiculopathy in a Professional Football Player." *Physician and Sportsmedicine* 15(1987):79.

Kamwendo, K., et al. "Neck and Shoulder Disorders in Medical Secretaries: Part II. Ergonomical Work Environment and Symptom Profile." *Scandinavian Journal of Rehabilitation Medicine* 23(1991): 135–142.

Kamwendo, K., et al. "Neck and Shoulder Disorders in Medical Secretaries. Part I: Pain Prevalence and Risk Factors." *Scandinavian Journal of Rehabilitation Medicine* 23(1991):127–33.

Kanders, B., et al. "Interaction of Calcium Nutrition and Physical Activity on Bone Mass in Young Women." *Journal of Bone Mineral Research* 3(1988):145.

Karkowsky, N. "Exercise with Care—Fitness Is Not Risk Free." *FDA Consumer* 23(1989):25.

Katch, F. I., and S. S. Drumm. "Effects of Different Modes of Strength Training on Body Composition and Anthropometry." *Clinics in Sports Medicine* 5(1986):413.

Katch, F. I., and W. D. McArdle. *Nutrition, Weight Control, and Exercise*. Philadelphia: Lea & Febiger, 1988.

Kavanaugh, T. "Does Exercise Improve Coronary Collateralization? A New Look at an Old Belief." *Physician and Sportsmedicine* 17(1989):96.

Keegan, A. "Mental Illness, Substance Abuse Cost U.S. $273.3 Billion in 1988, ADAMHA Study Says." *NIDA Notes*. Washington, DC: National Institutes on Drug Abuse; U.S. Department of Health and Human Services; Public Health Service; Alcohol Drug Abuse and Mental Health Administration (Winter 1990/1991):22.

Keeler, E., et al. "The External Costs of a Sedentary Life-Style." *American Journal of Public Health* 79(1989): 975.

Keim, H. A., and W. H. Kirkaldy-Willis. "Low Back Pain." *Clinical Symposia* 32(1980):6.

Kellie, S. E. "Tobacco Use: Women, Children and Minorities." In E. M. Blakeman, ed., *Final Report and Recommendations from the Health Community to the 101st Congress and the Bush Administration*. From the Tobacco Use in America Conference, Houston, Texas. Washington, DC: American Medical Association, 1989.

Kelly, D. L. "Exercise Prescription and the Kinesiological Imperative." *JOPERD* 53(1982):18.

Kemnitz, J. W. "Body Weight Set Point Theory." *Contemporary Nutrition* 10(1985):2.

Kendall, F. P., and E. K. McCreary. *Muscles: Testing and Function*. 3d ed. Baltimore: Williams & Wilkins, 1983.

Kennedy, J. F. "The Soft American." *Sports Illustrated* 13(1960):15.

Kenyon, G. S. "Six Scales for Assessing Attitudes Toward Physical Activity." *Research Quarterly* 39(1968):566.

Kibele, A. "Stress Factors in Leg Strength Training With Maximal Loads." *International Journal of Sports Medicine* 12(1991):93.

Kibler, W. "Musculoskeletal Adaptations and Injuries Due to Overtraining." *Exercise and Sport Sciences Reviews* 20(1992):99.

Kicman, A. T., et al. "Human Chorionic Gonadotrophin and Sport." *British Journal of Sports Medicine* 25(1991):73–78.

Kimiecik, J. "Predicting Vigorous Physical Activity of Corporate Employees." *Journal of Sport and Exercise Psychology* 14(1992):192.

King, A. C., et al. "Determinants of Physical Activity and Interventions in Adults." *Medicine and Science in Sports and Exercise* 24(1992):S221 (Supplement).

Kipp, D. "Stress and Nutrition." *Contemporary Nutrition* 9:7(1984).

Kisner, C., and L. A. Colby. *Therapeutic Exercise: Foundations and Techniques.* 2d ed. Philadelphia: F. A. Davis, Company, 1990.

Klatz, R. M., et al. "Effects of Gravity Inversion on Hypertensive Subjects." *Physician and Sportsmedicine* 13(1985):85.

Klein, K. K. "The Deep Squat as Utilized in Weight Training for Athletics and Its Effect on the Ligaments of the Knee." *Journal of Physical and Mental Rehabilitation* 15(1961):10.

Kleiner, S. "Fiber Facts." *Physician and Sportsmedicine* 18(1990):19.

Kleiner, S. "Vegetarian Vitality." *Physician and Sportsmedicine* 20(1992):15.

Klerman, G. L. "Clinical Epidemiology of Suicide." *Journal of Clinical Psychiatry* 48(1987):33.

Klingshirn, L. A., et al. "Iron Status of Habitual Female Aerobic Dancers." *Medicine and Science in Sports and Exercise* 21(1989):Supplement, 78.

Knox, R. A. "Smoke Gets in Your Eyes—Along with Cataracts." Santa Ana, CA: *Orange County Register,* August 26, 1992.

Kohrt, W., et al. "Body Composition of Healthy Sedentary and Trained, Young and Older Men and Women." *Medicine and Science in Sports and Exercise* 24(1992):832.

Koplan, J. P., et al. "The Risk of Exercise: A Public Health View of Injuries and Hazards." *Public Health Reports* 199(1985):189.

Koss, L. G. "The Papanicolaou Test for Cervical Cancer Detection: A Triumph and a Tragedy." *Journal of the American Medical Association* 261(1989):737.

Koszuta, L. E. "Low Impact Aerobics: Better Than Traditional Aerobic Dance?" *Physician and Sportsmedicine* 14(1986):156.

Kottke, F. J., et al. *Krusen's Handbook of Physical Medicine and Rehabilitation.* 4th ed. Philadelphia: W. B. Saunders Co., 1990.

Kraemer, W. J. "Endocrine Responses to Resistance Exercise." *Medicine and Science in Sports and Exercise* 20(1988):S152.

Kraus, H., and W. Raab. *Hypokinetic Disease.* Springfield, Ill.: Charles C. Thomas, 1961.

Kreighbaum, E., and Barthels, K. M. *Biomechanics.* Minneapolis: Burgess Publishing Co., 1985.

Kroll, W. P., et al. "Muscle Fiber Type Composition and Knee Extension Isometric Strength Fatigue Patterns in Power and Endurance Trained Males." *Research Quarterly for Exercise and Sport* 51(1980):323.

Krotkiewski, M. "Can Body Fat Patterning Be Changed." *Acta Medica Scandinavica* (Supplement) 723(1988):231.

Kubiak, R. J., et al. "Changes in Quadricep Femoris Muscle Strength Using Isometric Exercise versus Electrical Stimulation." *Journal of Orthopaedic and Sports Physical Therapy* 8(1987):537.

Kuipers, H., et al. "Influence of Anabolic Steroids on Body Composition, Blood Pressure, Lipid Profile and Liver Functions in Body Builders." *International Journal of Sports Medicine* 12(1991):413–18.

Kusserow, R. P. "Do They Know What They Are Drinking?" *Youth and Alcohol: A National Survey.* Washington, DC: Office of Inspector General, Department of Health and Human Services, June 1991.

Kusserow, R. P. "Drinking Habits, Access, Attitudes and Knowledge." *Youth and Alcohol: A National Survey.* Washington, DC: Office of Inspector General, Department of Health and Human Services, June 1991.

LaBree, M. "A Review of Anabolic Steroids: Uses and Effects." *Journal of Sports Medicine and Physical Fitness* 32(1991):618–26.

Laitner, B. "Doctors Criticize Tanning Salons." Santa Ana, CA: *Orange County Register* (Mar. 18 1991):E6.

Lake, D. A. "Neuromuscular Stimulation: An Overview and Its Implications in the Treatment of Sports Injuries." *Sports Medicine* 13(1992):320–36.

Lamanaca, J., and E. Haymes. "Effects of Dietary Iron Supplementation on Endurance." *Medicine and Science in Sports and Exercise* 21(1989): Supplement, 22.

Lampman, R., et al. "Effects of Exercise Training on Glucose Control, Lipid Metabolism, and Insulin Sensitivity in Hypertriglyceridemia and Non-Insulin Dependent Diabetes Mellitus." *Medicine and Science in Sport and Exercise* 23(1991):703.

Lance, L. M. "Leisure Time of U. S. Adults—A Look into the Future." *Journal of Physical Education, Recreation and Dance* 59(1988):43.

Lander, J. E., et al. "The Effectiveness of Weight-Belts During the Squat Exercise." *Medicine and Science in Sports and Exercise* 22(1990): 117–26.

Laseter, J. T., and J. A. Russell. "Anabolic Steroid-Induced Tendon Pathology: A Review of the Literature." *Medicine and Science in Sports and Exercise* 23(1991):1–3.

Leach, R. "The Impingement Syndrome." In Zarins, B., et al. (eds.) *Injuries to the Throwing Arm.* Philadelphia: W. B. Saunders Co., 1985.

Leaf, D. A. "Omega-3 Fatty Acids and Coronary Artery Disease." *Postgraduate Medicine* 85(1989):237.

Leatt, P., et al. "Seven-year Follow-up of an Employee Fitness Program." *Canadian Journal of Public Health* 79(1988):20.

Leatz, C. A. *Unwinding.* Englewood Cliffs, N.J.: Prentice-Hall, 1981.

Lee, C. K. "The Use of Exercise and Muscle Testing in the Rehabilitation of Spinal Disorders." *Clinics in Sports Medicine: Injuries to the Spine* 5(1986):271.

Lee, I., et al. "Change in Body Weight and Longevity." *Journal of the American Medical Association* 268(1992):2045.

Lee, I., et al. "Physical Activity and Risk of Developing Colorectal Cancer Among College Alumni." *Journal of the National Cancer Institute* 83(1991):1324.

Lee, I., et al. "Time Trends in Physical Activity Among College Alumni 1962–1988." *American Journal of Epidemiology* 135(1992):915.

Lehmkuhl, L. D., and L. K. Smith. *Brunnstrom's Clinical Kinesiology.* Philadelphia: F. A. Davis, Co., 1983.

Lemon, P. W. R. "Protein and Exercise: Update 1987." *Medicine and Science in Sports and Exercise* 19(1987): Supplement, 179.

Lemon, P. W. R. "Response to Letter to the Editor." *Medicine and Science in Sports and Exercise* 21(1989):416.

Lentell, G., et al. "The Use of Thermal Agents to Influence the Effectiveness of a Low Load Prolonged Stretch." (Platform presentation 1992 APTA Combined Sections Meeting, San Francisco.) Abstract. *Journal of Orthopaedic and Sports Physical Therapy* 15(Jan. 1992):48.

Leon, A., et al. "Leisure-time Physical Activity Levels and Risk of Coronary Health Disease and Death." *Journal of the American Medical Association* 258(1987):2388.

Lerman, C. "Reducing Avoidable Cancer through Prevention and Early Detection Regimens." *Cancer Research* 49(1989):4955.

Levine, M., et al. "An Analysis of Individual Stretching Programs of Intercollegiate Athletes." *Physician and Sportsmedicine* 15(1987):130.

Levy, M., et al. *Life and Health: Targeting Wellness.* New York: McGraw Hill, 1992.

Liemohn, W. "Flexibility and Muscular Strength." *Journal of Physical Education, Recreation and Dance* 59(1988):37.

Liemohn, W. S., et al. "Unresolved Controversies in Back Management." *Journal of Orthopaedic and Sports Physical Therapy* 9(1988):239.

Lightsey, D., and J. Attaway. "Deceptive Tactics Used in Marketing Purported Ergogenic Aids." *National Strength and Conditioning Association Journal* 14(1992):26.

Lindeman, A. "Eating for Endurance or Ultraendurance." *Physician and Sportsmedicine* 20(1992):87.

Lindsey, R. "Figure Wrapping: Would You Believe It?" *Fitness For Living.* March/April 1972.

Lindsey, R. *The Reducing Racket.* Unpublished book manuscript.

Lindsey, R., and C. Corbin. "Questionable Exercise—Some Alternatives." *Journal of Physical Education, Recreation and Dance* 60(1989):26.

Lindsey, R., and D. D. Gorrie. *Survival Kit for Those Who Sit.* Laguna Beach, Calif.: Publictec Editions, 1989.

Lindsey, R., et al. *Fitness for the Health of It.* 6th ed. Dubuque, Iowa: Wm. C. Brown Publishers, 1989.

Little, D. R. *Easy Stress-Reducing Strategies.* North Hollywood, CA: D. R. Little and Health Fair Expo, 1992.

Little, J. C. "The Athlete's Neurosis—A Deprivation Crisis." In Sacks, M. H., and M. L. Sachs. *Psychology of Running.* Champaign, Ill.: Human Kinetics Publishers, 1981.

Lohman, T. G., et al., eds. *Anthropometric Standardization Reference Manual.* Champaign, Ill.: Human Kinetics Publishers, 1988.

Long, B. C., and C. J. Haney. "Long-Term Follow-Up of Stressed Working Women: A Comparison of Aerobic Exercise and Progressive Relaxation." *Journal of Sport and Exercise Psychology* 10(1988):461.

Lord, J. P., et al. "Isometric and Isokinetic Measurement of Hamstring and Quadriceps Strength." *Archives of Physical Medicine and Rehabilitation* 73(1992):324–30.

Lowman, C., and C. Young. *Postural Fitness, Significance and Variance.* Philadelphia: Lea & Febiger, 1960.

Lubell, A. "Potentially Dangerous Exercises: Are They Harmful to All?" *Physician and Sportsmedicine* 17(1989):187.

Lucas, A. "Update and Review of Anorexia Nervosa." *Contemporary Nutrition* 14(1989):9.

Lucas, D. B. "Biomechanics of the Shoulder Joint." *Archives of Surgery* 107(1973):425.

Lundin, P., and W. Berg. "A Review of Plyometric Training." *National Strength and Conditioning Association Journal* 13(1991):22–30.

Luttgens, K., et al. *Kinesiology: Scientific Basis of Human Motion.* 8th ed. Dubuque, IA: Wm. C. Brown Publishers, 1992.

Madding, S. W., et al. "Effect of Duration of Passive Stretch on Hip Abduction Range of Motion." *Journal of Orthopaedic and Sports Physical Therapy* 8(1987):409–16.

Magill, R. A. *Motor Learning: Concepts and Applications.* 4th ed. Dubuque, Iowa: Wm. C. Brown Communications, Inc., 1993.

Maitland, G. D. *Vertebral Manipulation.* Boston: Bitterworth, 1984.

Makalous, S. L., et al. "Energy Expenditure during Walking with Hand Weights." *Physician and Sportsmedicine* 16(1988):139.

Marcus, B., et al. "Motivational Readiness, Self-Efficacy and Decision-making for Exercise." *Journal of Applied Social Psychology* 22(1992):3.

Marcus, B., et al. "Self-Efficacy and the Stages of Exercise Behavior Change." *Research Quarterly for Exercise and Sport* 63(1992):60.

Marcus, B., et al. "Using the Stages of Change Model to Increase the Adoption of Physical Activity Among Community Participants." *American Journal of Health Promotion* 6(1992):424.

Marcus, R., et al. "Osteoporosis and Exercise in Women." *Medicine and Science in Sports and Exercise* 24(1992):S301 (Supplement).

Martin, J. "Controlled Trial of Aerobic Exercise in Hypertension." *Circulation* 81(1990):1560.

Martin, M. J., et al. "Serum Cholesterol, Blood Pressure, and Mortality: Implications from a Cohort of 361,662 Men." *Lancet* 2(1986):933.

Mason, J. *Guide to Stress Reduction.* Culver City, Calif.: Peace Press, Inc., 1980.

McAuley, E., et al. "Self-Efficacy and Exercise Participation in Adult Females." *American Journal of Health Promotion* 5(1991):185.

McCarthy, P. "How Much Protein Do Athletes Really Need?"*Physician and Sportsmedicine* 17(1989):170.

McCunney, R. J. "Fitness, Heart Disease, and High-Density Lipoproteins: A Look at Relationships." *Physician and Sportsmedicine* 15(1987):67.

McDermott, R. J., and P. J. Marty. "Dipping and Chewing Behavior Among University Students: Prevalence and Patterns of Use." *Journal of School Health 56* 5(1986):175.

McGee, D., et al. "Leg and Hip Endurance Adaptations to Three Weight Training Programs." *Journal of Applied Sport Science Research* 6(1992):92–95.

McGinnis, J. M. "The Public Health Burden of a Sedentary Lifestyle." *Medicine and Science in Sports and Exercise* 24(1992):S196 (Supplement).

McGovern, P., et al. "Trends in Mortality, Morbidity and Risk Factor Levels for Stroke from 1960 to 1990." *Journal of the American Medical Association* 268(1992):753.

McIntosh, M. *Lifetime Aerobics.* Dubuque, Iowa: Wm. C. Brown Publishers, 1990.

McKenzie, R. *The Lumbar Spine: Mechanical Diagnosis and Therapy.* Upper Hutt, New Zealand: Spinal Publications, Ltd., 1981.

McKenzie, R. *Treat Your Own Back.* Waikanae, New Zealand: Spinal Publications, 1980.

McKenzie, R. *Treat Your Own Neck.* Waikanae, New Zealand: Spinal Publications, 1983.

McMaster, W. C. "Painful Shoulder in Swimmers: A Diagnostic Challenge." *Physician and Sportsmedicine* 12(1986):108.

Meacham, A. "Potent Pot Causes More Health Problems." *U.S. Journal of Drug and Alcohol Dependence 14* 1(1990):13.

"Media Action Alert. Issue: Industry Touts Alcohol as Heart Disease Cure-All." San Rafael, CA: The Marin Institute for the Prevention of Alcohol and Other Drug Problems, February 4, 1992.

"Medical Fraud/Quackery Rampant in U.S.A." *Food For Thought* (Orange County Nutrition Council) 12:2(1986):7.

"Medical Update: Kick Those Butts." *Golden Years* (Nov./Dec. 1991):34.

Melton, L., et al. "Epidemiology of Age-Related Fractures." In L. Avioli, ed., *The Osteoporetic Syndrome.* New York: Grune & Stratton, 1987.

Meredith, M. D. "Activity or Fitness: Is the Process or the Product More Important for Public Health?" *Quest* 40(1988):180.

Merten, T., and J. A. Potteiger. "Strength Training: Proper Techniques for the Big Three." *Athletic Training* 26(1991):295–309.

Mest, A., et al. "Long-term Morbidity and Mortality of Overweight Adolescents." *New England Journal of Medicine* 327(1992):1350.

Meyers, C. *Aerobic Walking.* New York: Random House, 1987.

Miko, C., et al. (eds.). *Opinions 90.* Detroit: Gale Research Inc., 1991.

Milgram, G. G. "Alcohol and Drug Education Programs." *Journal of Drug Education* 17(1987):43.

Miller, R. W. "Critiquing Quack Ads." *FDA Consumer,* November 1982 (reprint).

Miller, W. "Introduction: Obesity, Diet Composition, Energy Expenditure, and Treatment of the Obese Patient." *Medicine and Science in Sports and Exercise* 23(1991):273.

"Miracle Cures and Other Frauds." *Johns Hopkins Medical Letter,* 1(1990).

Mirkin, G. "Overtraining of Athletes: A Round Table." *Physician and Sportsmedicine* 11(1983):93.

Misner, J. E., et al. "Sex Differences in Static Strength and Fatigability in Three Different Muscle Groups. *Research Quarterly for Exercise and Sport* 61(1990):238–42.

Mitchell, J. "Bulimia Nervosa." *Contemporary Nutrition* 14(1989):10.

Mitchell, J. B., et al. "Effects of Carbohydrate Ingestion on Gastric Emptying and Exercise Performance." *Medicine and Science in Sports and Exercise* 20(1988):110.

Mochizuki, R. M., and K. J. Richter. "Cardiomyopathy and Cerebrovascular Accident Associated with Anabolic-Androgenic Steroid Use." *Physician and Sportsmedicine* 16(1988):109.

Moffatt, R. J., et al. "Effects of Anabolic Steroids on Lipoprotein Profiles of Female Weight Lifters." *Physician and Sportsmedicine* 18(1990):106–15.

Moffet, B. "Smoking: Implications for Lipids." San Francisco, CA: NASPE Session, AAHPERD National Convention, 1991.

Moffroid, M. T., and J. E. Kusial. "The Power Struggle—Definition and Evaluation of Power and Muscular Performance." *Physical Therapy* 55(1975):1098.

Moffroid, M. T., and R. H. Whipple. "Specificity of Speed of Exercise." *Journal of Orthopaedic and Sports Physical Therapy* 12(1990):72–78.

Mole, P. A., et al. "Exercise Reverses Depressed Metabolic Rate Produced by Severe Caloric Restriction." *Medicine and Science in Sports and Exercise* 21(1989):29.

Monahan, T. "Exercise and Depression: Swapping Sweat for Serenity." *Physician and Sportsmedicine* 14(1986):192.

Monahan, T. "Perceived Exertion: An Old Exercise Tool Finds New Applications." *Physician and Sportsmedicine* 16(1988):174.

Mooney, V., ed. "Evaluation and Care of Lumbar Spine Problems." *The Orthopedic Clinics of North America* 14(1983):701.

Moran, G., and G. McGlynn. *Dynamics of Strength Training.* Dubuque, Iowa: Wm. C. Brown Publishers, 1990.

Morgan, W. P. "Affective Beneficence of Vigorous Physical Activity." *Medicine and Science in Sports and Exercise* 17(1985):94.

Morgan, W. P., and Goldston, S. E., eds. *Exercise and Mental Health.* New York: Hemisphere, 1987.

Morgan, W. P., and P. J. O'Connor. "Exercise and Mental Health." In Dishman, R. K., *Exercise Adherence.* Champaign, Ill.: Human Kinetics Publishers, 1988.

Morris, J., et al. "Exercise in Leisure Time: Coronary Attack and Death Rates." *British Heart Journal* 63(1990):325.

Morton, M. B. *Growing Up Drug Free: Teachers' Manual and Resource Book.* Glenview, IL: Scott, Foresman and Company, 1991.

Munnings, F. "Exercise and Estrogen in Women's Health: Getting a Clearer Picture." *Physician and Sportsmedicine* 16(1988):152.

Munson, W. W., and F. E. Pettigrew. "Cooperative Strength Training." *Journal of Physical Education, Recreation and Dance* 59(1988):61.

Murphy, E., and R. Schwarzkoph. "Effects of Standard Set and Circuit Weight Training on Excess Post-exercise Oxygen Consumption." *Journal of Applied Sport Science Research* 6(1992):88–91.

Murphy, P. "Office Stress: Is a Solution Shaping Up?" *Physician and Sportsmedicine* 12(1984):114.

Mutoh, Y., et al. "Aerobic Dance Injuries among Instructors and Students." *Physician and Sportsmedicine* 16(1988):81.

Myburgh, K. H., et al. "Factors Associated with Shin Soreness in Athletes." *Physician and Sportsmedicine* 16(1988):129.

Myers, J. L., and J. L. Knight. "General and Specific Habituation to Electrical Muscle Stimulation during Three Weeks of Training." (Abstracts) *Athletic Training* 24(1989):115.

Nachemson, A. L. "Advances in Low Back Pain." *Clinical Orthopaedics and Related Research* 200(1985):266.

Nafziger, N. A., et al. "Passive Exercise System: Effect on Muscle Activity, Strength, and Lean Body Mass." *Archives of Physical Medicine and Rehabilitation* 73(1992):184–89.

Nash, H. J. "Can Exercise Make Us Immune to Disease?" *Physician and Sportsmedicine* 14(1986):250.

Nash, H. L. "Reemphasizing the Role of Exercise in Preventing Heart Disease." *Physician and Sportsmedicine* 17(1989):219.

Nathan, R. "Effects of a Stress Management Course on Grades and Health of First Year Medical Students." *Journal of Medical Education* 62(1987):514.

National Goals for Education. Washington, DC: U.S. Department of Education, 1990.

"National High School Senior Survey: Trends in Drug Use by High School Seniors." Washington, DC: National Institute on Drug Abuse; U.S. Department of Health and Human Services; Public Health Service; Alcohol, Drug Abuse and Mental Health Administration, Spring 1991.

National Institute of Health. "Consensus Statement: Preventing the Kidney Disease of Diabetes Mellitus." *American Journal of Kidney Disease* 13(1989):2.

National Institute of Occupational Safety and Health. *National Strategies for the Ten Leading Work-Related Diseases and Injuries.* Washington, DC: Department of Health and Human Services, 1989.

National Institute on Alcohol Abuse and Alcoholism. *Seventh Special Report to the U.S. Congress on Alcohol and Health.* Washington, DC: U.S. Department of Health and Human Services, 1990.

National Research Council. *Diet and Health: Implications for Reducing Chronic Disease Risk.* Washington, D.C.: National Academy of Sciences, 1989.

National Strength Coaches Association. "The Squat Exercise in Athletic Conditioning: A Position Statement." *National Strength and Conditioning Association Journal* 13(1991):51.

Neck Exercises for a Healthy Neck. Daly City, Calif.: Krames Communications, 1987.

Neck Owner's Manual. Daly City, Calif.: Krames Communications, 1985, 16 pp.

Nelson, A. G., et al. "Consequences of Combining Strength and Endurance Training Regimens." *Physical Therapy* 70(1990):287–94.

Nelson, K. C., and W. L. Cornelius. "The Relationship Between Isometric Contraction Durations and Improvement in Shoulder Joint Range of Motion." *Journal of Sports Medicine and Physical Fitness* 63(Sept. 1991):385–88.

"New Shades of Risk at Tanning Salons." *Consumer Reports,* February 1986, 73.

Newport, F., and L. DeStefano. "Football Top Sport Among Fans; Basketball Gains Support." *The Gallup Poll Monthly* 295(1990):17.

Nigg, B., et al. "Biomechanical and Orthopedic Concepts in Sport Shoe Construction." *Medicine and Science in Sports and Exercise* 24(1992):595.

Nirschl, R. P. "Health Clubs Are a Great Source of Business for Orthopedists." *Physician and Sportsmedicine* 14(1986):54.

Noble, E. P. "What the Doctor Orders." San Rafael, CA: The Marin Institute for the Prevention of Alcohol and Other Drug Problems (Summer 1991):7.

Noble, E. P., ed. *Third Report to the U.S. Congress on Alcohol and Health from the Secretary of HEW.* Washington, DC: National Institute on Alcohol Abuse and Alcoholism, 1978.

Norkin, C., and P. Levangie. *Joint Structure and Function: A Comprehensive Analysis.* Philadelphia: F. A. Davis, Co., 1983.

North, T., et al. "Effect of Exercise on Depression." *Exercise and Sport Sciences Reviews* 18(1990):379.

Novello, A. "Another Disease of Women: AIDS." *Arizona Republic,* July 22, 1992:A9.

Nutrition and Your Health: Dietary Guidelines for Americans. Hyattsville, MD: USDA, 1992, No. HG–232.

O₂ Max or Percent Body Fat." *Medicine and Science in Sports and Exercise* 20(1988):150.

O'Keefe, J. H. "Dietary Prevention of Coronary Artery Disease." *Postgraduate Medicine* 85(1989):243.

Office of Smoking and Health. *The Health Consequences of Smoking: Nicotine Addiction. A Report of the Surgeon General.* Washington, DC: Superintendent of Documents, 1988. (Department of Human Services Publication no. (CDC) 88-8406.)

Oldridge, N., et al. "The Health Belief Model: Predicting Compliance and Dropout in Cardiac Rehabilitation." *Medicine and Science in Sports and Exercise* 22(1990):678.

Olridge, N. B. "Compliance with Exercise Programs." In M. L. Pollack and D. H. Schmidt, eds. *Heart and Disease Rehabilitation.* New York: John Wiley & Sons, 1986.

"One in Nine American Women Will. . . ." *The University of California at Berkeley Wellness Letter.* Fernandina Beach, FL: Health Letter Associates, 8(1992):1.

Osbourne, R. "Turn Your Weight Room into a Body Composition Lab." *Fitness Management* 3(1987):40.

Oscai, L. B. "Exercise or Food Restriction: Effect of Adipose Cellularity." *American Journal of Physiology* 27(1974):902.

Osternig, L. R., et al. "Differential Responses to Proprioceptive Neuromuscular Facilitation (PNF) Stretch Techniques." *Medicine and Science in Sports and Exercise* 22(1990):106–11.

Otten, A. "Women's Growing Role in the Workforce." *Wall Street Journal* 7(1989):B1.

Owen, M. D., et al. "Effects of Ingesting Carbohydrate Beverages during Exercise in the Heat." *Medicine and Science in Sports and Exercise* 18(1986):568.

Owsley, H. K. "Altered Tennis Ball Exercises for Hand and Wrist Rehabilitation." *Athletic Training* 23(1988):361.

Pacelli, L. C. "To Fortify Bones, Use Calcium and Exercise." *Physician and Sportsmedicine* 17(1989):27.

Pacelli, L. S. "Straight Talk on Posture." *Physician and Sportsmedicine* 19(Feb. 1991):124–27.

Paffenbarger, R., et al. "Physical Activity and Physical Fitness as Determinants of Health and Longevity." In Bouchard, C., et al., *Exercise, Fitness and Health.* Champaign, IL: Human Kinetics, 1990.

Paffenbarger, R. S. "Contributions of Epidemiology to Exercise Science and Cardiovascular Health." *Medicine and Science in Sports and Exercise* 20(1988):426.

Paffenbarger, R. S., and R. T. Hyde. "Exercise Adherence, Coronary Heart Disease, and Longevity." In Dishman, R. K., *Exercise Adherence.* Champaign, Ill.: Human Kinetics Publishers, 1988.

Paffenbarger, R. S., et al. "Physical Activity, All-Cause Mortality, and Longevity of College Alumni." *New England Journal of Medicine* 314(1986):605.

Paffenbarger, R. S., et al. "Physical Activity and Incidence of Cancer in Diverse Populations: A Preliminary Report." *American Journal of Clinical Nutrition* 45(1987):312.

Paffenbarger, R. S., et al. "The Association of Changes in Physical-Activity Level and Other Lifestyle Characteristics with Mortality Among Men." *The New England Journal of Medicine* 328(1993):538.

Paliwal, Y., et al. "Stress and Cardiovascular Disease." *Hospital Medicine* n.d., 12, 16.

Parker, D., et al. "Juvenile Obesity." *Physician and Sportsmedicine* 19(1991):113.

Parry, C. W. "Stretching." In J. V. Basmajian, ed. *Manipulation, Traction and Massage.* Baltimore: Williams & Wilkins, 1985, 157.

Passer, M. W., and M. D. Seese. "Life Stress and Athletic Injury: Examination of Positive versus Negative Events and Three Moderator Variables." *Journal of Human Stress* 9(1983):11.

Pate, R., et al. "Physical Activity and Associated Behaviors in American Adolescents." *Medicine and Science in Sports and Exercise* 24(1992): Supplement, 124.

Pate, R. R. "The Evolving Definition of Physical Fitness." *Quest* 40(1988): 174.

Peota, C. "Studies Counter Myths about Iron in Athletes." *Physician and Sportsmedicine* 17(1989):26.

Perez, H., and S. Famasoli. "Benefit of Proprioceptive Neuromuscular Facilitation on the Joint Mobility of Youth-Aged Female Gymnasts with Correlations for Rehabilitation." *American Corrective Therapy Journal* 38:6(1984):142.

Perrine, J. J., and R. V. Edgerton. "Muscle Force-Velocity and Power Velocity Relationships under Isokinetic Loading." *Medicine and Science in Sports and Exercise* 10(1978):159.

Perry, C. L., and D. M. Murray. "The Prevention of Adolescent Drug Abuse: Implications from Etiological, Developmental, Behavioral, and Environmental Models." *Etiology of Drug Abuse: Implications for Prevention.* Washington, DC: National Institute on Drug Abuse, 1985. Superintendent of Documents, Research Monograph 56, DHHS Publication (ADM) 85-1335.

Perry, P. "You Can Relax on the Job." *American Health* 7(1986):42.

Perry, P. J. "Illicit Anabolic Steroid Use in Athletes: A Case Series Analysis." *American Journal of Sports Medicine* 18(1990):422–28.

Petersen, S. R., et al. "The Effects of Concentric Resistance Training on Eccentric Peak Torque and Muscle Cross-Sectional Area." *Journal of Orthopaedic and Sports Physical Therapy* 13(1991):132–33.

Petersen, S. R., et al. "The Influence of Velocity-Specific Resistance Training on the In Vivo Torque-Velocity Relationship and the Cross Sectional Area of the Quadriceps Femoris." *Journal of Orthopaedic and Sports Physical Therapy* 10(1989):456.

Peterson, P. *Drug Facts.* Santa Cruz, CA: ETR Associates, n.d.

Peterson, P. G. *About Steroids.* Santa Cruz, CA: ETR Associates, Network Publications, 1990.

Peterson, S. "Ca1-Ban 3000 Diet Aid Labeled a Health Risk." *Orange County Register,* July 27, 1992.

Peterson, S., et al. "Influence of Concentric Resistance Training on Concentric and Eccentric Strength." *Archives of Physical Medicine and Rehabilitation* 71(1990):101–5.

Petruzzello, S. J., et al. "A Meta-Analysis on the Anxiety-Reducing Effects of Acute and Chronic Exercise: Outcomes and Mechanisms." *Sports Medicine* 11(1991):143–82.

Philen, R., et al. "Survey of Advertising for Nutritional Supplements in Health and Body Building Magazines." *Journal of the American Medical Association* 268(1992):1008.

Physician and Sportsmedicine, published monthly, contains articles of all kinds on exercise, sports, and fitness.

Pickens, R. W., and D. S. Svikis. *Biological Vulnerability to Drug Abuse.* Washington, DC: National Institute on Drug Abuse Research Monograph 89, U.S. Department of Health and Human Services, Public Health Service, 1988.

Pickett, B., et al. "Bench Aerobics." *Strategies* 4(1990):28.

Plowman, S. "Physical Activity, Physical Fitness, and Low Back Pain." *Exercise and Sport Sciences Reviews* 20(1992):221.

Poehlman, E. "A Review: Exercise and Its Influence on Resting Energy Metabolism in Man." *Medicine and Science in Sports and Exercise* 21(1989):515.

Pollock, C. "Breaking the Risk of Falls: An Exercise Benefit for Older People." *Physician and Sportsmedicine* 20(1992):146.

Pollock, M., et al. "Exercise Prescription." *Journal of Physical Education and Recreation* 52(1981): 30.

Pollock, M. L., et al. "Measurement of Cardiorespiratory Fitness and Body Composition in the Clinical Setting." *Comprehensive Therapy* 6(1980):12.

Ponte, D. J., et al. "A Preliminary Report on the Use of the McKenzie Protocol versus Williams Protocol in the Treatment of Low Back Pain." *Journal of Orthopaedic and Sports Physical Therapy* 6(1984):130.

Poor Posture Hurts: Good Posture Works. Daly City, Calif.: Krames Communications, 1986, 7 pp.

Powell, K. E. "Habitual Exercise and Public Health: An Epidemiological View." In Dishman, R. K., *Exercise Adherence.* Champaign, Ill.: Human Kinetics Publishers, 1988.

Powell, K. E., et al. "An Epidemiological Perspective on the Cause of Running Injuries." *Physician and Sportsmedicine* 14(1986):100.

Powell, K. E., et al. "Physical Activity and Chronic Diseases." *American Journal of Clinical Nutrition* 49(1989):999.

Powell, K. E., et al. "Physical Activity and the Incidence of Coronary Heart Disease." *Annual Review of Public Health* 8(1987):253.

Powell, K. E., et al. "The Status of the 1990 Objectives for Physical Fitness and Exercise." *Public Health Reports* 101(1986):15.

Powles, A. C. P. "The Effect of Drugs on the Cardiovascular Response to Exercise." *Medicine and Science in Sports and Exercise* 13(1981):252.

Prapavessis, H., and A. V. Carron. "Learned Helplessness in Sport." *The Sport Psychologist* 2(1988):189.

President's Council on Physical Fitness and Sports. *Adult Physical Fitness* (Publication No. 017–000–00172–1). Washington, D.C.: U.S. Government Printing Office. Copies available from Superintendent of Documents.

President's Council on Physical Fitness and Sports. *Aquadynamics.* Washington, D.C.: U. S. Government Printing Office, publication no. 040–000–00360–6. Copies available from Superintendent of Documents.

Prevention Resource Guide: College Youth Put on the Brakes. Rockville, MD: National Clearinghouse for Alcohol and Drug Information, 1991. Produced for the Office for Substance Abuse Prevention; U.S. Department of Health and Human Services; Public Health Service; Alcohol, Drug Abuse and Mental Health Administration.

Public Health Service. *Healthy People 2000: National Health Promotion and Disease Prevention Objectives.* Washington, DC: U. S. Government Printing Office, 1991. (DHHS Pub. No. PHS 91–50212.)

Pugliese, M. T., et al. "Fear of Obesity: A Cause of Short Stature and Delayed Puberty." *New England Journal of Medicine* 309(1983):513.

"Pyramid Scheme Foiled." *Nutrition Action Health Letter* 19(1992):3.

Raithel, K. S. "Chronic Pain and Exercise Therapy." *Physician and Sportsmedicine* 17(1989):203.

Ramsey, M. L. "Pseudomonas Folliculitis Associated with Use of Hot Tubs and Spas." *Physician and Sportsmedicine* 17(1989):150.

Rasch, P. J. *Weight Training.* 5th ed. Dubuque, Iowa: Wm. C. Brown Publishers, 1990.

Recker, R., et al. "Bone Gain in Young Adult Women." *Journal of the American Medical Association* 268(1992):2403.

"Red Wine No 'Magic Bullet' for Heart Disease." *Health Digest* (July/August 1992):9.

Reid, I. R., et al. "Effects of Calcium Supplementation on Bone Loss in Post Menopausal Women." *New England Journal of Medicine* 328(1993):460.

Reiger, D. A., et al. "One-Month Prevalence of Mental Disorders in the United States." *Archives of General Psychiatry* 45(1988):977.

Reiken, G. B. "Negative Effects of Alcohol on Physical Fitness and Athletic Performance." *Journal of Physical Education, Recreation and Dance* (October 1991):64.

Rejeski, W. J., and E. A. Kenney. *Fitness Motivation: Preventing Participant Dropout.* Champaign, Ill.: Human Kinetics Publishers, 1988.

"Report of the National Cholesterol Education Program Expert Panel on Detection, Evaluation and Treatment of High Blood Cholesterol in Adults." *Archives of Internal Medicine* 148(1988):36.

Ricci, B., et al. "Biomechanics of Sit-Up Exercises." *Medicine and Science in Sports and Exercise* 13(1981):54.

Rice, D. P., et al. *The Economic Costs of Alcohol and Drug Abuse and Mental Illness: 1985.* Report submitted to U.S. Department of Health and Human Services, 1990. San Francisco, CA: Institute for Health and Aging, University of California, San Francisco, 1990.

Richie, D. H. "Aerobic Dance Injuries: A Retrospective Study of Instructors and Participants." *Physician and Sportsmedicine* 13(1985):130.

Rider, R. A., and J. Daly. "Effects of Flexibility Training on Enhancing Spinal Mobility in Older Women." *Journal of Sports Medicine and Physical Fitness* 31(1991):213–17.

Riebe, D., et al. "The Blood Pressure Response to Exercise in Anabolic Steroid Users." *Medicine and Science in Sports and Exercise* 24(1992): 633–37.

Rimer, B., et al. "Why Women Resist Screening Mammography." *Radiology* 172(1989):243.

Rippe, J., et al. "Walking for Health and Fitness." *Journal of the American Medical Association* 259(1988):2720.

Rizzo, T. H. "Join the Office Ergonomic Revolution." *Idea Today* (Mar. 1992): 42.

Robbins, S., et al. "Athletic Footwear: Unsafe Due to Perceptual Illusions." *Medicine and Science in Sports and Exercise* 23(1991):217.

Roberts, M. "The Well Done Stretch." *U.S. News and World Report* (Mar. 5, 1990):65–67.

Roberts, R., et al. "Effects of Warm-Up on Muscle Glycogenesis During Intense Exercise." *Medicine and Science in Sports and Exercise* 23(1991):37.

Roberts, W. "Managing Heatstroke." *Physician and Sportsmedicine* 20(1992):17.

Robertson, J. "Preventing Heat Injury in Sports." *Physician and Sportsmedicine* 19(1991):31.

Robinson, W., et al. "Competing With the Cold." *Physician and Sportsmedicine* 20(1992):61.

Rogan, A. "Domestic Violence and Alcohol: Barriers to Cooperation." *Alcohol Health and Research World.* Rockville, MD: National Institute on Alcohol Abuse and Alcoholism, Winter 1985/86.

Roper, W. L. "Current Approaches to Prevention of HIV Infections." *Public Health Reports* 106(1991):111.

Rossi, F., and S. Dragoni. "Lumbar Spondylolysis Occurrence in Competitive Athletes." *Journal of Sports Medicine and Physical Fitness* 30(Dec. 1990):450–52.

Round Table. "The Health Benefits of Exercise—Part II." *Physician and Sportsmedicine* 15(1987):121.

Round Table. "The Health Benefits of Exercise." *Physician and Sportsmedicine* 15(1987):115.

Rousseau, P. "Exercise in the Elderly." *Postgraduate Medicine* 85(1989):113.

Rovere, G. D. "Low Back Pain among Athletes." *Physician and Sportsmedicine* 15(1987):105.

Roy, S. H., et al. "Fatigue, Recovery, and Low Back Pain in Varsity Rowers." *Medicine and Science in Sports and Exercise* 22(1990):463–69.

Royal Canadian Air Force. *Exercise Plans for Physical Fitness.* Ottawa, Ontario, Canada: Queen's Printer. Rev. U.S. ed. published by Simon and Schuster, Inc., by special arrangement with *This Week Magazine.* Copies available from *This Week Magazine,* P.O. Box 77–E, Mt. Vernon, N.Y.

Rozenek, R., et al. "Physiological Responses to Resistance-Exercise in Athletes Self-Administering Anabolic Steroids." *Journal of Sports Medicine and Physical Fitness* 30(1990): 354–60.

Rubal, B. J., et al. "Effects of Physical Conditioning on the Heart Size and Wall Thickness of College Women." *Medicine and Science in Sports and Exercise* 19(1987):423.

"Running Shoes: The Sneaker Grows Up." *Consumer Reports* 57(1992):308.

Runyan, C., et al. "Epidemiology and Prevention of Adolescent Injury." *Journal of the American Medical Association* 262(1989):2273.

Ryan, B. E., and J. F. Mosher. "Media Action Alert. Issue: Study Finds Reduced Alcohol Industry Presence on College Campuses: Some Promotions Persist." *Progress Report: Alcohol Promotion on Campus.* San Rafael, CA: The Marin Institute for the Prevention of Alcohol and Other Drug Problems, December 16, 1991.

Ryan, L. M., et al. "Velocity Specific and Mode Specific Effects of Eccentric Isokinetic Training of the Hamstrings." *Journal of Orthopaedic and Sports Physical Therapy* 13(1991):33–39.

Ryan, M. E., et al. "A Research-Based HIV/AIDS Education Program via the University Computer System: Bridge to Prevention." *Health Education* 23(1992):198.

Saavedra, T. "Would-Be Quitters Learn That Patch Is No 'Magic Bullet' For Smoking." Santa Ana, CA: *Orange County Register,* Aug. 23, 1992.

Sady, S. P., et al. "Flexibility Training: Ballistic, Static or Proprioceptive Neuromuscular Facilitation." *Archives of Physical Medicine and Rehabilitation* 63(1982):261.

Safran, M., et al. "Warm-Up and Muscle Injury Prevention." *Sports Medicine* 8(1989):239.

Safran, M. R., et al. "The Role of Warm-up in Muscular Injury Prevention." *American Journal of Sports Medicine* 16(1988):123.

Sale, D. G. "Neural Adaptation to Resistance Training." *Medicine and Science in Sports and Exercise* 20(1988):Supplement, 135.

Sallade, J. "Variation on Robin McKenzie's Technique for Correction of Lateral Shift." *Journal of Orthopaedic and Sports Physical Therapy* 8(1987):417.

Sallis, J., et al. "Determinants of Physical Activity and Interventions in Youth." *Medicine and Science in Sports and Exercise* (Supplement) 24(1992): Supplement, 248.

Sallis, J., et al. "Determinants of Exercise Behavior." *Exercise and Sport Sciences Reviews* 18(1990):307.

Sallis, J., et al. "Distance Between Homes and Exercise Facilities Related to Frequency of Exercise among San Diego Residents." *Public Health Reports* 105(1990):179.

Samford, B. "Creeping Obesity." *Physician and Sportsmedicine* 16(1988):143.

Sapega, A. A., et al. "Biophysical Factors in Range of Motion Exercise." *Physician and Sportsmedicine* 9(1981):57.

Sarason, I. G., et al. "Assessing the Impact of Life Changes: Development of the Life Experiences Survey." *Journal of Consulting and Clinical Psychology* 46(1978):932.

Sargent, R., and M. L. Trexler. "Nutrition for Exercise." *Fitness Management* 5(1989):21.

Saudek, C. E., and K. A. Palmer. "Back Pain Revisited." *Journal of Orthopaedic and Sports Physical Therapy* 8(1987):556

Sawka, M. "Current Concepts Concerning Thirst, Dehydration, and Fluid Replacement: An Overview." *Medicine and Science in Sports and Exercise* 24(1992):643.

Schatz, M. P. "Exercises You Can Take to Work." *Physician and Sportsmedicine* 20(Jan. 1992):165–66.

Schenkman, M., and V. R. DeCartaya. "Kinesiology of the Shoulder Complex." *Journal of Orthopaedic and Sports Physical Therapy* 8(1987):438.

Schettler, J. *HIV: Get the Answers.* Santa Cruz, CA: ETR Associates, 1992.

Schipplein, O. D., et al. "Relationship Between Moments at the L5/S1 Level, Hip and Knee Joints When Lifting." *Journal of Biomechanics* 23(1990):907–12.

Schmidt, G., et al. "Sport Commitment: A Model Integrating Enjoyment, Dropout, and Burnout." *Journal of Sport and Exercise Psychology* 13(1991):254.

Schneider, D., et al. "Choice of Exercise: A Predictor of Behavioral Risks." *Research Quarterly for Exercise and Sport* 63(1992):231.

Schoenborn, C. A. "Health Habits of U. S. Adults." *Public Health Reports* 101(1986):571.

Schon, L., et al. "Chronic Exercise-Induced Leg Pain in Active People." *Physician and Sportsmedicine* 20(1992):100.

Sedlock, D. A., et al. "Accuracy of Subject-Palpated Carotid Pulse after Exercise." *Physician and Sportsmedicine* 11(1983):106.

Seiger, L. H., and J. Hesson. *Walking for Fitness*. Dubuque, Iowa: Wm. C. Brown Publishers, 1990.

Sekiya, C. *Help Your Child Succeed*. Los Angeles, CA: Asian American Drug Abuse Program, 1991.

Selby, G. "When Does an Athlete Need Iron?" *Physician and Sportsmedicine* 19(1991):96.

Selby, G. B., and E. R. Eichner. "Age-Related Increases of Iron Stores in Athletes." *Medicine and Science in Sports and Exercise* 21(1989): Supplement, 78.

Sellers, J. S. *Steroids in Athletes*. Phoenix, AZ: Center for Sports Medicine and Orthopedics, 1992.

Sellers, T., et al. "Effect of Family History, Body-Fat Distribution, and Reproductive Factors in the Risk of Postmenopausal Breast Cancer." *New England Journal of Medicine* 326(1992):1323.

Selye, H. "Secret of Coping with Stress." *U.S. News and World Report,* March 21, 1977, p. 51.

Selye, H. *Stress without Distress*. Philadelphia: J. B. Lippincott Co., 1975.

Selye, H. *The Stress of Life*. 2d ed. New York: McGraw-Hill, 1978.

Sex, Drugs, and Your Health: When You're Both a Kid and an Adult. San Bruno, CA: Krames Communications, 1988.

Shaffers, D., et al. *Prevention in Child and Adolescent Psychiatry: The Reduction of Risk of Mental Disorders*. Washington, DC: American Academy of Child and Adolescent Psychiatry, 1990.

Sharpe, G. L., et al. "Exercise Prescription and the Low Back." *JOPERD* 59(1988):74.

"Shearing the Suckers." *Consumer Reports,* February 1986, 87.

Sheehan, G. "Running Away from Smoking." *Physician and Sportsmedicine* 19(1991):55.

Shepard, R. J. "Does Cardiac Rehabilitation after Myocardial Infarction Favorably Affect Prognosis?" *Physician and Sportsmedicine* 16(1988):116.

Shepard, R. J. "Fitness Boom or Bust—A Canadian Perspective." *Research Quarterly for Exercise and Sport* 59(1988):265.

Shephard, R. "PAR-Q, Canadian Home Fitness Test and Exercise Screening Alternatives." *Sports Medicine* 5(1988):185.

Shephard, R., et al. "The Canadian Home Fitness Test." *Sports Medicine* 11(1991):358.

Shephard, R. J. *Physical Activity and Aging*. Chicago: Croom Helm Books. Distributed by YearBook Medical Publishers, Inc. (1978):117; 134.

Shockey, G. L. "Hydration and Health: Meeting the Athletes' Fluid Needs." *Sportcare and Fitness* 3(1988):43.

Shyne, K. "Richard H. Dominguez, M.D.: To Stretch or Not to Stretch." *Physician and Sportsmedicine* 10(1982):137.

Siegel, B. S. *Love, Medicine, and Miracles*. New York: Harper and Row, 1986.

Siff, M. C. "Modified PNF as a System of Physical Conditioning." *National Strength and Conditioning Association Journal* 13(1991):73–77.

Sihvonen, T., et al. "Electric Behavior of Low Back Muscles During Lumbar Pelvic Rhythm in Low Back Pain Patients and Healthy Controls." *Archives of Physical Medicine and Rehabilitation* 72 (Dec. 1991): 1080–1084.

Silverberg, E., et al. "Cancer Statistics—1987." *Cancer Journal for Clinicians* 37(1987):2.

Silverman, J. L., et al. "Quantitative Cervical Flexor Strength in Healthy Subjects and in Subjects with Mechanical Neck Pain." *Archives of Physical Medicine and Rehabilitation* 72 (Aug. 1991):679–81.

Simon, H. B. "Exercise and Infection." *Physician and Sportsmedicine* 15(1987):135.

Simons-Morton, D. G., et al. "Health-Related Physical Fitness in Childhood: Status and Recommendations." *Annual Review of Public Health* 9(1988):403.

Simons-Morton, D. G., et al. *Promoting Physical Activity among Adults*. Atlanta, GA: Centers for Disease Control, 1988.

Simopoulos, A. P. "Nutrition and Fitness." *Journal of the American Medical Association* 261(1989):2862.

Singh, A., et al. "Chronic Multivitamin-Mineral Supplementation Does Not Enhance Physical Performance." *Medicine and Science in Sports and Exercise* 24(1992):726.

Siskovic, D. S., et al. "The Disease-Specific Benefits and Risks of Physical Activity and Exercise." *Public Health Reports* 100(1985):180.

Slaby, A. E. *60 Ways to Make Stress Work for You*. New York: Bantam Books, 1991.

Slava, S., et al. "The Long-Term Effects of a Conceptual Physical Education Program." *Research Quarterly for Exercise and Sports* 55(1984):161.

Slavin, J. L., et al. "Amino Acid Supplements: Beneficial or Risky?" *Physician and Sportsmedicine* 16(1988):221.

"Slipped Disc." *Orange County Medical Association Health Letter* 2(1987):2.

Smith, B. J., et al. "National Adolescent Student Health Survey." *Health Education* 19(1988):4.

Smith, E. L., and C. Gilligan. "Effects of Inactivity and Exercise on Bone." *Physician and Sportsmedicine* 15(1987):91.

Smith, E. L., and S. L. Zook. "The Aging Process: Benefits of Regular Physical Activity." *JOPERD* 57(1986):32.

Smith, L. "Acute Inflammation: The Underlying Mechanism in Delayed Onset Muscle Soreness." *Medicine and Science in Sports and Exercise* 23(1991):542.

Smith, L. L., et al. "The Effects of Static and Ballistic Stretching on Delayed Onset Muscle Soreness and Creatine Kinase." *Research Quarterly for Exercise and Sport* 64(1993):103.

Smoke Signals. Santa Ana, CA: Orange County Health Care Agency Tobacco Use Prevention Program, Vol. 2, No. 2 (May/June 1991) and Vol. 3, No. 1 (Winter 1992).

Snow-Harter, C., et al. "Exercise, Bone Mineral, and Osteoporosis." *Exercise and Sport Sciences Reviews* 19(1991): 351.

Snyder, A. C., et al. "Influence of Dietary Iron Sources on Measures of Iron Status among Female Runners." *Medicine and Science in Sports and Exercise* 21(1989):7.

Soderberg, G. "Exercises for the Abdominal Muscles." *JOPERD* 37(1966):67.

Soderberg, G. L. *Kinesiology: Application to Pathological Motion*. Baltimore: Williams & Wilkins, 1986.

Solis, K., et al. "Aerobic Requirements for and Heart Rate Response to Variations in Rope Jumping Technique." *Physician and Sportsmedicine* 16(1988):121.

Solomon, M. Z., and W. DeJong. "Preventing AIDS and Other STDs Through Condom Promotion: A Patient Education Intervention." *American Journal of Public Health* 79(1989):453.

Spence, W. R. *Drugs and You: A Guide for Teenagers*. Waco, TX: Health EDCO, 1991.

Spence, W. R. *Hallucinogens: Trip or Trap?* Waco, TX: Health EDCO, 1991.

Spence, W. R. *Heroin: Highway to Oblivion.* Waco, TX: Health EDCO, n.d.

Spence, W. R. *Smokeless Tobacco: A Chemical Time Bomb.* Waco, TX: Health EDCO, n.d.

Spence, W. R. *Substance Abuse in the Workplace: Strung Out on the Job.* Waco, TX: Health EDCO, n.d.

Stamford, B. "Caffeine and Athletes." *Physician and Sportsmedicine* 17(1989):193.

Stamford, B. "Exercise and Air Pollution." *Physician and Sportsmedicine* 18(1990):153.

Stamford, B. "Isometric Exercise." *Physician and Sportsmedicine* 15(1987):191.

Stamford, B. "Posture Perfect Performance." *Physician and Sportsmedicine* 14(1986):197.

Stamford, B. "Saunas, Steam Rooms and Hot Tubs." *Physician and Sportsmedicine* 17(1989):188.

Stamford, B. "The Differences between Strength and Power." *Physician and Sportsmedicine* 13(1985):155.

Stamford, B. "Warming Up." *Physician and Sportsmedicine* 15(1987):168.

Stand, L. *Alcohol! Marta and Sean Talk to Teens.* Santa Cruz, CA: ETR Associates/Network Publications, 1990.

Stanistski, C. L. "Low Back Pain in Young Athletes." *Physician and Sportsmedicine* 10(1982):77.

Stanton, P., and C. Purdam. "Hamstring Injuries in Sprinting—The Role of Eccentric Exercise." *Journal of Orthopaedic and Sports Physical Therapy* 10(1989):343–49.

Staying Flexible: The Full Range of Motion. Alexandria, VA: Time-Life Books, 1987.

Steiner, M. E. "Hypermobility and Knee Injuries." *Physician and Sportsmedicine* 15(1987):159–68.

Stephens, T. "Exercise and Mental Health in the United States and Canada: Evidence from Four Population Surveys." *Preventive Medicine* 17(1988):195.

Stephens, T., et al. "A Descriptive Epidemiology of Leisure-Time Physical Activity." *Public Health Reports* 100(1985):147.

Sternfeld, B. "Cancer and the Protective Effect of Physical Activity." *Medicine and Science in Sports and Exercise* 24(1992):1195.

"Steroids: Not Just for Athletes Anymore." *Physician and Sportsmedicine* 14(1986):48.

Stevenson, E. "Double Leg Raising." *CAHPERD Journal Times* 44(1982):18.

Stevenson, E. "Hamstring Stretcher." *CAHPERD Journal Times* 46(1984):10.

Stevenson, E. "Hamstring Stretches." *CAHPERD Journal Times* 48(1986):6.

Stevenson, E. "Head Circling." *CAHPERD Journal Times* 45(1983):6.

Stevenson, E. "Hurdle Stretch." *CAHPERD Journal Times* 46(1984):16.

Stevenson, E. "Shoulder Stand." *CAHPERD Journal Times* 45(1983):19.

Stevenson, E. "Side Leg Raises." *CAHPERD Journal Times* 47(1985):10.

Stevenson, E. "Specificity of Exercise." *CAHPERD Journal Times* 44(1982):16–17.

Stevenson, E. "Stretches." *CAHPERD Journal Times* 48(1986):16.

Stevenson, E. "The Mad Cat." *CAHPERD Journal Times* 44(1982):23.

Stevenson, E. "The Sit-Up." *CAHPERD Journal Times* 44(1982):17.

Stevenson, E. "Trunk Circling." *CAHPERD Journal Times* 45(1983):20.

Stone, M. A. "Implications for Connective Tissue and Bone Alterations Resulting from Resistance Exercise Training." *Medicine and Science in Sports and Exercise* 20(1988):Supplement, 162.

Stone, M. H., "Muscle Conditioning and Muscle Injuries." *Medicine and Science in Sports and Exercise* 22(1990):457–61.

Stone, M. H., et al. "Health and Performance-Related Potential of Resistance Training." *Sports Medicine* 11(1991):210–31.

Stratton, J., et al. "Effects of Physical Conditioning of Fibrinolytic Variables and Fibrinogen in Young and Old Healthy Subjects." *Circulation* 83(1991):1692.

Straus, R. H. "Spittin' Image: Breaking the Sports-Tobacco Connection." *Physician and Sportsmedicine* 19(1991):46.

"Stress on Job Affects Health." *Orange County Register,* Jan. 1, 1990.

Stevenson, E. "Bench Press." *CAHPERD Journal Times* 45(1983):14.

Strickler, T., et al. "Effects of Passive Warming on Muscle Injury." *American Journal of Sports Medicine* 18(1990):141.

Stunkard, A., and R. Berkowitz. "Treatment of Obesity in Children." *Journal of the American Medical Association* 264(1990):2550.

Stunkard, A. J. "An Adoption Study of Human Obesity." *The New England Journal of Medicine* 314(1986):193.

"Substance Abuse Quiz." Downey, CA: Department of Health Services, Rancho Los Amigos Medical Center, n.d.

Substance Abuse Report. Washington, DC: National Institutes on Drug Abuse; U.S. Department of Health and Human Services; Public Health Service; Alcohol, Drug Abuse and Mental Health Administration, January 1, 1992:4.

Summerfield, L. M. "Adolescents and Aids." *ERIC Digest.* Washington, DC: ERIC Clearinghouse on Teacher Education, 1992. EDO-SP:8–89.

Summerfield, L. M. "Drug and Alcohol Prevention Education." *ERIC Digest.* Washington, DC: ERIC Clearinghouse on Teacher Education, 1991.

Superko, H. R. "Exercise Training, Serum Lipids, and Lipoprotein Particles: Is There a Change Threshold?" *Medicine and Science in Sport and Exercise* 23(1991):677.

Superko, H. R. "The Role of Diet, Exercise, and Medication in Blood Lipid Management of Cardiac Patients." *Physician and Sportsmedicine* 16(1988):65.

Surburg, P. R. "Neuromuscular Facilitation Techniques in Sports Medicine." *Physician and Sportsmedicine* 9(1981):115.

Tanji, J. "Hypertension: How Exercise Helps." *Physician and Sportsmedicine* 18(1990):77.

"Tanning the Hard Way." *Consumer Reports* (1986):285.

Tarnopolsky, M. A., et al. "Influence of Protein Intake and Training Status on Nitrogen Balance and Lean Body Mass." *Journal of Applied Physiology* 64(1988):187.

Taylor, C. B. "The Relation of Physical Activity and Exercise to Mental Health." *Public Health Reports* 100(1985):195.

Taylor, D. C., et al. "Viscoelastic Properties of Muscle-Tendon Units: The Biomechanical Effects of Stretching." *American Journal of Sports Medicine* 18(1990):300–309.

Taylor, L. P. *Electromyographic Biofeedback Therapy.* Los Angeles: Biofeedback Advanced Therapy Institute, 1981.

Taylor, W. N. *Hormonal Manipulation: A New Era of Monstrous Athletes.* Jefferson, N.C.: McFarland and Co., Inc., Publishers, 1985.

"Teenagers and AIDS." *Newsweek,* August 3, 1992:44.

Teitz, C. C., and D. M. Cook. "Rehabilitation of Neck and Low Back Injuries." *Clinics in Sports Medicine: Rehabilitation of Injured Athletes* 4(1985):456.

Tesch, P. A. "Skeletal Muscle Adaptations Consequent to Long Term Heavy Resistance Exercise." *Medicine and Science in Sports and Exercise* 20(1988):S132.

Tesch, P. A., and J. Karlsson. "Muscle Fiber Types and Sizes in Trained and Untrained Elite Athletes." *Journal of Applied Physiology* 59(1985):1716.

Thanepohn, S. G. "How to Kick the Butts." *U.S. Journal of Drug and Alcohol Dependence 14* 1(1990):1.

The Alcoholism Report. Newsletter for Professionals in the Fields of Alcoholism and Drug Dependence. Washington, D.C.: N.p., Vol. 9, No. 8. (March 1991).

The Foot Book. Daly City, Calif.: Krames Communications, 1985, 16 pp.

The Rockport Company. *The Rockport Guide to Fitness Walking.* Marlboro, MA: The Rockport Company, 1990.

"The Squat Exercise in Athletic Conditioning: A Position Statement and Review of the Literature." *National Strength and Conditioning Association Journal* 13(1991):51.

"The Supplement Story: Can Vitamins Help?" *Consumer Reports* 57(1992): 12.

"The Vitamin Pushers." *Consumer Reports* (March 1986):170.

The Wellness Way: Managing Stress. Daly City, Calif.: Krames Communications.

Thein, L. A. "Impingement Syndrome and Its Conservative Management." *Journal of Orthopaedic and Sports Physical Therapy* 11(Nov. 1989): 183–90.

Thompson, M. L. *Growing Up Drug Free.* Glenview, IL: Scott, Foresman, 1991.

Thompson, M. L. *Growing Up Drug Free.* Glenview, IL: Scott, Foresman & Co., 1991.

Thompson, P. D., et al. "Incidence of Death during Jogging in Rhode Island from 1975 through 1980." *Journal of the American Medical Association* 247(1982):2535.

Tichauer, E. R. *Biomechanical Basis of Ergonomics.* New York: John Wiley & Sons, 1978.

Tipton, C. "Exercise, Training, and Hypertension: An Update." *Exercise and Sport Sciences Reviews* 19(1991): 447.

Tittel, K. "The Loadability and Relievability of the Lumbo-sacral Transition in Sports." *Journal of Sports Medicine and Physical Fitness* 30 (June 1990):113–21.

"To Your Health: The Effects of Alcohol on Body Functions." *Reflections in a Glass.* Arlington, VA: National Center for Alcohol Education, 1977. Prepared under contract to The National Institute on Alcohol Abuse and Alcoholism; Alcohol, Drug Abuse and Mental Health Administration; Public Health Service; U.S. Department of Health, Education and Welfare.

"Tobacco Use Among Youth." *Tobacco Free America.* Washington, DC: Legislative Clearinghouse, August 1989.

Tobacco's Toll on America. New York, NY: American Lung Association, 1987.

"Toning Tables Fail Test." *NCAF Newsletter* 13(Nov./Dec. 1990).

Travell, J., and D. G. Simons. *Myofascial Pain and Dysfunction: The Trigger Point Manual.* Baltimore: Williams & Wilkins, 1983.

Travell, J. G., and D. G. Simons. *Myofascial Pain and Dysfunction: The Trigger Point Manual.* Baltimore: Williams & Wilkins, 1983.

Trzaskoma, Z., et al. "Investigation of an Experimental Weight-Training Program." *Journal of Sports Sciences* 10(1992):109–17.

Tucker, L. A., and Friedman, G. M. "Television Viewing and Obesity in Adult Males." *American Journal of Public Health* 79(1989):516.

Turia, P. A., and K. L. Hawkins. "Coping with Crises." *Success* 30(1983):13.

Understanding Anabolic Steroids: For Parents, Teachers and Coaches. San Diego, CA: San Diego County Office of Education, n.d.

"USDA Adopts New Pyramid Graphic for Nutrition Guide." *Food Production Management* 115(1992):8.

Vakos, J., et al. "EMG Activity of Selected Trunk and Hip Muscles During a Squat Lift: Effect of Varying the Lumbar Posture." (Abstract of platform presentation at the 1991 Section Meeting of APTA.) *Journal of Orthopaedic and Sports Physical Therapy* 13 (May 1991):257.

Van Camp, S. P. "Exercise-Related Sudden Death: Risks and Causes." *Physician and Sportsmedicine* 16(1988):97.

Van Camp, S. P., and J. L. Boyer. "Cardiovascular Aspects of Aging." *Physician and Sportsmedicine* 17(1989):121.

Van Camp, S. P., and J. L. Boyer. "Exercise Guidelines for the Elderly." *Physician and Sportsmedicine* 17(1989):83.

Van De Graaff, K. M., and S. I. Fox. *Concepts of Human Anatomy and Physiology.* 3d ed. Dubuque, Iowa: Wm. C. Brown Publishers, 1992.

Van Duser, B. L., and P. B. Raven. "The Effects of Oral Smokeless Tobacco on the Cardiorespiratory Response to Exercise." *Medicine and Science in Sports and Exercise* 24(1992):389.

Van Itallie, T. B. "Topography of Body Fat: Relationship to Risk of Cardiovascular and Other Diseases." In Lohman, T. G., et al., eds. *Anthropometric Standardization Reference Manual.* Champaign, Ill.: Human Kinetics Publishers, 1988.

Vena, J. E., et al. "Occupational Exercise and Risk of Cancer." *American Journal of Clinical Nutrition* 45(1987):318.

Vickers, B. J. *Swimming.* 5th ed. Dubuque, Iowa: Wm. C. Brown Publishers, 1989.

"Vitamins: New RDAs." *Newsweek* (November 6, 1989):84.

Volski, R. V., et al. "Lower Spine Screening in the Shooting Sports." *Physician and Sportsmedicine* 14(1986):101.

Voy, R. O. "Water-Soluble Vitamins Not Safe in Megadoses." *Physician and Sportsmedicine* 14(1986):52.

Walker, J. M. "Exercise and Its Influence on Aging in Rat Knee Joints." *Journal of Orthopaedic and Sports Physical Therapy* 8(1986):310.

Wallberg-Henriksson, H. "Exercise and Diabetes Mellitus." *Exercise and Sport Sciences Reviews* 20(1992):339.

Washburn, K. B., and M. A. Swanson. *Neck Care.* Redmon, Wash.: Medic Publishing Co., 1979.

Wathen, D. "Flexibility, Strength and Conditioning." *Strength and Conditioning Association Journal* 6(1984):71.

Weinstock, C. P. "The Grazing of America: A Guide to Healthy Snacking." *FDA Consumer* 23 (1989):8.

Wells, K. B., et al. "The Functioning and Well-Being of Depressed Patients." *Journal of the American Medical Association* 262(1989):914.

Weltman, A., and B. Stamford. "Is Excessive Sweating Healthy?" *Physician and Sportsmedicine* 11(1983):195.

West, R. R. "Changes in Life-Style After Early or Late Mobilization Following Acute Myocardial Infarction: A Ten-Year Follow-Up of a Randomized Controlled Trial." *Journal of Cardiopulmonary Rehabilitation* 6(1986):113.

What is Your Alcohol I.Q.? Skill Builder. St. Rose, LA: SYNDISTAR, INC., 1991.

What You Should Know About Smoking and Cancer. New York, NY: American Lung Association, n.d.

Wheeler, K. B. "Sport Nutrition for the Primary Care Physician: Importance of Carbohydrate." *Physician and Sportsmedicine* 17(1989):106.

White, G. W., et al. "Preventing Steroid Abuse in Youth: The Health Educator's Role." *Health Education 18* 4(1987):32.

White, G. W., et al. "Preventing Growth Hormone Abuse: An Emerging Concern." *Health Education 22* 4(1989):4.

Wichmann, S. "Exercise Excess: Treating Patients Addicted to Fitness." *Physician and Sportsmedicine* 20(1992):193.

Wichmann, S. A., and D. R. Martin. "Sports and Tobacco: The Smoke Has Yet to Clear." *Physician and Sportsmedicine* 19(1991):125–31.

Wilford, H. N., and J. F. Smith. "A Comparison of Proprioceptive Neuromuscular Facilitation and Static Stretching Techniques." *American Corrective Therapy Journal* 39:2(1985):30.

Wilks, B. "Stress Management for Athletes." *Sports Medicine* 11(1991):289–99.

Willett, W., et al. "Dietary Fat and Fiber in Relation to Risk of Breast Cancer." *Journal of the American Medical Association* 268(1992):2037.

Williams, M. H. *Nutrition for Fitness and Sport.* 3d ed. Dubuque, Iowa: Wm. C. Brown Publishers, 1992.

Williams, P. C. *Low Back and Neck Pain: Causes and Conservative Treatment.* Springfield, Ill: Charles C. Thomas, 1974.

Williford, H. N., et al. "Is Low-Impact Aerobic Dance an Effective Cardiovascular Workout?" *Physician and Sportsmedicine* 17(1989):95.

Willis, J. "About Body Wraps, Pills and Other Magic Wands for Losing Weight." *FDA Consumer,* November 1982 (reprint).

Willis, J. "Diet Books Sell Well But. . . ." *FDA Consumer,* March 1985 (reprint).

Willmore, J. H., et al. "Alterations in Body Size and Composition Consequent to Astro Trimmer and Slim Skins Training Programs." *Research Quarterly for Exercise and Sport* 56:1(1985):90.

Wilmore, J. H., and D. L. Costill. *Training for Sport and Activity: The Physiological Basis of the Conditioning Process.* 3d ed. Dubuque, Iowa: Wm. C. Brown Publishers, 1988.

Wilmore, J. H., et al. "Body Breadth Equipment and Measurement Techniques." In Lohman, T. G., et al., eds. *Anthropometric Standardization Reference Manual.* Champaign, Ill.: Human Kinetics Publishers, 1988.

Wilmore, J. H., et al. "Body Composition: A Round Table." *Physician and Sportsmedicine* 14(1986):144.

Wilson, G. J., et al. "Stretch Shorten Cycle Performance Enhancement Through Flexibility Training." *Medicine and Science in Sports and Exercise* 24(1992):116–23.

Wilson, G. J., et al. "The Relationship Between Stiffness of the Musculature and Static Flexibility: An Alternative Explanation for the Occurrence of Muscular Injury." *International Journal of Sports Medicine* 12(1991):403–7.

Wilst, W. H. "A Cholesterol Primer for Health Educators." *Health Education* 20(1989):24.

Wilterdink, E. "Amount of Exercise Per Day and Weeks of Training: Effects on Body Weight and Daily Energy Expenditure." *Medicine and Science in Sports and Exercise* 24(1992):396.

Windsor, R. E., and D. Dumitru. "Anabolic Steroid Use by Athletes." *Postgraduate Medicine* 84(1988):37.

Winningham, M. L., and M. G. MacVicar. "Response of Cancer Patients on Chemotherapy to a Supervised Exercise Program." (abs.) *Medicine and Science in Sports and Exercise* 17(1985):292.

Winningham, M. L., et al. "Exercise for Cancer Patients: Guidelines and Precautions." *Physician and Sportsmedicine* 14(1986):125.

Wooden, M. J., et al. "Effects of Strength on Throwing Velocity and Shoulder Muscle Performance in Teenage Baseball Players." *Journal of Orthopaedic and Sports Physical Therapy* 15(1992):223–27.

Woodhouse, M. L., "Isokinetic Trunk Rotation Parameters of Athletes Utilizing Lumbar/Sacral Supports." *Athletic Training* 25(1990):240–43.

Woodhouse, M. L., et al. "Selected Isokinetic Lifting Parameters of Adult Male Athletes Utilizing Lumbar/Sacral Supports." *Journal of Orthopaedic and Sports Physical Therapy* 11(1990):467–72.

Work, J. "Exercise for the Overweight Patient." *Physician and Sportsmedicine* 18(1990):113.

Work, J. A. "How Healthy Are Corporate Fitness Programs?" *Physician and Sportsmedicine* 17(1989):226.

Work, J. A. "Is Weight Training Safe during Pregnancy?" *Physician and Sportsmedicine* 17(1989):257.

Wright, J. E., and V. S. Cowart. *Anabolic Steroids.* Carmel, Ind.: Benchmark Press, 1990.

Yarber, W. L. *AIDS: What Young Adults Should Know. Instructor's Guide.* 2d ed. Reston, VA: AAHPERD, 1989.

Yesalis, C. *Anabolic Steroids in Sport and Exercise.* Champaign, Ill.: Human Kinetics Publishers, 1993.

Yesalis, C. E. "Winning and Performance-Enhancing Drugs: Our Dual Addiction." *Physician and Sportsmedicine* 18(1990):161–67.

Yessis, M. "Latest Strength Techniques You Can Offer Your Clients." *Fitness Management* 5(1989):36.

Yessis, M. "More Facts about Plyometrics." *Physician and Sportsmedicine* 16(1988):20.

Yessis, M. "Speaking of Strength." *Fitness Management* 5(1989):36.

Zacharkow, D. *The Healthy Lower Back: Laying a Foundation Through Proper Lifting, Sitting and Exercise.* Springfield, Ill.: Charles C. Thomas, Publisher, 1984, pp. 66–78.

Zahrawi, F. "Strength Gain without Back Pain." *Sportcare and Fitness* 1(1988):40.

Zamula, E. "Back Talk: Advice for Suffering Spines." *FDA Consumer* 23(1989):28.

CREDITS

Illustrations

Carlyn Iverson: 3.3, 3.4, 3.5, 6.2, 6.3
Cyndie C. H.-Wooley: 3.7, 4.1, 4.2, 4.3, 4.4, 4.5, 4.6, 8.1g&i, 10.1a–c, 11.3, 16.7, 16.8, 16.9, 16.10, 18.1, 18.2, 18.3, 18.4, 18.5, 18.6a–b, 18.7, 18.8, 18.9, 18.10, 18.11, 18.12, 18.13, 18.14, 18.15, 18.16, 18.17, 18.18, 18.19, 18.20, 18.21, 18.22, 18.23, 18.24, 18.25, 18.26, 18.27, 18.28, 18.29, 18.30, p. 84, p. 85, p. 87, p. 88, p. 89, p. 90, p. 91, p. 92, p. 93, p. 94, p. 95, p. 96, p. 110, p. 111, p. 112, p. 113, p. 121, p. 124, p. 125, p. 126, p. 127, p. 128, p. 129, p. 130, p. 131, p. 132, p. 133, p. 134, p. 135, p. 136, p. 137, p. 138, p. 139, p. 140, p. 141, p. 142, p. 143, p. 144, p. 145, p. 197, p. 198, p. 199, p. 200, p. 201, p. 202, p. 203, p. 204, p. 205, p. 206, p. 260, p. 261
Diane Nelson: 3.6
Robert Margulies/Tom Waldrop: p. 52
Precision Graphics: 1.1, 1.2, 2.1, 3.1, 6.4, 10.2, 16.1, 19.1, 21.1, 21.2, 22.4, 22.5, 25.1, 26.1, 27.1, 28.1, 29.1, p. 35, p. 67, p. L-60
Robert Margulies: 4.7
Rolin Graphics: 1.3, 3.2, 5.1, 5.2, 8.1a–f&h, 11.1, 11.2, 14.1, 16.2, 16.3, 16.4a–b, 16.5, 16.6a–b, 21.3, 22.1, 22.2, 23.1, 23.2, p. 17, p. 18, p. 19, p. 40, p. 41, p. 58, p. 156, p. 157, p. 160, p. 180, p. 181, p. 182, p. 193, p. 194, p. A-11, p. A-12, p. A-13, p. A-14, p. A-15, p. A-16
pages 33 and L-6: Adapted from CAD Risk Assessor, W. J. Stone, *Adult Fitness Programs,* 1987.
Chart 6B.1 (pages 65 and A-2): *The Aerobic Program for Total Well-Being* © 1982 by Kenneth H. Cooper. Used by permission of Bantam, a division of Bantam Doubleday Dell Publishing Group, Inc.
Table 7.4 (pages 72 and A-2): *The New Aerobics* © 1970 by Kenneth H. Cooper. Used by permission of Bantam, a division of Bantam Doubleday Dell Publishing Group, Inc.
Figure 12.51: Exer-Genie Physical Fitness Systems, division of Quick Innovations, Ltd., 680 Paseo Vista, Thousand Oaks, CA 91320. Reprinted by permission.

Photographs

Section Openers
Section 1: © Rick Rusing/Leo de Wys; **Section 2:** © David Stoecklein/Adstock; **Section 3:** © Rick Rusing/Leo de Wys; **Section 4:** © Tim Davis/Photo Researchers; **Section 5:** © Bill Bachmann/Adstock; **Section 6:** © Randy Taylor/Leo de Wys, Inc.

Chapter 1
Opener: © Rick Rusing/Leo de Wys

Chapter 2
Opener: © Tim Davis/Photo Researchers; **p. 9 bottom left:** © Mark Miller/First Image West; **p. 9 top right:** © Vic Bider/PhotoEdit; **p. 9 bottom right:** © Paul E. Loven/First Image West; **p. 10 top left:** © Tim W. Fuller/First Image West; **p. 10 bottom left:** © Dirk Gallian/First Image West; **p. 10 top right:** © Richard Anderson; **p. 10 bottom right:** © James Marshall/First Image West; **p. 11 top right:** © Dennis McDonald/Unicorn Stock Photos; **p. 11 bottom left:** © Scott Stallard/The Image Bank; **p. 11 top right:** © E. Bordis/Leo de Wys, Inc.; **p. 14:** © James G. White; **p. 15:** © Scott T. Baxter/First Image West

Chapter 3
Opener: © David Stoecklein/Adstock; **p. 29:** © David Young-Wolff/PhotoEdit

Chapter 4
Opener: © Brian Drake/Adstock; **p. 40:** © Dave Lyons/Unicorn Stock Photos

Chapter 5
Opener: © Christine & Hannah/Adstock; **p. 47:** © David Madison 1992

Chapter 6
Opener: © Ken Akers/Visual Images West, Inc.

Chapter 7
Opener: © Melanie Carr/Visual Images West, Inc.; **p. 69:** © Ken Akers/First Image West; **p. 73:** © Melanie Carr/First Image West

Chapter 8
Opener: © Vic Bider/PhotoEdit; **p. 80:** © David R. Laurie

Chapter 9
Opener: © Bob Krist/Leo de Wys

Chapter 10
Opener: © Kelly Ericson/Adstock; **p. 108:** © Rick Rusing/Leo de Wys, Inc.

Chapter 11
Opener: © David Stoecklein/Adstock

Chapter 12
Opener: © James W. Kay/Adstock

Chapter 14
Opener: © Rick Rusing/Leo de Wys; **p. 168:** © Richard Anderson

Chapter 15
Opener: © James W. Kay/Adstock; **p. 174:** © Mary E. Messenger; **p. 177:** © James Marshall/First Image West

Chapter 16
Opener: © James W. Kay/Adstock

Chapter 17
Opener: © Lew Long/Stock Market

Chapter 18
Opener: Index Stock

Chapter 19
Opener: © Tony Freeman/PhotoEdit; **p. 222:** © Reed Kaestner/First Image West; **p. 223:** © David R. Laurie

Chapter 20
Opener: © Tony Freeman/PhotoEdit; **p. 228:** © Rick Rusing/Leo de Wys, Inc.

Chapter 21
Opener: © James W. Kay/Adstock; **p. 235:** © James L. Shaffer; **p. 238:** © David R. Laurie

Chapter 22
Opener: © Richard Anderson; **p. 251:** © Ken Akers/First Image West

Chapter 23
Opener: © Richard Maack/Adstock; **p. 259:** © Larry Woodall/First Image West

Chapter 24
Opener: © Brian Drake/Adstock; **p. 269:** © James G. White; **p. 271:** © Deneve Feigh Bunde/Unicorn Stock Photos; **p. 273:** © Martha McBride/Unicorn Stock Photos

Chapter 25
Opener: © Murray Alcosser/The Image Bank; **p. 278:** © Dennis MacDonald/PhotoEdit; **p. 282:** © D & I MacDonald/PhotoEdit

Chapter 26
Opener: © Mike Howell/Leo de Wys, Inc.; **p. 288:** © Tony Freeman/PhotoEdit; **26.2:** Courtesy of Partnership for a Drug Free America © Richard Hutchings/PhotoEdit

Chapter 27
Opener: © David R. Frazier Photolibrary; **p. 297:** © Jeff Greenberg/Photo Researchers, Inc.; **p. 298:** CDC, Atlanta, GA

Chapter 28
Opener: © Bill Bachmann/Leo de Wys, Inc.; **p. 302:** © Larry Mulvehill/Photo Researchers, Inc.; **p. 306:** © James Prince/Photo Researchers, Inc.

Chapter 29
Opener: © David Stoecklein/Adstock; **p. 309:** © David Lissy/Leo de Wys, Inc.; **p. 311:** © Paul Gerda/Leo de Wys, Inc.

Chapter 30
Opener: © Myrleen Ferguson Cate/PhotoEdit

INDEX

C

Caffeine, beverages with, 247–248
Calisthenics, 71–72, 102, 125
Caloric balance, 154
  meaning of, 148
Calories
  calorie guide, A-4–A-6
  empty calories, 164, 166
  and losing weight, 154–155
  nature of, 148
  of protein/carbohydrates/fats,
    A-7–A-10
  weekly calorie count and exercise, 58
Cancer
  early warning signs, 302
  and exercise, 28
  incidence of, 301
  most prevalent types of, 301
  nature of, 300
  prevention of, 302, 303
  risk factors in, 301, L-83
  screening tests, types of, 303
  and tobacco use, 277–276
Capillaries, 56
Carbohydrate loading
  meaning of, 242
  and physical performance, 250–251
Carbohydrates
  calories of common foods, A-7–A-10
  dietary recommendations, 245–246
  simple and complex, 245
Carbon monoxide, 41
Carcinogen, nature of, 300, 302
Carcinoma
  nature of, 300, 301
  See also Cancer
Cardiovascular disease
  heart disease risk factor questionnaire,
    33, L-6
  heart disease risk factors, L-5
  research related to, 22–23
  risk factors, 23
  types of diseases, 22
Cardiovascular fitness, 55–62
  designing program for, 57–59
  evaluation of, 64, L-13
  maximal heart rate, calculation of,
    60–61
  maximal oxygen intake, 61–62
  meaning of, 9, 55
  pulse count in, 59–60
  working heart rate range, calculation
    of, 60
Cardiovascular system, components of,
  56–57
Cellulite, 268
Cellulose, 245
  nature of, 242
Center of gravity, meaning of, 183
Cervical lordosis, 188
  meaning of, 183
Chancre, nature of, 294, 298
Chewing tobacco, 278
Chlamydia, 299
  nature of, 294
Chronic disease, 20
  meaning of, 21

Chronic fatigue, meaning of, 255, 257
Cigarette smoking
  and addiction, 277
  dosage, factors in, 277
  effects of, 236, 277
  quitting, guidelines for, 279–280
  and sidestream smoke, 278
  teenager use of, 279
  withdrawal symptoms, 279
Cigars, 278
Circuit resistance training, 71, 119, L-31
Clothing, for exercise, 35, 39–40
Cocaine, 288
Cold, exercise in cold environment, 40–41
Collateral circulation, meaning of, 21
College students, alcohol use, 281, 283
Committed time, meaning of, 307, 308
Congestive heart failure, 22
  meaning of, 21
Continuous passive motion tables, 269
Contract-relax-antagonist-contract
  (CRAC), 81
Contract-relax (CR), 81
Cool-down exercises, 36–38, L-9
  meaning of, 34
Cooper, Dr. Kenneth, 71
Cooper's aerobics, 71
Coordination, meaning of, 10
Coronary occlusion, 22
  meaning of, 21
Corporate fitness programs, 13, 222
Crack, 288
Cross-country skiing, 72
Cureton, Dr. Thomas, 72
Cycles, exercise cycles, 269

D

Dance aerobics, 72–73
  cautions about, 218
  routine for, A-11–A-13
Death, early, factors in, 4
Dehydration, meaning of, 34, 39
Dependence
  physical dependence, 286
  psychological dependence, 287
Depressant drugs, 287, 288
  types of, 288
Depression, 305
  and exercise, 28
Designer drugs, 290
  types of, 290
Diabetes
  complications of, 304
  and exercise, 27
  incidence of, 304
  reducing risk of, 304
  Type I, 300, 304
  Type II, 300, 304
Diet, meaning of, 148
Dietary fat
  calories of common foods, A-7–A-10
  dietary recommendations, 245
  saturated fat, 243, 244
  unsaturated fat, 243, 244–245
Dietary habits questionnaire, 254, L-64
Dieting. *See* Body fat reduction
Diet record, L-65

Disease/illness prevention, 20, 234
  meaning of, 21
Disease/illness treatment, 20, 234
  meaning of, 21
Distress, meaning of, 255, 256
Driving, and alcohol use, 281–282
Drug, meaning of, 276
Drug abuse
  effects of, 236
  evaluation for potential abuse,
    L-81–L-82
Drugs
  and addiction, 291, 292
  anabolic steroids, 291
  common forms of abuse, 290–291
  depressant drugs, 287, 288
  designer drugs, 290
  hallucinogenic drugs, 288, 289
  help for abusers, 292–293
  narcotic drugs, 288
  and pregnancy, 291
  reasons for use of, 292
  stimulant drugs, 289

E

Eating disorders, 151–152
  anorexia athletica, 152
  anorexia nervosa, 151
  bulimia, 151–152
  fear of obesity, 152
Effectiveness, meaning of, 183
Electrical muscle stimulators, 270
Emotional storm, meaning of, 21
Emotional stressors, 256
Emotional wellness, meaning of, 232
Employee Assistance Programs, 316
Empty calories, 164, 166
Enabling factors
  and exercise adherence, 221–222
  meaning of, 219
Environment, protection of, 238
Environmental stressors, 256
Ergogenic aid, nature of, 242, 252
Eustress, meaning of, 255, 256
Exercise
  benefits of, 20, 22, 30
  choosing activity, criteria for, 14
  cold-related problems, 40–41
  exercise program, planning guidelines,
    228–229, L-55
  heat-related problems, 39–40
  lack of, reasons for, 14–15
  meaning of, 3
  most popular activities, 13
  pre-exercise guidelines, 35–36
  reasons for exercising, 15–16
  rehabilitative, 24
  for stress management, 258–259
  warm-up and cool down, 36–38
  weekly program, example of, 229
Exercise adherence
  and enabling factors, 221–222
  meaning of, 219
  and positive addiction to exercise, 224
  and predisposing factors, 220–221
  questionnaire on, 225–226, L-53
  and reinforcing factors, 223–224
  and stage of exercise, 224–225